Sixth Edition

PHARMACOTHERAPY
Casebook

a patient-focused approach

Sixth Edition

PHARMACOTHERAPY
Casebook

a patient-focused approach

Edited by
Terry L. Schwinghammer, PharmD, FCCP, FASHP, BCPS
Professor of Pharmaceutical Sciences
School of Pharmacy, University of Pittsburgh
Pittsburgh, Pennsylvania

A companion workbook to: *Pharmacotherapy: A Pathophysiologic Approach. 6th ed. DiPiro JT, Talbert RL, Yee GC, Matzke GR, Wells BG, Posey ML, eds. New York, NY: McGraw-Hill, 2005.*

McGraw-Hill
Medical Publishing Division

New York Chicago San Francisco Lisbon London
Madrid Mexico City Milan New Delhi San Juan Seoul
Singapore Sydney Toronto

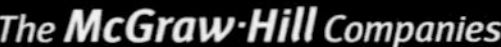

Pharmacotherapy Casebook: A Patient-Focused Approach, Sixth Edition

3 4 5 6 7 8 9 0 QPDQPD 0 9 8 7 6

ISBN 0-07-143360-0

This book was set in Garamond by Rainbow Graphics.
The editors were Michael Brown, Karen Edmonson, and Barbara Holton.
The production supervisor was Richard Ruzycka.
The cover designer was Mary McKeon.
Quebecor World Dubuque was printer and binder.
This book is printed on acid-free paper.

Please tell the author and publisher what you think of this book by sending your comments to pharmacotherapy@mcgraw-hill.com. Please put the author and title of the book in the subject line.

Contributors

Marie A. Abate, PharmD, Professor and Director of the West Virginia Center for Drug and Health Information, Department of Clinical Pharmacy, School of Pharmacy, West Virginia University, Morgantown, West Virginia

Cesar Alaniz, PharmD, Clinical Pharmacist and Clinical Associate Professor, Department of Pharmacy, University of Michigan Health System and College of Pharmacy, Ann Arbor, Michigan

Peter L. Anderson, PharmD, Assistant Professor, Department of Clinical Pharmacy, School of Pharmacy, University of Colorado Health Sciences Center, Denver, Colorado

Edward P. Armstrong, PharmD, BCPS, FASHP, Associate Professor, Department of Pharmacy Practice and Science, University of Arizona College of Pharmacy, Tucson, Arizona

Jacquelyn L. Bainbridge, PharmD, FCCP, Associate Professor, School of Pharmacy Department of Clinical Pharmacy, and School of Medicine Department of Neurology, University of Colorado Health Sciences Center, Denver, Colorado

Leslie L. Barton, MD, Professor of Pediatrics; Director, Pediatric Residency Program, University of Arizona Health Sciences Center, Tucson, Arizona

Susan D. Bear, BS, PharmD, Director of Clinical Pharmacy Services, Carolinas Healthcare System, Charlotte, North Carolina

Reina Bendayan, PharmD, Associate Professor, Department of Pharmaceutical Sciences, Leslie Dan Faculty of Pharmacy, University of Toronto, Toronto, Ontario, Canada

William H. Benefield, Jr., PharmD, BCPP, FASCP, Clinical Assistant Professor of Pharmacology, The University of Texas Health Science Center at San Antonio; Clinical Assistant Professor of Pharmacy, The University of Texas at Austin; Consultant, Pharmerica, San Antonio, Texas

Robert W. Bennett, MS, RPh, Associate Professor, Department of Pharmacy Practice; Director of Pharmacy Continuing Education, Purdue University School of Pharmacy and Pharmacal Sciences, West Lafayette, Indiana

Tina Penick Brock, MS, Clinical Associate Professor and Director of Student Services, Office of Professional Education, University of North Carolina at Chapel Hill School of Pharmacy, Chapel Hill, North Carolina

Gretchen M. Brophy, PharmD, BCPS, FCCP, Associate Professor, Departments of Pharmacy and Neurosurgery, Virginia Commonwealth University, Medical College of Virginia Campus, Richmond, Virginia

Karim Anton Calis, PharmD, MPH, BCPS, BCNSP, FASHP, FCCP, Clinical Specialist, Endocrinology & Women's Health; Coordinator, Drug Information Service, Warren G. Magnuson Clinical Center, National Institutes of Health, Bethesda, Maryland; Clinical Professor, University of Maryland, Baltimore; Associate Clinical Professor, Medical College of Virginia, Virginia Commonwealth University, Richmond; Clinical Professor, Shenandoah University, Winchester, Virginia

Bruce R. Canaday, PharmD, BCPS, FAPhA, FASHP, Clinical Professor and Vice Chair, Division of Pharmacotherapy, School of Pharmacy, University of North Carolina, Chapel Hill; Director, Department of Pharmacotherapy, Coastal AHEC, Wilmington, North Carolina

Bruce C. Carlstedt, PhD, Professor, Department of Pharmacy Practice, Purdue University School of Pharmacy and Pharmacal Sciences, West Lafayette, Indiana

Daniel T. Casto, PharmD, FCCP, Health Science Advisor, Merck Vaccine Division, Arlington, Texas

Juliana Chan, PharmD, Clinical Assistant Professor, Department of Pharmacy Practice, College of Pharmacy and Department of Medicine, Sections of Digestive and Liver Diseases, University of Illinois at Chicago, Chicago, Illinois

Marie A. Chisholm, PharmD, FCCP, Associate Professor of Pharmacy, University of Georgia College of Pharmacy; Associate Clinical Professor of Medicine, Medical College of Georgia; Director, Medication Access Program (MAP), Augusta, Georgia

Kerry A. Cholka, PharmD, was Clinical Pharmacist, University of Wisconsin Hospital and Clinics; Clinical Instructor, University of Wisconsin School of Pharmacy, Madison, Wisconsin at the time of this writing.

Susan K. Chuck, PharmD, BCPS, was Infectious Disease Clinical Pharmacist Specialist, Grady Health System, Atlanta, Georgia at the time of this writing.

Kevin W. Cleveland, PharmD, Pharmacy Resident, Idaho Drug Information Service, Idaho State University, Pocatello, Idaho

Sandy J. Close, PharmD, BCPS, Fellow in Infectious Disease and Critical Care Pharmacotherapy, The University of Toledo College of Pharmacy, Toledo, Ohio

Lawrence J Cohen, PharmD, BCPP, FASHP, FCCP, Chairman and Professor, Department of Pharmacotherapy, College of Pharmacy, Washington State University—Spokane

Travis W. Cooper, PharmD, BCPS, Assistant Professor, The University of Oklahoma College of Pharmacy, Oklahoma City, Oklahoma

John R. Corboy, MD, Associate Professor, Department of Neurology, School of Medicine, University of Colorado Health Sciences Center, Denver, Colorado

James D. Coyle, PharmD, Assistant Professor, Pharmacy Practice and Administration Division, College of Pharmacy, The Ohio State University, Columbus, Ohio

Brian L. Crabtree, PharmD, BCPP, Associate Professor of Pharmacy Practice, University of Mississippi School of Pharmacy; Clinical Associate Professor of Psychiatry, University of Mississippi Medical Center, Jackson; Psychopharmacologist, Mississippi State Hospital, Whitfield, Mississippi

Simon Cronin, PharmD, MS, Clinical Assistant Professor, University of Michigan School of Pharmacy, Ann Arbor, Michigan

Holly S. Divine, PharmD, CGP, CDE, Assistant Professor, Department of Pharmacy Practice & Science, University of Kentucky College of Pharmacy, Lexington, Kentucky

John M. Dopp, PharmD, Assistant Professor (CHS), Pharmacy Practice Division, University of Wisconsin School of Pharmacy, Madison, Wisconsin

Kimberly A. Dornbrook-Lavender, PharmD, BCPS, Fellow of Cardiorenal Therapeutics, Department of Pharmacotherapy, University of North Carolina School of Pharmacy, Chapel Hill, North Carolina

Victor G. Dostrow, MD, Clinical Assistant Professor, Department of Neurology and Department of Psychiatry, University of Mississippi Medical Center; Adjunct Associate Professor, Department of Pharmacy Practice, University of Mississippi School of Pharmacy, Jackson, Mississippi; Service Chief, Neurology, Mississippi State Hospital, Whitfield, Mississippi

Scott R. Drab, PharmD, CDE, BC-ADM, Assistant Professor of Pharmaceutical Sciences, Director of Professional Experience Programs, University of Pittsburgh School of Pharmacy, Pittsburgh, Pennsylvania

Tia D. Eddy, PharmD, Resident in Pulmonary Research, McGuire Research Institute, Hunter Holmes McGuire Veterans Affairs Medical Center, Richmond, Virginia

Brian L. Erstad, PharmD, FCCM, FASHP, FCCP, BCPS, Professor, Department of Pharmacy Practice and Science, College of Pharmacy, University of Arizona, Tucson, Arizona

Elizabeth J. Ewing, PharmD, Nutrition Support Specialty Resident, University of Arizona Medical Center, Tucson, Arizona

Patricia Fan-Havard, PharmD, Associate Professor, Division of Pharmacy Practice and Administration, The Ohio State University College of Pharmacy; HIV High-Risk Pregnancy Clinic Program Coordinator, Department of Obstetrics and Gynecology, Ohio State University Outpatient Clinic, Columbus, Ohio

Martha P. Fankhauser, MS Pharm, BCPP, FASHP, Clinical Associate Professor, Department of Pharmacy Practice and Science, University of Arizona College of Pharmacy, Tucson, Arizona

Jonathan D. Ference, PharmD, Clinical Instructor, Department of Pharmacy and Therapeutics, University of Pittsburgh School of Pharmacy; Family Medicine Clinical Pharmacist, University of Pittsburgh Medical Center—St. Margaret, Pittsburgh, Pennsylvania

Charles W. Fetrow, PharmD, Clinical Pharmacy Specialist, Pharmacy Services, University of Pittsburgh Medical Center—Passavant Hospital, Pittsburgh, Pennsylvania

Courtney V. Fletcher, PharmD, Professor and Chairman, Department of Clinical Pharmacy, University of Colorado Health Sciences Center, School of Pharmacy, Denver, Colorado

Pamela A. Foral, PharmD, BCPS, Assistant Professor, Department of Pharmacy Practice, Creighton University School of Pharmacy and Health Professions; Clinical Pharmacist in Critical Care, Alegent Health Bergan Mercy Medical Center, Omaha, Nebraska

Rex W. Force, PharmD, FCCP, BCPS, Associate Professor, Departments of Family Medicine and Pharmacy Practice; Director, Family Medicine Clinical Research Center, Idaho State University, Pocatello, Idaho

Michelle D. Furler, BScPhm, PhD, Department of Pharmaceutical Sciences, Leslie Dan Faculty of Pharmacy, University of Toronto, Toronto, Ontario, Canada

Marie E. Gardner PharmD, BCPP, CGP, Clinical Associate Professor, Department of Pharmacy Practice and Science, The University of Arizona College of Pharmacy, Tucson, Arizona

William R. Garnett, PharmD, FCCP, Professor of Pharmacy, Medical College of Virginia, College of Pharmacy, Richmond, Virginia

Patrick P. Gleason, PharmD, BCPS, Senior Clinical Pharmacist, Prime Therapeutics, Inc, Eagan, Minnesota; Clinical Assistant Professor, Department of Pharmaceutical Care and Health Systems, University of Minnesota, Minneapolis, Minnesota

Jean-Venable R. Goode, PharmD, BCPS, FAPhA, Associate Professor, Department of Pharmacy, Virginia Commonwealth University School of Pharmacy, Richmond, Virginia

John D. Grabenstein, EdM, PhD, CPHP, Deputy Director for Military Vaccines, U.S. Army Medical Command, Falls Church, Virginia

A. Christie Graham, PharmD, Clinical Assistant Professor of Pharmacy Practice, College of Health Sciences—School of Pharmacy, Wyoming Medical Center, Casper, Wyoming

Paige Robbins Gross, RPh, Staff Pharmacist II, Drug Use and Disease State Management Program, Department of Pharmacy and Therapeutics, School of Pharmacy, University of Pittsburgh Medical Center Health System, Pittsburgh, Pennsylvania

Amy J. Guenette, PharmD, BCPS, Director, Department of Pharmacy Services, Security Health Plan of Wisconsin, Inc., Marshfield, Wisconsin

Wayne P. Gulliver, MD, FRCPC, Associate Professor of Medicine (Dermatology), Faculty of Medicine, Memorial University of Newfoundland, St. John's, Newfoundland, Canada

John G. Gums, PharmD, Professor of Pharmacy and Medicine, Departments of Pharmacy Practice and Community Health & Family Medicine, University of Florida, Gainesville, Florida

Deanne L. Hall, PharmD, Assistant Professor, Department of Pharmacy and Therapeutics, University of Pittsburgh School of Pharmacy; Clinical Pharmacy Specialist, University of Pittsburgh Medical Center, Pittsburgh, Pennsylvania

Shawn R. Hansen, PharmD, Clinical Pharmacist—Cardiology Services, St. Joseph's Hospital, Marshfield; Clinical Instructor, University of Wisconsin School of Pharmacy, Madison, Wisconsin

R. Donald Harvey III, PharmD, BCPS, BCOP, Senior Clinical Specialist in Hematology/Oncology/Coagulation, Department of Pharmacy, University of North Carolina Health Systems; Clinical Assistant Professor, University of North Carolina School of Pharmacy, Chapel Hill, North Carolina

Keith A. Hecht, PharmD, Assistant Professor of Pharmacy Practice, University of Southern Nevada, Nevada College of Pharmacy; Clinical Pharmacy Specialist, Hematology/Oncology, University Medical Center of Southern Nevada, Henderson, Nevada.

Richard N. Herrier, PharmD, Clinical Associate Professor, Department of Pharmacy Practice and Science, The University of Arizona College of Pharmacy, Tucson, Arizona

Catherine A. Heyneman, PharmD, MS, FASCP, CGP, Associate Professor, Department of Pharmacy Practice and Administrative Sciences, Idaho State University College of Pharmacy; Director of Drug Information, Idaho Drug Information Service, Pocatello, Idaho

Tina M. Hisel, PharmD, BCPS, Assistant Professor (Clinical), Division of Clinical and Administrative Pharmacy, University of Iowa College of Pharmacy, Iowa City; Clinical Pharmacist, Broadlawns Medical Center Family Practice Residency Program, Des Moines, Iowa

Mark T. Holdsworth, PharmD, BCOP, Associate Professor of Pharmacy and Pediatrics, College of Pharmacy, University of New Mexico, Albuquerque, New Mexico

Jon D. Horton, Pharm.D, CACP, Critical Care Specialist, Director of Pharmacy Residency Programs, York Hospital—a Division of WellSpan Health, York, Pennsylvania

Denise L. Howrie, PharmD, Associate Professor of Pharmacy and Pediatrics, Schools of Pharmacy and Medicine, University of Pittsburgh; Clinical Specialist, Oncology & Pediatrics, Pharmacy Services, Children's Hospital of Pittsburgh, Pittsburgh, Pennsylvania

Beata A. Ineck, PharmD, BCPS, CDE, Department of Pharmacy Practice, University of Nebraska Medical Center; Ambulatory Care Pharmacist, Veterans Affairs Nebraska Western Iowa Health Care System, Omaha, Nebraska

Timothy J. Ives, PharmD, MPH, BCPS, FCCP, Associate Professor of Pharmacy and Medicine, Schools of Pharmacy and Medicine, University of North Carolina, Chapel Hill, North Carolina

Mark W. Jackson, MD, FACG, Private Practice in Gastroenterology, Knoxville, Tennessee

Donna M. Jermain, PharmD, BCPP, Director, Regional Medical & Research Specialist, Pfizer, Inc., Georgetown, Texas

Steven V. Johnson, PharmD, BCPS, Emerging Therapeutics Manager, Prime Therapeutics, Eagan Minnesota; Clinical Assistant Professor, University of Minnesota College of Pharmacy, Minneapolis, Minnesota

Kelly P. Jones, PharmD, was Community Pharmacy Practice Resident and Clinical Instructor, Virginia Commonwealth University, School of Pharmacy and Ukrop's Pharmacy, Richmond, Virginia at the time of this writing

Melanie S. Joy, PharmD, Assistant Professor, Division of Nephrology, University of North Carolina, Chapel Hill, North Carolina

Laura L. Jung, PharmD, Assistant Professor of Pharmacy and Therapeutics, University of Pittsburgh School of Pharmacy; Clinical Oncology Pharmacy Specialist, Magee-Womens Hospital, Pittsburgh, Pennsylvania

Daniel T. Kennedy, PharmD, BCPS, Clinical Director of Pulmonary Research, Group Practice Clinics; Director of Inpatient/Outpatient Smoking Cessation Clinic, Hunter Holmes McGuire Veterans Affairs Medical Center, Richmond, Virginia

Kinnari Khorana, PharmD, was Research Fellow, University of Illinois at Chicago College of Pharmacy, Chicago, Illinois at the time of this writing

Tien T. Kiat-Winarko, PharmD, BSc, Clinical Assistant Professor of Ophthalmology, Department of Ophthalmology, University of Southern California Keck School of Medicine, Los Angeles, California

Cynthia K. Kirkwood, PharmD, BCPP, Associate Professor, Vice Chair for Education, Department of Pharmacy, Virginia Commonwealth University, Richmond, Virginia

Jennifer J. Kiser, PharmD, Antiretroviral Clinical Pharmacology Fellow, University of Colorado Health Sciences Center School of Pharmacy, Denver, Colorado

Julie C. Kissack, PharmD, BCPP, Associate Professor of Clinical and Administrative Sciences, Mercer University Southern School of Pharmacy, Atlanta, Georgia

Daren L. Knoell, PharmD, FCCP, Associate Professor of Pharmacy and Internal Medicine; Director of the Dorothy M. Davis Heart and Lung Research Institute Lung Cell Isolation Program, The Ohio State University College of Pharmacy, Columbus, Ohio

Julia M. Koehler, PharmD, Associate Professor and Chair, Department of Pharmacy Practice, Butler University College of Pharmacy and Health Sciences; Clinical Pharmacist, Family Practice, Clarian Health Partners, Indianapolis, Indiana

Cynthia P. Koh-Knox, PharmD, Associate Director, Pharmacy Continuing Education, Department of Pharmacy Practice, Purdue University School of Pharmacy, West Lafayette, Indiana

Michael D. Kraft, PharmD, Clinical Assistant Professor, Department of Clinical Sciences, University of Michigan College of Pharmacy; Clinical Pharmacist in Surgery/Surgical ICU/Nutrition Support, University of Michigan Health System, Ann Arbor, Michigan

Robert J. Kuhn, PharmD, Professor and Vice Chair of Ambulatory Services, Division of Pharmacy Practice and Science, University of Kentucky College of Pharmacy, Lexington, Kentucky

Poh Gin Kwa, MD, FRCPC, Clinical Associate Professor of Pediatrics, Faculty of Medicine, Memorial University of Newfoundland, St. John's Newfoundland, Canada

Nancy P. Lam, PharmD, BCPS, Senior Manager, Medical Research, Medical Affairs, Amgen Inc., Thousand Oaks, California

Grace D. Lamsam, PharmD, PhD, was Assistant Professor for Research, Department of Pharmaceutical Sciences, University of Pittsburgh School of Pharmacy, Pittsburgh, Pennsylvania at the time of this writing

Rebecca M. Law, BS, PharmD, Associate Professor of Clinical Pharmacy, School of Pharmacy, Memorial University of Newfoundland, St. John's, Newfoundland, Canada

Cherokee Layson-Wolf, PharmD, Assistant Professor, Department of Pharmacy Practice and Science, University of Maryland School of Pharmacy, Baltimore, Maryland

W. Greg Leader, PharmD, Assistant Dean of Student and Professional Affairs, School of Pharmacy, The University of Louisiana at Monroe, Monroe, Louisiana

Mary Lee, PharmD, BCPS, FCCP, Dean and Professor, Pharmacy Practice, Midwestern University Chicago College of Pharmacy, Downers Grove, Illinois

Christine Lesch, PharmD, Clinical Pharmacy Manager, CT-SAICU, New York–Presbyterian Hospital, Columbia Presbyterian Campus, New York, New York

Cara L. Liday, PharmD, Assistant Professor, Department of Pharmacy Practice and Administrative Sciences, College of Pharmacy, Idaho State University, Pocatello, Idaho

William D. Linn, PharmD, Clinical Coordinator, South Texas Veterans Health Care System, San Antonio, Texas

Sherry A. Luedtke, PharmD, Associate Professor, Department of Pharmacy Practice and Associate Dean of Professional Affairs, Texas Tech University Health Sciences Center School of Pharmacy, Amarillo, Texas

Amy M. Lugo, PharmD, CDM, Clinical Assistant Professor of Pharmacy Practice, University of North Carolina School of Pharmacy, Chapel Hill; Associate Director of Pharmacotherapy, Mountain Area Health Education Center, Asheville, North Carolina

Robert L. Maher Jr., PharmD, BCPS, Vice-President of Clinical Services, Professional Specialized Pharmacies, LLC, Plum Boro, Pennsylvania

Henry J. Mann, PharmD, FCCP, FCCM, FASHP, Professor and Director, Center for Excellence in Critical Care, University of Minnesota College of Pharmacy, Minneapolis, Minnesota

Margery H. Mark, MD, Associate Professor, Department of Neurology, UMDNJ-Robert Wood Johnson Medical School, New Brunswick, New Jersey

Steven J. Martin, PharmD, BCPS, FCCM, Associate Professor and Director of the Infectious Disease Research Laboratory, The University of Toledo College of Pharmacy, Toledo, Ohio

Barbara J. Mason, PharmD, FASHP, Professor and Vice Chair of Pharmacy Practice, Ambulatory Care Clinical Pharmacist, Idaho State University and Veterans Affairs Medical Center, Boise, Idaho

James W. McAuley, PhD, Associate Professor of Pharmacy Practice and Neurology, The Ohio State University, Columbus, Ohio

Alex K. McDonald, PharmD, BCPS, Clinical Pharmacist, Pharmacy Clinical Support Services, Spartanburg Regional Healthcare System, Spartanburg, South Carolina; Clinical Assistant Professor, Department of Pharmacy Practice, Medical University of South Carolina, Charleston, South Carolina

Elaine McGhee, MD, Clinical Assistant Professor, Department of Pediatrics, University of Pittsburgh School of Medicine, Pittsburgh, Pennsylvania

William McGhee, PharmD, Clinical Pharmacy Specialist, Children's Hospital of Pittsburgh; Adjunct Assistant Professor, Department of Pharmacy and Therapeutics, University of Pittsburgh School of Pharmacy, Pittsburgh, Pennsylvania

Sarah T. Melton, PharmD, BCPP, Clinical Pharmacist, Melton Healthcare Consulting, LLC, Lebanon, Virginia

Renee-Claude Mercier, PharmD, BCPS, Associate Professor of Pharmacy, University of New Mexico College of Pharmacy, Albuquerque, New Mexico

Joette M. Meyer, PharmD, Clinical Reviewer, Division of Special Pathogen and Immunologic Drug Products, Center for Drug Evaluation and Research, US Food and Drug Administration, Rockville, Maryland

Laura Boehnke Michaud, PharmD, BCOP, Clinical Pharmacy Specialist—Breast Oncology, Division of Pharmacy, The University of Texas M.D. Anderson Cancer Center, Houston, Texas

Pamela J. Murray, MD, MHP, Associate Professor of Pediatrics and Obstetrics, Gynecology and Reproductive Sciences, University of Pittsburgh School of Medicine, Pittsburgh, Pennsylvania

James J. Nawarskas, PharmD, BCPS, Associate Professor, University of New Mexico College of Pharmacy; Assistant Professor of Internal Medicine, University of New Mexico School of Medicine, Albuquerque, New Mexico

Amy S. Nicholas, PharmD, CDE, Assistant Professor, Department of Pharmacy Practice and Science, Pharmacy REACH Program, University of Kentucky College of Pharmacy, Lexington, Kentucky

Thomas D. Nolin, PharmD, PhD, Clinical Pharmacologist, Department of Pharmacy Services and Division of Nephrology and Renal Transplantation, Maine Medical Center, Portland, Maine

Kimberly J. Novak, PharmD, Pediatric Pharmacy Practice Resident, University of Kentucky Medical Center, Lexington, Kentucky

Kelly K. Nystrom, PharmD, BCOP, Assistant Professor, Department of Pharmacy Practice, Creighton University School of Pharmacy and Health Professions; Clinical Pharmacist in Oncology, Alegent Health Bergan Mercy Medical Center, Omaha, Nebraska

Cindy L. O'Bryant, PharmD, BCOP, Assistant Professor, University of Colorado School of Pharmacy; Clinical Oncology Pharmacist, University of Colorado Health Sciences Center, Denver, Colorado

Dannielle C. O'Donnell, PharmD, BCPS, Primary Care Medical Liaison, Roche Laboratories, Inc., Nutley, New Jersey; Clinical Assistant Professor, College of Pharmacy, The University of Texas, Austin, Texas

Christine K. O'Neil, PharmD, BCPS, FCCP, Associate Professor, Department of Social, Clinical, and Administrative Sciences, Mylan School of Pharmacy, Duquesne University, Pittsburgh, Pennsylvania

Robert A. O'Rourke, MD, FACP, FACC, Charles Conrad Brown Distinguished Professor in Cardiovascular Disease, The University of Texas Health Science Center at San Antonio, San Antonio, Texas

Michael A. Oszko, PharmD, FASHP, BCPS, Associate Professor, Schools of Pharmacy, Medicine, and Nursing, The University of Kansas Medical Center, Kansas City, Kansas

Christopher T. Owens, PharmD, Assistant Professor, Department of Pharmacy Practice and Administrative Science, Idaho State University College of Pharmacy, Pocatello, Idaho

Manjunath P. Pai, PharmD, Assistant Professor, College of Pharmacy, University of New Mexico, Albuquerque, New Mexico

Nicole M. Paolini, PharmD, Clinical Assistant Professor/Rite Aid Liaison, Department of Pharmacy Practice, University at Buffalo, School of Pharmacy and Pharmaceutical Sciences, Buffalo, New York

Robert B. Parker, PharmD, FCCP, Associate Professor, Department of Pharmacy, University of Tennessee College of Pharmacy, Memphis, Tennessee

Tejal Patel, PharmD, Clinical Pharmacy Specialist, Neurosciences, Regina Qu'Appelle Health Region, Regina, Saskatchewan, Canada

Elizabeth Gray Paulson, PharmD, BCOP, was Clinical Pharmacy Specialist, Hematology/Oncology, University of Virginia Health Systems, Charlottesville, Virginia at the time of this writing.

Beth Bryles Phillips, PharmD, BCPS, Clinical Pharmacy Specialist, Ambulatory Care and Assistant Professor (Clinical), The University of Iowa Hospitals and Clinics and College of Pharmacy, Iowa City, Iowa

Bradley G. Phillips, PharmD, BCPS, Associate Professor and Assistant Head for Research and Faculty Development, Division of Clinical and Administrative Pharmacy, University of Iowa College of Pharmacy; Director, College of Medicine GCRC Laboratory Core, Iowa City, Iowa

Charles D. Ponte, PharmD, CDE, BCPS, BC-ADM, FASHP, FCCP, FAPhA, Professor, Departments of Clinical Pharmacy and Family Medicine, Robert C. Byrd Health Sciences Center, Schools of Pharmacy and Medicine, West Virginia University, Morgantown, West Virginia

Brian A. Potoski, PharmD, Assistant Professor, Department of Pharmacy and Therapeutics University of Pittsburgh School of Pharmacy; Clinical Pharmacist, Antibiotic Management Program, University of Pittsburgh Medical Center, Pittsburgh, Pennsylvania

Jane Pruemer, PharmD, BCOP, FASHP, Associate Professor of Clinical Pharmacy Practice, University of Cincinnati College of Pharmacy; Oncology Clinical Pharmacy Specialist, University Hospital, Health Alliance, Cincinnati, Ohio

Pat S. Rafferty, PharmD, BCPS, CDE, was Primary Care Clinical Pharmacy Specialist, Kaiser Permanente Colorado Region, Denver; and Assistant Professor of Pharmacy Practice (Adjoint), University of Colorado School of Pharmacy, Denver, Colorado at the time of this writing

Alicia M. Reese, PharmD, BCPS, Clinical Instructor, College of Pharmacy, University of Texas at Austin and University of Texas Health Science Center at San Antonio, San Antonio, Texas

Kristie C. Reeves, PharmD, BCPS, Clinical Pharmacist–SICU/CSICU, Department of Pharmacy Services, University of Miami/Jackson Memorial Hospital, Miami, Florida

Richard S. Rhodes, PharmD, Associate Professor, Department of Pharmacy Practice, Idaho State University College of Pharmacy, Pocatello, Idaho

Denise H. Rhoney, PharmD, Associate Professor, Department of Pharmacy Practice, Eugene Applebaum College of Pharmacy and Health Sciences, Wayne State University, Detroit, Michigan

Ted L. Rice, MS, BCPS, Associate Professor, Department of Pharmacy and Therapeutics, University of Pittsburgh School of Pharmacy; Clinical Pharmacist, University of Pittsburgh Medical Center, Pittsburgh, Pennsylvania

Anya Rockwell, PharmD, BCPS, was Infectious Disease Clinical Specialist, Parkland Health and Hospital System, Dallas, Texas at the time of this writing.

Keith A. Rodvold, PharmD, FCCP, Professor of Pharmacy Practice and Associate Professor of Medicine in Pharmacy, Colleges of Pharmacy and Medicine, University of Illinois at Chicago, Chicago, Illinois

Kelly C. Rogers, PharmD, Cardiology Clinical Specialist, Baptist Memorial Hospital—Memphis; Assistant Professor, Department of Pharmacy, University of Tennessee College of Pharmacy; Clinical Assistant Professor, Department of Pharmacy Practice, University of Mississippi School of Pharmacy

Carol J. Rollins, MS, RD, PharmD, BCNSP, Clinical Associate Professor, Department of Pharmacy Practice and Science, College of Pharmacy, University of Arizona; Coordinator, Nutrition Support Team and Clinical Pharmacist for Home Infusion Therapy, Arizona Health Sciences Center, Tucson, Arizona

Meredith L. Rose, PharmD, Assistant Professor, Department of Pharmacy and Therapeutics, University of Pittsburgh School of Pharmacy; Ambulatory Care Clinical Pharmacist, University of Pittsburgh Medical Center, Pittsburgh, Pennsylvania

Laurajo Ryan, PharmD, BCPS, Clinical Assistant Professor, College of Pharmacy, University of Texas at Austin; Clinical Assistant Professor, Division of Pharmacotherapy, University of Texas Health Science Center at San Antonio, San Antonio, Texas

Eric G. Sahloff, PharmD, Assistant Professor, Department of Pharmacy Practice, The University of Toledo College of Pharmacy, Toledo, Ohio

Libby S. Schindler, PharmD, BCPP, Director of Clinical Pharmacy, Pharmacy Practice Residency Program Director, Neuropsychiatric Clinical Pharmacist, Wilford Hall Medical Center, San Antonio, Texas

Christina E. Schober, PharmD, Ambulatory Care Specialty Resident, University of Pittsburgh Medical Center; Clinical Instructor, Department of Pharmacy and Therapeutics, University of Pittsburgh School of Pharmacy, Pittsburgh, Pennsylvania

Kristine S. Schonder, PharmD, Assistant Professor, Department of Pharmacy and Therapeutics University of Pittsburgh School of Pharmacy; Clinical Pharmacist in Ambulatory Care and Transplantation, University of Pittsburgh Medical Center and Thomas E. Starzl Transplantation Institute, Pittsburgh, Pennsylvania

Rowena N. Schwartz, PharmD, BCOP, Coordinator of Pharmacy Programs, University of Pittsburgh Cancer Institute; Associate Professor, Department of Pharmacy and Therapeutics, University of Pittsburgh School of Pharmacy; Pittsburgh, Pennsylvania

Terry L. Schwinghammer, PharmD, FCCP, FASHP, BCPS, Professor of Pharmaceutical Sciences, University of Pittsburgh School of Pharmacy; Ambulatory Care Clinical Pharmacist, University of Pittsburgh Medical Center, Pittsburgh, Pennsylvania

Mollie Ashe Scott, PharmD, BCPS, CPP, Director of Pharmacotherapy, Mountain Area Health Education Center, Asheville NC; Clinical Associate Professor of Pharmacy Practice and Assistant Professor of Family Medicine, University of North Carolina, Chapel Hill, North Carolina

Amy L. Seybert, PharmD, Assistant Professor, Department of Pharmacy and Therapeutics, University of Pittsburgh School of Pharmacy; Pharmaceutical Care Coordinator—Critical Care, Cardiovascular Clinical Pharmacist, University of Pittsburgh Medical Center, Pittsburgh, Pennsylvania

Amy Heck Sheehan, PharmD, Clinical Associate Professor, Department of Pharmacy Practice, Purdue University School of Pharmacy, Indianapolis, Indiana

Justin J. Sherman, PharmD, MCS, Assistant Professor of Clinical Pharmacy Practice, Department of Clinical and Administrative Sciences, University of Louisiana College of Health Sciences, Monroe, Louisiana

Carrie A. Sincak, PharmD, Assistant Professor, Pharmacy Practice Department, Chicago College of Pharmacy, Midwestern University, Downers Grove, Illinois

Susan J. Skledar, RPh, MPH, Assistant Professor, Department of Pharmacy and Therapeutics, University of Pittsburgh School of Pharmacy; Director, Drug Use and Disease State Management Program, University of Pittsburgh Medical Center; Pittsburgh, Pennsylvania

Douglas Slain, PharmD, BCPS, Assistant Professor, Department of Clinical Pharmacy, West Virginia University School of Pharmacy, Morgantown, West Virginia

Ralph E. Small, PharmD, FAPhA, FASHP, FCCP, Professor of Pharmacy and Medicine, Virginia Commonwealth University, Medical College of Virginia Campus, Richmond, Virginia

Courtney F. Smith, PharmD, BCOP, Clinical Pharmacy Specialist in Oncology, Department of Pharmacy, The University Hospital, Cincinnati, Ohio

Judith A. Smith, PharmD, BCOP, Assistant Professor, Department of Gynecologic Medical Oncology, Division of Cancer Medicine and Department of Gynecologic Oncology, Division of Surgery, University of Texas M.D. Anderson Cancer Center, Houston, Texas

Renata Smith, PharmD, Clinical Assistant Professor of Pharmacy Practice, College of Pharmacy, University of Illinois at Chicago, Chicago, Illinois

Denise R. Sokos, PharmD, BCPS, Assistant Professor, Department of Pharmacy and Therapeutics, University of Pittsburgh School of Pharmacy; Clinical Coordinator, Internal Medicine Pharmacy Services, University of Pittsburgh Medical Center, Pittsburgh, Pennsylvania

Melissa A. Somma, PharmD, CDE, Assistant Professor, Department of Pharmacy and Therapeutics, University of Pittsburgh School of Pharmacy; Director of Outpatient Pharmacologic Education, University of Pittsburgh Medical Center—St. Margaret Family Practice Residency Program, Pittsburgh, Pennsylvania

Suellyn J. Sorensen, PharmD, BCPS, Clinical Pharmacist, Infectious Diseases and Clinical Pharmacy Manager, Indiana University Hospital of Clarian Health Partners, Indianapolis, Indiana

Kelly Sprandel, PharmD, Research Fellow, University of Illinois at Chicago College of Pharmacy, Chicago, Illinois

William J Spruill, PharmD, FASHP, Associate Professor, Department of Clinical and Administrative Pharmacy, University of Georgia, College of Pharmacy, Athens, Georgia

Mary K. Stamatakis, PharmD, Assistant Dean for Academic Programs and Associate Professor of Clinical Pharmacy, West Virginia University School of Pharmacy, Morgantown, West Virginia

Monica A. Summers, PharmD, Clinical Research Fellow, The Ohio State University College of Pharmacy, Columbus, Ohio

Chris M. Terpening, PhD, PharmD, Assistant Professor, Departments of Clinical Pharmacy and Family Medicine, West Virginia University-Charleston Branch, Charleston, West Virginia

Colleen Terriff, PharmD, Clinical Assistant Professor, Washington State University College of Pharmacy; Deaconess Medical Center Pharmacy Department, Spokane, Washington

Margaret E. Tonda PharmD, Director, Clinical Development, ALZA Corporation (a subsidiary of Johnson & Johnson), Mountain View, California

Sharon M. Tramonte, PharmD, Clinical Assistant Professor, Department of Pharmacology, University of Texas Health Sciences Center at Austin, San Antonio, Texas

Tate N. Trujillo, PharmD, BCPS, Clinical Pharmacist Trauma / Critical Care, Department of Pharmacy, Clarian Health Partners, Indianapolis, Indiana

J. Michael Vozniak, PharmD, Hematology/Oncology Clinical Pharmacy Specialist, Hospital of the University of Pennsylvania, Philadelphia, Pennsylvania

William E. Wade, PharmD, FCCP, FASHP, Professor and Associate Head, Department of Clinical and Administrative Pharmacy, University of Georgia College of Pharmacy, Athens, Georgia

Mary Louise Wagner, MS, PharmD, Associate Professor, Department of Pharmacy Practice, Ernest Mario School of Pharmacy, Rutgers, The State University of New Jersey, Piscataway, New Jersey

Christine M. Walko, PharmD, Hematology/Oncology Resident, Department of Pharmacy, University of North Carolina Hospitals, Chapel Hill, North Carolina

Donna S. Wall, PharmD, BCPS, Critical Care Clinical Pharmacist, Indiana University Hospital, Clarian Health Partners, Indianapolis, Indiana

Amy L. Whitaker, PharmD, Assistant Professor, Department of Pharmacy, Virginia Commonwealth University—Medical College of Virginia School of Pharmacy, Richmond, Virginia

Dennis M. Williams, PharmD, FASHP, FAPHA, FCCP, BCPS, Associate Professor, Department of Pharmacotherapy, School of Pharmacy, University of North Carolina; Clinical Specialist, Pulmonary Medicine, UNC Hospitals, Chapel Hill, North Carolina

Susan R. Winkler, PharmD, BCPS, Clinical Associate Professor/Pharmacotherapist, Department of Pharmacy Practice, University of Illinois at Chicago College of Pharmacy, Chicago, Illinois

Maria Bulich Yaramus, PharmD, Clinical and Research Education Coordinator, Integrative Medicine, University of Pittsburgh Cancer Institute; Clinical Instructor, Department of Pharmacy and Therapeutics, University of Pittsburgh School of Pharmacy, Pittsburgh, Pennsylvania

Peggy C. Yarborough, PharmD, MS, BC-ADM, CDE, FAPP, FASHP, NAP Professor, Department of Pharmacy Practice, Campbell University School of Pharmacy; Pharmacist Clinician, Wilson Community Health Center, Wilson, North Carolina

Nancy Yunker, PharmD, Assistant Professor of Pharmacy, Department of Pharmacy, Virginia Commonwealth University School of Pharmacy—MCV Campus; Clinical Specialist in Adult Internal Medicine, Virginia Commonwealth University Health System—Medical College of Virginia Hospitals, Richmond, Virginia

William C. Zamboni, PharmD, Assistant Member of the Program of Molecular Therapeutics and Drug Discovery, University of Pittsburgh Cancer Institute; Assistant Professor, Department of Pharmaceutical Sciences, School of Pharmacy; Assistant Professor, Department of Medicine, School of Medicine, University of Pittsburgh, Pittsburgh, Pennsylvania

Basil J. Zitelli, MD, FAAP, Professor of Pediatrics, Department of Pediatrics, Children's Hospital of Pittsburgh, Pittsburgh, Pennsylvania

Contents

Preface xix
Acknowledgments xxi

SECTION 1
Principles of Patient-Focused Therapy

Chapter 1 Introduction: How to Use This Casebook 1
Terry L. Schwinghammer

Chapter 2 Active Learning Strategies 9
Gretchen M. Brophy, Cynthia K. Kirkwood

Chapter 3 Case Studies in Patient Communication 13
Marie E. Gardner, Richard N. Herrier

Chapter 4 Care Planning: A Component of the Patient Care Process 25
Grace D. Lamsam, Terry L. Schwinghammer

Chapter 5 Documentation of Pharmacist Interventions 33
Bruce R. Canaday, Peggy C. Yarborough, Timothy J. Ives

SECTION 2
Cardiovascular Disorders

Chapter 6 Cardiopulmonary Resuscitation 39
Tate N. Trujillo, Donna S. Wall

Chapter 7 Hypertension 42
Alicia M. Reese, Laurajo Ryan

Chapter 8 Obstructive Sleep Apnea and Hypertension 45
John M. Dopp, Bradley G. Phillips

Chapter 9 Hypertensive Urgency/Emergency 47
James J. Nawarskas

Chapter 10 Heart Failure 49
Jon D. Horton

Chapter 11 Ischemic Heart Disease and Acute Coronary Syndrome 53
Shawn R. Hansen, Amy J. Guenette

Chapter 12 Acute Myocardial Infarction 56
Kelly C. Rogers, Robert B. Parker

Chapter 13 Ventricular Tachycardia 58
Amy L. Seybert

Chapter 14 Atrial Fibrillation 61
Bradley G. Phillips

Chapter 15 Hypertrophic Cardiomyopathy 63
William D. Linn, Robert A. O'Rourke

Chapter 16 Deep Vein Thrombosis 65
Deanne L Hall, Meredith L. Rose

Chapter 17 Pulmonary Embolism 68
Amy L. Seybert, Ted L. Rice

Chapter 18 Chronic Anticoagulation 72
Beth Bryles Phillips

Chapter 19 Ischemic Stroke 74
Susan R. Winkler.

Chapter 20 Hyperlipidemia: Primary Prevention 76
Laurajo Ryan, Alicia M. Reese

Chapter 21 Hyperlipidemia: Secondary Prevention 79
Tina M. Hisel

Chapter 22 Peripheral Vascular Disease 81
Susan D. Bear

Chapter 23 Hypovolemic Shock 83
Brian L. Erstad

SECTION 3
Respiratory Disorders

Chapter 24 Acute Asthma 87
Tia D. Eddy, Daniel T. Kennedy, Ralph E. Small

Chapter 25 Chronic Asthma 90
Dennis M. Williams

Chapter 26 Chronic Obstructive Lung Disease 93
Daren L. Knoell

Chapter 27 Cystic Fibrosis 95
Robert J. Kuhn, Kimberly J. Novak

SECTION 4
Gastrointestinal Disorders

Chapter 28 Gastroesophageal Reflux Disease 99
Meredith L. Rose

Chapter 29 Peptic Ulcer Disease 102
Marie A. Chisholm, Mark W. Jackson

Chapter 30 NSAID-Induced Ulcer Disease 104
Cherokee Layson-Wolf, Ralph E. Small

Chapter 31 Stress Ulcer Prophylaxis/Upper GI Hemorrhage 106
Kristie C. Reeves, Henry J. Mann

Chapter 32 Crohn's Disease 109
Kerry A. Cholka

Chapter 33 Ulcerative Colitis 111
Nancy S. Yunker, Ralph E. Small

Chapter 34 Nausea and Vomiting 114
Kelly K. Nystrom, Pamela A. Foral

Chapter 35 Diarrhea 116
Marie A. Abate, Charles D. Ponte

Chapter 36 Irritable Bowel Syndrome 118
Nancy S. Yunker, William R. Garnett

Chapter 37 Pediatric Gastroenteritis 120
William McGhee, Basil J. Zitelli

Chapter 38 Constipation 122
Beth Bryles Phillips

Chapter 39 Ascites Management in Portal Hypertension and Cirrhosis 124
Joette M. Meyer

Chapter 40 Esophageal Varices 126
Cesar Alaniz

Chapter 41 Hepatic Encephalopathy 128
Carrie A. Sincak

Chapter 42 Acute Pancreatitis 130
Charles W. Fetrow, Maria B. Yaramus

Chapter 43 Chronic Pancreatitis 133
Susan D. Bear, Donna S. Wall

Chapter 44 Viral Hepatitis A Vaccination 135
Juliana Chan

Chapter 45 Viral Hepatitis B 137
Juliana Chan

Chapter 46 Viral Hepatitis C 139
Cesar Alaniz, Nancy P. Lam

SECTION 5
Renal Disorders

Chapter 47 Drug-Induced Acute Renal Failure 143
Mary K. Stamatakis

Chapter 48 Acute Renal Failure 145
Reina Bendayan, Michelle D. Furler

Chapter 49 Progressive Renal Disease 147
Reina Bendayan, Michelle D. Furler

Chapter 50 End-Stage Renal Disease 149
James D. Coyle

Chapter 51 Chronic Glomerulonephritis 151
Melanie S. Joy

Chapter 52 Syndrome of Inappropriate Antidiuretic Hormone Release 154
Rex W. Force

Chapter 53 Hyperkalemia, Hyperphosphatemia, and Hypercalcemia 156
Mary K. Stamatakis

Chapter 54 Hypercalcemia of Malignancy 158
Laura L. Jung, Rowena N. Schwartz

Chapter 55 Hypokalemia and Hypomagnesemia 161
Denise R. Sokos, W. Greg Leader

Chapter 56 Metabolic Acidosis 163
Kimberly A. Dornbrook-Lavender, Melanie S. Joy

Chapter 57 Metabolic Alkalosis 165
Thomas D. Nolin

SECTION 6
Neurologic Disorders

Chapter 58 Multiple Sclerosis 169
Jacquelyn L. Bainbridge, John R. Corboy

Chapter 59 Complex Partial Seizures 171
James W. McAuley

Chapter 60 Generalized Tonic-Clonic Seizures 173
Monica A. Summers, Sharon M. Tramonte

Chapter 61 Status Epilepticus 175
Monica A. Summers, Sharon M. Tramonte

Chapter 62 Acute Management of the Brain Injury Patient 177
Denise H. Rhoney

Chapter 63 Parkinson's Disease 179
Mary Louise Wagner, Margery H. Mark

Chapter 64 Pain Management 181
Christine K. O'Neil

Chapter 65 Headache Disorders 184
Tejal Patel, Susan R. Winkler

SECTION 7
Psychiatric Disorders

Chapter 66 Attention-Deficit Hyperactivity Disorder 187
William H. Benefield, Jr.

Chapter 67 **Eating Disorders: Anorexia Nervosa** 189
Libby S. Schindler

Chapter 68 **Alzheimer's Disease** 191
Cynthia P. Koh-Knox, Robert W. Bennett

Chapter 69 **Alcohol Withdrawal** 193
Robert L. Maher, Jr.

Chapter 70 **Nicotine Dependence** 195
Julie C. Kissack

Chapter 71 **Schizophrenia** 197
William H. Benefield, Jr., Lawrence J. Cohen

Chapter 72 **Major Depression** 200
Brian L. Crabtree, Victor G. Dostrow

Chapter 73 **Bipolar Disorder** 202
Lawrence J. Cohen, William H. Benefield, Jr.

Chapter 74 **Generalized Anxiety Disorder** 205
Sarah T. Melton, Cynthia K. Kirkwood

Chapter 75 **Obsessive-Compulsive Disorder** 208
Sarah T. Melton, Cynthia K. Kirkwood

Chapter 76 **Insomnia** 210
Mollie Ashe Scott, Amy M. Lugo

SECTION 8
Endocrinologic Disorders

Chapter 77 **Type 1 Diabetes Mellitus and Ketoacidosis** 213
Amy S. Nicholas, Holly S. Divine

Chapter 78 **Type 2 Diabetes Mellitus: New Onset** 216
Scott R. Drab

Chapter 79 **Type 2 Diabetes Mellitus: Existing Disease** 218
Kelly P. Jones, Jean-Venable R. Goode

Chapter 80 **Hyperthyroidism: Graves' Disease** 221
Kristine S. Schonder

Chapter 81 **Hypothyroidism** 223
Michael A. Oszko

Chapter 82 **Cushing's Syndrome** 225
Christopher M. Terpening, John G. Gums

Chapter 83 **Addison's Disease** 227
Cynthia P. Koh-Knox, Bruce C. Carlstedt

Chapter 84 **Hyperprolactinemia** 228
Amy Heck Sheehan, Karim Anton Calis

SECTION 9
Gynecologic Disorders

Chapter 85 **Contraception** 231
Julia M. Koehler

Chapter 86 **Premenstrual Dysphoric Disorder** 233
Martha P. Fankhauser, Donna M. Jermain

Chapter 87 **Managing Menopausal Symptoms** 236
Melissa A. Somma, Jonathan D. Ference

SECTION 10
Urologic Disorders

Chapter 88 **Erectile Dysfunction** 239
Cara L. Liday

Chapter 89 **Benign Prostatic Hyperplasia** 241
Kevin W. Cleveland, Catherine A. Heyneman, Richard S. Rhodes

Chapter 90 **Neurogenic Bladder & Urinary Incontinence** 244
Mary Lee

SECTION 11
Immunologic Disorders

Chapter 91 **Systemic Lupus Erythematosus** 247
Ralph E. Small, Nicole M. Paolini

Chapter 92 **Solid Organ Transplantation** 249
Kristine S. Schonder

SECTION 12
Bone and Joint Disorders

Chapter 93 **Osteoporosis** 253
Julia M. Koehler

Chapter 94 **Rheumatoid Arthritis** 255
Amy L. Whitaker, Ralph E. Small

Chapter 95 **Osteoarthritis** 257
Michael A. Oszko

Chapter 96 **Gout and Hyperuricemia** 260
Ralph E. Small

SECTION 13
Disorders of the Eyes, Ears, Nose and Throat

Chapter 97 **Glaucoma** 263
Tien T. Kiat-Winarko

Chapter 98 **Allergic Rhinitis** 265
W. Greg Leader

SECTION 14
Dermatologic Disorders

Chapter 99 **Acne Vulgaris** 269
Rebecca M. Law, Wayne P. Gulliver

Chapter 100 **Psoriasis** 271
Rebecca M. Law, Wayne P. Gulliver

Chapter 101 **Atopic Dermatitis** 273
Rebecca M. Law, Poh Gin Kwa

Chapter 102 **Cutaneous Reaction to Drugs** 275
Rebecca M. Law, Wayne P. Gulliver

SECTION 15
Hematologic Disorders

Chapter 103 **Iron Deficiency Anemia** 277
William J. Spruill, William E. Wade

Chapter 104 **Vitamin B_{12} Deficiency** 280
Barbara J. Mason, Beata Ineck

Chapter 105 **Folic Acid Deficiency** 282
Beata Ineck, Barbara J. Mason

Chapter 106 **Sickle Cell Anemia** 284
Christine M. Walko, R. Donald Harvey III

SECTION 16
Infectious Diseases

Chapter 107 **Using Laboratory Tests in Infectious Disease** 289
Steven J. Martin, Eric G. Sabloff

Chapter 108 **Bacterial Meningitis** 291
Sherry Luedtke

Chapter 109 **Pediatric Cough Illness/Acute Bronchitis** 293
Justin J. Sherman, W. Greg Leader

Chapter 110 **Prevention and Treatment of Influenza** 295
Christina E. Schober, Meredith L. Rose

Chapter 111 **Community-Acquired Pneumonia** 297
Patrick P. Gleason

Chapter 112 **Otitis Media** 300
Patrick P. Gleason, Steven V. Johnson

Chapter 113 **Streptococcal Pharyngitis** 301
Denise L. Howrie, Elaine McGhee

Chapter 114 **Rhinosinusitis** 303
Steven V. Johnson, Patrick P. Gleason

Chapter 115 **Pressure Sores** 304
Richard S. Rhodes, Catherine A. Heyneman, Christopher T. Owens

Chapter 116 **Diabetic Foot Infection** 307
Renee-Claude Mercier, A. Christie Graham

Chapter 117 **Infective Endocarditis** 309
Manjunath P. Pai, Renata Smith, Keith A. Rodvold

Chapter 118 **Pulmonary Tuberculosis** 311
Tina Penick Brock, Dennis M. Williams

Chapter 119 **Clostridium Difficile-Associated Diarrhea** 314
Eric G. Sabloff, Steven J. Martin

Chapter 120 **Intra-Abdominal Infection** 316
Renee-Claude Mercier, A. Christie Graham

Chapter 121 **Lower Urinary Tract Infection** 318
Kelly A. Sprandel, Christine A. Lesch, Keith A. Rodvold

Chapter 122 **Acute Pyelonephritis** 320
Brian A. Potoski

Chapter 123 **Pelvic Inflammatory Disease and Other Sexually-Transmitted Diseases** 324
Denise L. Howrie, Pamela J. Murray

Chapter 124 **Syphilis** 327
Alex K. McDonald, Dennis M. Williams

Chapter 125 **Genital Herpes and Chlamydial Infections** 328
Suellyn J. Sorensen

Chapter 126 **Osteomyelitis and Septic Arthritis** 330
Edward P. Armstrong, Leslie L. Barton

Chapter 127 **Gram-Negative Sepsis** 333
Steven J. Martin, Sandy J. Close

Chapter 128 **Dermatophytosis** 335
Robert Maher, Jr.

Chapter 129 **Bacterial Vaginosis** 337
Charles D. Ponte

Chapter 130 **Candida Vaginitis** 339
Rebecca M. Law

Chapter 131 **Systemic Fungal Infection** 341
Travis W. Cooper, Anya Rockwell

Chapter 132 **Infections in Immunocompromised Patients** 344
Douglas Slain

Chapter 133 **Antimicrobial Prophylaxis for Surgery** 346
Susan J. Skledar, Paige Robbins Gross

Chapter 134 **Pediatric Immunization** 348
John D. Grabenstein, Daniel T. Casto

Chapter 135 **Adult Immunization** 350
Pat S. Rafferty

Chapter 136 **Cytomegalovirus (CMV) Retinitis** 352
Patricia Fan-Havard

Chapter 137 **HIV Infection** 354
Susan Chuck, Keith A. Rodvold, Kinnari Khorana

Chapter 138 **HIV and Hepatitis C Coinfection** 357
Jennifer J. Kiser, Peter L. Anderson, Courtney V. Fletcher

SECTION 17
Oncologic Disorders

Chapter 139 **Breast Cancer** 361
Laura Boehnke Michaud

Chapter 140 **Non-Small Cell Lung Cancer** 364
Courtney F. Smith, Jane M. Pruemer

Chapter 141 **Colon Cancer** 367
Elizabeth Gray Paulson

Chapter 142 **Prostate Cancer** 369
Judith A. Smith

Chapter 143 **Non-Hodgkin's Lymphoma** 371
Keith A. Hecht

Chapter 144 **Hodgkin's Disease** 373
Cindy L. O'Bryant

Chapter 145 **Ovarian Cancer** 376
William C. Zamboni, Laura L. Jung, Margaret E. Tonda

Chapter 146 **Acute Lymphocytic Leukemia** 378
Mark T. Holdsworth

Chapter 147 **Chronic Myelogenous Leukemia** 382
R. Donald Harvey III, Christine Walko

Chapter 148 **Melanoma** 384
J. Michael Vozniak, Rowena N. Schwartz

Chapter 149 **Hematopoietic Stem Cell Transplantation** 386
Simon Cronin

SECTION 18
Nutrition and Nutritional Disorders

Chapter 150 **Parenteral Nutrition** 391
Michael D. Kraft

Chapter 151 **Adult Enteral Nutrition** 394
Carol J. Rollins, Elizabeth J. Ewing

Chapter 152 **Obesity** 397
Dannielle C. O'Donnell

SECTION 19
Emergency Preparedness and Response

Chapter 153 **Chemical Exposure** 401
Colleen Terriff

SECTION 20
Complementary and Alternative Therapies
Charles W. Fetrow, Maria B. Yaramus

Appendix A: Conversion Factors and Anthropometrics 409

Appendix B: Common Laboratory Tests 415

Appendix C: Medical Abbreviations 421

Appendix D: Samples Responses to Case Questions 431

Preface

The purpose of the *Pharmacotherapy Casebook* is to help students in the health professions develop the skills required to identify and resolve drug therapy problems through the use of patient case studies. Case studies can actively involve students in the learning process, engender self-confidence, and promote the development of skills in independent self-study, problem analysis, decision making, oral communication, and teamwork. Patient case studies can also be used as the focal point of discussions about pathophysiology, medicinal chemistry, pharmacology, and pharmacotherapeutics of individual diseases. By integrating the biomedical and pharmaceutical sciences with pharmacotherapeutics, case studies can help students appreciate the relevance and importance of a sound scientific foundation in preparation for practice.

The patient cases in this book are intended to complement the scientific information presented in the Sixth Edition of the textbook *Pharmacotherapy: A Pathophysiologic Approach.* This edition of the casebook contains 148 unique patient cases, 33 more than the first edition. The case chapters are organized into organ system sections that correspond to those of the Pharmacotherapy textbook. Students should read the relevant textbook chapter to become thoroughly familiar with the pathophysiology and pharmacotherapy of each disease state before attempting to make "decisions" about the care of patients described in this casebook. By using these realistic cases to practice creating, defending, and implementing pharmaceutical care plans, students can begin to develop the skills and self-confidence that will be necessary to make the real decisions required in professional practice.

The cases vary in the knowledge and experience required to answer the questions associated with each patient presentation. Some cases deal with a single disease state, whereas others have multiple diseases and drug-related problems. As a guide for instructors, each case is identified as being one of three complexity levels; this classification system is described in more detail in Chapter 1.

The sixth edition has five introductory chapters:

- Chapter 1 describes the format of case presentations and the means by which students and instructors can maximize the usefulness of the casebook. A systematic approach is consistently applied to each case. The steps involved in this approach include:

    1. Identification of real or potential drug therapy problems
    2. Determination of the desired therapeutic outcome
    3. Determination of therapeutic alternatives
    4. Design of an optimal individualized pharmacotherapeutic plan
    5. Development of methods to evaluate the therapeutic outcome
    6. Provision of patient education
    7. Communication and implementation of the pharmacotherapeutic plan

- In Chapter 2, the philosophy and implementation of active learning strategies is presented. This chapter sets the tone for the casebook by describing how these approaches can enhance student learning. The chapter offers a number of useful active learning strategies for instructors and provides advice to students on how to maximize their learning opportunities in active learning environments.
- Chapter 3 presents an efficient method of patient counseling developed by the Indian Health Service. The information can be used as the basis for simulated counseling sessions related to the patient cases.
- Chapter 4 describes the patient care process and delineates the steps necessary to create care plans that can help to ensure that the drug-related needs of patients are met. A blank care plan form is included at the end of the chapter. Students should be encouraged to practice using this form (or a similar one) when completing the case studies in this casebook.
- Chapter 5 describes two methods for documenting clinical interventions and communicating recommendations to other health care providers. These include the traditional SOAP note and the more pharmacy-specific FARM note. Student preparation of SOAP or FARM notes for the patient cases in this book will be excellent practice for future documentation in actual patient records.

It should be emphasized that the focus of classroom discussions about these cases should be on the process of solving patient problems as much as it is on finding the actual answers to the questions themselves. Isolated scientific facts learned today may be obsolete or incorrect tomorrow. Health care providers who can identify patient problems and solve them using a reasoned approach will be able to adapt to the continual evolution in the body of scientific knowledge and contribute in a meaningful way to improving the quality of patients' lives.

We are grateful for the broad acceptance that previous editions of the casebook have received. In particular, it has been adopted by many schools of pharmacy and nurse practitioner programs. It has also been used in institutional staff development efforts and by individual pharmacists wishing to upgrade their pharmaceutical care skills. It is our hope that this new edition will be even more valuable in assisting health care practitioners to meet society's need for safe and effective drug therapy.

Acknowledgments

I would like to thank the 183 case and chapter authors from 82 schools of pharmacy, health care systems, and other institutions in the United States and Canada who contributed their scholarly efforts to this casebook. I am especially appreciative of their diligence in meeting deadlines, adhering to the unique format of the casebook, and providing the most current drug therapy information available. The next generation of pharmacists will benefit from the willingness of these authors to share their expertise.

My sincere appreciation is also extended to the other Section Editors of this casebook, whose support and guidance contributed to the quality of the final product.

I am indebted to the following colleagues for their assistance in obtaining and interpreting illustrations to assist in the learning process: Lydia C. Contis, MD; William Pasculle, MD; Orlando F. Gabriele, MD; Terence W. Starz, MD; Philip J. Nerti, RPh; and Jason Lazar, MD. The expertise of the Creative Services/Medical Photography Department at UPMC is also gratefully acknowledged.

I would also like to thank Michael Brown, Executive Editor, and Barbara Holton, Senior Editing Supervisor, Medical Publishing Division of McGraw-Hill, Inc. Their cooperation, advice, and commitment were instrumental in maintaining the high standards of this publication.

Finally, I am grateful to my wife, Donna, and children, Amanda and Steven, for their understanding, support, and encouragement during the preparation of this book.

This book is dedicated to my grandson "Joey."

Terry L. Schwinghammer, PharmD, FCCP, FASHP, BCPS

Sixth Edition

PHARMACOTHERAPY

Casebook

a patient-focused approach

SECTION 1

Principles of Patient-Focused Therapy

CHAPTER 1

Introduction: How to Use This Casebook

Terry L. Schwinghammer, PharmD, FCCP, FASHP, BCPS

USING CASE STUDIES TO ENHANCE STUDENT LEARNING

The primary goals of the case method are to develop the skills of self-learning, critical thinking, and decision making. When case studies are used in the formal curricula of the health care professions or for independent study by practitioners, the focus of attention should be on learning the process of solving drug therapy problems, rather than simply on finding the scientific answers to the problems themselves. Students do learn scientific facts during the resolution of case study problems, but they usually learn more of them from their own independent study and from discussions with their peers than they do from the instructor. Working on subsequent cases with similar problems reinforces information recall. Traditional programs in the health care professions that rely heavily on the lecture format tend to concentrate on scientific content and the rote memorization of facts, rather than on the development of higher-order thinking skills.

Case studies in the health sciences provide the personal history of an individual patient and information about one or more health problems that must be solved. The learner's job is to work through the facts of the case, analyze the available data, gather more information, develop hypotheses, consider possible solutions, arrive at the optimal solution, and consider the consequences of the learner's decisions.[1] The role of the teacher is to serve as coach and facilitator rather than as the source of "the answer." In fact, in many cases there is more than one acceptable answer to a given question. Because instructors do not need to possess the correct answer, they need not be experts in the field being discussed. Rather, the students become teachers and learn from each other through thoughtful discussion of the case.

FORMAT OF THE CASEBOOK

Background Reading

The patient cases in this casebook should be used as the focal point for independent self-learning by individual students and for in-class problem-solving discussions by student groups and their instructors. If meaningful learning and discussion are to occur, students must come to discussion sessions prepared to discuss the case material rationally, to propose reasonable solutions, and to defend their pharmacotherapeutic plans. This requires a strong commitment to independent self-study prior to the session. The cases in this book were prepared to correspond with the scientific information contained in the sixth edition of *Pharmacotherapy: A Pathophysiologic Approach.*[2] For this reason, thorough familiarity with the corresponding textbook chapter is recommended as the principal method of student preparation. Other primary and tertiary literature should also be consulted as necessary to supplement the textbook readings.

Most of the cases in the casebook represent common diseases likely to be encountered by generalist pharmacy practitioners. As a result, not all of the *Pharmacotherapy* textbook chapters have an associated patient case in the casebook. On the other hand, some of the textbook chapters that discuss multiple disease entities have several corresponding cases in the casebook.

Levels of Case Complexity

Each case is identified at the top of the first page as being one of three levels of complexity. Instructors may use this classification system to select cases for discussion that correspond to the experience level of the student learners. These levels are defined as follows:

Level I—An uncomplicated case; only the single textbook chapter is required to complete the case questions. Little prior knowledge of the disease state or clinical experience is needed.
Level II—An intermediate-level case; several textbook chapters or other reference sources may be required to complete the case. Prior clinical experience may be helpful in resolving all of the issues presented.
Level III—A complicated case; multiple textbook chapters and substantial clinical experience are required to solve all of the patient's drug therapy problems.

Developing Ability Outcomes

Several ability outcomes are included at the beginning of each case for student reflection. The focus of these outcomes is on achieving competency in the clinical arena, not simply on learning isolated scientific facts. These items indicate some of the functions that the student should strive to perform in the clinical setting after reading the textbook chapter, studying the case, preparing a pharmacotherapeutic plan, and defending his or her recommendations.

The ability outcomes provided are meant to serve as a starting point to stimulate student thinking, but they are not meant to be all-inclusive. In fact, students should also generate their own personal ability outcomes and learning objectives for each case. By so doing, students take greater control of their own learning, which serves to improve personal motivation and the desire to learn.

PATIENT PRESENTATION

The format and organization of cases reflect those usually seen in actual clinical settings. The patient's medical history and physical examination findings are provided in the following standard outline format.

Chief Complaint

The chief complaint is a brief statement of the reason why the patient consulted the physician, stated in the patient's own words. In order to convey the patient's symptoms accurately, medical terms and diagnoses are generally not used.

HPI

History of present illness is a more complete description of the patient's symptom(s). Usually included in the HPI are:

- Date of onset
- Precise location
- Nature of onset, severity, and duration
- Presence of exacerbations and remissions
- Effect of any treatment given
- Relationship to other symptoms, bodily functions, or activities (e.g., activity, meals)
- Degree of interference with daily activities

PMH

The past medical history includes serious illnesses, surgical procedures, and injuries the patient has experienced previously. Minor complaints (e.g., influenza, colds) are usually omitted.

FH

The family history includes the age and health of parents, siblings, and children. For deceased relatives, the age and cause of death are recorded. In particular, heritable diseases and those with a hereditary tendency are noted (e.g., diabetes mellitus, cardiovascular disease, malignancy, rheumatoid arthritis, obesity).

SH

The social history includes the social characteristics of the patient as well as the environmental factors and behaviors that may contribute to the development of disease. Items usually included are the patient's marital status, number of children, educational background, occupation, physical activity, hobbies, dietary habits, and use of tobacco, alcohol, or other drugs.

Meds

The medication history should include an accurate record of the patient's current prescription and nonprescription medication use. Because pharmacists possess extensive knowledge of the thousands of prescription and nonprescription products available, they can perform a valuable service to the health care team by obtaining a complete medication history that includes the names, doses, schedules, and duration of therapy for all medications, including dietary supplements and other alternative therapies.

All (Allergies)

Allergies to drugs, food, pets, and environmental factors (e.g., grass, dust, pollen) are recorded. An accurate description of the reaction that occurred should also be included. Care should be taken to distinguish adverse drug effects ("upset stomach") from true allergy ("hives").

ROS

In the review of systems, the examiner questions the patient about the presence of symptoms related to each body system. In many cases, only the pertinent positive and negative findings are recorded. In a complete ROS, body systems are generally listed starting from the head and working toward the feet and may include the skin, head, eyes, ears, nose, mouth and throat, neck, cardiovascular, respiratory, gastrointestinal, genitourinary, endocrine, musculoskeletal, and neuropsychiatric systems. The purpose of the ROS is to evaluate the status of each body system and to prevent the omission of pertinent information. Information that was included in the HPI is not repeated in the ROS.

PE

The exact procedures performed during the physical examination vary depending upon the chief complaint and the patient's medical history. In some practice settings, only a limited and focused physical examination is performed. In psychiatric practice, greater emphasis is usually placed on the type and severity of the patient's symptoms than on physical findings. A suitable physical assessment textbook should be consulted for the specific procedures that may be conducted for each body system. The general sections for the PE are outlined as follows:

Gen (general appearance)
VS (vital signs)—blood pressure, pulse, respiratory rate, temperature (weight and height are usually included in this casebook, although they are not technically considered to be vital signs)
Skin (integumentary)

HEENT (head, eyes, ears, nose, and throat)
Lungs/Thorax (pulmonary)
Cor or CV (cardiovascular)
Abd (abdomen)
Genit/Rect (genitalia/rectal)
MS/Ext (musculoskeletal and extremities)
Neuro (neurologic)

Labs

The results of laboratory tests are included with almost all cases in this casebook. **Appendix A** contains a number of commonly used conversion factors and anthropometric information that will be helpful in solving many case answers. Normal ranges for the laboratory tests used throughout the casebook are included in **Appendix B.** The normal range for a given laboratory test is generally determined from a representative sample of the general population. The upper and lower limits of the range usually encompass two standard deviations from the population mean, which includes a range within which about 95% of healthy persons would fall. The term *normal range* may be misleading, because a test result may be abnormal for a given individual even if it falls within the "normal" range. Furthermore, given the statistical methods used to calculate the range, about 1 in 20 normal, healthy individuals may have a value for a test that lies outside the range. For these reasons, the term *reference range* is preferred over normal range. Reference ranges differ among laboratories, so the values given in Appendix B should be considered only as a general guide. Institution-specific reference ranges should be used in actual clinical settings.

All of the cases include some physical examination and laboratory findings that are within normal limits. For example, a description of the cardiovascular examination may include a statement that the point of maximal impulse is at the fifth intercostal space; laboratory evaluation may include a serum sodium of 140 mEq/L. The presentation of actual findings (rather than simple statements that the heart examination and the serum sodium were normal) reflects what will be seen in actual clinical practice. More importantly, listing both normal and abnormal findings requires students to carefully assess the complete database and identify the pertinent positive and negative findings for themselves. A valuable portion of the learning process is lost if students are only provided with findings that are abnormal and are known to be associated with the disease being discussed.

The patients described in this casebook have fictitious names in order to humanize the situations and to encourage students to remember that they will one day be caring for patients, not treating disease states. However, in the actual clinical setting, patient confidentiality is of utmost importance, and patient names should not be used during group discussions in patient care areas unless absolutely necessary. To develop student sensitivity to this issue, instructors may wish to avoid using these fictitious patient names during class discussions. In this casebook, patient names are usually given only in the initial presentation; they are seldom used in subsequent questions or other portions of the case.

The issues of race, ethnicity, and gender also deserve thoughtful consideration. The traditional format for case presentations usually begins with a description of the patient's age, race, and gender, as in: "The patient is a 65-year-old white male. . . ." Single-word racial labels such as "black" or "white" are actually of limited value in many cases and may actually be misleading in some instances.[3] For this reason, racial descriptors are excluded from the opening line of each presentation. When ethnicity is pertinent to the case, this information is presented in the social history or physical examination. Patients in this casebook are referred to as men or women, rather than males or females, to promote sensitivity to human dignity.

The patient cases in this casebook include medical abbreviations and drug brand names, just as medical records do in actual practice. Although these customs are sometimes the source of clinical problems, the intent of their inclusion is to make the cases as realistic as possible. **Appendix C** lists the medical abbreviations used in the casebook. This list is limited to commonly accepted abbreviations; thousands more exist, which makes it difficult for the novice practitioner to efficiently assess patient databases. Most institutions have an approved list of accepted abbreviations; these lists should be consulted in practice to facilitate one's understanding and to avoid using abbreviations in the medical record that are not on the official approved list. Appendix C also lists abbreviations and designations that should be avoided. Given the immense human toll resulting from medical errors, this section should be considered "must" reading for all students.

The casebook also contains some photographs of commercial drug products. These illustrations are provided as examples only and are not intended to imply endorsement of those particular products.

Pharmaceutical Care and Drug Therapy Problems

Modern drug therapy plays a crucial role in improving the health of people by enhancing the quality of life and by extending life expectancy. The advent of biotechnology has led to the introduction of unique compounds for the prevention and treatment of disease that were unheard of a decade ago. Each year the US Food and Drug Administration approves approximately two dozen new drug products that contain active substances that have never before been marketed in the United States. Although the cost of new therapeutic agents has received intense scrutiny in recent years, drug therapy actually accounts for a relatively small proportion of overall health care expenditures. Appropriate drug therapy is cost-effective and may actually serve to reduce total expenditures by decreasing the need for surgery, preventing hospital admissions, and shortening hospital stays.

Several studies have indicated that improper use of prescription medications is a frequent and serious problem. Based on a decision analytic model, one study estimated that the cost of drug-related morbidity and mortality was more than $177 billion in 2000. Hospital admissions accounted for almost 70% ($121.5 billion) of total costs; long-term-care admissions were responsible for 18% of costs ($32.8 billion).[4] In 1999, the National Institute of Medicine estimated that 7,000 patients die each year from medication errors that occur both within and outside hospitals. A societal need for better use of medications clearly exists. Widespread implementation of pharmaceutical care has the potential to positively impact this situation by the design, implementation, and monitoring of rational therapeutic plans to produce defined outcomes that improve the quality of patients' lives.[5]

The mission of the pharmacy profession is to render pharmaceutical care. Schools of pharmacy have implemented innovative instructional strategies to prepare future pharmacists to provide pharmaceutical care. Doctor of Pharmacy programs have an increased emphasis on patient-centered care, as evidenced by more experiential training, especially in ambulatory care. Many programs are structured to promote self-directed learning, to develop problem-solving and communication skills, and to instill the desire for lifelong learning.

In its broadest sense, pharmaceutical care involves the identification, resolution, and prevention of potential drug therapy problems. A drug therapy problem has been defined as "any undesirable event experienced by a patient which involves, or is suspected to involve, drug therapy and that interferes with achieving the desired goals of therapy."[5] Seven distinct types of drug therapy problems have been identified that may potentially lead to an undesirable event that has physiologic, psychological, social, or economic ramifications.[6] These categories of drug therapy problems include:

1. Unnecessary drug therapy
2. Needs additional drug therapy
3. Ineffective drug
4. Dosage too low
5. Adverse drug reaction
6. Dosage too high
7. Noncompliance

These drug therapy problems are discussed in more detail in Chapter 4 of the casebook. Because this casebook is intended to be used in conjunction with the *Pharmacotherapy* textbook, one of its purposes is to serve as a tool for learning about the pharmacotherapy of disease states. For this reason, the primary problem to be identified and addressed for most of the patients in the casebook is the need for additional drug treatment for a specific medical indication (problem #2 above). Other actual or potential drug therapy problems may coexist during the initial presentation or may develop during the clinical course of the disease.

Patient-Focused Approach to Case Problems

In this casebook, each patient presentation is followed by a set of patient-centered questions that are similar for each case. These questions are applied consistently from case to case to demonstrate that a systematic patient care process can be successfully applied regardless of the underlying disease state(s). The questions are designed to enable students to identify and resolve problems related to pharmacotherapy. They help students recognize what they know and what they do not know, thereby guiding them in determining what information must be learned to satisfactorily resolve the patient's problems.[7] A description of each of the steps involved in solving drug therapy problems is included in the following paragraphs.

1. Identification of real or potential drug therapy problems

The first step in the patient-focused approach is to collect pertinent patient information, interpret it properly, and determine whether drug therapy problems exist. Some authors prefer to divide this process into two or more separate steps because of the difficulty that inexperienced students may have performing these complex tasks simultaneously.[8] This step is analogous to documenting the subjective and objective patient findings in the SOAP format. It is important to differentiate the process of identifying the patient's drug therapy problems from making a disease-related medical diagnosis. In fact, the medical diagnosis is known for the majority of patients seen by pharmacists. However, pharmacists must be capable of assessing the patient's database to determine whether drug therapy problems exist that warrant a change in drug therapy. In the case of preexisting chronic diseases such as asthma or rheumatoid arthritis, one must be able to assess information that may indicate a change in severity of the disease. This process involves reviewing the patient's symptoms, the signs of disease present on physical examination, and the results of laboratory and other diagnostic tests. Some of the cases require the student to develop complete patient problem lists. Potential sources for this information in actual practice include the patient or his or her advocate, the patient's physician or other health care professionals, and the patient's medical chart or other records.

After the drug therapy problems are identified, the clinician should determine which of them are amenable to pharmacotherapy. Alternatively, one must also consider whether any of the problems could have been caused by drug therapy. In some cases (both in the casebook and in real life), not all of the information needed to make these decisions is available. In that situation, providing precise recommendations for obtaining additional information needed to satisfactorily assess the patient's problems can be a valuable contribution to the patient's care.

2. Determination of the desired therapeutic outcome

After pertinent patient-specific information has been gathered and the patient's drug therapy problems have been identified, the next step is to define the specific goals of pharmacotherapy. The primary therapeutic outcomes include:

- Cure of disease (e.g., bacterial infection)
- Reduction or elimination of symptoms (e.g., pain from cancer)
- Arresting or slowing of the progression of disease (e.g., rheumatoid arthritis, HIV infection)
- Preventing a disease or symptom (e.g., coronary heart disease)

Other important outcomes of pharmacotherapy include:

- Not complicating or aggravating other existing disease states
- Avoiding or minimizing adverse effects of treatment
- Providing cost-effective therapy
- Maintaining the patient's quality of life

Sources of information for this step may include the patient or his or her advocate, the patient's physician or other health care professionals, medical records, and the *Pharmacotherapy* textbook or other literature references.

3. Determination of therapeutic alternatives

After the intended outcome has been defined, attention can be directed toward identifying the kinds of treatments that might be beneficial in achieving that outcome. The clinician should ensure that all feasible pharmacotherapeutic alternatives available for achieving the predefined therapeutic outcome(s) are considered before choosing a single therapeutic regimen. Nondrug therapies (e.g., diet, exercise, psychotherapy) that might be useful should be included in the list of therapeutic alternatives when appropriate. Useful sources of information on therapeutic alternatives include the *Pharmacotherapy* textbook and other references, as well as the clinical experience of the health care provider and other involved health care professionals.

There has been a resurgence of interest in dietary supplements and other alternative therapies in the past decade. The public spends billions of dollars each year on supplements to treat diseases for which there is little scientific evidence of efficacy. Some products are hazardous, and others may interact with a patient's prescription medications or aggravate concurrent disease states. Conversely, there is scientific evidence of efficacy for some dietary supplements (e.g., glucosamine for osteoarthritis). Health care providers must be knowledgeable about these products and prepared to answer patient questions regarding their efficacy and safety. The casebook contains a separate section devoted to this important topic (**Section 20**). This portion of the casebook contains nine fictitious patient vignettes that are directly related to a patient case that was presented earlier in this book. Each scenario involves one or more questions asked by a patient about a specific remedy. Additional follow-up questions are then asked to help the reader provide a scientifically based answer to the patient's question(s). Ten different dietary supplements are included in this section: garlic, omega-3 fatty acids, Ginkgo biloba, St. John's wort, valerian, black cohosh, saw palmetto, glucosamine, kava kava, and Echinacea.

4. Design of an optimal individualized pharmacotherapeutic plan

The purpose of this step is to determine the drug, dosage form, dose, schedule, and duration of therapy that are best suited for a given patient. Individual patient characteristics should be taken into consideration when weighing the risks and benefits of each available therapeutic alternative. For example, an asthma patient who requires new drug therapy for hypertension might better tolerate treatment with a thiazide diuretic rather than treatment with a β-blocker. On the other hand, a hypertensive patient with gout may be better served by use of a β-blocker rather than by use of a thiazide diuretic.

The reason for avoiding specific drugs should be stated in the therapeutic plan. Some potential reasons for drug avoidance include drug allergy, drug–drug or drug–disease interactions, patient age, renal or hepatic impairment, adverse effects, poor compliance, pregnancy, and high treatment cost.

The specific dose selected may depend upon the indication for the drug. For example, the dose of aspirin used to treat rheumatoid arthritis is much higher than that used to prevent myocardial infarction. The likelihood of adherence with the regimen and patient tolerance come into play in the selection of dosage forms. The economic, psychosocial, and ethical factors that are applicable to the patient should also be given due consideration in design of the pharmacotherapeutic regimen. An alternative plan should also be in place that would be appropriate if the initial therapy fails or cannot be used.

5. Identification of parameters to evaluate the outcome

One must identify the clinical and laboratory parameters necessary to assess the therapy for achievement of the desired therapeutic outcome and for detection and prevention of adverse effects. The outcome parameters selected should be specific, measurable, achievable, directly related to the therapeutic goals, and have a defined end point. As a means of remembering these points, the acronym SMART has been used (*S*pecific, *M*easurable, *A*chievable, *R*elated, and *T*ime bound). If the goal is to cure a bacterial pneumonia, one should outline the subjective and objective clinical parameters (e.g., relief of chest discomfort, cough, and fever), laboratory tests (e.g., normalization of white blood cell count and differential), and other procedures (e.g., resolution of infiltrate on chest x-ray) that provide sufficient evidence of bacterial eradication and clinical cure of the disease. The intervals at which data should be collected are dependent upon the outcome parameters selected and should be established prospectively. It should be noted that expensive or invasive procedures may not be repeated after the initial diagnosis is made.

Adverse effect parameters must also be well defined and measurable. For example, it is insufficient to state that one will monitor for potential drug-induced "blood dyscrasias." Rather, one should identify the likely specific hematologic abnormality (e.g., anemia, leukopenia, or thrombocytopenia) and outline a prospective schedule for obtaining the appropriate parameters (e.g., obtain monthly hemoglobin/hematocrit, white blood cell count, or platelet count).

Monitoring for adverse events should be directed toward preventing or identifying serious adverse effects that have a reasonable likelihood of occurrence. For example, it is not cost-effective to obtain periodic liver function tests in all patients taking a drug that causes mild hepatic abnormalities only rarely, such as omeprazole. On the other hand, serious patient harm may be averted by outlining a specific screening schedule for drugs associated more frequently with hepatic abnormalities, such as methotrexate for rheumatoid arthritis.

6. Provision of patient education

The concept of pharmaceutical care is based on the existence of a covenantal relationship between the patient and the provider of care. Patients are our partners in health care, and our efforts may be for naught without their informed participation in the process. For chronic diseases such as diabetes mellitus, hypertension, and asthma, patients may have a greater role in managing their diseases than do health care professionals. Self-care is becoming more widespread as increasing numbers of prescription medications receive over-the-counter status. For these reasons, patients must be provided with sufficient information to enhance compliance, ensure successful therapy, and minimize adverse effects. **Chapter 3** describes patient interview techniques that can be used efficiently to determine the patient's level of knowledge. Additional information can then be provided as necessary to fill in knowledge gaps. In the questions posed with individual cases, students are asked to provide the kind of information that should be given to the patient who has limited knowledge of his or her disease. Under the Omnibus Budget Reconciliation Act (OBRA) of 1990, for patients who accept the offer of counseling, pharmacists should consider including these items:

- Name and description of the medication (which may include the indication)
- Dosage, dosage form, route of administration, and duration of therapy
- Special directions or procedures for preparation, administration, and use
- Common and severe adverse effects, interactions, and contraindications (with the action required should they occur)
- Techniques for self-monitoring
- Proper storage
- Prescription refill information
- Action to be taken in the event of missed doses

Instructors may wish to have simulated patient-interviewing sessions for new and refill prescriptions during the case discussions to practice medication education skills. Factual information should be provided as concisely as possible to enhance memory retention. An excellent source for information on individual drugs is the USP-DI Volume II, *Advice for the Patient: Drug Information in Lay Language.*[9]

7. Communication and implementation of the pharmacotherapeutic plan

The most well-conceived plan is worthless if it languishes without implementation because of inadequate communication with prescribers or other health care providers. Permanent, written documentation of significant recommendations in the medical record is important to ensure accurate communication among practitioners. Oral communication alone can be misinterpreted or transferred inaccurately to others. This is especially true because there are many drugs that sound alike when spoken but that have different therapeutic uses.

The SOAP format (*S*ubjective, *O*bjective, *A*ssessment, *P*lan) has been used by clinicians for many years to assess patient problems and to communicate findings and plans in the medical record. However, writing SOAP notes may not be the optimal process for learning to solve drug therapy problems because several important steps taken by experienced clinicians are not always apparent and may be overlooked. For example, the precise therapeutic outcome desired is often unstated in SOAP notes, leaving others to presume what the desired treatment goals are. Health care professionals using the SOAP format also commonly move directly from an assessment of the patient (diagnosis) to outlining a diagnostic or therapeutic plan, without necessarily conveying whether careful consideration has been given to all available feasible diagnostic or therapeutic alternatives. The plan itself as outlined in SOAP notes may also give short shrift to the monitoring parameters that are required to ensure successful therapy and to detect and prevent adverse drug effects. Finally, there is often little suggestion provided as to the treatment information that should be conveyed to the most important individual involved: the patient. If SOAP notes are used for documenting drug therapy problems, consideration should be given to including each of these components.

In **Chapter 5** of this casebook, the FARM note (*F*indings, *A*ssessment, *R*ecommendations, *M*onitoring) is presented as a useful method of consistently documenting therapeutic recommendations and implementing plans.[10] This method can be used by students as an alternative to the SOAP note to practice communicating pharmacotherapeutic plans to other members of the health care team. Although preparation of written communication notes is not included in written form with each set of case questions, instructors are encouraged to include the composition of a SOAP or FARM note as one of the requirements for successfully completing each case study assignment.

In addition to communicating with other health care professionals, practitioners of pharmaceutical care must also develop a personal record of each patient's drug therapy problems and the health care provider's plan for resolving them, interventions made, and actual therapeutic outcomes achieved. A pharmaceutical care plan is a well-conceived and scientifically sound method of documenting these activities. **Chapter 4** of this casebook discusses the philosophy of care planning and describes their creation and use. A sample care plan document is included in that chapter for use by students as they work through the cases in this book.

Clinical Course

The process of pharmaceutical care entails an assessment of the patient's progress in order to ensure achievement of the desired therapeutic outcomes. A description of the patient's clinical course is included with many of the cases in this book to reflect this process. Some cases follow the progression of the patient's disease over months to years and include both inpatient and outpatient treatment. Follow-up questions directed toward ongoing evaluation and problem solving are included after presentation of the clinical course.

Self-Study Assignments

Each case concludes with several study assignments related to the patient case or the disease state that may be used as independent study projects for students to complete outside class. These assignments generally require students to obtain additional information that is not contained in the corresponding *Pharmacotherapy* textbook chapter.

Literature References and Internet Sites

Selected literature references that are specific to the case at hand are included at the end of the cases. These references may be useful to students for answering the questions posed. The *Pharmacotherapy* textbook contains a more comprehensive list of references pertinent to each disease state.

Some cases list Internet sites as sources of drug therapy information. The sites listed are recognized as authoritative sources of information, such as the US Food and Drug Administration (www.fda.gov) and the Centers for Disease Control and Prevention (www.cdc.gov). Students should be advised to be wary of information posted on the Internet that is not from highly regarded health care organizations or publications. The uniform resource locators (URLs) for Internet sites sometimes change, and it is possible that not all sites listed in the casebook will remain available for viewing.

DEVELOPING ANSWERS TO CASE QUESTIONS

The use of case studies for independent learning and in-class discussion may be unfamiliar to many students. For this reason, it may initially be difficult for students to devise complete answers to the case questions. **Appendix D** contains the answers to three cases in order to demonstrate how case responses might be prepared and presented. The authors of the cases contributed the recommended answers provided in the appendix, but they should not be considered the sole "right" answer. Thoughtful students who have prepared well for the discussion sessions may arrive at additional or alternative answers that are also appropriate.

With diligent self-study, practice, and the guidance of instructors, students will gradually acquire the knowledge, skills, and self-confidence to develop and implement pharmaceutical care plans for their own future patients. The goal of the casebook is to help students progress along this path of lifelong learning.

References

1. Herreid CF. Case studies in science: A novel method of science education. J College Sci Teaching 1994;23:221–229.

2. DiPiro JT, Talbert RL, Yee GC, et al., eds. Pharmacotherapy: A Pathophysiologic Approach, 6th ed. New York, McGraw-Hill, 2005.
3. Caldwell SH, Popenoe R. Perceptions and misperceptions of skin color. Ann Intern Med 1995;122:614–617.
4. Ernst FR, Grizzle AJ. Drug-related morbidity and mortality: Updating the cost-of-illness model. J Am Pharm Assoc 2001;41:192–199.
5. Cipolle RJ, Strand LM, Morley PC. Pharmaceutical care practice: The clinician's guide, 2nd ed. New York, McGraw-Hill, 2004.
6. Strand LM, Morley PC, Cipolle RJ, et al. Drug-related problems: Their structure and function. Drug Intell Clin Pharm 1990;24:1093–1097.
7. Delafuente JC, Munyer TO, Angaran DM, Doering PL. A problem-solving active-learning course in pharmacotherapy. Am J Pharm Educ 1994;58:61–64.
8. Winslade N. Large-group problem-based learning: A revision from traditional to pharmaceutical care-based therapeutics. Am J Pharm Educ 1994; 58:64–73.
9. Advice for the patient: Drug information in lay language (USP-DI volume II), 24th ed. Greenwood Village, CO; Thomson Micromedex, 2004.
10. Canaday BR, Yarborough PC. Documenting pharmaceutical care: Creating a standard. Ann Pharmacother 1994;28:1292–1296.

CHAPTER 2

Active Learning Strategies

Gretchen M. Brophy, PharmD, BCPS, FCCP
Cynthia K. Kirkwood, PharmD, BCPP

Students in the health professions are faced with situations daily that require use of problem-solving skills—for example, trying to prioritize what courses they need to study for that day and developing a plan to use their time efficiently. Also, if they are involved in student professional organizations, they may need to do a service project that requires identifying an idea, developing a project plan, assigning tasks to different group members, and, finally, finishing the project and evaluating the results. On a practice rotations, students often need to determine if a drug is causing an adverse event in a particular patient. To solve problems, we call upon our previous experiences with similar situations and we observe, investigate, ask appropriate questions, and finally come to a conclusion or resolution.

Students who finish their formal training in health care must recognize that learning is a lifelong process. Scores of new drugs are approved every year, and innovative research changes the way that many diseases are treated. Drug use practices have changed dramatically in the last 20 years, and students will have the opportunity to pursue many different career paths. They must be prepared to take direct responsibility for patient outcomes by practicing pharmaceutical care. Health care professionals are working in multidisciplinary environments that require active participation in patient care. They will need to use their skills in communications, problem solving, independent learning, drug information retrieval, and knowledge of disease state management.[1–3] To prepare students to practice in this manner, many health care educators are using active learning strategies in the classroom.[4] In many therapeutics courses, students are given actual written patient cases as the basis for learning. Students may be asked to identify the significant subjective and objective findings; to develop a drug therapy problem list; to create an assessment statement; to consider all feasible therapeutic alternatives; to make therapeutic recommendations; to develop a monitoring plan; to formulate a written communication note for other health care providers; and to decide how they would educate the patient about his/her new drug therapies. This process actively engages students in problem solving because it requires them to integrate knowledge gained in other areas of the curriculum with specific patient information. As a result, students learn skills that they will use on a daily basis in their future practice sites.

TRADITIONAL TEACHING

Most students are taught using a teacher-centered approach before entering professional programs. At the beginning of the course, students are given a massive course syllabus packet that contains "everything they need to know" for the semester. In class, the teacher lectures on a predetermined subject that does not require student preparation. Students are passive recipients of information, and the testing method is usually a written examination that employs a multiple-choice or short-answer format. With this method, students are tested primarily on their ability to recall isolated facts that the teacher has identified as being important and do not learn to apply their knowledge to situations that they will ultimately encounter in pharmacy practice. The reward is an external one (i.e., exam or course grade) that may or may not reflect a student's actual ability to use knowledge to improve patient care. To teach students to be lifelong learners, it is essential to stimulate them to be inquisitive and actively involved with the learning that takes place in the classroom. This requires that teachers move away from more comfortable teaching methods and learn new techniques that will help students "learn to learn."

ACTIVE LEARNING STRATEGIES

Active learning has numerous definitions, and various methods are described in the educational literature. Simply put, active learning means involving students in the learning process.[5] In classes with active learning formats, students are involved in much more than listening. The transmission of information is deemphasized and replaced with the development of skills. Most proponents agree that active learning allows students to become engaged in the learning process while developing cognitive skills. Learning is reinforced when students actually apply their knowledge to new situations.[6] Willing students, innovative teachers, and administrative support within the school are required for active learning to be successful.[7] Control of learning must be shifted from the teacher to the students; this provides an opportunity for students to become active participants in their own learning. Although it sounds frightening at first, students can take control of their own learning. Knowledge of career and life goals can help students make decisions about how to spend their educational time. Warren[8] identifies several traits that prepare students for future careers:

- Analytical thinking
- Polite assertiveness
- Tolerance
- Communication skills
- Understanding of one's own physical well-being
- The ability to continue to teach oneself after graduation

After going through the active learning process, most students realize that knowledge is easily acquired, but developing critical thinking skills aids in lifelong learning.[7]

Teachers implement active learning exercises into classes in a variety of ways. Some of the active learning strategies give students the opportunity to pause and recall information, cooperate and collaborate in groups, solve problems, and generate questions.[9] More advanced methods include use of simulation, role-playing, debates, peer teaching, problem-based learning, and case studies.[10] Tests and quizzes evaluate student comprehension of material. Each of these strategies allows students to demonstrate their skills.

Didactic lectures can be enhanced by several active learning strategies. The "pause procedure" is designed to enhance student retention and comprehension of material.[11] It involves 15- to 20-minute mini-lectures with 2- to 3-minute pauses for students to rework their notes, discuss the material with their peers for clarification, and develop questions.[12] This strategy can be incorporated into a 50-minute lecture up to three times. Students are able to assess their understanding of the material and formulate opinions. The pause procedure is a useful method for classes that require retention of factual information.[10] With the "think-pair-share" exercise, students are asked to write down the answer to a question and turn to a classmate to compare answers. This method provides immediate feedback to students.[13] The"quick-thinks" technique allows students to quickly process the information they have learned.[14] Examples of "quick-thinks" include completing a sentence presented by the teacher on the treatment of a disease state, comparing and contrasting drug treatment strategies for a specific patient, drawing conclusions on the best treatment strategies for a disease state, and identifying and correcting errors in a case presentation.

Another active learning technique for classroom sessions is to involve the students in short writing assignments. Writing helps students identify knowledge deficits, clarify understanding of the material, and organize thoughts in a logical manner. Students can be asked to write questions related to the reading assignment and submit them for discussion at the next class session. Alternatively, students can formulate questions and answers before class, and then discuss them in small groups. The "shared paragraph" exercise requires students to write a paragraph at the end of class summarizing the major concepts that were presented. The paragraph is then shared with a partner to clarify the material and receive feedback.[10] Students can be asked to write a "minute paper" or "half-sheet response" to a question or issue raised in class to stimulate discussion.[15] Discussions of any misconceptions can be conducted in class or one-on-one with the teacher.

Students benefit by having access to pre- or postclass quizzes. Sample test questions can also be used to assess student comprehension of the presentation and facilitate class discussion. The Active Learning Centre (http://www.med.jhu.edu/medcenter) is an educational website designed to provide interactive exercises that engage students in active learning.[16]

Tests and quizzes are effective tools to help students review the class presentations or reading assignments. Quizzes can be administered several times during class and may or may not be graded. Quizzes given at the beginning of class help stimulate students to review information they did not know and listen for clarification during class lecture. Quizzes at the end of the class session allow students to use their problem-solving skills by applying what they have just learned to a patient case or problem.

Problem-solving skills can be developed during a class period by applying knowledge of pharmacotherapy to a patient case. Application reinforces the previously learned material and helps students understand the importance of the topic in a real-life situation. Problem-based learning (PBL) is a teaching and learning method in which a problem is used as the stimulus for developing critical thinking and problem-solving skills for acquiring new knowledge. The process of PBL starts with the student identifying the problem in a case. The student spends time either alone or in a group exploring and analyzing the problem and identifying learning resources needed to solve the problem. After acquiring the knowledge, the student applies it to solve the problem.[17] Small or large groups can be established for case discussions to help students develop communication skills, respect for other students' opinions, satisfaction for contributing to the discussion, and the ability to give and accept criticism.[17] Interactive PBL computer tools and the use of real patients also stimulate learning both outside and inside the classroom.[18–20] Computer technology can be used creatively in PBL cases as a tool for problem solving.[21]

Cooperative or collaborative learning strategies involve students in the generation of knowledge.[10] Students are randomly assigned to groups of four to six at the beginning of the school term. Several times during the term, each group is given a patient case and a group leader is selected. Each student in the group volunteers to work on a certain portion of the case. The case is discussed in class and each member receives the same grade. After students have finished working in their small groups or during large group sessions, the teacher serves as a facilitator of the discussion rather than as a lecturer. The students actively participate in the identification and resolution of the problem. The integration of this technique helps with development of skills in decision making, conflict management, and communication.[9] Group discussions help students develop concepts from the material presented, clarify ideas, and develop new strategies for clinical problem solving. These skills are essential for lifelong learning and will be used by the students throughout their careers.

CASE STUDIES

Case studies are used by a number of professional schools to teach pharmacotherapy.[1,19,22,23] Case studies are a written description of a real-life problem or situation. Only the facts are provided, usually in chronologic sequence similar to what would be encountered in a patient care setting. Many times, as in real life, the information given is incomplete or important details are not available. When working through a case, the student must distinguish between relevant and irrelevant facts and become accustomed to the fact that there is no single "correct" answer. The use of cases actively involves the student in the analysis of facts and details of the case, selection of a solution to the problem, and defense of his or her solution through discussion of the case.[24]

Students enrolled in such courses find that the case study method requires a large amount of preparation time outside of class. During class, active participation is essential for the maximum learning benefit to be achieved. Because of their various backgrounds, students learn different perspectives when dealing with patient problems. Some general steps proposed by McDade[24] for students when preparing cases for class discussion include:

- Skim the text quickly to establish the broad issues of the case and the types of information presented for analysis.
- Reread the case very carefully, underlining key facts as you go.
- Note on scratch paper the key issues and problems. Next, go through the case again and sort out the relevant considerations and decisions for each problem.
- Prioritize problems and alternatives.
- Develop a set of recommendations to address the problems.
- Evaluate your decisions.

EXPECTATIONS OF STUDENTS AND TEACHERS

Active learning provides students with an opportunity to take a dynamic role in the learning process. Students are expected to participate in class discussions and be creative in formulating their own opinions. This method also requires that students listen and be respectful of the thoughts and opinions of their classmates. Assigned readings and homework must be completed before class in order to use class time efficiently for questions that are not answered in other reference material. To prepare answers or appropriate therapeutic recommendations, students may have to look beyond the reference materials provided by the teacher; they may have to perform literature searches and use the library or Internet to retrieve additional information. It is important for students to justify their recommendations. The active learning strategies outlined previously allow students to comprehend the material presented, participate in peer discussions, and formulate opinions as in real-life situations.

To implement active learning strategies in the classroom, teachers must overcome the anxiety that change often creates. Experimenting with active learning methods such as the pause technique and slowly implementing a change in the classroom may work best. Using any of the active learning strategies requires teachers to encourage as much classroom discussion as possible instead of lecturing. Use of a wireless microphone is helpful in encouraging student participation in large classrooms. Teachers should make an effort to learn the names of all students so they can more easily interact with them. In addition, teachers should have a preconceived plan for how the class discussion will go and stick to it. Hutchings recommends envisioning what the chalkboard should look like at the end of the session before beginning.[25]

MAXIMIZING ACTIVE LEARNING OPPORTUNITIES: ADVICE TO STUDENTS

Taking initiative is the key to deriving the benefits of active learning. It is crucial to recognize the three largest squelchers of initiative: laziness, fear of change, and force of habit.[26] You will find that time management is important. Be sure to schedule adequate time for studying, prepare for class by reading ahead, use transition times wisely, identify the times of day that you are most productive, and focus on the results rather than the time to complete an activity.[8]

In active learning, you are expected to talk about what you are learning, write about it, relate it to previous patient cases, and apply it to the current case. In a sense, you repeatedly manipulate the information until it becomes a part of you. Some techniques to use when studying are to compare, contrast, and summarize similarities and differences among disease states, drug classes, and appropriate pharmacotherapy. In class, take advantage of every opportunity to present your own work. Attempt to relate personal experiences or outside events to topics discussed in class, and always be an active participant in class or group discussions; lively debates about pharmacotherapy issues allow more therapeutic options to be discussed.[27]

When reading assignments, summarize the information using tables or charts and take notes. These will be your personal set of notes to study for the course exams and to review for the pharmacy state board examination. While taking notes in class, leave a wide margin on the left to write down questions that you generate later when reviewing the notes.[13] Alternatively, make lists of questions from class or readings to discuss with your colleagues or faculty or try to answer them on your own. When time allows, seek out recent information on subjects that interest you. Use Web-based cases and other online resources to extend your knowledge on a particular disease state and drug therapy.[16] In class, always try to determine the "big picture."[27]

Some other methods for maximizing active learning are to review corrected assignments and exams for information that you do not understand and seek clarification from faculty. Complete assignments promptly and minimize short-term memorization. Attend class regularly and ask questions when you do not understand something. Give others a chance to contribute and try not to embarrass fellow classmates.[27]

In active learning, much of what you learn you will learn on your own. You will probably find that you read more, but you will gain understanding from reading. At the same time, you are developing a critical lifelong learning skill. Your reading will become more "depth processing" in which you focus on:

- The intent of the article
- Actively integrating what you read with previous parts of the text
- Using your own ability to make a logical construction
- Thinking about the functional role of the different parts of an argument

In writing, consider summarizing the major points of each class. Writing about a topic develops critical thinking, communication, and organization skills. In classes that involve active learning, you may write for "think-pair-share" exercises, quizzes, summary paragraphs, and other activities. Stopping to write allows you to reflect on the information you have just heard and reinforces learning. Discussions may occur in large or small groups.

Discussing material helps you to apply your knowledge, verbalize the medical and pharmacologic terminology, engage in active listening, think critically, be a leader or a follower, and develop interpersonal skills. When working in groups, all members should participate in problem solving. Teaching others is an excellent way to learn the subject matter.[8]

HOW TO USE THE CASEBOOK

This casebook was prepared to assist in the development of each student's understanding of a disease and its management as well as problem-solving skills. It is important for students to realize that learning and understanding the material is guided through problem solving. Students are encouraged to solve each of the cases individually or with others in a study group before discussion of the case and topic in class. Being prepared for class is essential!

As cases are solved, the student begins to understand that each case may not have a single solution or answer; this may be frustrating initially but reflects real-world situations. The student will begin to appreciate the variety and complexity of diseases that are encountered in different patient populations. In some cases, more detailed information from the patient will play a pivotal role in drug therapy selection and monitoring. In others, most of the diagnoses may be resolved through use of laboratory analysis or specific medical tests. Some cases may require a much more in-depth assessment of the patient's disease state and treatment rendered so far. Other cases may involve initiation of both non-pharmacologic and pharmacologic therapy, ranging from single to multiple drug regimens.

Regardless of disease and/or treatment complexity, students must rely on knowledge previously learned in other courses (e.g., anatomy, biochemistry, microbiology, physiology, pathophysiology, chemistry, pharmacology, pharmacokinetics, pharmacoeconomics, drug literature evaluation, ethics, physical assessment). As a consequence, students may need to review previous notes, handouts, or textbooks. Students can use MEDLINE searches for primary literature, drug reference books, the Internet, and faculty experts as information sources. These resources, the textbook *Pharmacotherapy: A Pathophysiologic Approach* and the website Pharmacotherapy Online at http://www.pharmacotherapyonline.com are essential in supporting each student's ability to solve the cases successfully. Understanding the usefulness and limitations of these resources will be beneficial in the future. Likewise, discussions in study groups and class should lead to a further understanding of disease states and treatment strategies.

SUMMARY

The use of case studies and other active learning strategies will enhance the development of essential skills necessary to practice in any setting, including community, ambulatory care, primary care, health-systems, long-term care, home health care, managed care, and the pharmaceutical industry. The role of the health care professional is constantly changing; thus, it is important for students to acquire knowledge and develop the lifetime skills required for continued learning. Teachers who incorporate active learning strategies into the classroom are facilitating the development of lifelong learners who will be able to adapt to change that occurs in their profession.

References

1. Winslade N. Large-group problem-based learning: A revision from traditional to pharmaceutical care-based therapeutics. Am J Pharm Educ 1994;58:64–73.
2. Kane MD, Briceland LL, Hamilton RA. Solving problems. US Pharmacist 1995;20:55–74.
3. Kaufman DM, Laidlaw TA, Macleod H. Communication skills in medical school: Exposure, confidence, and performance. Acad Med 2000;75(10 Suppl):S90–S92.
4. Brandt BF. Effective teaching and learning strategies. Pharmacotherapy 2000;20:307S–316S.
5. Tanenbaum BG, Cross DS, Tilson ER, et al. How to make active learning work for you. Radiol Technol 1998;69:374–376.
6. Moffett BS, Hill KB. The transition to active learning: a lived experience. Nurs Educator 1997;22:44–47.
7. Rangachari PK. Active learning: in context. Adv Physiol Educ 1995; 13:S75–S80.
8. Warren G. Carpe Diem: A Student Guide to Active Learning. Landover, MD, University Press of America, 1996.
9. Bonwell CC, Eison JA. Active Learning: Creating Excitement in the Classroom. ASHE-ERIC Higher Education Report no. 1. Washington, DC, George Washington University, School of Education and Human Development, 1991.
10. Shakarian DC. Beyond lecture: Active learning strategies that work. JOPERD May–June 1995, 21–24.
11. Ruhl KL, Hughs CA, Schloss PJ. Using the pause procedure to enhance lecture recall. Teacher Educ Spec Educ 1987;10:14–18.
12. Rowe MB. Pausing principles and their effects on reasoning in science. New Directions for Community Colleges 1980;8:27-34.
13. Elliot DD. Promoting critical thinking in the classroom. Nurs Educator 1996;21:49–52.
14. Johnson SP, Cooper J. Quick-thinks: Active-thinking tasks in lecture classes and televised instruction. Cooperative Learning and College Teaching 1997;8:2–6.
15. McKeachie WJ. Teaching large classes (You can still get active learning!). In: McKeachie WJ, ed. Teaching Tips: Strategies, Research, and Theory for College and University Teachers, 10th ed. Boston, Houghton Mifflin, 1999:209–215.
16. Turchin A, Lehmann CU. Active Learning Centre: Design and evaluation of an educational World Wide Web site. Med Inform 2000;25:195–206.
17. Walton HJ, Matthews MB. Essentials of problem-based learning. Med Educ 1989;23:542–558.
18. Fukuchi SG, Offutt LA, Sacks J, et al. Teaching a multidisciplinary approach to cancer treatment during surgical clerkship via an interactive board game. Am J Surg 2000;179:337–340.
19. Raman-Wilms L. Innovative enabling strategies in self-directed, problem-based therapeutics: Enhancing student preparedness for pharmaceutical care. Am J Pharm Educ 2001;65:56–64.
20. Dammers J, Spencer J, Thomas M. Using real patients in problem-based learning: Students' comments on the value of using real, as opposed to paper cases, in a problem-based learning module in general practice. Med Educ 2001;35: 27–34.
21. Lowther DL, Morrison GR. Integrating computers into the problem-solving protocol. New Directions Teaching and Learning 2003;95:33–38.
22. Hartzema AG. Teaching therapeutic reasoning through the case-study approach: Adding the probabilistic dimension. Am J Pharm Educ 1994;58: 436–440.
23. Delafuente JC, Munyer TO, Angaran DM, et al. A problem-solving active-learning course in pharmacotherapy. Am J Pharm Educ 1994;58:61–64.
24. McDade SA. An Introduction to the Case Study Method: Preparation, Analysis, and Participation. New York, Teachers College Press, 1988.
25. Hutchings P. Using Cases to Improve College Teaching. Washington, DC, American Association of Higher Education, 1993.
26. Robbins A. Awaken the Giant Within. New York, Simon & Schuster, 1991.
27. Chickering AW, Gamson ZF, Barsi LM. Seven Principles for Good Practice in Undergraduate Education. Racine, WI, The Johnson Foundation, 1989.

CHAPTER 3

Case Studies in Patient Communication

Marie E. Gardner, PharmD
Richard N. Herrier, PharmD

Pharmaceutical care has always been founded on strong technical and people skills. Although all pharmacists are well versed in the technical aspects of the profession, most are not so well prepared regarding interpersonal communication within the clinical context. In contemporary pharmacy practice, good communication skills are critical for achieving optimal patient outcomes and increasing pharmacists' satisfaction with their professional roles. This chapter summarizes some of the communication skills required to provide quality pharmaceutical care and highlights cases that illustrate these skills. The focus is limited to the essential skills needed for symptom assessment and medication consultation and strategies to improve compliance and monitor clinical progress. Readers are encouraged to review aspects of basic communication skills in other sources.[1–5]

BASIC MEDICATION CONSULTATION

Consultation on medication use is a fundamental and important activity of the pharmacist, whether care is provided in a community pharmacy, clinic, or institutional site. Consultation on new medications is mandated by the Omnibus Budget Reconciliation Act of 1990, and most states require counseling for all patients on either new or both new and refill prescriptions.[6,7]

The traditional method of consulting involves providing information: the pharmacist "tells" and the patient "listens." There is little true dialogue or exchange of information. Pharmacists often ask closed-ended questions such as, "Do you understand?" or, "Do you have any questions?" These closed-ended questions, which can be answered with a yes or no, provide little or no information about what the patient knows about the medication or what concerns the patient may have. When the pharmacist merely provides information and the conversation is essentially one-way, there is no opportunity to ascertain what the patient may know or think about the medication.

The pharmacist–patient consultation techniques used by the Indian Health Service for decades, and further refined in collaboration with colleagues around the country, teach an interactive method of consultation that seeks to verify what the patient knows about the medication and "fill in the gaps" of knowledge only when needed.[2] Research shows that people forget 90% of what is heard within 60 minutes of hearing it.[1] Counseling techniques based on the pharmacist speaking most of the time are ineffective, because patients almost immediately forget what they heard. By making the patient an active participant in the process, increased learning will occur. Engaging patient participation in the exchange requires the use of specific, open-ended questions that seek to understand what the patient already knows about the medication, followed with new information and a summary at the end of the consultation. The specific techniques will now be discussed in more detail.

Basic Medication Consultation Skills

Interactive techniques for consulting on medications use open-ended questions that start with who, what, where, when, why, and how. The patient's answers should provide specific information rather than a simple yes or no. In fact, if the patient answers with a yes or no, one should be suspicious of a language barrier or problem with cognition.

Two sets of open-ended questions are used in the consultation. One is for new prescriptions *(Prime Questions),* and the other is for refill prescriptions *(Show-and-Tell Questions),* as shown in Table 3–1. These open-ended questions make the patient an active participant in the learning process. They provide an organized approach to ascertain what the patient already knows about the medication. Using a systematic approach has been associated with improved recall of prescription instructions.[8] The pharmacist can praise the patient for correct information recalled, clarify points misunderstood, and add new information as needed. It spares the pharmacist from repeating information already known by the patient, which is an inefficient use of time. The steps in the consultation process are described next.

TABLE 3–1. Medication Consultation Skills

Prime Questions
1. What did your doctor tell you the medication is for?
or
What were you told the medication is for?
What problem or symptom is it supposed to help?
What is it supposed to do?
2. How did your doctor tell you to take the medication?
or
How were you told to take the medication?
How often did your doctor say to take it?
How much are you supposed to take?
What did your doctor say to do when you miss a dose?
What does three times a day mean to you?
3. What did your doctor tell you to expect?
or
What were you told to expect?
What good effects are you supposed to expect?
What bad effects did your doctor tell you to watch for?
What should you do if a bad reaction occurs?
Show-and-Tell Questions
1. What do you take the medication for?
2. How do you take it?
3. What kind of problems are you having?

1. Open the Consultation

When the patient is called for counseling, establish rapport by introducing yourself by name and stating the purpose of the consultation. Then verify the patient's identity, either by asking for identification or at least by asking, "And you are . . . ?" If the patient is non-English speaking, hard of hearing, or otherwise unable to provide his or her name, you have identified a barrier in the consultation that must be overcome before discussing the medication.

If time permits and a private space is available, suggest that the consultation be conducted there and move to that area. This will be important for patients who have hearing problems or those needing extra privacy, such as patients receiving vaginal creams or those with AIDS. Sit facing the patient, and maintain the appropriate interpersonal distance (1.5 to 2 feet) during the consultation.

2. Conduct the Counseling Session

Begin by asking the *Prime Questions* if the prescription is a new one, or use the *Show-and-Tell* method for a refill prescription. If the patient is able to tell you what the medication is for, you may choose to probe further or move to the next question. Probing further may be helpful when the patient answers in broad or vague terms. As an example, if a patient who is receiving a β-blocker tells you that the medication is for "my heart," you may wish to ask in an open-ended fashion, "What is it supposed to do for your heart?" Avoid asking, "Is it for chest pains?" or similar closed-ended questions, because you may alarm the patient by your suggestions, and you might waste time if multiple questions have to be asked. If the patient does not know what the medication is for, or if the patient says, "Don't you know?", you should ask why the patient visited the physician. The patient may describe symptoms of a condition known to be treatable with the medication in question. If so, indicate what symptoms the medication will help. If the patient is totally unaware of the medication's purpose, a referral back to the physician is indicated, lest the pharmacist judge in error the indication for the medication.

After verifying that the patient knows what the medication is for, ask the second prime question. Often, patients are unaware of the dosage instructions or indicate, "It's on the label, isn't it?" Be aware of the optimal dosing instructions, because the patient may correctly respond "twice a day," but you may need to advise on exact timing, or whether to take the drug with meals. Other questions to include under the second prime question are addressed to these areas of concern: (a) how long to take the medication; (b) exactly how much or how often to take it when the medication is prescribed as needed; (c) what to do when a dose is missed; and (d) how to store the medication. Rather than providing facts, consider asking the patient, "What did the doctor say about how long to take this medication?" or, "What will you do if you miss a dose?" Asking a question of the patient prompts the patient's attention, whereas "telling" the information is more passive for the patient and the patient may not listen as well. Think of the counseling session as an opportunity to find out what the patient knows, rather than a place to showcase your knowledge. Keep the information you provide brief and to the point.

After verifying patient understanding about how to take the medication, proceed to the third prime question. Often, patients have been told nothing about beneficial or adverse effects. On the other hand, patients may describe anticipated results from the medication. If beneficial effects are mentioned, follow with, "What side effects were you warned about?" to determine the patient's knowledge of potential side effects. Other questions subsumed under this third prime question relate to how the patient will know if the medication is working, what precautions to take while taking the medication, and what to do if the medication does not work.

If the patient is unaware of potential adverse effects from the drug therapy, mention the most common or most serious adverse effects, and describe what to do if they occur. Research shows that patients want information about their medications, especially adverse effects, and that providing such information does not lead to the development of those reactions in most cases.[9–12] Recent work on communicating about the risk of drug reactions suggests a four-quadrant model in which each quadrant requires specific communication skills.[13] The quadrants contain a combination of either high or low probability of occurrence with high or low levels of severity or magnitude. An example of high probability and high magnitude is cancer chemotherapy, which entails frequent and severe toxicities. Empathic communication should be the lead skill in discussing the risk of therapy in this case. The combination of high probability and low magnitude is exemplified by gastric complaints from erythromycin. Pharmacists often encounter patients with common, bothersome side effects. Useful communication skills include providing information about how the medication will work and why it is a good therapy for them, as well as how to manage expected side effects.

When there is low probability but high magnitude (e.g., stroke from an oral contraceptive), careful attention to and assessment of the patient's perceptions about the possible side effects are needed. Be aware of how the patient's perceptions may differ from your own. Because the patient may only hear, "This is unlikely to happen but . . ." and tune out the specifics about the toxicity, it is helpful to ask the patient for feedback on the discussion of toxicity. In the final quadrant, the low probability and low magnitude of risk may be associated with a perception that the medication may have little value to the patient. Heavy-handed tactics to convince, frighten, or otherwise threaten the patient will not be effective. Questioning patients to determine their view of what benefits might be accrued from taking the medication is necessary. Follow with comments to match their assessment. For example, when a patient says, "Well, I could get an allergic reaction to this," the issue of the adverse effect is first and foremost in her mind, whereas the pharmacist may think, "I have never seen anyone allergic to this." Rather than try to convince the patient that no one becomes allergic to it, one might say, "Yes, that is possible. Which do you think is worse—putting up with the pain or taking a chance on the medication?" This brings into the open the discussion of both the risks and benefits of treatment. If the pharmacist can bring the patient along the thought continuum with a discussion of potential benefits, the patient may decide to give it a try. At times, the authors have found it useful to "contract" with the patient. For example, "Sam, we have discussed both the good and bad about taking this medicine, and I know you still have concerns about side effects. I really think this medicine is best for you. Would you be willing to try it for a week, and I will check in with you after a few days to see how things are going?" More often than not, the anticipated adverse effects do not appear.

Using the skills described in the sections above for confronting adverse reactions or the fear of them will set the stage for better patient compliance. However, just the act of having to take a medication when one is not used to doing so poses compliance problems. When a patient has a new medication, and after using the prime questions to counsel the patient, it may be helpful to raise compliance concerns. A *universal statement* is a useful opener. It describes the situation for a group and then narrows to focus on the individual. For example, "Mrs. Green, many patients have trouble fitting medications into their daily schedule. What problems do you foresee in taking this medicine?" It may be necessary to probe into their daily habits and to help them find a way to tie medication taking into a particular activity. For instance, if the patient always makes coffee in the morning, having the medication nearby may be sufficient reminder to promote compliance. Be sure to use a partnership approach. Additional compliance-enhancing skills are discussed later in this chapter.

3. Close the Consultation

Most consultations are a combination of the patient knowing some information and the pharmacist providing additional information as the prime questions are reviewed. Because of this, it is important to close the consultation with the *final verification.* Think of the final verification as asking the patient to "play back" everything learned in order to check that the information is complete and accurate. Say to the patient, "Just to make sure I didn't leave anything out, please go over with me how you are going to use the medication." Avoid saying "Just to make sure you've got this . . ." as the patient may feel embarrassed if he or she does not recall important facts. At this point, the patient should describe correct use of the medication. Any errors can be corrected and any omissions clarified. Then ask the patient if there is anything else he or she needs and offer assistance as required.

A similar process is used for refill prescriptions. The *Show-and-Tell Questions* verify patient understanding of proper use of chronic medications or medications that the patient has used in the past. The pharmacist begins the process by showing the medication to the patient; that is, by opening the bottle and displaying the contents. Then, the patient tells the pharmacist how he uses the medication by answering the questions listed in Table 3–1. Note that the doctor is omitted as a reference, because the patient should have been counseled properly by the pharmacist before this and should have all information needed for proper medication usage. The show-and-tell technique enables the pharmacist to detect problems with compliance or unwanted drug effects. If the patient answers incorrectly to the second question, the patient may be non-compliant or the physician may have changed the dosage. The pharmacist will need to further define the reason for the discrepancy. The second show-and-tell question also allows the pharmacist to ask the patient to demonstrate use of an inhaler or injectable medication or how to measure liquid doses to assure proper usage.

Some pharmacists have difficulty asking the third question, fearing that they may arouse suspicion in the patient. However, research discounts this notion, as previously discussed. If potential adverse effects were discussed when the patient was initially counseled, it seems natural, and certainly relevant and important, to query the patient about adverse effects at the refill visit. If new symptomatology is present, explore this further using the *Key Symptom Questions.* Because it is important to evaluate new symptoms critically, we will describe this in detail next.

Exploring Symptoms

At the prescription counter, over the telephone, or at a bedside visit, the patient may mention symptoms that could be related to drug therapy. Knowing how to explore the patient's symptoms and how to evaluate their relationship to either the disease or its treatment is a key assessment skill. The first step is to get the patient to reveal more information about the symptom. An introductory statement such as "Tell me more about it" encourages the patient to provide more specific details. After this, the *Key Symptom Questions* should be used. These seven focused, open-ended questions, based on medical interviewing techniques, seek specifics that will help to define whether the symptom is related to drug therapy.[14,15] The seven questions are:

1. *Onset/timing:* When did you notice this? *or* When did it start?
2. *Duration:* How long have you had this problem?
3. *Context:* Under what circumstances does this symptom appear?
4. *Quality:* What does it feel like?
5. *Quantity:* How much and how often do you notice it?
6. *Treatment:* What makes it better? *or* What have you done about it?
7. *Associated symptoms:* What other symptoms are you having?

Without proper attention to detail, many pharmacists make assumptions that the symptom expressed is caused by a disease state and do not adequately address it. Or they may jump to conclusions about the cause of the symptom and recommend a treatment without knowing the true cause. For example, a patient taking a nonsteroidal anti-inflammatory drug who complains of fatigue might be recommended a vitamin if the pharmacist thinks the patient is tired from inadequate nutrition. Probing the symptom of fatigue with the questions listed above may reveal that the fatigue started after the medication was begun and is accompanied by gastric distress, suggesting anemia from gastrointestinal blood loss as a possible cause for the fatigue.

The *Key Symptom Questions* are also important when there is a tendency to attribute every symptom to a medication, as patients are sometimes inclined to do. For instance, a pharmacy student reviewed the chart of a patient with bipolar illness, seizures, and parkinsonism. The patient was receiving several medications, including carbamazepine and carbidopa/levodopa. The patient complained of blurred vision and insomnia, which the student initially felt were caused by the medications. However, using all the key symptom questions disclosed that the patient had blurred vision only out of the left eye and that she had insomnia "since the day I was born." Her answers suggested that the symptoms were unlikely to be related to her drug therapy.

Knowledge of each drug's side effect profile and the disease state symptomatology is essential to discern whether the symptom results from drug therapy or a disease state. In some cases, it could be either, in which case it is important to ascertain the onset of the symptom. If the symptom began or worsened after starting a new medication, then there is a higher likelihood that the problem is drug related.

Students and new practitioners are often confused about what to do once the symptom has been explored. Determining the seriousness of the problem is sometimes difficult. It is helpful to ask yourself, "What is the worst thing that can happen in this case? If this is an adverse reaction to the medication, what will happen if the medication is continued? What will happen to the patient (and disease process) if the medication is stopped?" Easily discernible side effects, such as dizziness from an antihypertensive, are managed by practical suggestions to the patient without discontinuation of drug therapy. Even so, the patient may elect to stop taking the medication, and the pharmacist must think ahead to those consequences and advise the patient accordingly. More serious toxicities require either calling the patient's physician or advising the patient to discuss the problem with the physician as soon as possible, rather than suggesting stopping the medication.

The most important point in addressing symptoms is to obtain enough information to make an informed clinical judgment. This is accomplished by using the *Key Symptom Questions* outlined earlier.

Barriers in the Consultation

The clinical skills described are easily applied in situations where there are few or no barriers in communication between patient and pharmacist. In reality, there are often obstacles to overcome in the environment or within the pharmacist or patient. Examples of problems within the pharmacy environment that deter patient consultation include lack of privacy, interruptions, high workload, and insufficient staff. Barriers present within the pharmacist include lack of desire or skills to adequately counsel patients, stereotyping patients and problems, and difficulty maintaining concentration while counseling, especially when stress is a factor. A detailed analysis of these barriers is beyond the scope of this discussion but can be found in the references.[3] Barriers that the patient brings to the encounter are discussed here insofar as overcoming them relates to the clinical communication skills discussed.

The structured approach for patient consultation can be likened to knowing the road on which you are traveling. However, unforeseen events happen on every path and may arise at any time. Just as one must remove or negotiate around the obstacle on the highway, the pharmacist must recognize and manage barriers brought by the patient during the encounter for the consultation to reach the desired end. There are two types of barriers: functional and emotional.

1. Functional Barriers

These barriers include problems with hearing and vision that make it difficult for the patient to absorb information during the consultation. Language barriers and illiteracy are formidable obstacles to proper consultation. Recognizing these barriers is usually not difficult, as the signs of poor vision are easy to observe. Language problems become apparent early in the counseling process provided you use open-ended questions that require more than a yes/no answer. Strategies specific to each barrier are needed when these problems are identified. For instance, moving to a quiet area, repeating information, and asking for feedback from the patient are important when hearing is a problem. Giving clear verbal instructions and using large-type print materials are helpful when the patient has vision difficulties. Using translators, picture diagrams, and involving English-speaking caregivers are important when language problems exist.

2. Emotional Barriers

Emotional barriers are common in everyday interactions, including pharmacist–patient communication. When not handled properly, they give rise to further aggravation and break down communication, inhibiting effective consultation. Patients may express anger, hostility, sadness, depression, fear, anxiety, or embarrassment directly or indirectly during consultation with the pharmacist. They may also give the attitude of a "know-it-all," be suspicious of medications, or seem unmotivated or uninterested. Some of these barriers might be momentary, such as the frustration experienced when the prescription cannot be filled because the medication is unavailable at that time. On the other hand, the patient with a chronic pain syndrome may be less attentive as a result of being uncomfortable or in pain. The attitude of the patient who "knows all" about his or her medications is unlikely to change over time. The patient with a terminal illness may be chronically depressed, uninterested, or feel hopeless about the benefits of therapy.

Unlike seeing the patient with a white cane and knowing that a vision problem exists, emotional barriers can be more difficult to discern. Because most patients will not say, "I'm angry and frustrated about feeling so ill," or, "I'm upset that my doctor didn't spend much time with me," their feelings surface in statements such as, "I don't know why it takes all day to put a few pills in the bottle!" or, "I don't know why I have to take this stupid medicine. Nothing seems to help anyway." Unfortunately, we usually respond to the content of the message (e.g., "I'll have this ready for you as soon as I can") without recognizing that there may be other issues behind the statement, issues that impact on the encounter and, more importantly, on the patient's decision to comply with therapy. It takes patience and practice to listen beyond the words, and this requires the skill of reflective responding.

When we respond with a reflection of what the patient is saying, thinking, or feeling, we let the person know we are truly listening and give the person the opportunity to admit to feelings, clarify thoughts, and bring forth information. Making a reflecting response is not natural for us because most of us have not been trained to use these skills. Reflective responding attempts to reflect in words what the patient is saying or feeling. The reflection may be based on the content or thought expressed by the patient, and/or the feelings associated with it that are often not outwardly expressed. Reflecting responses are especially called for when the patient is demonstrating emotions. Angry looks, pounding fists, averted eye contact, and head drooping all convey certain emotional states. Hesitating gestures or remarks such as, "Well . . . I guess I could try it," call for reflecting responses to bring concerns to light.

The first step in effective reflective responding is to identify and label the emotional state. The four basic emotional states are mad, sad, glad, and scared. As you observe the patient during consultation, certain non-verbal or verbal signs (e.g., hesitating words) may suggest one of the four feeling states. The second step is to put the word describing the feeling state into a sentence to use as a response to the patient. Some basic structures for sentences include, "It sounds as if you are (frustrated, mad, happy)," or, "I can see that you are (happy, confused, mad)." These remarks indicate to patients that you are truly attempting to understand their concerns; thus, the patient and his or her concerns remain the focus of the encounter.

To the patient who remarked, "I don't know why I have to take this. Nothing helps anyway," the pharmacist might determine that the non-verbal tone of voice and choice of words indicate the patient is disappointed with results of his therapy. Alternatively, he may be feeling hopeless about getting better. One reflecting response is, "It sounds as if you have been frustrated with the things you have tried." This statement neither judges nor advises. It gives the patient an opportunity to open discussion of a difficult topic, if the patient so chooses. Contrast this with, "This is a good medicine, Joe, and I really think it will help." Although this may be true, maintaining the consultation on a technical, information-providing level avoids dealing with the underlying issues of the patient's fears.

Emotional barriers can occur at any time throughout the consultation, and they must be dealt with in order to put the patient in a receptive frame of mind. Embarrassment is a factor when vaginal preparations, condom use, and similar topics are the subject of the consultation. Observe for signs of embarrassment such as averted gaze or fidgeting, and respond with, "This can be hard to talk about, but it's important that we discuss. . . ." Also, be matter-of-fact, move to a private space, and speak in a normal tone of voice to help alleviate the embarrassment.

When faced with patients' emotional outbursts, acknowledge their expressed feelings before continuing with the consultation. The initial use of reflecting responses will allow the consultation to proceed with both parties devoting attention to the primary issues of drug therapy and usage, rather than to interpersonal difficulties. Remember, though, that reflecting responses will not work in every situation nor with every type of patient.

COMPLIANCE AND DISEASE MONITORING

In no other situation is the pharmacist's role in monitoring and managing medication usage more vital than in the case of patients requiring chronic drug therapy, especially for diseases that are asymptomatic. Many factors contribute to the pharmacist's success in assuring beneficial outcomes. Among them are practice site, pharmacist competence, support of administration, and breadth of responsibilities, including, in some cases, prescriptive authority. An increasing amount of literature attests to the beneficial patient outcomes from pharmaceutical care. Hatoum and Akhras and the Indian Health Service practitioners have documented extensively the value of pharmacists' contributions to ambulatory care practices.[16–19]

Contemporary pharmacy practice continues to evolve direct patient-care roles for pharmacists. The monitoring and management of common, chronic diseases such as hypertension, asthma, and diabetes are now being done in partnership between pharmacists and medical professionals. Models of community pharmacy practice now include private consultations and advanced practice techniques that were formerly limited to sites such as the Indian Health Service. Several states have regulations that allow pharmacists to assess and prescribe.[17] Although all these advances are important to providing good pharmaceutical care, pharmacists must remain cognizant of the most fundamental point in managing chronic disease: it is the patient's responsibility.

Whose Disease Is It Anyway?

A common misperception that is held by health care professionals regarding a patient with a chronic disease is that the professional manages the patient's disease. Nothing could be further from the truth, and this medical myth is probably a major contributor to compliance problems among patients with chronic diseases. In the traditional medical care model, health care professionals perceive their roles to be in the diagnosis, treatment, and management of disease. As drug therapy managers, clinical pharmacists focus on blood levels, kinetic dosage calculations, and drug interactions. Guided by this focus on technical aspects of patient care, health care professionals often become frustrated and angry when patients do not follow instructions, or, despite the provider's best efforts, achieve only partial results. In reality, the only time the professional manages the treatment is during an office visit or while the patient is institutionalized in a hospital or long-term care facility. Almost all of the time, the patient controls the treatment of his or her disease, especially those that require continuous medication. Failure to recognize this basic truth has created: (a) considerable tension in patient–provider relationships; (b) provider frustration and anger; (c) poor communication; (d) negative provider attitudes toward individual patients; (e) poor patient outcomes; (f) patient distrust of providers; and (g) legal consequences that have been a major contributor to rising health care costs.[20–23]

One author strongly suggests that non-compliance in diabetes mellitus is due in large part to the failure of providers to recognize that their goal is not to treat the disease, but *helping the patient to treat the disease.*[24] That contention is supported by current medical literature on compliance that links good communication and a partnership style of provider–patient relationship to increased satisfaction, compliance, and better patient outcomes.[23–26]

To be successful in assisting patients to achieve good outcomes, the provider and pharmacist must adopt a partnership approach, with health professionals acting as facilitators to help patients manage their disease. That is, it is the patient's disease; the providers' job is *to help them manage it.*

Go Slow/Use Interactive Techniques

Patients can absorb only a limited amount of new information at each encounter. In an attempt to do a thorough job, health care professionals often overwhelm the patient with information at or near the time of diagnosis or treatment initiation. Patients' active listening abilities last less than a minute during a monologue presentation, and they retain only a few pieces of information from a prolonged discussion and may miss key facts. In addition, a large volume of technical information may confuse or frighten patients, leading to the poor outcome that educational efforts are intended to prevent.[25] Also, newly diagnosed patients may not have accepted their diagnosis or the need for treatment.

Successful patient educators do three things: (a) they give patients information in small manageable increments, (b) they actively involve the patient in the educational process by creating an interactive dialogue and using other hands-on approaches that are consistent with adult learning principles,[26] and (c) they understand patient readiness for information. For the pharmacist dispensing the initial prescription, this entails verifying that the patient understands how to take the medicine and its most common side effects. For example, with hydrochlorothiazide 25 mg daily for hypertension, the pharmacist should verify that the patient knows what it is for, knows to take it once daily in the morning to prevent nighttime voiding, knows that it takes a while before any changes in blood pressure occur, and knows that there will be a noticeable increase in urination the first week, which should lessen thereafter. Discussions about diet, exercise, and related issues can wait until later visits. Giving the patient a handout on hypertension and diuretics is appropriate and can lead to questions and subsequent education at later visits or during a follow-up phone call.

Set the Stage for Future Encounters

Many providers explain to patients what follow-up visits will entail so that patients view subsequent laboratory tests and examinations as a normal part of their care. However, few providers follow a similar process regarding medication compliance. Patients then perceive questions about compliance to be intrusive and, fearing parental-type sanctions from the provider, lie about being compliant. Using specific strategies during the *initial* patient visit when follow-up care is discussed can prevent this all-too-common problem. Explain that compliance is very important to successful outcomes, but that you know how hard it is to remember to take medication every day. Tell the patient that you expect that he or she will be like all patients and experience some difficulty remembering to take the medication. Ask the patient to keep track of those instances if possible, and further explain that you will be asking at each visit about the problems the patient has had with the medication so you can assist the patient to better remember to take the medication.

Monitoring and Education of the Patient at Return Visits

Organizing an effective approach to evaluating and educating patients with chronic diseases at return visits may be problematic in a busy practice setting. One simple way to look at all patients returning for follow-up of chronic diseases is to use the three Cs: *Control, Complications,* and *Compliance.* To evaluate the *control* of the chronic disease, couple objective findings (e.g., blood pressure or range of motion) with subjective findings from the consultation (e.g., reports of dizziness, nocturnal voiding, or degree of morning joint stiffness). *Complications* can occur both from disease progression and drug effects. As with the control parameters, a combination of subjective findings (e.g., symptoms) and objective findings from the health record or patient profile can disclose the presence of potential complications. For example, a patient with hypertension, diabetes mellitus, and osteoarthritis who takes captopril, chlorpropamide, and ibuprofen can be queried about the presence of cough, difficulty sleeping, and exercise tolerance. These questions are primarily directed at detecting congestive heart failure or renal failure caused by hypertension and/or diabetes, but also will help detect drug-related problems such as cough caused by the angiotensin-converting enzyme (ACE) inhibitor and renal effects from ibuprofen. Checking recent laboratory values for serum creatinine, electrolytes, and blood glucose will help assess diabetes and hypertension control and complications such as non-steroidal antiinflammatory drug (NSAID)-induced renal impairment, excessive chlorpropamide dosage, and ACE inhibitor-induced hyperkalemia.

With regard to *compliance* problems, the pharmacist's actions can be divided into three steps: (a) *recognize* potential compliance problems; (b) *identify* probable causes of non-compliance; and (c) *manage* the problem with specific steps. This RIM model is a process that can be used by pharmacists to enhance patient compliance.[27] In this model (Table 3–2), subjective and objective findings are used to detect potential compliance problems. First, the health record or patient profile is reviewed for objective evidence of potential non-compliance before talking with the patient. During profile review, three items should alert the pharmacist to potential compliance problems. The first and most common item is a discrepancy between the number of doses that should have been taken and the number of doses dispensed. Second, patients with incomplete refill requests (e.g., only one or two of multiple chronic medications due at the same time) raise suspicion for non-compliance. Third, the prescribing of a new medication for the same condition or one that may unknowingly be prescribed to offset adverse effects from another medication may indicate compliance problems. Patients often present to medical providers with new complaints. If the provider does not make the connection between the new symptom and the side effect, compliance or therapeutic problems may eventually occur. If patients taking ACE inhibitors present with new or repeat prescriptions for cough suppressants, the pharmacist should consider the potential for ACE inhibitor-induced cough. In extreme cases, patients may stop the needed drug and continue with the drug used to treat the side effects, which is unnecessary and could pose risks in itself.

Potential compliance problems found during profile or chart review call for further exploration before a definite compliance problem can be ascertained. There may be rational explanations for the objective findings. Gaps in refills may be a result of patients obtaining refills at another location, or the doctor may have told the patient to change the dosage schedule or to stop the drug altogether.

When the profile indicates potential non-compliance, begin the consultation using the *Show-and-Tell* technique for refill prescriptions. The patient may provide one or more clues during consultation to confirm your suspicions. If not, the pharmacist must initiate a more direct approach using a *supportive compliance probe.* This is a specific type of statement that uses "I" language to describe what the profile shows and to probe the discrepancy. For example, "I noticed when I reviewed your profile that you hadn't had your prednisone refilled in about 2 weeks. I was concerned that there might have been some changes that I'm not aware of." This combination of "I noticed . . . and I'm concerned . . ." can be very effective in getting a dialogue started in a non-threatening manner. Another useful approach is the *universal statement,* such as, "Most of my patients have problems remembering to take every dose of their medication. What kinds of problems are you having?" Open the discussion of compliance problems with non-threatening language, and there is a greater likelihood that the patient will disclose problems.

Supportive compliance probes and universal statements are useful strategies for the pharmacist when profile review suggests noncompliance. Very often, the patient may provide clues to compliance problems. Patients who tell the pharmacist during the *Show-and-Tell* questioning that they are taking their medication differently than prescribed are providing evidence of a potential compliance problem. Some clues are obvious, such as

TABLE 3–2. Steps in the RIM Model for Compliance Counseling

Recognize Potential Non-Compliance
• For objective evidence, use supportive compliance probes. Examples: *I noticed that this refill was due. I'm concerned that you will not get the full benefits from your medication if it's not taken as prescribed.* • For subjective evidence, use reflecting responses. Examples: *It sounds as if you are worried about side effects. So you feel that your medication is not working.*
Identify/Categorize the Non-Compliance
• *Knowledge deficits* are evidenced through a patient's statements, indicating a misunderstanding or lack of information. • *Practical impediments* are revealed by a patient's description of lack of funds, inability to access the medication, forgetfulness, difficulty with a complicated dosing schedule, or an adverse reaction. • *Attitudinal barriers* are disclosed by a patient's statements that highlights his or her lack of faith in medication.
Manage the Non-Compliance
• *Knowledge deficits* are resolved by providing both verbal and written information, verifying the patient's understanding. • *Practical impediments* are dealt with by providing corrective actions individualized for the problem (e.g., providing a dosing calendar developed with the patient, working with the physician to find easier dosing regimens, or using pill boxes). Adverse reactions require the use of the *Key Symptom Questions.* • *Attitudinal barriers* are rectified by maintaining an understanding of the patient's view using empathy, open-ended questions, and universal statements.

when a patient asks, "Why do I have to keep taking this medicine?" This is a "red flag" because it is clear that the patient wishes not to take the prescription. However, many statements are more subtle. Examples of these vague clues, called "pink flags," include: "My doctor says I *should* take it . . .," or "My doctor *wants* me to. . .," or "I'm *supposed* to be taking. . . ." These are usually detected when the pharmacist asks the first two *Show-and-Tell* questions. "What kinds of problems are you having with the medication?" may prompt the following "pink flag" responses: "Well . . . none, really," or a hesitation before saying "No, none." Reflecting responses discussed earlier in this chapter are appropriate in this situation. Responses include, "It seems as if you are not too sure about taking that," or "It sounds as if you think the medicine is causing a problem." These responses open the dialogue in a non-threatening manner and focus on the patient's perceptions or suggestion that a problem exists.

Patients may ask, "Does this medicine have any side effects?" or "What kind of side effects does this have?" or "Is this anything like (another specific drug)?" More often than not, pharmacists simply answer the question without really listening to the underlying concern. "Why do you ask?" is an appropriate response, especially if the patient looks hesitant or the intonation of the question suggests doubt about taking the medication. When the authors use this question, patients often disclose that a relative had it (or a similar medication) or the media has reported problems with the drug. These indirect experiences create enough doubt such that the patient wavers about taking the medication. Obviously, if the pharmacist uses the *Show-and-Tell* technique alone and does not recognize these "pink flags," the consultation will be in vain, for the patient will leave not having the underlying doubt resolved. Therefore, it is crucial to develop keen active listening skills to denote the presence of the "pink flags" and then use reflecting responses to probe into the problem.

During the *Show-and-Tell* questioning, patients may disclose symptoms that may indicate an adverse effect. This is sometimes a reason for stopping treatment or skipping doses. When symptoms are mentioned, use the *Key Symptom Questions* to identify the exact nature of the problem. Resolution of the problem will be dictated by its clinical urgency.

Once the presence of the compliance problem has been confirmed, additional skills are needed. Compliance problems can be categorized within three groups. The first is a *knowledge* deficit. In these cases, patients have insufficient information or skills or misinformation that prevents compliance. An example is the patient who put contraceptive jelly on toast, or the patient who was never shown or has forgotten how to use an inhaler. The second group involves *practical impediments* or barriers, such as complex drug regimens involving multiple drugs and/or different dosage schedules, difficulty in developing routines that facilitate medication compliance, difficulty in opening containers, or insufficient mental aptitude to comply. The final category is *attitudinal barriers.* Among the most difficult to identify and manage, these include patient beliefs about health, disease, and/or treatment that are inconsistent with the prescribed regimen. These may reflect differences in cultural beliefs.[28–30] As outlined by the health belief model, the patient's perceived severity of risk compared to the perceived benefit of treatment plays a large role in determining medication compliance.[29] Other factors such as patient desire to be in control and patient belief that he or she can successfully implement the recommended treatment also strongly influence compliance.[25] Finally, the most prevalent and potentially the most difficult belief differences to overcome are patients' *lay theories.*[29] Common lay theories held by patients include, "You need to give your body a rest from medicine or it will become immune to it," or "You only need to take medicine when you feel sick, not when you feel okay," or "If one dose is good, then two must be better."

Once the specific cause is identified, a specific strategy to manage that problem can be attempted. Most knowledge and skill deficiencies can be successfully corrected with education and/or training. Practical impediments respond well to specific measures such as simplifying regimens, use of easy-open containers, and enlisting the aid of a spouse or caregiver. Attitudinal issues tend to be the most complex and difficult to solve. Even lay theories, which would seem easily fixed by correcting misinformation, are extremely difficult to overcome because the nature of lay theories makes them highly resistant to change. Again, it takes practice, careful listening, repeated conversations with the patient, and a supportive climate for the patient to acknowledge one of these barriers. Patients will only do so when they feel the pharmacist will not denigrate them or argue against their beliefs. Partnership language and gentle confrontation on the facts are indicated. Repeated efforts to enlighten may, over time, change the view of the patient.

CONCLUSION

Contemporary pharmacy practice is changing at a very rapid pace. Pharmaceutical care, which focuses on the outcomes of drug therapy, is the founding principle for today's practitioners. The delivery of quality pharmaceutical care involves the skills and techniques discussed in this chapter and many others that support the pharmacist–patient interaction and medication use process. As direct patient contact and responsibility for drug therapy outcomes become the main task for the pharmacist, the skills of interpersonal communication, medication history taking, patient consultation, plus compliance monitoring and enhancement become the "tools of the trade." The consistent application of a high level of interpersonal and applied clinical skills by the pharmacist will lead to optimal outcomes for the patient.

References

1. Bolton R. People Skills. New York, Simon & Schuster, 1979.
2. Gardner M, Boyce RW, Herrier RN. Pharmacist–Patient Consultation Program, Unit 1: An Interactive Approach to Verify Patient Understanding. New York, Pfizer, 1991.
3. Pharmacist–Patient Consultation Program, Unit 2: Counseling Patients in Challenging Situations. New York, Pfizer, 1993.
4. Meldrum H. Interpersonal Communication in Pharmaceutical Care. New York, Haworth Press, 1994.
5. Muldary TW. Interpersonal Relations for Health Professionals: A Social Skills Approach. New York, Macmillan, 1983.
6. Meade V. OBRA '90: How has pharmacy reacted? Am Pharm 1995;NS35:12–16.
7. Pugh CB. Pre-OBRA '90 Medicaid survey: How community pharmacy practice is changing. Am Pharm 1995;NS35:17–23.
8. Gardner M, Hurd PD, Slack M. Effect of information organization on recall of medication instructions. J Clin Pharm Ther 1989;14:1–7.
9. Morris LA, Grossman R, Barkdoll GL, et al. A survey of patient sources of prescription drug information. Am J Public Health 1984;74:1161–1162.
10. Lamb GC, Green SS, Heron J. Can physicians warn patients of potential side effects without fear of causing those side effects? Arch Intern Med 1994;154:2753–2756.
11. Howland JS, Baker MG, Poe T. Does patient education cause side effects? A controlled trial. J Fam Pract 1990;31:62–64.
12. Gardner ME, Rulien N, McGhan WF, Mead RA. A study of patients' perceived importance of medication information provided by physicians in a health maintenance organization. Drug Intell Clin Pharm 1988;22:596–598.
13. Meldrum H, Hardy M. Challenges in communicating about risk. In: Communicating Risk to Patients: Proceedings of the Conference. Rockville, MD, United States Pharmacopeial Convention, 1995:36–49.
14. Billings JA, Stoeckle JD. The Clinical Encounter. Chicago, Year Book Medical Publishers, 1989.
15. Boyce RW, Herrier RN. Obtaining and using patient data. Am Pharm 1991;NS31:65–71.
16. Hatoum HT, Akhras K. 1993 Bibliography: A 32-year literature review on the value and acceptance of ambulatory care provided by pharmacists. Ann Pharmacother 1993;27:1106–1119.
17. Church RM. Pharmacy practice in the Indian Health Service. Am J Hosp Pharm 1987;44:771–775.
18. Herrier RN, Boyce RW, Apgar DA. Pharmacist-managed patient-care services and prescriptive authority in the US Public Health Service. Hosp Formul 1990;25:67–68, 76–78, 80.
19. Ellis SL, Carter BL, Malone DC, et al. Clinical and economic impact of ambulatory care clinical pharmacists in management of dyslipidemia in older adults: The IMPROVE study. Impact of managed pharmaceutical care on resource utilization and outcomes in Veterans Affairs Medical Centers. Pharmacotherapy 2000;20:1508–1516.
20. Beckman HS, Markakis KM, Suchman AL, Frankel RM. The doctor–patient relationship and malpractice: Lessons from plaintiff depositions. Arch Intern Med 1994;154:1365–1370.
21. Anderson LA, Zimmerman MA. Patient and physician perceptions of their relationship and patient satisfaction: A study of chronic disease management. Patient Educ Couns 1993;20:27–36.
22. DiMatteo MR. The physician–patient relationship: Effects on the quality of health care. Clin Obstet Gynecol 1994;37:149–161.
23. Viinamaki H. The patient–doctor relationship and metabolic control in patients with type 1 (insulin dependent) diabetes mellitus. Int J Psychiatry Med 1993;23:265–274.
24. Anderson RM. Is the problem of noncompliance all in our heads? Diabetes Educ 1985;11:31–34.
25. Herrier RN, Boyce RW. Compliance with prescribed drug regimens. In: Bressler R, Katz M, eds. Geriatric Pharmacology. New York, McGraw-Hill, 1993:63–77.
26. Eraker SA, Kirscht JP, Becker MH. Understanding and improving patient compliance. Ann Intern Med 1984;100:258–268.
27. Pharmacist–Patient Consultation Program, Unit 3: Counseling to Enhance Compliance. New York, Pfizer, 1995.
28. Becker MH. Patient adherence to prescribed therapies. Med Care 1985;23:539–555.
29. Leventhal H. The role of theory in the study of adherence to treatment and doctor–patient interactions. Med Care 1985;23:556–563.
30. Kübler-Ross E. On Death and Dying. New York, Macmillan, 1969.

PATIENT CASES

This section includes three scenarios with patient profiles and prescriptions that require counseling. First, review the profile and prescription and think about issues that may arise during the consultation. Then provide written answers to the questions asked. Use concepts from the preceding material on counseling strategies, as well as any other techniques you think are useful or have found useful through your own experience or by observing others in practice.

Sally comes to the pharmacy alone to pick up the tamoxifen prescription. You have reviewed the profile and are ready to counsel her on the medication.

Case No. 1: Sally M. Johnson

NAME Johnson, Sally M. ADDRESS 1862 Briar Court Lansdale, PA 18018	DATE 2/20/05 AGE IF CHILD
FULL DIRECTIONS FOR USE	Rx No. 148647
R_x	Date filled
Tamoxifen 10 mg	Cost
#60	Fee
Sig: i po BID	Total Price
	☐ Do not refill No. of refills authorized: 6
☐ IDENTIFY CONTENTS ON LABEL UNLESS CHECKED	
☐ NON-PROPRIETARY EQUIVALENT UNLESS CHECKED	
S. Mayer M.D.	

Patient Medication Profile

Name: Sally M. Johnson	Known Diseases	Allergies and Sensitivities	Additional Information
Address: 1862 Briar Court	s/p hysterectomy 9/00 with	Sulfa: rash	
Lansdale, PA 18018	estrogen replacement		
Telephone: 832-7358	s/p surgery, CA breast 2/05		
Date of Birth: 4/15/48			

Date	Rx No.	Medication	Strength	Quantity	Dosage Regimen	R.Ph.	Physician
07/18/04	83104	Premarin	0.625 mg	#100	1 QD	JD	Hepler
10/25/04	89436	Premarin	0.625 mg	#100	1 QD	HV	Hepler
12/04/04	145922	Tylox		#12	1–2 Q4H PRN	JD	Cavanaugh
12/04/04	145923	Dicloxacillin	250 mg	#40	2 QID	JD	Cavanaugh

1. Before talking with the patient, what functional/emotional barriers would you expect during the consultation? What else would you like to know about your patient?
2. How are you going to begin the consultation?
3. Listed below are three different responses by the patient to the first *Prime Question.* For each statement, consider what each statement reveals about what the patient knows or feels, and state what should happen next in the consultation.

   Patient Response A:* *"He gave it to me after my surgery."*
   Patient Response B: *"I just had surgery for breast cancer."*
   Patient Response C: *"I know what it's for."*

4. Listed below are three different responses to the second *Prime Question.* Consider what each tells you, and state what you would do next in the consultation.

   Patient Response A: *"I'm going to take it twice a day."*
   Patient Response B: *"It's on the label, isn't it?"*
   Patient Response C: *"I don't remember. He didn't tell me."*

5. Listed below are three different responses to the third *Prime Question.* Consider what each tells you, and state what you would do next in the consultation.

   Patient Response A: *"I hope it will keep my cancer in check."*
   Patient Response B: *"The doctor says things look good, but I thought I heard something about uterine cancer?"*
   Patient Response C: *"Nothing. I'm not sure anything is going to help me now."*

Case No. 2: Thomas Gordon

Tom is a 53-year-old man with type 2 diabetes mellitus who is picking up an antibiotic for an infected cut on his arm. He owns his own construction company and is always "on the go." You are ready to counsel him about his antibiotic prescription.

NAME Gordon, Thomas ADDRESS 38 Main Street Muncie, IL	DATE 2/15/02 AGE IF CHILD
FULL DIRECTIONS FOR USE Rx Cephalexin 500 mg #40 Sig: i po QID	Rx No. 82695 Date filled Cost Fee Total Price ☐ Do not refill No. of refills authorized: 0
☐ IDENTIFY CONTENTS ON LABEL UNLESS CHECKED ☐ NON-PROPRIETARY EQUIVALENT UNLESS CHECKED	
B. Higley M.D.	

1. What concerns do you have based on review of the patient's medication profile? What else would you like to know about your patient? Before talking with the patient, what functional/emotional barriers would you expect during consultation? What are the goals of the consultation?
2. How are you going to begin the consultation?
3. Listed below are Tom's responses to the *Prime Questions.* Consider what each response reveals about what the patient knows or feels, and state how you would address any concerns you detect.

   Pharmacist: "What did the doctor tell you the medication was for?"
   Tom: "He said he was giving me an antibiotic for this infection on my arm. It started as just a scratch, but it's gotten really bad."
   Pharmacist: "How did the doctor tell you to take the medicine?"
   Tom: "I don't know. He said it was on the label. I know I'm supposed to take it all."
   Pharmacist: "What did the doctor tell you to expect?"
   Tom: "I guess it will kill the infection and make the cut heal."

4. You have decided to ask about glipizide. Listed next is Tom's answer to your inquiry about the glipizide. Consider what the statement reveals, and state how you would address his concerns.

   Tom: "Yeah, well, I'm really busy with my business and it's hard to remember to take it."

* Patient statements A, B, and C do not necessarily correspond throughout the consultation.

Patient Medication Profile

Name: Thomas Gordon		**Known Diseases:**		**Allergies/Sensitivities**			
Date of Birth: 01/10/52		Diabetes since 1997			NKA		
Address: 38 Main Street, Muncie, IL					Telephone: 542-5016		
Additional Information:							
Notes:							
Date	**Rx No.**	**Medication**	**Strength**	**Quantity**	**Dosage**	**R.Ph.**	**M.D.**
01/10/04	75243	Glipizide	10 mg	100	1 Q AM	EM	B. Higley
06/20/04	75243R	Glipizide	10 mg	100	1 Q AM	EM	B. Higley
10/28/04	75243R	Glipizide	10 mg	100	1 Q AM	JR	B. Higley

Case No. 3: William Hodges

NAME Hodges, William ADDRESS 4212 W. Mission Lane Albuquerque, NM 87546	DATE 7/12/05 AGE IF CHILD
Rx FULL DIRECTIONS FOR USE	Rx No. 27021
1. Digoxin 0.125 mg #45	Date filled
Sig: 1 tab po Q AM on Sat M W F	Cost
2 tab po Q AM on Tues Thurs Sun	Fee
	Total Price
2. Captopril 25 mg #180	☐ Do not refill
Sig: 2 po TID	No. of refills authorized: 6
☐ IDENTIFY CONTENTS ON LABEL UNLESS CHECKED	
☐ NON-PROPRIETARY EQUIVALENT UNLESS CHECKED	
Ames M.D.	

Bill is a 65-year-old man with an 8-year history of congestive heart failure secondary to an anterior wall myocardial infarction. Shortly after his recovery, he had a four-vessel coronary artery bypass graft performed. In addition to his prescription medications, he takes one baby aspirin daily to prevent re-infarction.

Bill has seen his physician today and brings in renewal prescriptions for digoxin and captopril (captopril replaced nifedipine due to lack of efficacy). His condition worsened enough that he had to cancel his June trip to Disneyland with his grandchildren.

1. Review the patient's profile. What concerns do you have based on your review of the patient profile? What are the goals of the consultation?
2. How are you going to begin the consultation?
3. Listed below are Bill's responses to *Show-and-Tell* questions. What do you notice?

a. Digoxin

Pharmacist: "What is this for?" (as he shows the patient the tablets)
Bill: "That's digoxin, my heart pill."
Pharmacist: "How do you take it?"
Bill: "I take it once a day in the morning."
Pharmacist: "What kind of problems are you having?"
Bill: "None. I'm doing great!"

b. Captopril

Pharmacist: "What is this for?" (as he shows the patient the tablets)
Bill: "Also for my heart."
Pharmacist: "How do you take it?"
Bill: "Uh . . . two, three times a day."
Pharmacist: "What kind of problems are you having?"
Bill: "None. . . . What kind of problems could this medicine cause?"

4. How should you respond to Bill's last question?
5. Bill tells you that captopril made him feel funny when he first started taking it. What should be your next response, and what technique should you now use?
6. The patient's response to your questions was:
   a. I felt real dizzy.
   b. It started about 24 hours after I started taking it.
   c. It was bad enough that I saw spots and almost fell.
   d. It happened primarily when I got up out of bed or from a chair.
   e. I tried getting up slowly and it only helped some, so I stopped it for a day and it went away. Then I started back at one pill twice a day for a couple of weeks. I'm back up to one pill three times a day and I'm not having any problems. I'm going to try to slowly increase it to what the doctor wants me to take. I mean to ask him about it, but I forget.
   f. I haven't noticed anything else except this new medicine seems to be working better than the other. I've got lots more energy and I can make that six-block walk to the store without getting winded.

Patient Medication Profile

Name: William Hodges	Known Diseases	Allergies and Sensitivities	Additional Information
Address: 4212 W. Mission Ln.	CABG s/p 1990	Penicillin	
Albuquerque, NM 87546	Angina		
Telephone: 555/425-7219	CHF		
Date of Birth: 3/22/39			

Date	Rx No.	Name of Med.	Strength	Quantity	Dosage Regimen	R.Ph.	Physician
04/20/05	18591	Digoxin	0.125 mg	45	1 Sat M W F 2 Sun T Th	BR	Ames
04/20/05	18592	K Tabs	10 mEq	60	2 QD	BR	Ames
04/20/05	18593	Furosemide	40 mg	15	½ tab QD	BR	Ames
04/20/05	18594	Nifedipine XL	30 mg	60	1 BID	BR	Ames
05/15/05	21052	Digoxin	0.125 mg	45	1 Sat M W F 2 Sun T Th	JC	Ames
05/15/05	21053	K Tabs	10 mEq	120*	2 QD	JC	Ames
05/15/05	21054	Furosemide	40 mg	30*	½ QD	JC	Ames
05/15/05	21055	Nifedipine XL	30 mg	60	1 BID	JC	Ames
6/16/05	24273	Digoxin	0.125 mg	45	1 Sat M W F 2 Sun T Th	DT	Ames
6/16/05	24274	K Tabs	10 mEq	60	2 QD	DT	Ames
6/16/05	24275	Furosemide	40 mg	15	½ QD	DT	Ames
6/16/05	24276	Captopril	25 mg	180	2 TID	DT	Ames

* Vacation supply

What clinical assessment do you make from these responses?

7. Before taking action to correct the problem, what should you do now in the consultation?
8. What about the problem with his digoxin?
9. You need to call Dr. Ames. How would you phrase your comments to Dr. Ames regarding the two problems you detected?
10. What would you recommend to Dr. Ames?

CHAPTER 4

Care Planning: A Component of the Patient Care Process

Grace D. Lamsam, PharmD, PhD
Terry L. Schwinghammer, PharmD, FCCP, FASHP, BCPS

THE PATIENT CARE PROCESS

The *patient care process* for pharmacists is a systematic and comprehensive method that is employed to identify, solve, and prevent drug therapy problems.[1] A drug therapy problem is "any undesirable event experienced by a patient which involves, or is suspected to involve, drug therapy and that interferes with achieving the desired goals of therapy."[1] The patient care process includes three essential elements: (a) assessment of the patient's drug-related needs; (b) creation of a care plan to meet those needs; and (c) follow-up evaluation to determine whether positive outcomes were achieved. Consequently, development of a patient care plan is only one component of the overall patient care process. Before developing a patient-specific care plan, it is important for the clinician to have an understanding of the comprehensive nature of the patient care process. This process offers a logical and consistent framework that can be most useful in care planning and serves as the framework for this chapter.

Assessment of Drug-Related Needs

The first step in assessment is to identify the patient's drug-related needs by collecting, organizing, and integrating pertinent patient, drug, and disease information. In the patient care process, as with all direct patient care services, the patient is the primary source of information. This involves asking patients what they *want* (expectations) and what they *don't want* (concerns) and by determining how well they understand their drug therapies. For example, the clinician may ask, "How can I help you today?" or, "What concerns do you have that I can address for you today?" In addition to speaking with the patient, data can also be obtained from family members or caretakers when appropriate, the patient's current and past medical records, and discussions with other health care providers. The types of information that may be relevant include:[1,2]

Patient information

- Demographics and background information: age, gender, race, height, weight
- Social history: living arrangements, occupation, special needs (e.g., physical abilities, cultural traits, drug administration devices)
- Family history: relevant health histories of parents and siblings
- Insurance/administrative information: name of health plan, primary care physician

Disease information

- Past medical history
- Current medical problems
- History of present illness
- Pertinent information from the review of systems, physical exam, laboratory results, x-ray/imaging results
- Medical diagnoses

Drug information

- Allergies, side effects (include the name of the medication and the reaction that occurred)
- Current prescription medications:
  - How the medication was prescribed
  - How the patient is actually taking the medication
  - Effectiveness and side effects of current medications
  - Questions or concerns about current medications
- Current nonprescription medications, vitamins, and alternative/complementary therapies
- Past prescription and nonprescription medications (i.e., those discontinued within the past 6 months)

The information obtained is then organized, analyzed, and integrated to: (a) determine whether the patient's drug therapy is appropriate, effective, safe, and convenient for the patient; (b) identify drug therapy problems that may interfere with goals of therapy; (c) identify potential drug therapy problems that require prevention. One method of organizing and integrating this information with appropriate pharmacotherapeutic knowledge has been described as the Pharmacotherapy Workup© (copyright 2003, the Peters Institute of Pharmaceutical Care).[1]

Drug therapy problems are uncovered through careful assessment of the patient, drug, and disease information to determine the appropriateness of each medication regimen. This process involves a logical sequence of steps. It begins with evaluating each medication regimen for appropriateness of indication; then optimizing the drug and dosage regimen to ensure maximum effectiveness; and, lastly, individualizing drug therapy to make it as safe as possible for the patient. After completing these three steps, the pharmacist considers other issues such as cost, compliance, and convenience.

Drug therapy problems can be placed into distinct categories, as summarized below. See Table 4–1 for a useful checklist that can be used in actual practice situations.[1]

1. *Inappropriate* indication for drug use
   a. The patient requires additional drug therapy
   b. The patient is taking unnecessary drug therapy
2. *Ineffective* drug therapy
   a. The patient is taking a drug that is not effective for his/her situation
   b. The medication dose is too low
3. *Unsafe* drug therapy
   a. The patient is experiencing an adverse drug reaction
   b. The medication dose is too high
4. Inappropriate *adherence* or *compliance*
   a. The patient is unable or unwilling to take the medication as prescribed

A drug therapy problem can be resolved or prevented only when the cause of the problem is clearly understood. Therefore, it is necessary to identify and categorize both the drug therapy problem and its cause (see Table 4–2).[1]

Creation of a Patient Care Plan

Care plan development is a cooperative effort that should involve the patient as an active participant. It may also involve an interdisciplinary team of care providers and the patient's family. Care planning involves establishing therapeutic goals and determining appropriate interventions to:

1. Resolve all existing drug therapy problems
2. Achieve the goals of therapy intended for each active medical problem

TABLE 4–1. Drug Therapy Problems to Be Resolved or Prevented

Assessment	Drug Therapy Problem	Assessment	Drug Therapy Problem
Indication	**Unnecessary Drug Therapy** No medical indication Duplicate therapy Nondrug therapy indicated Treating avoidable ADR Addictive/recreational use **Needs Additional Drug Therapy** Untreated condition Preventive/prophylactic Synergistic/potentiating	**Safety**	**Adverse Drug Reaction** Undesirable effect Unsafe drug for patient Drug interaction Dose administered or changed too rapidly Allergic reaction Contraindications present **Dosage Too High** Wrong dose Frequency too short Duration too long Drug interaction Incorrect administration
Effectiveness	**Needs Different Drug Product** More effective drug available Condition refractory to drug Dosage form inappropriate Not effective for condition **Dosage Too Low** Wrong dose Frequency too long Duration too short Drug interaction Incorrect administration	**Compliance**	**Nonadherence** Directions not understood Patient prefers not to take Patient forgets to take Drug product too expensive Cannot swallow or administer Drug product not available

Adapted with permission from Cipolle RJ, Strand LM, Morley PC. Pharmaceutical care practice: A clinician's guide, 2nd ed. New York, McGraw-Hill, 2004:168.

TABLE 4–2. Causes of Drug Therapy Problems

Drug Therapy Problem	Possible Causes of Drug Therapy Problems
Unnecessary drug therapy	No valid medication indication for the drug at this time. Multiple drug products are used when only single-drug therapy is required. The condition is better treated with nondrug therapy. Drug therapy is used to treat an avoidable adverse drug reactions associated with another medication. The medical problem is caused by drug abuse, alcohol use, or smoking.
Need for additional drug therapy	A medical condition exists that requires initiation of new drug therapy. Preventive therapy is needed to reduce the risk of developing a new condition. A medical condition requires combination therapy to achieve synergism or additive effects.
Ineffective drug	The drug is not the most effective one for them medical problem. The drug product is not effective for the medical condition. The condition is refractory to the drug product being used. The dosage form is inappropriate.
Dosage too low	The dose is too low to product the desired outcome. The dosage interval is too infrequent. A drug interaction reduces the amount of active drug available. The duration of therapy is too short.
Adverse drug reaction	The drug product causes an undesirable reactions that is not dose-related. A safer drug is needed because of patient risk factors. A drug interaction causes an undesirable reaction that is not dose-related. The regimen was administered or changed too rapidly. The product causes an allergic reaction. The drug is contraindicated because of patient risk factors.
Dosage too high	The dose is too high for the patient. The dosing frequency is too short. The duration of therapy is too long. A drug interaction causes a toxic reaction to the drug product. The dose was administered too rapidly.
Noncompliance	The patient does not understand the instructions. The patient prefers not to take the medication The patient forgets to take the medication. Drug product is too expensive. The patient cannot swallow or self-administer the medication properly. The drug product is not available for the patient.

Adapted with permission from Cipolle RJ, Strand LM, Morley PC. Pharmaceutical care practice: A clinician's guide, 2nd ed. New York, McGraw-Hill, 2004:178–179.

3. Prevent future drug therapy problems that have a potential to develop

Although care plans have been a standard component of the practice of other health professionals (e.g., nurses, physical therapists, respiratory therapists) for many years, there is still no standard, widely accepted method of care planning in pharmacy. In 1995, the Joint Commission on Accreditation of Healthcare Organizations (JCAHO) made pharmaceutical care planning a requirement for accreditation in all settings that it accredits. This requirement mandates that pharmaceutical care planning be included in the overall plan of care for the patient.[3] Implementation of a systematic care planning process serves to organize the pharmacist's practice, to communicate activities to other health care professionals, and to provide a record of drug therapy interventions in the event that questions arise regarding the standard of care provided to a patient.

It cannot be overemphasized that a plan of care is not merely a document; rather, it is a systematic, ongoing process of planning, action, and documentation. It is a dynamic instrument that reflects the continuing care that is modified according to the patient's changing needs.[4] The most essential element to remember is that the needs of the patient drive the plan, regardless of the care-planning format used. In short, the plan must be tailored to the needs of each unique patient. All care providers and the patient should agree on the care plan because each participant has a responsibility for implementing a portion of the plan. In the ambulatory care setting, the patient often assumes much of the responsibility for plan implementation.

Organization of a care plan is important, and each medical problem should be addressed separately and in its entirety so that the drug therapy problems associated with each condition and the plans for intervention are logically organized and implemented. The elements of a care plan include:

- *Medical condition:* List the disease state for which the patient has drug-related needs.
- *Drug therapy problems:* State the drug therapy problems by including the patient's problem or condition, the drug therapy involved, and the association between the drug(s) and the patient's condition(s).
- *Goals of therapy:* State the goals in the future tense. Goals should be realistic, measurable and/or observable, specific, and associated with a definite time frame.
- *Interventions:* In collaboration with the patient, the practitioner develops and prioritizes a list of activities to address the patient's drug-related needs. The patient's input is important because the plan should adequately address the patient's unique concerns, needs, and preferences. The list of activities may be stated in the past, present, or future tense. Include the recommendations made to the patient, the caregiver on the patient's behalf, or to the prescriber to resolve (or prevent) the patient's drug therapy problems.
- *Follow-up plan:* Determine when the patient should return for follow-up and what will occur at that subsequent visit.

An example of how each of these components might be incorporated into a care plan is given in the following case vignette:

> *Patrick Murphy is a 73-year-old man who underwent coronary artery bypass grafting 2 months ago and was started on simvastatin 10 mg po once daily 6 weeks ago for dyslipidemia. The results of this week's fasting lipid profile revealed total cholesterol 230 mg/dL, LDL cholesterol 141 mg/dL, HDL cholesterol 45 mg/dL, and triglycerides 220 mg/dL. He continues to smoke 1.5 packs of cigarettes per day.*

- *Medical condition:* Dyslipidemia
- *Drug therapy problems:* Dyslipidemia treated with an inadequate dose of a lipid-lowering agent.
- *Goals of therapy:* The patient's LDL cholesterol will be lowered to <100 mg/dL within 6 weeks. (Note: Because the patient has known coronary artery disease, his goal LDL cholesterol is <100 mg/dL.[5])
- *Interventions:* The maximum dose of simvastatin is 80 mg, so the dose should be increased in an attempt to achieve the target LDL level. Increase simvastatin to 20 mg po once daily; #30 dispensed. Reviewed possible side effects of simvastatin with patient (constipation, rare muscle weakness) and monitoring for liver injury (serum ALT measurements). Recommended that the patient consider stopping smoking—advised to keep a log of smoking habits, including # of cigarettes, time of day, and trigger events.
- *Follow-up plan:* Patient will return to clinic in 6 weeks for a repeat fasting lipid profile, questioning about potential adverse effects, and discussion of a plan for smoking cessation.

Follow-Up Evaluation

The purpose of a follow-up evaluation is to evaluate the positive and negative impact of the care plan on the patient, to uncover new drug therapy problems, and to take appropriate action to address new problems or adjust previous therapies as needed. Follow-up evaluation requires direct contact with the patient to obtain feedback including benefits of therapy, problems such as side effects, or concerns about treatment. Additionally, relevant data is gathered from current clinical assessments, laboratory tests, radiographs, or other procedures. The practitioner evaluates and documents the patient's progress in achieving the goals of therapy.

The evaluation involves comparing goals of therapy with the patient's current status. Cipolle, Strand, and Morley developed terminology to describe the patient's status, the medical conditions, and the comparative evaluation of that status with the previously determined therapeutic goals.[1] These terms also describe the actions taken as a result of the follow-up evaluation:

STATUS	DEFINITION
Resolved	Therapeutic goals achieved for acute condition, discontinue therapy
Stable	Therapeutic goals achieved, continue same therapy for chronic disease management
Improved	Progress is being made in achieving goals, continue same therapy as more time is required to assess the full benefit of therapy
Partial improvement	Progress is being made, but minor adjustments in therapy are required to fully achieve the therapeutic goals before the next assessment
Unimproved	Little or no progress has been made, but continue the same therapy to allow additional time for benefit to be observed
Worsened	A decline in health is observed despite an adequate duration using the optimal drug; modify drug therapy (e.g., increase the dose of the current medication, add a second agent with additive or synergistic effects)
Failure	Therapeutic goals have not been achieved despite an adequate dose and duration of therapy; discontinue current medication(s) and start new therapy
Expired	The patient died while receiving drug therapy; document possible contributing factors, especially if they may be drug related

Example: If the patient Mr. Murphy described above returns in six weeks with a repeat fasting LDL cholesterol of 120 mg/dL without complaints of side effects, the outcome status of this patient would be partial improvement. Another adjustment in therapy is indicated to further reduce his LDL cholesterol (e.g., increase the simvastatin dose to 40 mg po once daily).

Example of Care Plan Documentation

Each step in the patient care process must be documented. Documentation should take place on an ongoing basis to provide an updated record of the patient's current and changing needs, care activities in response to those needs, the patient's progress, and plans for future care and follow-up evaluation. This document provides a means for communication among health care providers and is now required for accreditation by JCAHO. What JCAHO requires is not merely a list of the patient's current medications but a document that reflects the systematic and dynamic process of patient care. The example provided in Figure 4–1 below is intended to demonstrate to students how a care plan might be created.

A blank care plan form is also included at the end of this chapter for use by students who are completing the cases for this casebook (see Figure 4–2). Students should practice using this form when completing the case studies in this casebook.

The vast amount of medical information available and the widespread computerization of patient records make the use of electronic pharmaceutical care records virtually mandatory. Consequently, use of this relatively simple form should be considered as only the first step in developing the

FIGURE 4–1. Sample pharmaceutical care patient record.

Pharmaceutical Care Patient Record

Patient Name: Donald Benferardo	**Gender:** M
Address: 621 E. Greene Street, Punxsutawney, PA 15767	**Race:** W
Telephone: 321-555-1950 **Age:** 64	**Actual Weight:** 177 lb. (80 kg)
Insurance: Metro United Health Plan #1234789	**Ideal Weight:** 166 lb. (75.3 kg)
Medical Conditions: Osteoarthritis left knee (stable)	**Allergies:** Penicillin → hives
Tobacco/Alchohol/Substance Use: occasional cigar 3X/week; EtOH 3X/wk; no caffeine	**Adverse Reactions:** Ibuprofen → dyspepsia

Medication Record

Start Date	Stop Date	Indication	Drug Name	Strength	Actual Regimen	Clinical Impressions
12/14/02		Osteoarthritis	Relafen	750 mg	2 tablets po QD	Tolerating well; min. knee pain
5/03/05	5/17/05	Hypertension	Hydrochlorothiazide	25 mg	1 tablet po QD	5/17/05: D/C due to hypokalemia
5/17/05		Hypertension	Triamterene/ Hydrochlorothiazide	37.5/25 mg	1 tablet po QD	5/31/05: K^+ WNL; HTN partially improved
5/31/05		Hypertension	Atenolol	50 mg	1 tablet po QD	

Assessment, Plan, and Follow-Up Evaluation

Date	Medical Condition	Drug Therapy Problem	Goal	Current Status	Interventions	Follow-Up Plan
5/3/05	Hypertension	Untreated HTN	Lower BP to 110–138/70–88 within 4 weeks	Untreated (BP 160/104)	Start hydrochlorothiazide 25 mg po QD × 4 weeks	Return for BP check and serum K^+ in 2 weeks
5/17/05	Hypertension	Hypokalemia secondary to hydrochlorothiazide	K^+ 3.5-5.0 mEq/L	Untreated (K 3.2 mEq/L)	Discontinue hydrochlorothiazide Begin triamterene/ hydrochlorothiazide 37.5/25 mg, 1 po QD	Recheck K^+ in 2 weeks
5/17/05	Hypertension	HTN inadequately treated with hydrochlorothiazide	BP 110-138/70-88	Partial improvement (BP 150/92)	Change to triamterene/ hydrochlorothiazide as above	Return in 2 weeks for BP and K^+ check
5/31/05	Hypertension	Hypokalemia requiring drug therapy	K^+ 3.5-5.0 mEq/L	Stable (K 3.6 + mEq/L)	Continue current therapy	Check symptoms of ↓ K^+ in 1 mo.
5/31/05	Hypertension	HTN inadequately treated with hydrochlorothiazide	Same as above	Partial improvement (BP 146/92)	Add atenolol 50 mg po QD × 4 weeks	Return for BP check in 1 mo.

student's ability to electronically organize and manage large volumes of complex medical information.

Example Case Vignette: Donald Benferardo is a 64-year-old man with osteoarthritis currently treated with Relafen. He has been diagnosed with hypertension based on the average of two blood pressure readings taken at three previous clinic visits.[6] The hypertension is presently untreated. What information must be included in the patient's care plan?

Patient Information

- *The patient's name* is essential to identify the patient to whom the record belongs. The name, Donald Benferardo, should be the first information placed on the chart. Although this guideline seems logical, it sometimes does not happen. When in a hurry, a care provider may grab a blank form and begin to make notes with the intention of placing the patient's personal information on it later, and in the midst of distractions, the name is not recorded.
- *Current address and phone number* are necessary for future contact and follow-up evaluation. The information should be complete (621 E. Greene Street, Punxsutawney, PA 15767), and the telephone number should include the area code (321-555-1950).
- *Insurance* information should include the name of the insurance plan and policy number (Metro United Health Plan #1234789) to ensure accurate billing of services.
- *Demographic* information including *age (birth date), gender, race, height, and weight* should be recorded for the purpose of individualizing drug therapy. Mr. Benferardo is a 64-year-old white man who is 5′11″ tall and weighs 177 lbs. Include weight information in both pounds (lb.) and kilograms (kg). The equation for converting lbs to kg is as follows: weight in lbs/2.2 = weight in kg. Mr. Benferardo weighs 177 lbs or 80.4 kg (177/2.2 = 80.4). This information is used to determine the appropriate drug and dosage regimens for treatment. *Ideal body weight (IBW)* is necessary for calculating appropriate dosage for medications that do not distribute into fatty tissues. IBW is calculated as follows: For men, IBW = 50 kg + [2.3 × (height in inches above 5 feet)]. For women, IBW = 45.5 kg + [2.3 × (height in inches above 5 feet)]. For Mr. Benferardo, 50 kg + (2.3 × 11) = 75.3 kg.
- *Allergies and adverse drug reactions* should be clearly documented with specific descriptions of the reactions. Reactions should be clearly identified as allergies or side effects. Mr. Benferardo has an allergic reaction to penicillin that resulted in hives. He also has experienced dyspepsia, a well-documented side effect of ibuprofen. This information is critical to avoiding patient harm. Allergies are distinct from side effects. An allergy is an immune-mediated reaction that often precludes future use of the medication except in rare cases in which the benefit of using the drug outweighs the risk of the reaction. However, a side effect may sometimes be self-limiting with continued use or it may be successfully managed with adjustments in the dosage regimen or dosage administration. For example, a drug that is taken once daily and causes drowsiness may be administered at bedtime. A drug that causes GI upset may be successfully managed by taking it with meals.
- *Tobacco/alcohol/substance use* information is important for appropriate drug selection, dosing calculation, and patient education. Include the name of the substance, the amount, and frequency, when possible. Mr. Benferardo occasionally smokes approximately three cigars each week and drinks 1 ounce of whiskey with each cigar. It is important to record pertinent negatives for substance use. For example, caffeine may increase blood pressure acutely, although tolerance to this effect develops quickly. Nevertheless, caffeine use may be relevant to this patient and should be recorded. Alcohol and tobacco may affect the metabolism of certain drugs and potentiate or counteract the benefits of other drugs. For example, tobacco enhances the metabolism of theophylline. Therefore, smokers generally require higher doses of theophylline to achieve therapeutic benefits. Substances such as cocaine, caffeine, or tobacco may enhance the sympathomimetic effect of some drugs while counteracting the sympatholytic effects of others, such as some antihypertensive medications.
- *Medical conditions* should be listed to offer a general overview of the patient's medical problems. The care plan is also organized according to the medical condition whereby all drug therapy problems associated with each medical condition are addressed separately and in their entirety.

Medication Record

- The list of medications should include the date each was started; the indication for use; and the drug name, strength, and regimen that the patient is actually taking. The *actual* regimen may differ from the *prescribed* regimen because patients don't always take medications as directed. Assessment of therapy must be made based upon the actual therapy the patient is receiving. Mr. Benferardo is currently taking Relafen (nabumetone) two 750-mg tablets by mouth daily. A stop date should be recorded for medications that have been discontinued. Relevant clinical impressions or comments can also be recorded, for example: "Discontinued ibuprofen secondary to dyspepsia that occurred even when taken with food." Also note the antihypertensive regimen, which was initiated with hydrochlorothiazide 25 mg po once daily and subsequently changed to triamterene/hydrochlorothiazide 37.5/25 mg po once daily. Atenolol 50 mg po once daily was added later because only partial improvement in hypertension was achieved with diuretic therapy.

Assessment, Plan, and Follow-up Evaluation

This section of the patient's chart provides a record of therapeutic interventions and the patient's responses to them. Information is documented as events occur, providing a "flow chart" of the patient's progress to date. The historical information contained in this chart is important to incorporate in therapeutic decision making.

- The *Date* should be recorded in the far-left column to document when each encounter occurred. Mr. Benferardo's chart shows that he has been seen three times: on May 3, May 17, and May 31, 2005.
- In the next column, *Medical Condition* specifies the medical diagnosis for which the medications are indicated. On May 3, Mr. Benferardo was diagnosed with hypertension; his subsequent visits also were for evaluation of hypertension.
- The *Drug Therapy Problem* is recorded in the next column to indicate the drug therapy problem(s) associated with each medical diagnosis. Each medical diagnosis may have one or more drug therapy problems associated with it. On May 3, Mr. Benferardo had one drug therapy problem—untreated hypertension. That is, he had an indication for drug therapy but was not receiving treatment. On May 17 and May 31, the dates were recorded twice because on these days he had two drug therapy problems that were being addressed. Each drug therapy problem should be recorded in a separate row. Although he had only one active diagnosis (hypertension), he had two drug therapy problems associated with that diagnosis as shown on May 17 and May 31. He had hypokalemia possi-

bly secondary to hydrochlorothiazide and hypertension inadequately treated with hydrochlorothiazide.

- The *Goal* of therapy is recorded in the next column. Using the SMART acronym, therapy goals should be ***Specific***, ***Measurable*** (or observable) and ***Achievable***. The goal should also be directly ***Related*** to the drug therapy problem. In this case, the systolic blood pressure goal should be less than 140 mm Hg with a diastolic pressure of less than 90 mm Hg. Treatment to lower levels may be useful if tolerated by the patient. For example, the clinician may establish an acceptable range of blood pressure control, such as systolic BP between 110 and 138 mm Hg and diastolic BP between 70 and 88 mm Hg. The ***Timeline*** to achieve the goal should also be specified. For example, his blood pressure should be reduced to within the indicated range within 4 weeks of therapy.
- The *Current Status* includes the patient's actual blood pressure at each encounter. In this case, Mr. Benferardo's blood pressure was 160/104 mm Hg on May 3 prior to starting drug therapy. Notice that his blood pressure continues to decline with treatment. On May 17 and 31, his blood pressures were 150/92 and 146/92 mm Hg, respectively. The status on May 31 (4 weeks after treatment) is considered partially improved because the blood pressure did decrease with treatment, but an adjustment in treatment is still required to achieve the blood pressure goal.
- *Interventions* that were implemented must be recorded. The drug name, dose, route, frequency, and duration of therapy should be documented. On May 3, hydrochlorothiazide was started at a dose of 25 mg orally once a day. As you look down this column, you can see that the therapy was adjusted on May 17 and May 31. These interventions were made in response to the patient's blood pressure as recorded in the previous column. By looking across the row, you can see the supportive evidence for the intervention: a clearly documented problem (hypertension) and the patient's status measured objectively (blood pressure). Looking down the columns, one can see what interventions have been made and also how the patient has responded over time.
- The *follow-up plan* specifies details of how the outcome of therapy will be assessed. This column should contain information about who will do what and when they will do it. The plan made on May 3 indicated that Mr. Benferardo was to return to the clinic in 2 weeks to have his blood pressure and serum potassium level measured. This flow chart provides an easy way to see whether the patient is appearing for the follow-up visits. Mr. Benferardo did return for follow-up in 2 weeks (May 17) according to the plan. There should continue to be a follow-up plan as long as a person is receiving drug therapy. After the patient's condition is stabilized, the follow-up intervals may be much longer, such as every 6 months or once a year. However, the assessment, plan, and follow-up must continue for the duration of drug therapy. In this case, after Mr. Benferardo's blood pressure is stabilized, he may be responsible for monitoring his own blood pressure and assessing the side effects by self-monitoring while keeping a twice-yearly appointments for a more formal evaluation at the clinic. The patient's care plan remains active and represents the ongoing and dynamic process of providing pharmaceutical care.

Patient Summary

Based on the information documented in the care plan, the practitioner providing care to this patient and other health care professionals who have access to this information should be able to extract the following summary of this patient's past and present status regarding hypertension treatment and response.

Mr. Benferardo is a 64-year-old man diagnosed with osteoarthritis and hypertension. He was seen on May 3, 2005, at which time his blood pressure was 160/104 mm Hg. His goal blood pressure range was set as systolic BP of 110–138 mm Hg and diastolic BP of 70–88 mm Hg. This was the standard against which future blood pressure measurements would be compared. He was started on hydrochlorothiazide 25 mg orally once daily for 2 weeks and was to return to clinic for a follow-up blood pressure check and serum potassium level 2 weeks later. He returned according to the plan, but the blood pressure reading of 152/98 indicated only a partial improvement. The blood pressure reduction had not yet reached the goal level; it may take 4 weeks for the full effect of diuretic therapy to be manifested. Consequently, no adjustment in therapy was made pending an adequate trial of single-agent diuretic therapy. However, the low serum potassium value of 3.2 mEq/L (reference range 3.5–5.0 mEq/L) indicated hypokalemia that required treatment. Because the hypokalemia may have resulted from the thiazide diuretic, hydrochlorothiazide 25 mg was discontinued and a combination product containing triamterene 37.5 mg + hydrochlorothiazide 25 mg, 1 tablet orally once daily, was begun. He returned 2 weeks later as planned and his blood pressure continued to show improvement (148/96 mm Hg), but it was not at the therapeutic goal that had been established 4 weeks earlier. This indicated partial improvement requiring further adjustment of his antihypertensive therapy. However, his potassium level had risen to within the normal range. Therefore, atenolol 50 mg orally once daily was added to the regimen. The patient was scheduled to return for a follow-up visit in 1 month.

Conclusion

Implementation of a care planning process is necessary for providing consistent pharmaceutical care and for documenting the outcomes of that care. It is also essential for obtaining compensation for care provided. Care planning captures past and current events occurring in a dynamic patient care process that is provided in response to changing patient needs. This process should be incorporated into the practice of each provider of pharmaceutical care, regardless of the practice setting.

References

1. Cipolle RJ, Strand LM, Morley PC. Pharmaceutical care practice: The clinician's guide, 2nd ed. New York, McGraw-Hill, 2004.
2. ASHP Council on Professional Affairs. ASHP Guidelines on a standard method for pharmaceutical care. Am J Hosp Pharm 1996;53:1713–1716.
3. Rich DS. JCAHO's pharmaceutical care plan requirements. Hosp Pharm 1995;30(4):315–319.
4. McCallian DJ, Carlstedt BC, Rupp MT. Elements of a pharmaceutical care plan. Am J Pharm Assoc 1999;39(1):82–83.
5. Expert Panel on Detection, Evaluation, and Treatment of High Blood Cholesterol in Adults. Executive summary of the third report of the National Cholesterol Education Program (NCEP) Expert Panel on detection, evaluation, and treatment of high blood cholesterol in adults (Adult Treatment Panel III). JAMA 2001:285; 2486–2497.

ACKNOWLEDGMENTS

The authors thank Linda M. Strand, PharmD, PhD for her thoughtful review of this chapter.

FIGURE 4–2. Sample pharmaceutical care patient record for creating a care plan.

Pharmaceutical Care Patient Record		
Patient Name:		**Gender:**
Address:		**Race:**
Telephone:	**Age:**	**Actual Weight:**
Insurance:		**Ideal Weight:**
Medical Conditions:		**Allergies:**
Tobacco/Alcohol/Substance Use:		**Adverse Reactions:**

Medication Record

Start Date	Stop Date	Indication	Drug Name	Strength	Actual Regimen	Clinical Impressions

Assessment, Plan, and Follow-Up Evaluation

Date	Medical Condition	Drug Therapy Problem	Goal	Current Status	Interventions	Follow-Up Plan

CHAPTER 5

Documentation of Pharmacist Interventions

Bruce R. Canaday, PharmD, BCPS, FASHP, FAPhA
Peggy C. Yarborough, PharmD, MS, CDE, FAPP, FASHP, NAPP
Timothy J. Ives, PharmD, MPH, FCCP, BCPS

If there is no documentation, then it didn't happen! This philosophy is the standard in all health care settings as physicians, nurses, respiratory therapists, physical therapists, social workers, and other health care providers generate and maintain detailed notes regarding the patient's situation and their efforts to achieve the best possible outcomes for the patient. Documentation chronologically outlines the care the patient received and serves as a form of communication among health care practitioners, an important element that contributes to the quality of care provided. Each practitioner involved knows what evaluation has occurred, what the plan for the patient's treatment is, and who will provide it. Furthermore, third-party payers require reasonable documentation from practitioners that assures that the services provided are consistent with the insurance coverage.[1] General components of documentation include:

- A complete and legible record;
- Documentation for each encounter with a rationale for the encounter, physical findings, prior test results, assessment, clinical impression (or diagnosis) and plan for care;
- Identified health risk factors, and an easily inferred rationale for ordering diagnostic tests or ancillary services; and
- The patient's progress, response to and changes in treatment, and revision of the original diagnosis/assessment.

PRINCIPLES OF DOCUMENTATION

Documentation in the record is required to record pertinent facts, findings, and observations about a patient's health history including past and present illnesses, examinations, tests, treatments, and outcomes. Particularly in an era of evolution of electronic databases,[2] it also facilitates:

- The ability of providers to evaluate and plan the patient's immediate treatment and monitor his/her health care over time;
- Communication and continuity of care among providers involved in the patient's care;
- Accurate and timely claims review and payment;
- Appropriate utilization review and quality of care evaluations;
- Collection of data that may be useful for research and education; and
- Appropriate coding (i.e., CPT [Current Procedural Terminology] and ICD-10-CM [International Classification of Diseases, Tenth Revision, Clinical Modification]) for use on health insurance claim forms should be supported by documentation in the patient record.

Much of this documentation is derived from a systematic patient care process of evaluation that is standardized within each discipline. For example, physicians are taught to perform a history and physical examination based upon a standardized review of body systems and to document their results using a universally accepted, standardized, systematic process.

Several evaluation/documentation systems have been suggested for health care professionals. More than 30 years ago, the use of a Problem-Oriented Medical Record was proposed[3] and most, if not all, physicians, nurse practitioners, physician associates, and other health care practitioners have been taught to write progress notes using the Subjective, Objective, Assessment, Plan (SOAP) format. Institutional consultant notes often use an abbreviated version of the SOAP format. This abbreviated version usually includes Findings (i.e., subjective and objective information), Assessment (or Impression), and Diagnosis (or Recommendations). Other variations of this standard exist,[4] such as SOAPER, which includes Education and Return instructions; SOAPIE, which includes Intervention and Evaluation; and SNOCAMP, which stands for Subjective, Nature of presenting problem, Objective, Counseling, Assessment, Medical decision making, and Plan. With the current documentation guidelines from the Centers for Medicare & Medicaid Services (CMS), older formats such as SOAP no longer meet minimal criteria for appropriate documentation in most cases.

Historically, pharmacy has not had a corresponding standard approach to the evaluation and documentation of the patient's pharmacotherapy that is applicable to all types of pharmacy practice settings. Thus, pharmacy has not been as active as other disciplines in documenting its contributions to patient care.

IMPORTANCE OF DOCUMENTATION

Pharmaceutical care uses a process through which a pharmacist cooperates with a patient and other health care professionals in designing, implementing, and monitoring a therapeutic plan that will produce specific therapeutic outcomes for the patient.[5] This process involves three major functions:

1. Identifying potential and actual drug-related problems
2. Resolving actual drug-related problems
3. Preventing potential drug-related problems

These functions aid in the provision of patient care through the identification of medication-related problems, development of a pharmacotherapeutic plan to address the problems, and the ultimate resolution or prevention of those problems.

As described in Chapter 1, a systematic approach is used in this casebook to identify and resolve the medication-related problems of patients. The steps can be summarized as follows:

1. Identification of real or potential medication-related problems
2. Determination of desired therapeutic outcomes and therapeutic endpoints
3. Determination of therapeutic alternatives
4. Design of an optimal pharmacotherapeutic plan for the patient
5. Identification of parameters to evaluate the outcome
6. Provision of patient education
7. Communication and implementation of the pharmacotherapeutic plan

Step 7 is crucial; the tenets of pharmaceutical care suggest that pharmacists should document, at the very least, the actual or potential medication-related problems identified, as well as the associated interventions that they desire to implement or have implemented. Pharmacists must adequately communicate their recommendations and actions to non-pharmacy health care practitioners (e.g., physicians, nurses), the patient or caregiver (e.g., parents), or other pharmacists. The goal is to provide a clear, concise record of the actual/potential problem,[6,7] the thought process that led the pharmacist to select an intervention, and the intervention itself. Additionally, the ability to receive remuneration for services provided necessitates an acceptable documentation strategy.

TRADITIONAL DOCUMENTATION FORMAT: SOAP NOTES

In the SOAP note format, subjective (S) and objective (O) data are recorded and then assessed (A) to formulate a plan (P). Subjective data include patient symptoms, things that may be observed about the patient, or information obtained about the patient. By its nature, subjective information is descriptive and generally cannot be confirmed by diagnostic tests or procedures. Much of the subjective information is obtained by speaking with the patient while obtaining the medical history, as described in Chapter 1 (i.e., chief complaint, history of present illness, past medical history, family history, social history, medications, allergies, and review of systems). Important subjective information may also be obtained by direct interview with the patient after the initial medical history has been performed (e.g., a description of an adverse drug effect, rating of pain severity using standard scales).

A primary source of objective information (O) is the physical examination. Other relevant objective information includes laboratory values, serum drug concentrations (along with the target therapeutic range for each level), and the results of other diagnostic tests (e.g., ECG, x-rays, culture and sensitivity tests). Risk factors that may predispose the patient to a particular problem should also be considered for inclusion. The communication note should include only the pertinent positive and negative findings. Pertinent negative findings are signs and symptoms of the disease or problem that are not present in the particular patient being evaluated.

The assessment (A) section outlines what the practitioner thinks the patient's problem is, based upon the subjective and objective information acquired. This assessment often takes the form of a diagnosis or differential diagnosis. This portion of the SOAP note should include all of the reasons for the clinician's assessment. This helps other health care providers reading the note to understand how the clinician arrived at his or her particular assessment of the problem.

The plan (P) may include ordering additional diagnostic tests or initiating, revising, or discontinuing treatment. If the plan includes changes in pharmacotherapy, the rationale for the specific changes recommended should be described. The drug, dose, dosage form, schedule, route of administration, and duration of therapy should be included. The plan should be directed toward achieving a specific, measurable, goal or endpoint, which should be clearly stated in the note. The plan should also outline the efficacy and toxicity parameters that will be used to determine whether the desired therapeutic outcome is being achieved and to detect or prevent drug-related adverse events. Ideally, information about the therapy that should be communicated to the patient should also be included in the plan. The plan should be reviewed and referred to in the note as often as necessary.

AN ALTERNATIVE APPROACH TO DOCUMENTING DRUG THERAPY PROBLEMS AND PLANS

There is a pharmacist equivalent of a physician's progress note in a systematized approach for the construction and maintenance of a record reflecting the pharmacist's contributions to care.[8] This process includes provisions for the identification and assessment of actual or potential medication-related problems, description of a therapeutic plan, and appropriate follow-up monitoring of the problems. Although there is no current uniform documentation system for the profession of pharmacy, students are encouraged to try this system as they learn to document patient interventions and compare its effectiveness with the SOAP format. In this system, problems that have been identified are addressed systematically in a pharmacist's note under the headings Findings, Assessment, Resolution, and Monitoring. The sections of the pharmacist's note can be easily recalled with the mnemonic F-A-R-M.

Identification of Drug Therapy Problems

The first step in the construction of a FARM note is to clearly state the nature of the drug-related problem(s). Each problem in the FARM note should be addressed separately and assigned a sequential number. Understanding the types of problems that may occur facilitates identification of pharmacotherapy problems. Seven types of medication-related problems have been identified (see Chapter 1):[9]

1. Unnecessary drug therapy
2. Needs additional drug therapy
3. Ineffective drug
4. Dosage too low
5. Adverse drug reaction
6. Dosage too high
7. Noncompliance

Use of a classification system such as this for the various types of medication-related problems offers at least two advantages. First, it presents a framework, applicable in any practice setting, to assure that the pharmacist has considered each possible type of problem. Second, categorization allows optimal data analysis and retrieval capabilities. Thus, problems as well as the interventions to resolve them can be stored in a standardized format in a computer. When an analysis of this information is needed at a later date, such as determining how much money was saved through an intervention, how outcomes were improved by the pharmacist, or how many problems of a certain type have occurred, the problems and interventions can be reviewed by groups rather than individually.

Documentation of Findings

Each statement of a drug-related problem should be followed by documentation of the pertinent findings (F) indicating that the problem may (potential) or does (actual) exist. Information included in this section should include a summary of the pertinent information obtained after collection and thorough assessment of the available patient information. Demographic data that may be reported include a patient identifier (e.g., name, initials, or medical record number), age, race (if pertinent), and gender. As noted earlier under the section on SOAP notes, medical information included in the note should include both subjective and objective findings that indicate a drug-related problem.

Assessment of Problems

The assessment (A) section of the FARM note includes the pharmacist's evaluation of the current situation (i.e., the nature, extent, type, and clinical significance of the problem). This part of the note should delineate the thought process that led to the conclusion that a problem did or did not exist and that an active intervention either was or was not necessary. If additional information is required to satisfactorily assess the problem and make recommendations, this data should be stated along with its source (e.g., the patient, pharmacist, physician). The severity or urgency of the problem should be indicated by stating whether the interventions that follow should be made immediately or within one day, one week, one month, or longer. The desired therapeutic endpoint or outcome should be stated. This may include both short-term goals (e.g., lower blood pressure to < 140/90 mm Hg in a patient with primary hypertension [therapeutic endpoint]) and long-term goals (e.g., prevent cardiovascular complications in that patient [therapeutic outcome]).

Problem Resolution

The resolution (R) section should reflect the actions proposed (or already performed) to resolve the drug-related problem based upon the preceding analysis. The note should convey that, after consideration of all appropriate therapeutic options, the option(s) considered to be the most beneficial was either carried out or suggested to someone else (e.g., the physician, patient, or caregiver). Recommendations may include nonpharmacologic therapy, such as dietary modification or assisting devices (e.g., canes, walkers); the rationale for this method of treatment should be described. If pharmacotherapy is recommended, a specific drug, dose, route, schedule, and duration of therapy should be specified. It is not sufficient to simply provide a list of choices for the prescriber. Importantly, the rationale for selecting the particular regimen(s) should be stated. It is reasonable to include alternative regimens that would be satisfactory if the patient is unable to complete treatment with the initial regimen because of adverse effects, allergy, cost, or other reasons. If patient education is recommended, the information that will be included in the session should be described. Conversely, if certain types of information will be withheld from the patient, the reasons for doing so should be stated. If no action is recommended or was taken, that should be documented as well. In this situation, the note serves as a record of the pharmacist's involvement in the patient's care. The pharmacist then has documentation that patient care activities were performed.

Monitoring for Endpoints and Outcomes

It is not enough, however, to only provide a clear, concise record of the nature of a problem, the assessment that led to the conclusion that a problem exists, and the selection of a plan for resolution of the problem. In the spirit of pharmaceutical care, the patient must not be abandoned after an intervention has been made. A plan for follow-up monitoring (M) of the patient must be documented and adequately implemented. This process is likely to include questioning the patient, gathering laboratory data, and performing the ongoing physical assessments necessary to determine the effect of the plan that was implemented to assure that it results in an optimal outcome for the patient.

Monitoring parameters to assess efficacy generally include improvement in or resolution of the signs, symptoms, and laboratory abnormalities that were initially assessed. The monitoring parameters used to detect or prevent adverse reactions are determined by the most common and most serious events known to be associated with the therapeutic intervention. Potential adverse reactions should be precisely described along with the method of monitoring. For example, rather than stating "monitor for GI complaints," the recommendation may be to "question the patient about the presence of dyspepsia, diarrhea, or constipation." The frequency, duration, and target endpoint for each monitoring parameter should be identified. The points at which changes in the plan may be warranted should be included. For example, in the case of a patient with dyslipidemia, one may recommend to "obtain fasting HDL, LDL, total cholesterol, and triglycerides after 3 months of treatment. If the goal LDL of < 100 mg/dL is not achieved with good compliance at 3 months, increase simvastatin to 40 mg po once daily. If goal LDL is achieved, maintain simvastatin 20 mg po once daily and repeat fasting lipoprotein profile annually."

SUMMARY

A SOAP or FARM progress note constructed in the manner described identifies each drug-related problem and states the pharmacist's Findings observed, an Assessment of the findings, the actual or proposed Resolution of the problem based upon the analysis, and the parameters and timing of follow-up Monitoring. Either form of note should provide a clear, concise record of process, activity, and projected follow-up. When written for each medication-related problem, these notes should provide data in a standardized, logical system. In particular, FARM notes provide a convenient format for progress notes for all pharmacists, applicable to any practice setting.

SAMPLE CASE PRESENTATION

The following case presentation illustrates how such a system can be used in practice.

History of Present Illness

Geraldine Johns is a 70-year-old woman seen Monday morning in clinic for her first visit. She has just moved to town to be near her son following the death of her husband. She has a history of atrial fibrillation, type 2 diabetes, COPD, mild CHF, and is s/p MI 4 years ago. She lives alone and maintains a good level of activity and self care. Denies pain in legs upon walking. She is maintained on metformin 500 mg po BID, glyburide 10 mg po Q AM, famotidine 20 mg po daily, digoxin 0.125 mg po Q AM, warfarin 5 mg po Q AM, aspirin 81 mg po Q AM, furosemide 80 mg po BID, and metoprolol XL 100 mg po Q AM.

Physical Examination

VS

BP 169/88, P 68 and regular, RR 13, T 99°F; Wt 100 lb., Ht 5′2″

Skin

Normal

Cardiac

No murmurs or rubs. (+) S_3 gallop; PMI in the 6th intercostal space 3 cm distal to the midclavicular line

Chest

Slight crackles at the right and left bases; no rales, e-to-a changes or tactile fremitus

Extremities

1–2+ pedal edema bilaterally. ABI (ankle brachial index) = 1.02 (negative)

HEENT

Slight AV nicking, otherwise unremarkable

GI, GU, & Neuro

Unremarkable

Laboratory values are unremarkable with the following exceptions:

INR 3.5
Glucose 198 mg/dL
HbA_{1c} 11.3%
Serum creatinine 1.3 mg/dL
Digoxin level 1.0 ng/mL

Chest x-ray

Some diffuse patchiness at the bases. Enlarged cardiac silhouette. Decreased density of the vertebrae consistent with mild osteoporosis.

ECG

Normal sinus rhythm

Medical Assessment

1. Mild to moderate CHF with pedal edema and slight pulmonary edema on digoxin and metoprolol
2. Type 2 DM, not optimally controlled on metformin and glyburide
3. Hypertension not optimally managed on metoprolol and furosemide
4. Atrial fibrillation, currently controlled on digoxin and metoprolol
5. Possible moderate renal insufficiency; SCr 1.3, estimated CLcr = 28 mL/min (Cockcroft & Gault)
6. Possible hyperlipidemia, as suggested by history of MI
7. Osteoporosis suggested by chest radiographs
8. COPD requiring no additional intervention at this time
9. S/P MI, on aspirin; lipid status unknown

Construction of a SOAP or FARM Note

NOTE: The Subjective and Objective findings of the SOAP note are combined into Findings for a FARM note. The Plan of the SOAP note is split into Recommendations/Resolution and Monitoring/Follow-up in the FARM note.

Findings

Subjective

70-year-old woman recently moved here after the death of her husband. Patient complains of slight shortness of breath when walking up stairs and long distances. She voices no other complaints. She has a history of atrial fibrillation, type 2 diabetes, COPD, mild CHF, and is s/p MI 4 years ago. She lives alone and maintains a good level of activity and self care. She is maintained on metformin 500 mg po BID, glyburide 10 mg po Q AM, famotidine 20 mg po daily, digoxin 0.125 mg po Q AM, warfarin 5 mg po Q AM, aspirin 81 mg po Q AM, furosemide 80 mg po BID, and metoprolol XL 100 mg po Q AM. She states that she takes her medications as prescribed, but she has some difficulty describing precisely how she takes them and is not quite certain what each medication does for her.

Objective

VS: BP 169/88, P 68 and regular, RR 13, T 99°F; Ht 5′2″, Wt 100 lb.
Cardiac: S_3 gallop, PMI in the 6th intercostal space 3 cm distal to the midclavicular line
Chest: Slight crackles at the right and left bases
Extremities: 1–2+ pedal edema bilaterally, ABI negative
HEENT: Slight AV nicking, otherwise unremarkable
Medications:
Metformin 500 mg po BID
Glyburide 10 mg po Q AM

Famotidine 20 mg po daily
Digoxin 0.125 mg po Q AM
Warfarin 5 mg po Q AM
Aspirin 81 mg po Q AM
Furosemide 80 mg po BID
Metoprolol XL 100 mg po Q AM

Labs:
INR 3.5
Glucose 198 mg/dL
HbA_{1c} 11.3%
Serum creatinine 1.3 mg/dL
Serum digoxin level 1.0 ng/mL

Chest x-ray: Some diffuse patchiness at the bases. Enlarged cardiac silhouette. Decreased density of the vertebrae consistent with mild osteoporosis.
ECG: NSR

Assessment

1. Possible non-adherence/concordance and lack of knowledge about medications.
2. Mild to moderate CHF as suggested by pedal edema, DOE, and cardiomegaly on chest x-ray. Maintained on a β-blocker and is not currently prescribed an ACE inhibitor.
3. Type 2 diabetes mellitus, not optimally controlled on metformin and glyburide; HbA_{1c} above goal of < 7%. Not prescribed either an ACE inhibitor or an ARB for renal protective effects.
4. Hypertension, not optimally controlled on metoprolol, as suggested by increased BP, elevated serum creatinine and AV nicking. The renal and ophthalmic findings are suggestive of significant, sustained hypertension. Repeated measurements will be necessary to confirm this assessment.
5. Atrial fibrillation
   a. Rate control: Rate currently under control with metoprolol and digoxin. No adjustment indicated.
   b. Anticoagulation: INR above target range of 2.0 to 3.0, without clinical complications at this time. No cause could be identified, although a change in diet associated with recent life events is suspected.
6. Possible moderate renal insufficiency as indicated by increased SCr. Renal dose adjustments may be necessary.
7. S/P MI on aspirin.
8. Possible hyperlipidemia as suggested by history of MI.
9. R/O Osteoporosis: Chest radiography suggestive of osteoporosis. Her petite frame and age are consistent with post-menopausal osteoporosis.
10. COPD: Mild DOE may suggest that the COPD is contributing to the CHF symptoms. COPD appears to be an untreated indication.
11. Adverse medication effects: although metoprolol may be considered appropriate for both the post-MI and CHF indications and is a β_1-selective β-blocker, its β_2-blocking properties (usually at higher doses) may contribute to worsening COPD and/or CHF due to bronchoconstriction, negative inotropic effects, or both.
12. Medication without indication (famotidine): On further questioning, the patient recalls being put on it while hospitalized for MI 4 years ago. She was given a prescription for it when she left the hospital. She has no complaints related to GERD or PUD. No need for famotidine can be identified.

Plan

RECOMMENDATIONS/RESOLUTION

1. Assess and reinforce adherence/concordance with recommended therapy. Educate on purpose of each medication.
2. Mild to moderate CHF: Continue both the β-blocker metoprolol and digoxin, pending evaluation by the Cardiology Service to determine appropriateness. Suggest initiation of an ACE inhibitor at low doses and increasing furosemide to 100 mg po BID until her return next week because of persistent pedal and pulmonary edema. No added dietary salt. May consider adding spironolactone at next visit.
3. Type 2 diabetes mellitus:
   a. Medication: Suggest initiation of an ACEI (as above) per current ADA guidelines. Suggest changing glyburide 10 mg to glipizide XL 10 mg po daily to improve control and enhance compliance/concordance. Continue to follow blood glucose readings and, if indicated, may supplement glyburide with insulin lispro for elevated pre-meal BG, based upon an estimated insulin sensitivity of 1 unit per 30 to 40 mg/dL:

If blood glucose:	Give insulin lispro:
180 mg/dL	2 units
220	3 units
260	4 units
300	5 units
340	6 units, and test for urinary ketones. Call MD if ketones moderate or large.

   b. Diet: Suggest 3 meals with bedtime snack, with no concentrated carbohydrate (CHO) choices. Limit CHO intake per meal to 60 g; snacks 15 to 20 g CHO. No added salt. Check blood glucose AC and HS.
4. Hypertension: Suggest initiation of an ACEI (as above), started at low doses. If repeated measurements confirm the diagnosis of hypertension, they may be titrated to maintain blood pressure control. Blood pressure goal is ≤ 130/80 mm Hg in patients with diabetes. Currently, the patient is stage 2, > 160/100 mm Hg.
5. Atrial fibrillation:
   a. Rate control: Suggest continuing metoprolol and digoxin unless Cardiology suggests otherwise. No adjustment indicated at this time.
   b. Anticoagulation: INR is above target range of 2.0 to 3.0. Recommend warfarin 2.5 mg today and then resume 5 mg po daily; dose to be adjusted as needed to maintain INR between 2.0 and 3.0.
6. Renal insufficiency: Suggest hydration regimen and repeat of serum creatinine. No medication dosage adjustments are indicated currently.
7. S/P MI: Recommend continuation of aspirin 81 mg po Q AM. Suggest initiation of ACEI/ARB as noted above, and a statin (e.g., pravastatin 10 mg po at bedtime). Continue metoprolol, if acceptable to Cardiology.
8. Possible hyperlipidemia: Treat based upon lipid panel; goal LDL is < 100 mg/dL in patient with existing CAD or diabetes; this patient has both.

9. Possible osteoporosis: If DXA scan indicates osteoporosis, begin a bisphosphonate (e.g., alendronate 70 mg po weekly) and calcium 1500 mg daily.
10. COPD: COPD appears to be an untreated indication. Suggest initiation of ipratropium 2 puffs QID.
11. Adverse medication effects: As noted above, will await Cardiology opinion on need for/appropriateness of β-blocker and digoxin to manage CHF.
12. Medication without indication: Suggest discontinuation of famotidine.

MONITORING/FOLLOW-UP

1. RTC in one week
2. Prior to RTC:
   a. Laboratory (slips given)
      i. Baseline electrolytes (K, Na, Ca, & Mg levels in light of unopposed furosemide therapy of unknown duration and use of digoxin) today
      ii. Serum creatinine today
      iii. Fasting lipid panel next week prior to RTC
      iv. INR next week prior to RTC
   b. DXA scan. Patient referred to Jones Pharmacy.
   c. Cardiology consult. Appointment made with Dr. Welford's office.
3. Patient instructed to monitor blood glucose AC and HS and bring information on RTC.
4. Prescribed medication after this visit:
   a. Enalapril 5 mg po daily for CHF, hypertension, & type 2 DM
   b. Metformin 500 mg po BID for type 2 DM
   c. Glipizide XL 10mg po daily for type 2 DM substituted for glyburide 10 mg po Q AM
   d. Lispro, as indicated
   e. Digoxin 0.125 mg po Q AM for CHF and rate control
   f. Furosemide 100 mg po BID for CHF
   g. Warfarin 5 mg po Q AM for s/p MI and CVA prevention
   h. Aspirin 81 mg po daily for s/p MI
   i. Metoprolol XL 100 mg po Q AM for s/p MI and rate control
   j. Pravastatin 10 mg po at bedtime for hyperlipidemia
   k. Ipratropium 2 puffs QID for COPD, and
   l. D/C Famotidine 20 mg po BID.

REFERENCES

1. Medicare Learning Network (Medlearn) Documentation Guidelines – Evaluation and Management Services. Washington, DC, Centers for Medicare & Medicaid Services, September 2003 (www.cms.hhs.gov/medlearn/emdoc.asp). Accessed August 25, 2004.
2. Shortliffe EH. The evolution of electronic medical records. Acad Med 1999;74: 414–419.
3. Weed LL. Medical records that guide and teach. N Engl J Med. 1968;278: 593–600, 652–657.
4. Larimore WL, Jordan EV. SOAP to SNOCAMP: Improving the medical record format. J Fam Pract 1995;41:393–398.
5. Hepler CD, Strand LM. Opportunities and responsibilities in pharmaceutical care. Am J Hosp Pharm. 1990;47:533–543.
6. Donnelly WJ. The language of medical case histories. Ann Intern Med 1997;127: 1045–1048.
7. Voytovich AE. Reduction of medical verbiage. Ann Intern Med 1999;131: 146–147.
8. Canaday BR, Yarborough PC. Documenting pharmaceutical care: Creating a standard. Ann Pharmacother. 1994;28:1292–1296.
9. Cipolle RJ, Strand LM, Morley PC. Pharmaceutical care practice: The clinician's guide. 2nd ed. New York, NY: McGraw-Hill; 2004.

SECTION 2

Cardiovascular Disorders

6 CARDIOPULMONARY RESUSCITATION

► A Near-Death Experience (Level II)

Tate N. Trujillo, PharmD, BCPS
Donna S. Wall, PharmD, BCPS

► After completing this case study, students should be able to:

- Discuss possible causes for cardiac arrest.
- Outline medications used to treat cardiac arrest.
- List the pharmacologic actions of medications used in cardioversion.
- Outline the Advanced Cardiac Life Support (ACLS) guidelines.
- Identify appropriate parameters to monitor a patient who has just been cardioverted.

PATIENT PRESENTATION

Chief Complaint

"I'm finally going to get my heart problem taken care of."

HPI

Jennifer Maple is a 62 yo woman who was admitted this morning for coronary artery bypass surgery. Recently while on vacation, she was hospitalized for unstable angina. Upon returning she underwent cardiac catheterization, which showed multiple-vessel CAD. The patient has been followed for some time for chronic renal insufficiency related to membranous nephropathy. While admitted for her cardiac catheterization, a right-sided Perma-Cath was placed followed by her first dialysis session. The Perma-Cath did not function during the second dialysis session. After trying to reposition the catheter, it was removed and replaced with another Perma-Cath.

PMH

ESRD (chronic membranous glomerulonephritis)
IV access difficulties
Anemia secondary to CRF
HTN
Hyperlipidemia
Type 2 DM—diet controlled
AMI × 2; coronary angioplasty 9 years ago
S/P appendectomy
S/P cholecystectomy
S/P hysterectomy

FH

Mother had HTN and died of an AMI at age 69; no information available for father; one brother at age 73 is alive with HTN and DM

SH

Smoker; quit 8 years ago; previously 1.5 ppd

ROS

Feels tired with frequent chest pain, fever, chills, nausea, and fatigue

Meds

Diltiazem CD 300 po at bedtime
Nephrocaps 1 po daily
Atorvastatin 20 mg po daily

Furosemide 160 mg po daily
EC ASA 325 mg po daily (hold until after CABG)
Prochlorperazine 10 mg po TID PRN nausea
Nitroglycerin 0.4 mg sublingual PRN chest pain
PhosLo 667 mg 2 po after meals
Nitroglycerin transdermal patch 0.4 mg daily at night and remove in AM
Acetaminophen 650 mg po QID PRN pain
Clonidine 0.2 mg po TID, but not before dialysis

All

IV Dye → worsened renal function (10 years ago)

PE

Gen

Obese white woman in NAD

VS

BP 168/106, P 86, RR 16, T 37.9°C; dry wt 76.5 kg

Skin

Warm, dry

HEENT

PERRLA; EOMI; arteriolar narrowing on funduscopic exam; no hemorrhages, exudates, or papilledema; oral mucosa clear

Neck/LN

Supple with no JVD or bruits; no lymphadenopathy or thyromegaly

Chest

Mild bibasilar rales

CV

RRR; S_1, S_2 normal; no S_3 or S_4; no murmurs or rubs

Abd

Obese, soft, non-tender; (+) BS; no HSM

Genit/Rect

Stool heme (–)

MS/Ext

2+ pedal edema with palpable pulses; capillary refill <2 sec; age-appropriate strength and ROM

Neuro

A & O × 3, decreased sensation in lower legs, CN II–XII intact

Labs

Na 134 mEq/L	Hgb 9.3 g/dL	Ca 6.7 mg/dL
K 3.9 mEq/L	Hct 28%	Mg 2.5 mg/dL
Cl 97 mEq/L	Plt 229 × 10^3/mm^3	Phos 5.5 mg/dL
CO_2 20 mEq/L	WBC 18.9 × 10^3/mm^3	Alb 2.5 g/dL
BUN 86 mg/dL	79% PMNs	
SCr 11.1 mg/dL	1% Bands	
Glu 88 mg/dL	17% Lymphs	
	3% Monos	

ECG

NSR at a rate of 86 bpm

▶ Clinical Course

The patient subsequently underwent CABG. Postoperatively she was given a morphine PCA for pain control (1 mg Q 10 min; 0.5 mg/hour basal rate), cefuroxime 1.5 g IV q 24 hr × 2 doses, and sliding-scale insulin. She had an unremarkable course for 24 hours and was restarted on all preoperative medications except for nitroglycerin patch. Approximately 36 hours S/P CABG the patient developed multifocal PVCs that quickly changed to ventricular fibrillation (Figure 6–1). A code was called.

▶ Questions

Problem Identification

1. a. *What actual and potential drug therapy problems does this patient have just prior to the development of ventricular fibrillation?*

   b. *Discuss the possible causes for the development of ventricular fibrillation.*

Desired Outcome

2. *What are the short-term goals of pharmacotherapy for this patient?*

Therapeutic Alternatives

3. a. *What nonpharmacologic maneuvers should be undertaken immediately in a patient with ventricular fibrillation?*

   b. *What pharmacotherapeutic agents are available for the acute therapy of this patient's condition?*

Optimal Plan

4. a. *A pharmacist was not available to participate in this resuscitation effort. Assess the appropriateness of the treatment used to obtain a cardiac conversion in this patient (see Clinical Course on page 41).*

   b. *Upon conversion to normal sinus rhythm, what is your pharmacotherapeutic plan to maintain the patient's stability?*

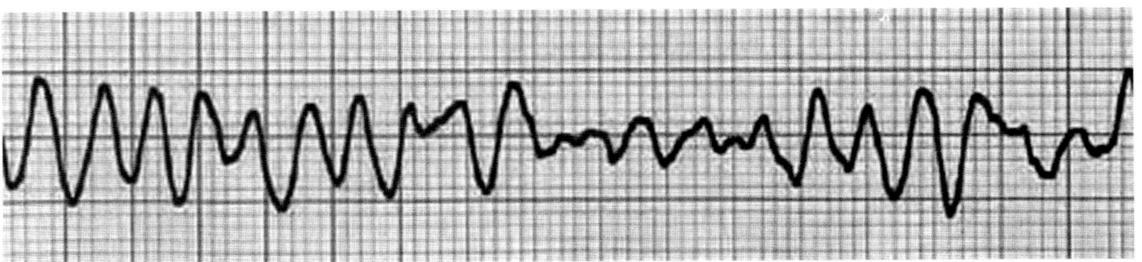

Figure 6–1. Electrocardiogram showing ventricular fibrillation.

▶ Clinical Course

Cardiopulmonary Resuscitation Record of Events and Orders

Time	BP	Spont. Resp.	Cardiac Rhythm	HR	Defib. (watt sec)	Rhythm after Defib.	Drugs Given
1320	188/56	10	VF (Figure 6–1)	98	100	Torsades (Figure 6–2)	
1321	150/46				200	Torsades	
1322	116/?				300	Agonal	
1325	88/?	10	Torsades		360	Agonal to Torsades	EPI 1 mg IVP Atropine 1 mg IVP Lidoc. 100 mg IVP
1332	302/133	10	SVT	160	360	SVT	
1338	160/84	10	SVT	180	360	NSR	Lidoc. 50 mg IVP
1347	133/50	10	NSR	96		Torsades to NSR with PVC	
1352						NSR with PVC	

Key: ?, not recorded; BP, blood pressure; Spont. Resp., spontaneous respirations; HR, heart rate; Defib., defibrillation; VF, ventricular fibrillation; EPI, epinephrine; IVP, intravenous push; Lidoc., lidocaine; SVT, supraventricular tachycardia; NSR, normal sinus rhythm; PVC, premature ventricular contraction.

Outcome Evaluation

5. *How should the patient be monitored to assess drug efficacy and to prevent and detect adverse effects? Describe how the therapy should be adjusted if adverse events occur.*

▶ Self-Study Assignments

1. Search the Internet for commercially available automated external defibrillator (AED) devices (see Figure 6–3 for one example). Explain how such a device would be used by a lay person during a cardiac arrest that occurred in the home or workplace.
2. Perform a literature search to determine the odds of surviving a cardiac arrest while hospitalized.
3. List medications that can be administered through an endotracheal tube.

▶ Clinical Pearl

During a cardiac arrest, a patient's serum potassium and glucose concentrations will increase dramatically due to the presence of acidosis; this may be further accentuated in the presence of renal failure.

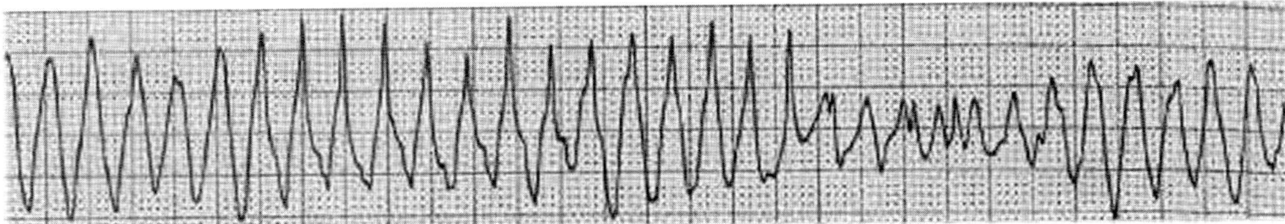

Figure 6–2. Electrocardiogram showing the abnormal rhythm of Torsades de Pointes.

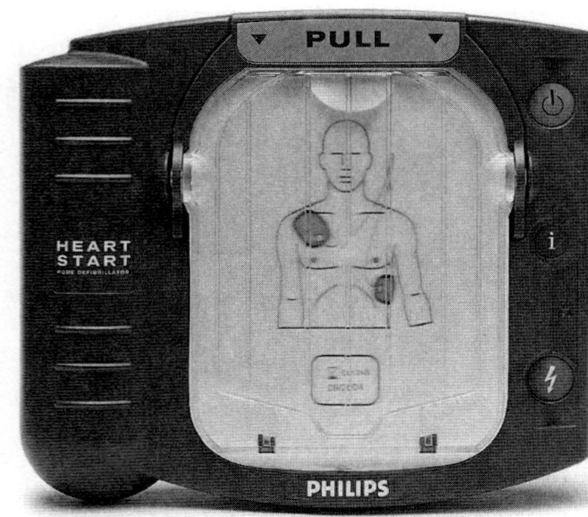

Figure 6–3. The Heartstart Home Defibrillator, an automated external defibrillator (AED) device approved by the FDA for home use. *(Photograph courtesy of Philips Medical Systems, Bothell, Washington.)*

References

1. International Liaison Committee on Resuscitation. Guidelines 2000 for cardiopulmonary resuscitation and emergency cardiovascular care. Circulation 2000;102(8):Suppl I.
2. Lopez LM, Scheife RT, eds. Acute management of ventricular arrhythmias: Focus on new developments. Pharmacotherapy 1997;17(2 Pt 2):56S–88S.
3. Wenzel V, Krismer AC, Arntz HR, et al. A comparison of vasopressin and epinephrine for out-of-hospital cardiopulmonary resuscitation. N Engl J Med 2004;350:105–13.

7 HYPERTENSION

▶ Mom's Medical Care is Mandatory (Level II)

Alicia M. Reese, PharmD, BCPS
Laurajo Ryan, PharmD, BCPS

▶ After completing this case study, students should be able to:

- Establish goals for the treatment of hypertension.
- Choose appropriate lifestyle modifications and antihypertensive regimens based on patient-specific characteristics and concurrent disease states.
- Design appropriate monitoring plans for patients receiving antihypertensive therapy, including laboratory parameters and time intervals.
- Modify pharmacotherapeutic regimens for patients who experience adverse events or do not have adequate blood pressure reduction on an initial regimen.
- Provide appropriate patient education for antihypertensive regimens.

PATIENT PRESENTATION

Chief Complaint

"I went to a blood pressure screening at the grocery store a couple of weeks ago and they said my blood pressure is still high. I haven't had time to come in because I've been so busy with my kids."

HPI

Rebecca Louise Thompson is a 43 yo woman who presents to internal medicine clinic for evaluation and follow-up of her medical problems. She has no complaints today. She attended a blood pressure screening three weeks ago, and her blood pressure at that time was 162/97 with a pulse of 74. She reports that her previous physician diagnosed her with high blood pressure several years ago, but she did not return for follow-up. At that time, she was instructed to exercise regularly and improve her eating habits, which she has tried to do. Since she had to stop running due to knee pain, she has recently started low-impact aerobics twice weekly to try to lose weight.

PMH

Seasonal allergic rhinitis
Hypertension
Arthroscopic surgery on left knee (10 years ago)
Cesarean section (4 years ago)

FH

Father died of heart disease at age 73, but his first MI was at age 41; mother died at age 69 and had HTN; brother (age 48) has HTN and high cholesterol; younger sister (age 35) has no known medical problems.

SH

She has been married for 19 years and has two sons who are healthy. She quit smoking cigarettes about 15 years ago. She occasionally drinks alcohol (1–2 drinks per week). She has been trying to "eat healthy."

Meds

Fluticasone nasal spray, 1 spray in each nostril twice daily
Ibuprofen 200 mg, 2–3 tablets po as needed for knee pain
Pseudoephedrine 30 mg, 1–2 tablets po TID PRN nasal congestion

All

NKDA

ROS

Patient states that overall she is doing well. She has noticed that her weight has been slowly increasing over the past three years. She denies headache, blurred vision, chest pain, SOB, or hemoptysis; no nausea, vomiting, abdominal pain, cramping, diarrhea, constipation, or blood in stool. She denies urinary frequency, dysuria, or nocturia. She has regular menstrual periods, approximately every 28–30 days. She complains of occasional knee pain which occurs primarily with extended exercise, for which she takes ibuprofen.

PE

Gen

The patient is a WDWN well-dressed and well-groomed woman in NAD.

VS

BP 164/108 mm Hg (right arm, seated) and 159/102 mm Hg (left arm, seated), HR 66, RR 16, T 37.1°C; Ht 5′7″, Wt 172 lb

HEENT

NCAT, PERRLA, EOMI. TMs clear throughout and without drainage; sclerae without icterus. Normal funduscopic exam.

Neck

Supple without masses or bruits, no thyroid enlargement or lymphadenopathy.

Lungs

Lung fields CTA bilaterally. No crackles or wheezes.

Heart

RRR; normal S_1 and S_2. No S_3 or S_4. PMI located at 5th ICS, MCL on the left.

Abd

Soft, NTND; no masses, bruits, or organomegaly. Normal BS.

Ext

No C/C/E. Several surgical scars surrounding left knee.

Neuro

No gross motor-sensory deficits present. CN II–XII intact. Negative Babinski.

Labs (fasting)

Na 142 mEq/L	Ca 9.7 mg/dL	*Fasting Lipid Profile*:
K 4.4 mEq/L	Mg 2.3 mEq/L	TC 198 mg/dL
Cl 101 mEq/L	AST 35 U/L	HDL 39 mg/dL
CO_2 27 mEq/L	ALT 28 U/L	LDL 134 mg/dL
BUN 16 mg/dL	T. bili 0.6 mg/dL	TG 122 mg/dL
SCr 0.9 mg/dL	T. prot 6.7 g/dL	
Glucose 92 mg/dL		

UA

Yellow, clear, SG 1.007, pH 5.5, (–) protein, (–) glucose, (–) ketones, (–) bilirubin, (–) blood, (–) nitrite, RBC 0/hpf, WBC 1/hpf, no bacteria, 1–5 epithelial cells

▶ Questions

Problem Identification

1. a. *Create a list of this patient's drug therapy problems.*
   b. *Outline the steps for obtaining an accurate blood pressure measurement. What are some potential sources of error?*
   c. *This patient has already been diagnosed with hypertension. What are her risk factors (modifiable and non-modifiable) for cardiovascular disease?*
   d. *Based on the data from the Framingham Heart Study, calculate this patient's 10-year cardiovascular risk.*
   e. *Based on the guidelines from JNC VII, classify this patient's hypertension.*

Desired Outcome

2. *List the goals of treatment for this patient.*

Therapeutic Alternatives

3. a. *What nonpharmacologic therapies are necessary for this patient to achieve and maintain adequate blood pressure reduction?*
   b. *What reasonable pharmacotherapeutic options are available for controlling this patient's blood pressure?*

Optimal Plan

4. a. *Outline specific lifestyle modifications for this patient.*
   b. *Outline a specific and appropriate pharmacotherapeutic regimen for this patient, including drug, dose, dosage form, and schedule.*

Outcome Evaluation

5. *Based on your recommendations, what parameters should be monitored after initiating this regimen and throughout the treatment course? At what time intervals should these parameters be monitored?*

Patient Education

6. *Based on your recommendations, provide appropriate education to this patient.*

▶ Clinical Course

At Mrs. Thompson's two-month follow-up appointment, she states that she has been walking 3 miles a day, following her dietary regimen, and has been adherent to her medications as prescribed. Now her average blood pressure is 132/84 mm Hg. Her fasting blood glucose is 98 mg/dL, and her fasting lipid profile is: TC 190 mg/dL, HDL 41 mg/dL, LDL 129 mg/dL, TG 107 mg/dL.

▶ Follow-Up Questions

1. *What instruction should you give the patient at this point in her therapy?*
2. *Suppose the patient now complains of intolerable adverse effects due to the current antihypertensive drug therapy. Outline an appropriate change to her current therapy.*
3. *Suppose the patient is tolerating the current drug therapy but has not achieved the desired BP control (average BP = 152/92 mm Hg). Outline an appropriate change to her current therapy.*

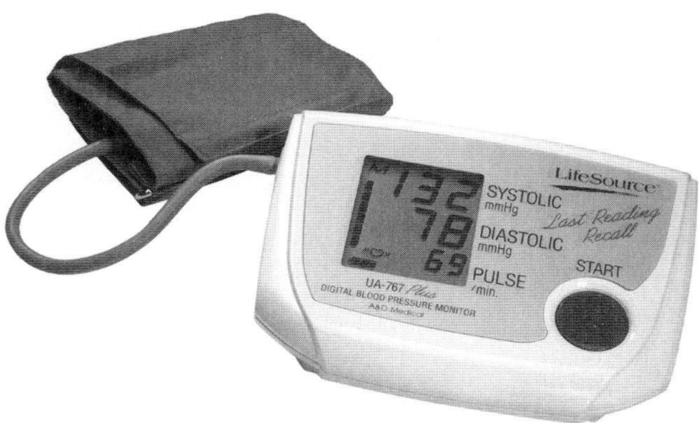

Figure 7–1. The LifeSource UA-767 Plus—One-Step Plus Memory digital home blood pressure monitor. *(Photograph courtesy of A&D Medical, Milpitas, California.)*

▶ Self-Study Assignments

1. Outline the changes, if any, you would make to the pharmacotherapeutic regimen for this patient if she had presented at the initial visit with each of the following characteristics:
   - African-American descent
   - 10 year history of asthma
   - Major depression for 2 years
   - History of severe coronary artery disease and angina pectoris
   - Diabetes mellitus, diagnosed during her last pregnancy
   - Frequent gouty attacks
   - A pregnant woman
   - Chronic renal failure, not yet on dialysis
   - End-stage renal disease, on hemodialysis three days of the week
   - Low fixed income
2. Describe how you would explain to a patient how to use a digital home blood pressure monitor such as the one shown in Figure 7–1.

▶ Clinical Pearl

Blood pressure self-monitoring by the patient can provide insight into the potential differences between measurements in and outside of the clinic. Patients who monitor their blood pressure at home should be advised on selection of an accurate device.

References

1. Jones DW, Appel LJ, Sheps SG, et al. Measuring blood pressure accurately: new and persistent challenges. JAMA 2003;289:1027–1030.
2. Chobanian AV, Bakris GL, Black HR, et al. The Seventh Report of the Joint National Committee on Prevention, Detection, Evaluation, and Treatment of High Blood Pressure: the JNC 7 report. Hypertension 2003;42:1206–1252.
3. Wilson PW, D'Agostino RB, Levy D, et al. Prediction of coronary heart disease using risk factor categories. Circulation 1998;97:1837–1847.
4. Expert Panel on Detection, Evaluation, and Treatment of High Blood Cholesterol in Adults. Third report of the National Cholesterol Education Program (NCEP) expert panel on detection, evaluation, and treatment of high blood cholesterol in adults (Adult Treatment Panel III): final report. Circulation. 2002;106:3143–3421.
5. Neal B, MacMahon S, Chapman N. Effects of ACE inhibitors, calcium antagonists, and other blood-pressure-lowering drugs: results of prospectively designed overviews of randomised trials. Blood Pressure Lowering Treatment Trialists' Collaboration. Lancet 2000;356:1955–1964.
6. ALLHAT Officers and Coordinators for the ALLHAT Collaborative Research Group. Major outcomes in high-risk hypertensive patients randomized to angiotensin-converting enzyme inhibitor or calcium channel blocker vs diuretic: The Antihypertensive and Lipid-Lowering Treatment to Prevent Heart Attack Trial (ALLHAT). JAMA 2002;288:2981–2997.

8 OBSTRUCTIVE SLEEP APNEA AND HYPERTENSION

▶ Asleep at the Wheel (Level III)

John M. Dopp, PharmD
Bradley G. Phillips, PharmD, BCPS

▶ After completing this case study, students should be able to:

- Recognize the signs, symptoms and characteristics of obstructive sleep apnea.
- Be familiar with the evaluation, treatment, and complications of obstructive sleep apnea.
- Recognize that obstructive sleep apnea is a risk factor for hypertension.
- Understand how obstructive sleep apnea can affect the medical management of concomitant diseases, specifically hypertension.
- Recognize the benefits of optimizing treatment of obstructive sleep apnea.

PATIENT PRESENTATION

Chief Complaint

"My blood pressure readings at home are still not in the good range."

HPI

Thomas Bradford is an obese 54 yo man who is seen in your hypertension clinic today. He recently reported for his annual physical and was found to have gained 12 kg in the last year. He has a history of refractory hypertension, requiring multiple medications without successful BP control. He presented three months ago with uncontrolled hypertension, daytime sleepiness, and forgetfulness, and he reported that his wife had to shake him to stop his loud snoring and unusual breathing during sleep. He subsequently underwent an overnight polysomnographic (sleep) study and was diagnosed with severe obstructive sleep apnea (OSA).

[*Note*: Severity of OSA is determined by the number of apneic episodes

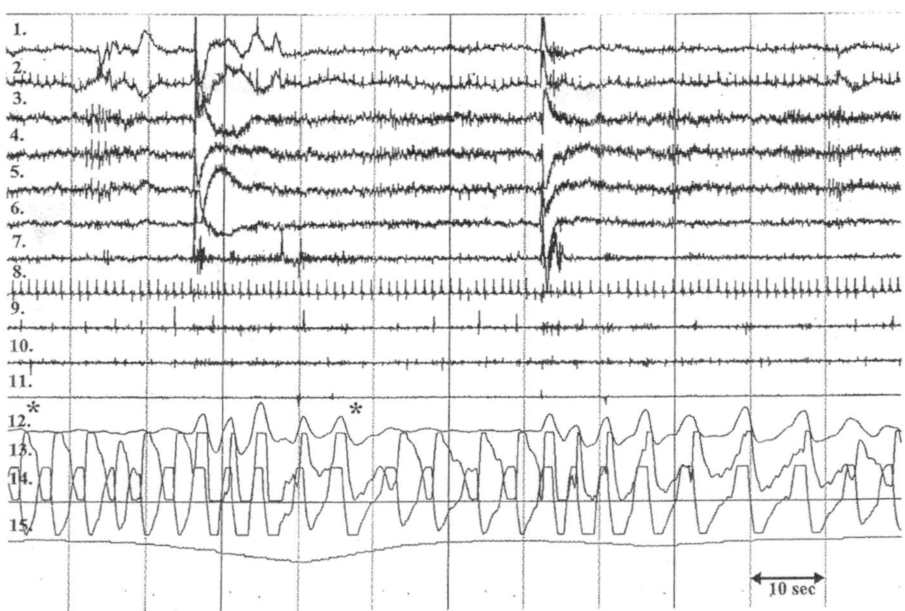

Figure 8–1. Polysomnogram obtained from this patient. The first 6 leads from the top of the figure are electroencephalographic recordings during sleep. The next four leads show the chin electromyogram, electrocardiogram, and left and right leg electromyograms, respectively. The remaining five leads at the bottom of the figure depict nasal airflow (11), oral airflow (12), chest effort (13), abdominal effort (14), and oxygen saturation (15). It is important to note two episodes of apnea, each lasting approximately 20 to 30 seconds. The beginning of each apnea is denoted with an asterisk (*) between leads that measure nasal and oral airflow. During these episodes there is no nasal (11) or oral (12) airflow but considerable chest and abdominal effort (13 and 14). At the end of the apneic episodes the patient arouses from sleep (movement in all electroencephalographic leads 1 to 6) and breathing resumes. Oxygen saturation (bottom lead) decreases significantly. This sequence of apnea, arousal from sleep, and oxygen desaturation occurs 84 times an hour in this patient.

the patient has during sleep. Patients with more than 30 episodes of apnea and hypopnea per hour or an apnea-hypopnea index (AHI) >30 have severe sleep apnea. An AHI of 15 to 30 events per hour is defined as moderate sleep apnea; 5 to 15 events per hour is considered mild sleep apnea.]

During polysomnography, Mr. Bradford experienced an average of 84 apneas per hour (AHI = 84). His polysomnogram is depicted in Figure 8–1. His baseline oxygen saturation prior to sleep was 96% and his minimum oxygen saturation was 75% during sleep.

At that time, he received a prescription for continuous positive airway pressure (CPAP) therapy and received his CPAP machine and nasal CPAP mask (see Figure 8–2). He later returned to the sleep laboratory for nasal CPAP titration and had successful alleviation of apneas at 13 cm H_2O (AHI = 2). [*Note*: Nasal CPAP produces a positive pressure column in the upper airway to maintain breathing during sleep.]

Today in hypertension clinic, Mr. Bradford's average seated clinic BP measurement is 158/95 mm Hg and his heart rate is 71 bpm. He has a home BP monitor but often forgets to perform his BP checks. One home BP measurement he has recorded is 165/96 mm Hg. He states that he tries to use his CPAP machine three or four nights per week but usually ends up pulling the mask off. He reports that his job schedule makes it difficult to use his mask when he is on the road and he feels trapped sometimes when wearing the mask. The compliance meter on his CPAP machine indicates it has been used at effective pressure (13 cm H_2O) for 145 hours over the previous 3 months. No changes have been made to his medications.

PMH

Type 2 DM × 8 years
HTN (uncontrolled) × 6 years
Depression
Hyperlipidemia
CAD (angina, S/P MI 3 years ago)

FH

Mother died at 60 years old with CAD; father died at 54 of MI. Married, lives with wife.

SH

19 pack-year history of smoking. Currently still smokes one-half pack per day. Occasional alcohol use. Patient is a truck driver and frequently is away on the road.

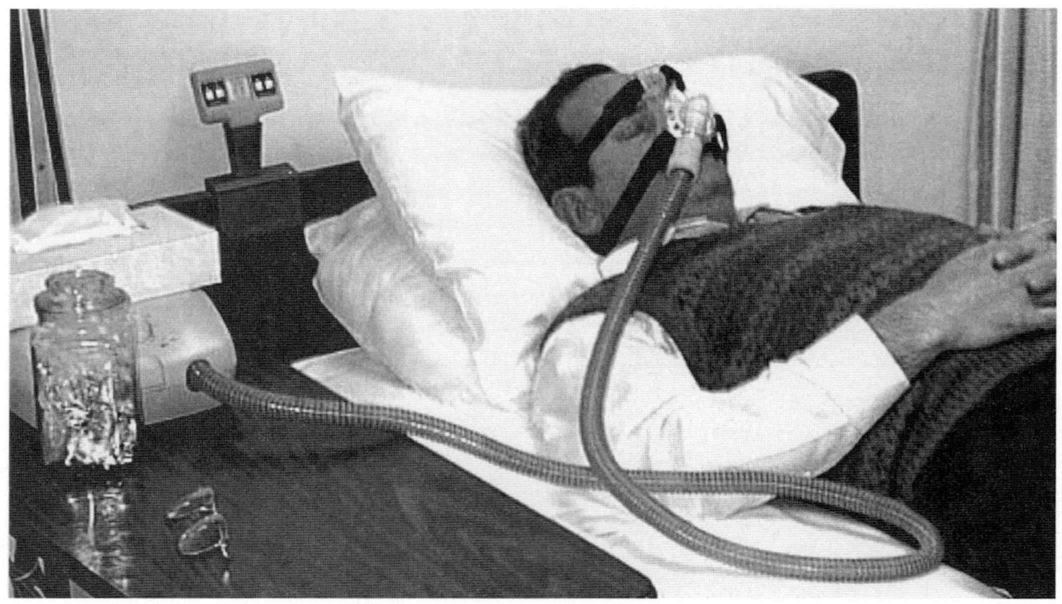

Figure 8–2. A sleep apneic patient (not this patient) sleeping with nasal continuous positive airway pressure (CPAP) therapy to alleviate sleep-disordered breathing. CPAP produces a positive pressure column in the upper airway to prevent airway collapse so that breathing can be maintained during sleep. The air pressure is adjusted so that the patient maintains oxygen saturation and has no episodes or fewer than 5 episodes of apnea or hypopnea per hour during sleep.

Meds

- NPH insulin 18 units SQ BID
- Rosiglitazone 8 mg po once daily
- Glipizide XL 10 mg po once daily
- ASA 325 mg po once daily
- Atenolol 50 mg po once daily
- Doxazosin 8 mg po at bedtime
- Amlodipine 10 mg po once daily
- Losartan 50 mg po BID
- Isosorbide mononitrate extended release 60 mg po once daily
- Atorvastatin 10 mg po once daily
- Sertraline 150 mg po once daily
- NTG 0.4 mg SL PRN chest pain

All

NKDA

ROS

He complains of persistent daytime sleepiness and lethargy. He reports that he still occasionally nods off while driving and reveals that he still has occasional morning headaches.

PE

Gen

Pleasant, obese white man in NAD. Patient appears older than stated age.

VS

BP 158/95, P 71, RR 18, T 36.9°C, Wt 129 kg, Ht 5′11″

Skin

No rashes or bruises.

HEENT

EOMI; PERRLA; fundi intact, no hemorrhages or exudates; TMs intact.

Neck

Supple and large, no adenopathy or thyromegaly. Neck circumference 49 cm.

Lungs

CTA, no crackles or rales noted upon auscultation.

CV

RRR, no m/r/g

Abd

Soft, obese, NT, ND, (+) BS

Ext

Normal ROM

Neuro

CNs intact, drowsy

Labs (from annual physical 3 months ago):

Na 141 mEq/L	Hgb 15.5 g/dL	*Fasting Lipid Profile*
K 4.2 mEq/L	Hct 48%	T. Chol 168 mg/dL
Cl 101 mEq/L	WBC $3.8 \times 10^3/mm^3$	HDL 45 mg/dL
CO_2 23 mEq/L	Plt $225 \times 10^3/mm^3$	LDL 95 mg/dL
BUN 12 mg/dL		TG 140 mg/dL
SCr 1.5 mg/dL		$HbgA_{1C}$ 10.2%
Glu 143 mg/dL		

Assessment

Resistant hypertension, likely due to noncompliance with CPAP therapy and consequent sleep apnea.

Questions

Problem Identification

1. a. *Identify this patient's drug therapy problems upon presentation to the clinic today.*
   b. *What factors cause resistant hypertension? Which of these conditions may be a likely cause of this patient's resistant hypertension?*
   c. *What characteristics place him at risk for obstructive sleep apnea?*
   d. *What are the common characteristics of obstructive sleep apnea? Which of these characteristics does this patient exhibit?*
   e. *Which of this patient's medical conditions place him at risk for cardiovascular disease?*
   f. *Could effective treatment of his sleep apnea improve any of this patient's concomitant diseases or complaints?*

Desired Outcome

2. *What are the treatment goals for this individual's hypertension, sleep apnea and other medical conditions?*

Therapeutic Alternatives

3. *What treatment measures are available for this patient's obstructive sleep apnea?*

Optimal Plan

4. *What recommendations would you make at this most recent visit with regard to the patient's non-drug and pharmacologic therapies?*

Outcome Evaluation

5. *How will you monitor this patient's therapy to assure optimal adherence and outcomes and to detect or prevent adverse effects?*

Patient Education

6. *What information should be provided to enhance adherence, ensure success, and minimize adverse effects of the patient's therapies?*

Clinical Pearl

Effective CPAP can decrease blood pressure in hypertensive patients with sleep apnea. Assessment of CPAP adherence and elimination of nocturnal hypoxemia should be evaluated when investigating causes of resistant hypertension in patients with OSA.

Self-Study Assignment

1. Describe the role of wake-promoting medications such as modafinil in managing patients with obstructive sleep apnea.

References

1. Peppard PE, Young, T, Palta M, et al. Prospective study of the association between sleep-disordered breathing and hypertension. N Engl J Med 2000;342: 1378–1384.
2. Nieto FJ, Young TB, Lind BK, et al. Association of sleep-disordered breathing, sleep apnea, and hypertension in a large community-based study. Sleep Heart Health Study. JAMA 2000;283:1829–1836.
3. Phillips BG, Kato M, Narkiewicz K, et al. Increases in leptin levels, sympathetic drive, and weight gain in obstructive sleep apnea. Am J Physiol Heart Circ Physiol 2000;279:H234–H237.
4. Millman RP, Fogel BS, McNamara ME, et al. Depression as a manifestation of obstructive sleep apnea: reversal with nasal continuous positive airway pressure. J Clin Psychiatry 1989;50:348–351.
5. Becker HF, Jerrentrup J, Ploch T, et al. Effect of nasal continuous positive airway pressure treatment on blood pressure in patients with obstructive sleep apnea. Circulation 2003;107:68–73.
6. Pack AI, Black JE, Schwartz JR, et al; the U.S. Modafinil in obstructive sleep apnea study group. Modafinil as adjunct therapy for daytime sleepiness in obstructive sleep apnea. Am J Respir Crit Care Med 2001;164:1675–1681.
7. Schwartz JR, Hirshkowitz M, Erman MK, et al; the United States modafinil in OSA study group. Modafinil as adjunct therapy for daytime sleepiness in obstructive sleep apnea: a 12-week, open-label study. Chest 2003;124:2192–2199.

9 HYPERTENSIVE URGENCY/EMERGENCY

My Doctor Made Me Do It (Level I)

James J. Nawarskas, PharmD

After completing this case study, students should be able to:

- Distinguish a hypertensive urgency from a hypertensive emergency
- Recognize signs and symptoms of target organ damage due to severely elevated blood pressure

- Identify treatment goals for a patient with a hypertensive urgency or emergency
- Develop appropriate treatment plans for patients with a hypertensive urgency or emergency
- List advantages and disadvantages of oral versus parenteral drug therapy for a patient with severely elevated blood pressure

PATIENT PRESENTATION

Chief Complaint
"My doctor told me to come here because of my blood pressure."

HPI
Carlos Sanchez is a 68 yo man with a history of HTN (well-controlled on medication), diabetes, and hypercholesterolemia who was at a routine clinic visit with his primary care physician when he was noted to have a BP of 240/137 mm Hg. Upon questioning, Mr. Sanchez stated that he felt "OK, I guess, but I've been having trouble seeing over the last few days and seem out of breath a lot." The patient was referred to the Emergency Department where he admitted to not taking any of his medications for a "couple of months" because he is not able to afford them.

PMH
HTN × 25 years
Diabetes × 15 years
Hypercholesterolemia × 10 years

FH
Father died in his 70's secondary to CHF, mother had HTN and diabetes and died in her 60's from a stroke. Two brothers, 59 and 70 years old, are alive and both have HTN and hypercholesterolemia. One sister with diabetes and hypercholesterolemia died at 62 years of age from a myocardial infarction. Two other sisters, 61 and 65 years of age are both alive; one with diabetes and HTN, the other with HTN and hypercholesterolemia.

SH
Married, retired construction worker. States he used to smoke cigarettes (1 ppd) for about 40 years before quitting 10 years ago, and used to drink "several" alcoholic beverages daily (mostly beer) before cutting back when his endocrinologist diagnosed him with diabetes. He says he completely stopped drinking about a year ago.

ROS
Complaints of blurred vision of about two weeks' duration, which is slowly worsening, and frequent headaches; denies nausea, dizziness, loss of muscle control, or other signs of CNS damage; does complain of a "tight" feeling in his chest that makes it difficult to breathe at times.

Meds (none taken for 2 months other than aspirin)
Aspirin 81 mg po once daily
Lovastatin 80 mg po at bedtime
Atenolol 100 mg po once daily
Enalapril 20 mg po BID
Metformin 1000 mg po BID
Glipizide XL 10 mg po once daily

All
NKDA

PE

Gen
The patient is a thin, elderly Hispanic man appearing to be in mild distress.

VS
BP 242/138, P 88, RR 24, T 36.8°C; Ht 5′7″, Wt 59 kg

Skin
Cool to touch, good turgor

HEENT
PERRLA; EOMI; funduscopic exam revealed focal narrowing of the retinal arteries, flame-shaped hemorrhages, cotton-wool spots, and macular swelling; oropharynx clear

Neck/LN
Neck supple, no JVD, no bruits, no thyromegaly

Chest
CTA

CV
RRR, II/VI SEM at right upper sternal border, $S_2 > S_1$, no S_3 or S_4

Abd
Soft, NT/ND, no guarding, (+) BS, liver span about 15 cm

Genit/Rect
Normal male genitalia, heme-negative stool

MS/Ext
Normal ROM, no CCE, pulses 3+ throughout

Neuro
A & O × 3, CN II–XII intact, motor/sensory normal, DTRs 2+

Labs

Na 141 mEq/L	Hgb 13.4 g/dL	AST 42 IU/L
K 4.1 mEq/L	Hct 43.1%	ALT 50 IU/L
Cl 102 mEq/L	WBC 8.9 × 10^3/mm^3	Troponin-I <0.5 ng/mL
CO_2 28 mEq/L	Plt 271 × 10^3/mm^3	CK 120 IU/L
BUN 44 mg/dL		CK-MB 2.0 ng/mL
SCr 2.1 mg/dL		
Glu 210 mg/dL		

UA
200 mg/g albumin/creatinine, negative for blood with 2–5 WBCs/hpf and 0 to 2 casts/lpf. Negative for recreational drugs.

CXR
Enlarged heart, no infiltrates

ECG

Normal sinus rhythm; LVH by voltage criteria. There is T-wave flattening in the anterolateral leads but there are no acute ST-segment changes.

Assessment

68 yo man with a history of HTN, diabetes, and hypercholesterolemia presents to the ED symptomatic with a BP of 242/138 which is likely caused by discontinuation of antihypertensive treatment.

▶ Questions

Problem Identification

1. a. *Did this patient's situation result from a drug-related problem? Why or why not?*
   b. *What signs and symptoms are present that may be related to this patient's hypertension?*
   c. *Is this a hypertensive urgency or an emergency? Explain your answer.*
   d. *Is hospitalization necessary for Mr. Sanchez? Why or why not?*

Desired Outcome

2. a. *What are the goals of pharmacotherapy for this patient's hypertension?*
   b. *How would the treatment goals differ if this patient was asymptomatic and had a normal physical exam and laboratory values?*

Therapeutic Alternatives

3. a. *What non-drug therapies might be useful for this patient?*
   b. *What feasible pharmacotherapeutic alternatives are available for the treatment of this patient's hypertension?*
   c. *As the pharmacist in the Emergency Department, you are approached by the medical resident who is treating this patient. She mentions that she has seen sublingual nifedipine used in this situation at other institutions where she has trained and asks for your opinion regarding this treatment for Mr. Sanchez. What is your response to her request?*

Optimal Plan

4. *What drug, dosage form, schedule, and duration of therapy are best for this patient?*

Outcome Evaluation

5. *Which clinical and laboratory parameters are necessary to evaluate your therapy for reducing this patient's blood pressure and monitoring for adverse events?*

Patient Education

6. *Following a 2-day admission, Mr. Sanchez's blood pressure is now averaging 140/90 mm Hg and discharge planning is in progress. The attending physician requests your help in counseling Mr. Sanchez regarding the importance of taking his medications as prescribed to prevent this from happening again. How can you help in this situation?*

▶ Self-Study Assignments

1. *Compare and contrast the multiple intravenous antihypertensives used for treating hypertensive emergencies with regard to: efficacy, cost, onset and duration of action, safety, and special indications (i.e., utility for different co-morbidities).*
2. *From a biochemical perspective, explain how cyanide and thiocyanate are generated from nitroprusside.*
3. *Define eclampsia and pre-eclampsia and relate these conditions to hypertensive emergencies.*

▶ Clinical Pearl

The distinction between a hypertensive urgency and a hypertensive emergency is based on medical history and clinical presentation, not on blood pressure readings.

References

1. Joint National Committee on Prevention, Detection, Evaluation, and Treatment of High Blood Pressure. The JNC 7 Report. JAMA 2003;289:2560–2572.
2. Varon J, Marik PE. The diagnosis and management of hypertensive crises. Chest 2000;118:214–227.
3. Mansoor GA, Frishman WH. Comprehensive management of hypertensive emergencies and urgencies. Heart Dis 2002;4:358–371.
4. Joint National Committee on Prevention, Detection, Evaluation, and Treatment of High Blood Pressure. Sixth report. Arch Intern Med 1997;157:2413–2446.
5. Thach AM, Schultz PJ. Nonemergent hypertension. New perspectives for the emergency medicine physician. Emerg Med Clin North Am 1995;13:1009–1035.
6. Marwick C. FDA gives calcium channel blockers clean bill of health but warns of short-acting nifedipine hazards. JAMA 1996;275:423–424.

10 HEART FAILURE

▶ The Pump Organist (Level III)

Jon D. Horton, PharmD

▶ After completing this case study, students should be able to:

- Recognize the signs and symptoms of heart failure.
- Develop a pharmacotherapeutic plan for treatment of heart failure.

- Outline a monitoring plan for heart failure that includes both clinical and laboratory parameters.
- Initiate, titrate, and monitor β-adrenergic blocker therapy in heart failure when indicated.

PATIENT PRESENTATION

Chief Complaint

"I think I might have the flu. I have been feeling run down, and I haven't been able to get up the stairs to my bedroom because I get winded."

HPI

Richard Anderson is a 65 yo man who was brought to the ED by ambulance upon request of his endocrinologist. The patient had called the physician's office this morning to cancel his routine visit for diabetes follow-up because he became short of breath and diaphoretic after attempting to climb a flight of stairs. When evaluated by the paramedics in his home, the diaphoresis had resolved and his heart rate was in the range of 120–140 bpm. The patient states that he has been gaining weight and having progressively worse dyspnea on exertion over the last 5 days. His shortness of breath is often worse at night, forcing him to "sit bolt upright." He began sleeping in his recliner about 3 days ago. He is unable to complete physical activities that he could do 2 weeks ago without difficulty. When he saw his continuing care physician 1 week ago, he was in atrial fibrillation and was started on digoxin for rate control.

PMH

Atrial fibrillation ×2 weeks
Type 2 DM × 15 years, untreated until 3 years ago; neuropathy × 2 years and retinopathy × 1 year
HTN × 20 years
Hypercholesterolemia (documented 6 months ago)
CVA's 2 and 3 years ago
Recurrent TIA's × 4 years resistant to ASA and clopidogrel; started on warfarin 7 months ago with improvement

FH

Father died at age 65 of a heart attack. Mother recently died in her 70's in an MVA. One brother age 70 alive with DM.

SH

Retired musician who lives alone. Prior to his CVA's, his hobby was repairing and playing antique pump organs. He has a 30 pack-year history of smoking but reports quitting 22 years ago. He has a positive history for alcohol use but states he "hasn't had a drop in 12 years."

Meds

Rosiglitazone 4 mg po once daily
Metformin 850 mg po TID
Glyburide 2.5 mg po BID
Pravastatin 10 mg po once daily (LDL 112 mg/dL 1 month ago)
Lisinopril 2.5 mg po once daily
Digoxin 0.125 mg po once daily
Warfarin 7.5 mg po once daily since his last admission 7 months ago because of repeated "mini-strokes." INR 1 week ago was 2.2

All

NKDA

ROS

Reports having headaches recently, but nothing that he would consider unusual or out of the ordinary. He is followed ophthalmologically and was told he had a small bleeding area in the back of one eye, but he states that this occurred prior to taking warfarin. Denies any recent chest pain. No chronic cough, but has had recent episodes of coughing spells without productivity. Complains of recent abdominal bloating and of being awakened the past four evenings to relieve his bladder. He reports some weakness in his right lower extremity but states that it is unchanged from his most recent stroke. He denies chronic joint pain.

PE

Gen

The patient is sitting up on the gurney in the ED in moderate distress.

VS

BP 150/95, P 100–150 (irregularly irregular), RR 22, T 35°C; Ht 5′11″; Wt 103 kg (usual weight 93 kg)

Skin

Color pale and diaphoretic; no unusual lesions noted

HEENT

PERRLA, EOMI, fundi were not examined. He has a complete upper denture and about two-thirds of the teeth in the lower jaw are remaining and are in fair repair.

Neck

(+) JVD at 30° (8 cm). Carotid bruit is not appreciated. No lymphadenopathy or thyromegaly.

Heart

Irregularly irregular rhythm, no rubs, variation in intensity of S_1 as expected. S_3 is appreciated at apex in lateral position. PMI displaced laterally and difficult to discern.

Thorax/Lungs

Respirations are even. There are fine crackles in both lung fields posteriorly noted two-thirds of the way up the lung fields. No CVAT.

Abd

Soft, NT/ND, (+) HJR, liver and spleen slightly enlarged, no masses, hypoactive bowel sounds

Genit/Rect

Guaiac (–), genital examination not performed

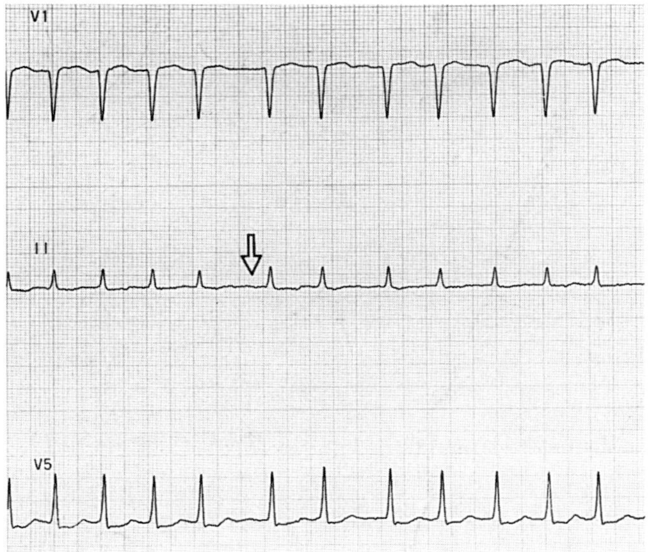

Figure 10–1. The ECG demonstrates low voltage in all leads. The arrow points out the absence of a P wave, which is observed in patients with atrial fibrillation. This ECG does not meet criteria for left ventricular hypertrophy (S in V1 + R in V5 > 35 mm).

MS/Ext

3+ pitting pedal edema bilaterally; radial and pedal pulses are of poor intensity bilaterally; grip strength greater on left than on right

Neuro

A & O × 3, CNs intact. Some sensory loss in both LE below the knee. DTR 1+

Labs

Na 139 mEq/L	Hgb 12.6 g/dL	Mg 1.2 mEq/L	CK 20 IU/L
K 3.4 mEq/L	Hct 39.5%	Ca 8.8 mg/dL	CK-MB 0.8 IU/L
Cl 99 mEq/L	Plt 339 × 10^3/mm^3	AST 36 IU/L	PT 20.6 sec
CO_2 27 mEq/L	WBC 8.6 × 10^3/mm^3	ALT 43 IU/L	INR 2.8
BUN 20 mg/dL	70% PMNs	Alk phos 150 IU/L	TSH 1.42 mIU/L
SCr 1.3 mg/dL	23% Lymphs	GGT 37 IU/L	Digoxin 1.0 ng/mL
Glucose 139 mg/dL	7% Monos	T. bili 0.2 mg/dL	HbA_{1c} 7.2%
BNP 1200 pg/mL	Troponin I 0.8 ng/mL		

ECG

Atrial fibrillation with a rapid ventricular response (see Figure 10–1); rate of 140, QRS 0.08. Diffuse nonspecific ST-T wave changes. Low voltage.

Chest X-Ray

PA and lateral views (see Figure 10–2) show evidence of congestive failure with cardiomegaly, interstitial edema, and some early alveolar edema. There is a small right pleural effusion.

Assessment

Diabetic patient with new-onset congestive heart failure and atrial fibrillation with rapid ventricular response.

► Clinical Course

The patient was admitted to a step-down unit and placed on telemetry. A 2D echocardiogram was obtained to evaluate LV and valvular function (see Figure 10–3). The results showed severe LV dilation and increased left atrial dimension, akinesia of the septum, and severe LV dysfunction. EF was estimated at 15% to 20%, with no visible clots.

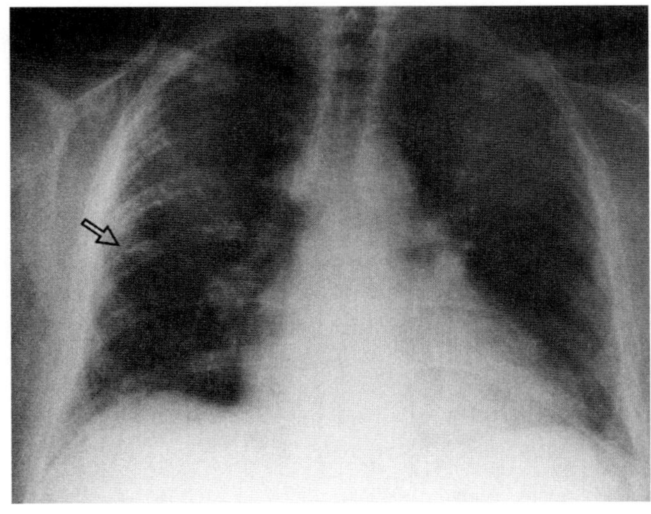

A

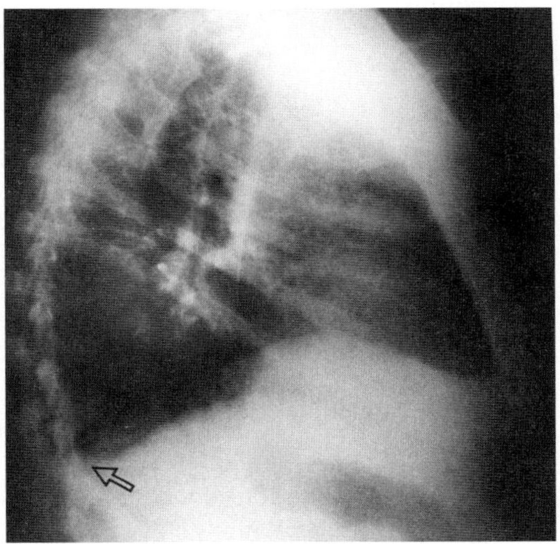

B

Figure 10–2. A. PA CXR demonstrates increased vascular markings representative of interstitial edema, with some early alveolar edema. The arrow points out fluid lying in the fissure of the right lung. Note the presence of cardiomegaly. **B.** Lateral view of CXR. Arrow points out the presence of pulmonary effusion.

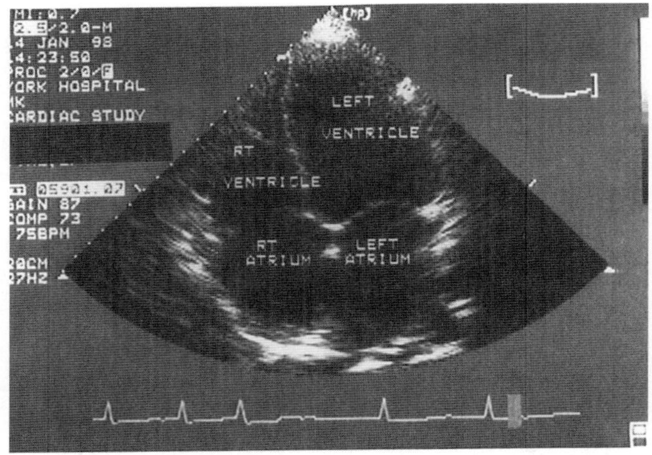

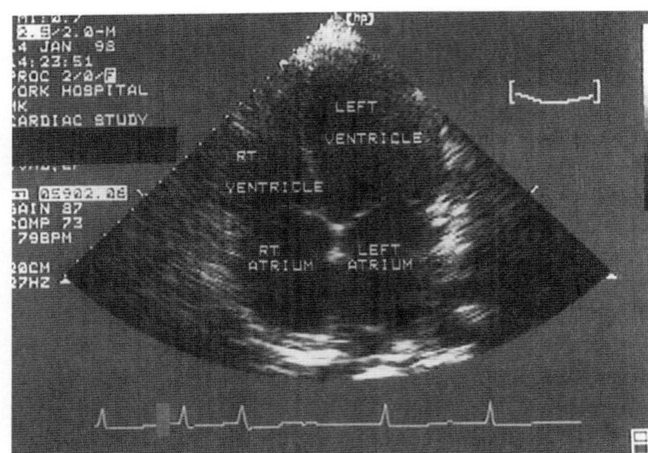

Figure 10–3. 2D echocardiogram. **A.** End systole. **B.** End diastole. Note the presence of severe left ventricular dilation and increased left atrial dimension in end diastole **(B)** that appear to be unchanged from the photographs of end systole **(A).** The ventricular septum appears to be in nearly the identical position in both films, thus representing akinesia.

▶ Questions

Problem Identification

1. a. *Create a list of this patient's drug therapy problems.*
   b. *What signs, symptoms, and other information indicate the presence and severity of the patient's heart failure?*
   c. *What functional classification and hemodynamic subset is this patient upon presentation?*
   d. *Could any of this patient's problems have been caused by drug therapy?*

Desired Outcome

2. a. *What are the goals for the pharmacologic management of heart failure in this patient?*
   b. *Considering his other medical problems, what other treatment goals should be established?*

Therapeutic Alternatives

3. *What medications are indicated in the long-term management of this patient's heart failure?*

Optimal Plan

4. *What drugs, doses, schedules, and duration are best suited for the management of this patient?*

Outcome Evaluation

5. *What clinical and laboratory parameters are needed to evaluate the therapy for achievement of the desired therapeutic outcome and to detect and prevent adverse events?*

▶ Clinical Course

Over the next 3 days, the patient received maximal drug therapy, and his condition improved. He was discharged on lisinopril 20 mg po daily, digoxin 0.25 mg po daily, furosemide 40 mg po daily, potassium chloride 40 mEq po daily, magnesium oxide 400 mg po daily, metformin 850 mg po TID, glyburide 2.5 mg po daily, warfarin 7.5 mg po daily, and pravastatin 20 mg po daily.

Patient Education

6. *What information should be provided to the patient about the medications used to treat his heart failure?*

▶ Clinical Course

Despite subsequent inpatient efforts to chemically convert the patient to sinus rhythm, he remained in atrial fibrillation. The Cardiology Service recommended outpatient DC cardioversion to try to improve cardiac output by reestablishing an effective atrial kick. An outpatient elective DC cardioversion failed. Despite 3 months of maximal drug therapy, the patient currently complains of episodic shortness of breath that he associates with "faster palpitations." A Holter monitor was placed, and the results suggested poor rate control. The current serum digoxin concentration is 1.8 ng/mL.

▶ Follow-Up Questions

1. *What medications could be used to provide better rate control, and which of these alternatives is most appropriate considering the patient's heart failure?*
2. *Outline a therapeutic plan for employing a β-blocking agent in this patient.*
3. *The patient was started on carvedilol at an appropriate starting*

dose. What information should be provided to the patient about common adverse effects? Describe how they should be managed if they occur.

▶ Clinical Course

The patient returns to your clinic site 3 weeks later stating that his palpitations seem to be better. However, he feels worse despite using the new medication as prescribed. You sense that there is potential for noncompliance with the carvedilol.

4. *What information should you convey to the patient about his current perspective on the usefulness of carvedilol?*

▶ Self-Study Assignments

1. Which vitamins and/or minerals should this patient consider supplementing because of chronic diuretic use?
2. This patient may develop diuretic resistance. Write a one-page essay describing what this phenomenon is and how it might be overcome.
3. Describe how you would evaluate and monitor this patient's quality of life.

▶ Clinical Pearl

The presence of pitting edema is associated with a substantial increase in body weight; it typically takes a weight gain of 10 pounds to result in the development of pitting edema.

References

1. Pitt B, Poole-Wilson PA, Segal R, et al. Effect of losartan compared with captopril on mortality in patients with symptomatic heart failure: randomised trial – the Losartan Heart Failure Survival Study ELITE II. Lancet 2000;355:1582–1587.
2. Cohn JN, Tognoni, G; Valsartan Heart Failure Trial Investigators. A randomized trial of the angiotensin-receptor blocker valsartan in chronic heart failure. N Engl J Med 2001; 345:1667–1675.
3. McMurray JJ, Ostergren J, Swedberg K, et al. Effects of candesartan in patients with chronic heart failure and reduced left ventricular systolic function taking angiotensin-converting-enzyme inhibitors: the CHARM-added trial. Lancet 2003;362:759–771.
4. Pitt B, Zannad F, Remme WJ, et. al. The effect of spironolactone on morbidity and mortality in patients with severe heart failure. Randomized Aldactone Evaluation Study Investigators. N Engl J Med 1999;341–709–717.
5. Pitt B, Remme W, Zannad F, et al. Eplerenone, a selective aldosterone blocker, in patients with left ventricular dysfunction after myocardial infarction. N Engl J Med 2003;348:1309–1321.
6. Colucci WS, Elkayam U, Horton DP, et al. Intravenous nesiritide, a natriuretic peptide, in the treatment of decompensated congestive heart failure. Nesiritide Study Group. N Engl J Med 2000;343:246–253.
7. Packer M, Poole-Wilson PA, Armstrong PW et al. Comparative effects of low and high doses of the angiotensin-converting enzyme inhibitor, lisinopril, on morbidity and mortality in chronic heart failure. ATLAS Study Group. Circulation 1999;100:2312–2318.
8. Svensson M, Gustafsson F, Galatius S, et al. Hyperkalaemia and impaired renal function in patients taking spironolactone for congestive heart failure: retrospective study. BMJ 2003;327:1141–1142.

11 ISCHEMIC HEART DISEASE AND ACUTE CORONARY SYNDROME

▶ Mrs. Hale is Not Hearty (Level III)

Shawn R. Hansen, PharmD
Amy J. Guenette, PharmD, BCPS

▶ After completing this case study, students should be able to:

- Identify modifiable risk factors for IHD and discuss the potential benefit to be derived by their modification in an individual patient.
- Optimize medical therapy in a patient with persistent angina considering response to present therapy and the presence of comorbidities.
- Assess clinical response to antianginal therapy by identifying relevant monitoring parameters for efficacy and adverse effects.
- Outline contemporary antiplatelet therapy in catheter-based intervention for acute coronary syndromes.

PATIENT PRESENTATION

Chief Complaint

Chest pain

HPI

Mary Hale is a pleasant 55 yo woman with a history of CAD who presents to the clinic today for an unscheduled visit. She has been experiencing episodes of chest pain in the past week. She suffered an MI two years ago and has since tried to minimize heavy lifting or over-exerting herself. She currently works as a truck driver for an asphalt company. Two days ago, while sweeping out her truck bed, she developed non-radiating, substernal chest pressure that she rates a 5 on a scale of 1 to 10. There was no associated dyspnea or diaphoresis. She immediately sat down and took two sublingual nitroglycerin tablets five minutes apart and the pain subsided. Yesterday, as she was climbing stairs at home, she developed similar chest pain that again responded to a single sublingual nitroglycerin tablet. These attacks are more intense and frequent than she has experienced in the past, and she is very concerned about having a recurrent heart attack. She does admit to occasionally missing afternoon doses of some of her medications while she is on the job site.

PMH

1. Acute anterior wall MI 2 years ago with moderately reduced overall LV dysfunction (LVEF 30% to 35% by echo). She underwent coronary angiography and her LAD coronary artery was found to be totally occluded distally with acute thrombus present. She also had a 60% stenosis in her proximal LAD. She was successfully revascularized with a single 3.0 mm stent to her distal LAD.
2. Asthma as a child, exercise-induced. She has been asthmatic for at least 45 years but has had no significant difficulties. Since her MI she has engaged in only moderate exercise and has needed to use her albuterol inhaler only a few times per month.

3. Hypertension
4. Dyslipidemia
5. Postmenopausal, mild vasomotor symptoms, on estrogen replacement therapy
6. Medication noncompliance

FH
Father had been quite healthy but died suddenly at age 62 of "a massive heart attack" while fighting a forest fire. Mother is alive and well. She has one brother who is older, age 61, and healthy. The patient is married and has two sons and a daughter, all healthy.

SH
Married, lives with husband, non-drinker, quit smoking 2 years ago

Meds
Aspirin 325 mg daily
Captopril 12.5 mg TID
Isosorbide dinitrate 20 mg TID
Diltiazem, extended-release 180 mg daily
Albuterol Inhaler 1–2 puffs PRN
Conjugated estrogen 0.625 mg daily
Atorvastatin 5 mg at bedtime (1/2 of a 10 mg tablet)
Nitroglycerin 0.4 mg SL PRN

All
NKDA; codeine intolerance (nausea/vomiting)

ROS
No fever, chills, or night sweats. No recent viral illnesses. No SOB; occasional cough with cold weather due to asthma. No nausea, vomiting, diarrhea, constipation, melena, or hematochezia. No dysuria or hematuria. No myalgias or arthralgias.

PE

VS
BP 155/92 (right, sitting, large arm cuff), BP 150/90 (left, sitting, large arm cuff), P 88, RR 22, T 36.4°C; Ht 5′5″; Wt 75 kg; waist circumference 33 inches

Gen
Pleasant, cooperative female in no acute distress.

Skin
Intact, no rashes or ulcers

HEENT
PERRL; EOMI; oropharynx is clear

Neck
Supple, no masses; no JVD, lymphadenopathy, or thyromegaly

Lungs
Bilateral air entry is clear. No wheezes.

CV
RRR, S_1, S_2 normal; no murmurs or gallops; PMI palpated at left 5th ICS, MCL

Abd
Soft, NT/ND; bowel sounds normoactive

G/U
Heme (–) stool

Ext
No CCE; pulses 2+ throughout

Neuro
A & O × 3, CN II–XII intact; speech is fluent; no motor or sensory deficit; no facial asymmetry; tongue midline

Labs

		Fasting Lipid Profile
Na 137 mEq/L	Hgb 11.8 g/dL	Chol 202 mg/dL
K 4.8 mEq/L	Hct 35.1%	LDL 125 mg/dL
Cl 103 mEq/L	Plt 187 × 10^3/mm^3	HDL 38 mg/dL
CO_2 21 mEq/L	WBC 7.9 × 10^3/mm^3	Trig 215 mg/dL
BUN 24 mg/dL	MCV 77 μm^3	
SCr 1.2 mg/dL	MCHC 29 g/dL	
Glu 98 mg/dL		

ECG
Sinus rhythm at 90 bpm, old AWMI, no ST–T wave changes noted

Impression:
1. Recurrent exertional angina, poorly controlled on present medications
2. Hypertension, poorly controlled
3. Dyslipidemia, poorly controlled
4. Asthma, mildly symptomatic

► Questions

Problem Identification

1. a. *What drug therapy problems appear to be present in this patient?*
   b. *Could any of these problems potentially be caused or exacerbated by her current therapy?*
   c. *What information presented in this case supports the diagnosis of ischemic heart disease and provides insight into the severity of this disease?*

Desired Outcome

2. *What are the goals of pharmacotherapy for IHD in this case?*

Therapeutic Alternatives

3. a. Does this patient possess any modifiable risk factors for IHD? If so, would addressing them improve her condition?

b. What pharmacotherapeutic options are available for treating this patient's IHD? Discuss the agents in each class with respect to their relative utility in her care.

Optimal Plan

4. Given the patient information provided, construct a complete pharmacotherapeutic plan for optimizing management of her IHD.

Outcome Evaluation

5. When the patient returns to the clinic in 2 weeks for a follow-up visit, how will you evaluate the response to her new antianginal regimen for efficacy and adverse affects?

Patient Education

6. What information will you communicate to the patient about her antianginal regimen to help her experience the greatest benefit and fewest adverse effects?

▶ Clinical Course

Two months later, the patient's cardiologist is notified of her arrival at the ED of the local hospital. She is complaining of severe substernal chest pain that came on at rest. She rated the pain as 10/10 on presentation and said that it radiated to her left arm. She has received only partial relief with IV NTG and morphine. An ECG revealed 1-mm ST segment depression consistent with anterior wall ischemia. A troponin level was drawn but is not yet available for interpretation. She is diagnosed with acute coronary syndrome and taken urgently to the cath lab. Cardiac catheterization revealed a high-grade lesion in the proximal LAD with acute thrombus present. The decision was made to perform percutaneous coronary intervention (PCI) with deployment of a 3.5 mm CYPHER™ sirolimus-eluting coronary stent. Immediately prior to PCI, a loading dose of heparin 50 units/kg IV was given and the patient was started on antiplatelet therapy with clopidogrel 300 mg orally × 1 and eptifibatide (Integrilin) 180 mcg/kg IV bolus followed by 2 mcg/kg/min infusion. A second bolus dose of eptifibatide 180 mcg/kg IV was given 10 minutes after the first.

▶ Follow-Up Questions

2. What role does antiplatelet therapy with glycoprotein IIb/IIIa receptor antagonists play in the setting of PCI?

▶ Self-Study Assignments

1. Based on current evidence, what is the role of drug-eluting stents in the prevention of restenosis in patients undergoing PCI? Compare the sirolimus-eluting stent to the paclitaxel-eluting stent as part of your answer.
2. What is the role of low-molecular-weight heparins in the management of acute coronary syndromes?
3. Describe the epidemiology and potential mechanisms of aspirin resistance and its relationship to clinical outcomes in primary and secondary prevention scenarios.
4. Discuss precautions related to the use of sildenafil, vardenafil, and tadalafil in the setting of ischemic heart disease, and assess the relative risk to patient subgroups based on disease and therapy considerations.

▶ Clinical Pearl

β blockers alter the natural history of cardiac disease and lead to reduced cardiac events and improved survival post-MI. The traditional contraindications of asthma, diabetes, and peripheral vascular disease should be considered relative contraindications and the risk and benefit of therapy carefully weighed for each patient.

References

1. ACC/AHA Guidelines for the Evaluation and Management of Chronic Heart Failure in the Adult. Executive Summary: A Report of the American College of Cardiology/American Heart Association Task Force on Practice Guidelines (Committee to Revise the 1995 Guidelines for the Evaluation and Management of Heart Failure). Circulation 2001;104:2996–3007.
2. Hulley S, Grady D, Bush T, et al, for the Heart and Estrogen/progestin Replacement Study (HERS) Research Group. Randomized trial of estrogen plus progestin for secondary prevention of coronary heart disease in postmenopausal women. JAMA 1998;280:605–613.
3. Herrington DM, Reboussin DM, Brosnihan KB, et al. Effects of estrogen replacement on the progression of coronary-artery atherosclerosis. N Engl J Med 2000;343:522–529.
4. The Seventh Report of the Joint National Committee on Prevention, Detection, Evaluation, and Treatment of High Blood Pressure. The JNC 7 Report. JAMA 2003;289:2560–2572.
5. Executive Summary of the Third Report of the National Cholesterol Education Program (NCEP) Expert Panel on Detection, Evaluation, and Treatment of High Blood Cholesterol in Adults (Adult Treatment Panel III). JAMA 2001;285: 2486–2497.
6. Antithrombotic Trialists' Collaboration. Collaborative meta-analysis of randomised trials of antiplatelet therapy for prevention of death, myocardial infarction, and stroke in high risk patients. BMJ 2002;324:71–86.
7. CAPRIE Steering Committee. A randomised, blinded, trial of clopidogrel versus aspirin in patients at risk of ischaemic events (CAPRIE). Lancet 1996;348: 1329–1339.
8. Yusuf S, Sleight P, Pogue J, et al. Effects of an angiotensin-converting-enzyme inhibitor, ramipril, on cardiovascular events in high-risk patients. The Heart Outcomes Prevention Evaluation Study Investigators. N Engl J Med 2000;342: 145–153.
9. ACC/AHA 2002 guideline update for the management of patients with chronic stable angina—summary article: a report of the American College of Cardiology/American Heart Association Task Force on practice guidelines (Committee on the Management of Patients with Chronic Stable Angina). J Am Coll Cardiol 2003;41:159–168.
10. Yusuf S, Zhao F, Mehta SR, et al. Effects of clopidogrel in addition to aspirin in patients with acute coronary syndromes without ST-segment elevation. N Engl J Med 2001;345:495–502.
11. Braunwald E, Antman EM, Beasley JW, et al. ACC/AHA guidelines update for the management of patients with unstable angina and non-ST-segment elevation myocardial infarction–2002: summary article: a report of the American College of Cardiology/American Heart Association Task Force on Practice Guidelines (Committee on the Management of Patients with Unstable Angina). Circulation 2002;106:1893–1900.

12. Kong DF, Hasselblad V, Harrington RA et al. Meta-analysis of survival with platelet glycoprotein IIb/IIIa antagonists for percutaneous coronary interventions. Am J Cardiol 2003;92:651–655.
13. Topol EJ, Moliterno DJ, Herrmann HC, et al; TARGET Investigators. Comparison of two platelet glycoprotein IIb/IIIa inhibitors, tirofiban and abciximab, for the prevention of ischemic events with percutaneous coronary revascularization. N Engl J Med 2001;344;1888–1894.

12 ACUTE MYOCARDIAL INFARCTION

▶ Not Just for Men Alone (Level II)

Kelly C. Rogers, PharmD
Robert B. Parker, PharmD, FCCP

▶ After completing this case study, students should be able to:

- Determine the goals of pharmacotherapy for acute MI patients.
- Design an optimal therapeutic plan for management of acute MI and describe how the selected drug therapy achieves the therapeutic goals.
- Identify appropriate parameters to assess the recommended drug therapy for both efficacy and adverse effects.
- Provide appropriate patient education information to an acute MI patient.

PATIENT PRESENTATION

Chief Complaint

"I'm having burning pain in my chest. It feels like really bad heartburn."

HPI

Lorraine Hunt is a 66 yo woman transported by paramedics to the ED of her local community hospital with severe burning, substernal chest pain for the last 3 hours. She states she was fine until about an hour after she ate breakfast. The pain radiates to her back and is accompanied by mild SOB, N/V, and a sense of impending doom. In the ambulance, her chest pain is unrelieved by 3 SL NTG tablets.

PMH

HTN × 20 years
Type 2 DM
Hyperlipidemia
Hysterectomy 20 years ago; ovaries intact

FH

Father died of an MI at age 54; mother died of breast CA at age 80. She has one sister who is 61 yo, alive and well, and one brother who is 58 yo with HTN.

SH

No tobacco × 15 years; occasional glass of wine with friends

ROS

Positive for some baseline CP for "some time"

All

NKDA

Meds

Amlodipine 10 mg po Q AM
Glyburide 10 mg po Q AM, 5 mg po Q PM
EC ASA 325 mg po once daily
Gemfibrozil 600 mg po BID

PE

Gen

WDWN woman A & O × 3, still with chest pain

VS

BP 145/89, P 89, RR 18, T 37.1°C; Ht 5′10″, Wt 86 kg

HEENT

PERRLA, EOMI, fundi benign, TMs intact

Neck

No bruits, mild JVD; no thyromegaly

Lungs

Few dependent inspiratory crackles, bibasilar rales, no wheezes

CV

PMI displaced laterally, normal S_1 and S_2, no S_3 or S_4, I/VI SEM @ LUSB

Abd

Soft, nontender, liver span ~10–12 cm, no bruits

MS/Ext

Normal ROM; muscle strength on right 5/5 UE/LE, on left 4/5 UE/LE; pulses 2+, no femoral bruits or peripheral edema

Neuro

CN II–XII intact; DTRs decreased on left; Babinski (–)

Labs

Na 134 mEq/L	Ca 9.8 mg/dL	Hgb 14.0 g/dL	*Fasting Lipid Profile*
K 4.4 mEq/L	Mg 2.0 mg/dL	Hct 44%	T. chol 214 mg/dL
Cl 102 mEq/L	PO_4 2.4 mg/dL	WBC 5.0 × 10^3/mm^3	Trig 175 mg/dL
CO_2 23 mEq/L	AST 22 U/L	Plt 268 × 10^3/mm^3	LDL 144 mg/dL
BUN 15 mg/dL	ALT 30 U/L	PT 12.5 sec	HDL 35 mg/dL
SCr 1.0 mg/dL	Alk Phos 75 U/L	aPTT 32.4 sec	
Glu 266 mg/dL (non-fasting)	Troponin I 0.3 ng/mL	INR 1.0	
		HbA_{1c} 1 mo ago 9.3%	

ECG

2–5 mm ST segment elevation in leads V2 to V6 (see Figure 12–1).

Assessment

Acute anterior ST-segment elevation myocardial infarction (STEMI)

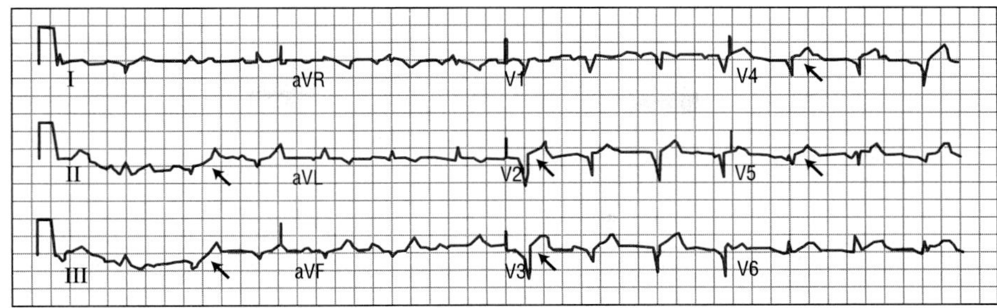

Figure 12–1. ECG taken on arrival in the ED showing ST segment elevation (arrows) in leads V2 to V6 consistent with acute anterior myocardial infarction.

Questions

Problem Identification

1. a. *Which findings in this patient's case history are consistent with acute STEMI?*
   b. *What risk factors for the development of coronary artery disease are present in this patient?*

Desired Outcome

2. *What are the goals of pharmacotherapy in this patient?*

Therapeutic Alternatives

3. a. *What feasible pharmacotherapeutic alternatives are available to treat this patient?*
   b. *What nonpharmacologic alternative therapies might be used in this patient?*

Optimal Plan

4. *Based on the history and presentation, what drug therapy is indicated in this patient?*

Outcome Evaluation

5. a. *How should the recommended therapy be monitored for efficacy and adverse effects?*

Clinical Course

The patient received aspirin, morphine, IV unfractionated heparin, IV nitroglycerin, IV metoprolol, and reteplase. Approximately 1 hour after initiation of reteplase therapy, the patient's chest pain and the ST segment elevation on the ECG resolved. The patient was stable until 2 days after admission, when she began to experience chest pain at rest. With the recurrent chest pain, she was transferred to another hospital with facilities to perform cardiac catheterization. The cath revealed a 70% proximal stenosis in the LAD coronary artery. The patient then received PCI, which consisted of PTCA of the vessel followed by successful placement of a coronary artery stent. After the stent was placed, the patient received an abciximab infusion. Ejection fraction by echocardiogram 3 days postinfarct was 45%. The remainder of the patient's hospital stay was uncomplicated, and she was discharged 5 days post-MI.

5. b. *What is the role of glycoprotein IIb/IIIa inhibitors in the setting of PCI with coronary artery stenting, and how should these drugs be used?*

5. c. *How should therapy with glycoprotein IIb/IIIa inhibitors be monitored?*

Patient Education

6. a. *What discharge medications would be most appropriate for this patient?*
   b. *What patient information should you provide to this patient?*

Follow-Up Questions

1. *This patient returns to the cardiology clinic in 4 weeks for a follow-up visit. She reports feeling fine. What interventions do you recommend at this time?*

Self-Study Assignments

1. The patient comes into your pharmacy and asks you whether taking vitamins would do her heart any good. What would you tell her about vitamins? Which ones would you recommend and why?
2. A 54 yo man is admitted to the CCU for an acute MI. He states that he heard on the news that taking fish oil supplements or eating fish might help his heart. How would you respond to him?
3. Perform a literature search and evaluate recent clinical trials comparing thrombolytic therapy with PCI in patients with ST-segment elevation MI.

Clinical Pearl

Signs of successful thrombolysis include disappearance of chest pain, reperfusion arrhythmias, resolution of ST segment changes, and early peak of cardiac isoenzymes.

References

1. Ryan TJ, Antman EM, Brooks NH, et al. ACC/AHA guidelines for the management of patients with acute myocardial infarction: 1999 update: A report of the American College of Cardiology/American Heart Association Task Force on Practice Guidelines (Committee on Management of Acute Myocardial Infarction). J Am Coll Cardiol 1999;34:890–911. Available at: www.acc.org; accessed August 15, 2003.
2. Braunwald E, Antman EM, Beasley JW, et al. ACC/AHA 2002 guideline update for the management of patients with unstable angina and non-ST-segment elevation myocardial infarction: A report of the American College of Cardiology/American Heart Association Task Force on Practice Guidelines (Committee on the Management of Patients with Unstable Angina). J Am Coll Cardiol 2002;40:1355–1374. Available at: www.acc.org; accessed August 15, 2003.
3. Armstrong PW, Collen D. Fibrinolysis for acute myocardial infarction: current status and new horizons for pharmacological reperfusion, part 1. Circulation 2001;103:2862–2866.
4. Armstrong PW, Collen D. Fibrinolysis for acute myocardial infarction: current status and new horizons for pharmacological reperfusion, part 2. Circulation 2001;103:2987–2992.
5. The EPISTENT Investigators. Randomised placebo-controlled and balloon-angioplasty-controlled trial to assess safety of coronary stenting with use of platelet glycoprotein-IIb/IIIa blockade. Lancet 1998;352:87–92.
6. O'Shea JC, Buller CE, Cantor WJ, et al; ESPRIT Investigators. Long-term efficacy of platelet glycoprotein IIb/IIIa integrin blockade with eptifibatide in coronary stent intervention. JAMA 2002;287:618–621.
7. Topol EJ, Moliterno DJ, Herrmann HC, et al. for the TARGET Investigators. Comparison of two platelet glycoprotein IIb/IIIa inhibitors, tirofiban and abciximab, for the prevention of ischemic events with percutaneous coronary revascularization. N Engl J Med 2001;344:1888–1894.
8. ACE Inhibitor Myocardial Infarction Collaborative Group. Indications for ACE inhibitors in the early treatment of acute myocardial infarction: systematic overview of individual data from 100,000 patients in randomized trials. Circulation 1998;97:2202–2212.
9. Yusuf S, Sleight P, Pogue J, et al. Effects of an angiotensin-converting-enzyme inhibitor, ramipril, on cardiovascular events in high-risk patients. The Heart Outcomes Prevention Evaluation Study Investigators. N Engl J Med 2000;342:145–153.
10. Cannon CP, Braunwald E, McCabe CH, et al. for the Pravastatin or Atorvastatin Evaluation and Infection Therapy–Thrombolysis in Myocardial Infarction 22 Investigators. Intensive versus moderate lipid lowering with statins after acute coronary syndromes. N Engl J Med 2004;350:1495–1504.
11. The Clopidogrel in Unstable Angina to Prevent Recurrent Events Trial Investigators. Effects of clopidogrel in addition to aspirin in patients with acute coronary syndromes without ST-segment elevation. N Engl J Med 2001;345:494–502.
12. Mehta SR, Yusuf S, Peters RJ, et al. Effects of pretreatment with clopidogrel and aspirin followed by long-term therapy in patients undergoing percutaneous coronary intervention: The PCI-CURE study. Lancet 2001;358:527–533.
13. Steinhubl SR, Berger PB, Mann JT, et al. for the CREDO Investigators. Early and sustained dual oral antiplatelet therapy following percutaneous coronary intervention: a randomized controlled trial. JAMA 2002;288:2411–2420.
14. Peters RJ, Mehta SR, Fox KA, et al. for the Clopidogrel in Unstable angina to prevent Recurrent Events (CURE) Trial Investigators. Effects of aspirin dose when used alone or in combination with clopidogrel in patients with acute coronary syndromes: observations from the Clopidogrel in Unstable angina to prevent Recurrent Events (CURE) Study. Circulation 2003;108:1682–1687.
15. Roussouw JE, Anderson GL, Prentice RL, et al; Writing Group for the Women's Health Initiative Investigators. Risks and benefits of estrogen plus progestin in healthy postmenopausal women: principal results from the Women's Health Initiative randomized controlled trial. JAMA 2002;288:321–333.
16. Manson JE, Hsia J, Johnson KC, et al. Estrogen plus progestin and the risk of coronary heart disease. N Engl J Med 2003;349:523–534.
17. Hodis HN, Mack WJ, Azen SP, et al. for the Women's Estrogen-Progestin Lipid-Lowering Hormone Atherosclerosis Regression Trial Research Group. Hormone therapy and the progression of coronary-artery atherosclerosis in postmenopausal women. N Engl J Med 2003;349:535–545.

Acknowledgement: This case was modified from the case written for the fifth edition by Rebecca L. Waltman, PharmD.

13 VENTRICULAR TACHYCARDIA

► Hello, 911 Operator? (Level III)

Amy L. Seybert, PharmD

► After completing this case study, students should be able to:

- Understand the risk factors for development of ventricular tachycardia (VT).
- Differentiate VT from other cardiac arrhythmias.
- Select appropriate first-line and second-line therapies for treatment of VT.
- Monitor antiarrhythmic and other therapies used to treat VT.
- Discuss long-term approaches to prevention of recurrent VT.

PATIENT PRESENTATION

Chief Complaint

"Operator, I've had pains in my chest twice that shoot down into my left arm. I think I need the paramedics."

HPI

Paul Gates is a 51 yo man who has had minor chest pains in the past. An exercise stress test done about 1 month ago was negative. Today, he was watching TV at home when he felt a crushing pain in his chest that radiated to the left arm that was relieved by lying down. A few minutes later, he developed recurrent chest pain, grade 7/10 in pain intensity that again radiated to the left arm. The chest pain was associated with shortness of breath and diaphoresis. He then called 911. Upon arrival of the paramedics, he had an episode of sustained VT that degenerated into VF, and he passed out. He was defibrillated × 1 by the paramedics and was successfully resuscitated (see Figure 13–1). He was taken by ambulance to the ED at a community hospital, where he was found to have an acute anterior wall MI. He was treated with 100 mg alteplase in an accelerated dose fashion. He still had recurrences of chest pain, grade 6/10 in pain intensity, which were not relieved with IV nitroglycerin. He was emergently transferred to a university hospital for cardiac catheterization. The cardiac cath showed 100% mid and proximal LAD occlusion and an estimated EF of 25%. He underwent rescue PTCA, and two coronary artery stents were placed in the mid and proximal LAD. He also received abciximab during PTCA/stent placement to prevent abrupt vessel closure. He was then admitted to the CCU.

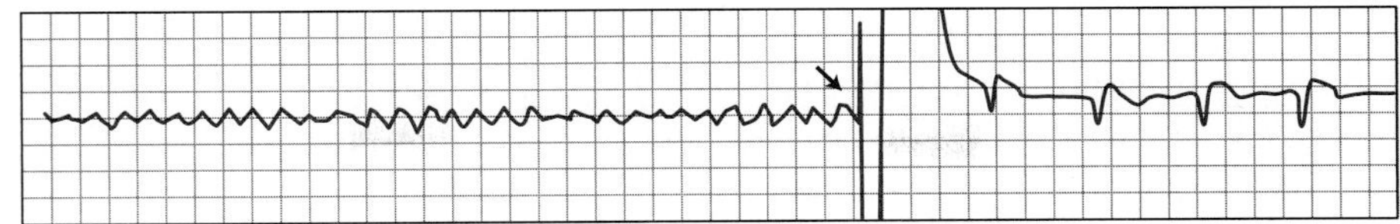

Figure 13–1. Rhythm strip showing ventricular fibrillation that was successfully defibrillated *(arrow)* to sinus rhythm. *(Photo courtesy of Jason Lazar, MD.)*

PMH
HTN × 10 years

PSH
Appendectomy

FH
Father alive, age 76 with angina; mother alive, age 72 with arthritis; both paternal grandparents had CAD at age 70

SH
Works as a systems analyst for a large corporation; occasional cigar smoker

ROS
Negative except for complaints noted above

Meds
Quinapril 20 mg po once daily (on admission)

All
NKDA

PE (Performed in the CCU)

Gen
WDWN male

VS
BP 155/95, P 89, RR 26, T 36.8°C

HEENT
PERRLA, EOMI, pink conjunctiva, AV nicking (Grade 1) on funduscopic exam

Neck
Supple, (–) JVD, no bruits

Chest
Significant bibasilar crackles

CV
S_1 and S_2 normal; no S_3. No m/r/g

Abd
Soft, NT/ND. (+) bowel sounds

Ext
Right groin lines in place, no hematomas, 2+ peripheral pulses

Neuro
No focal neurologic deficits. CN II–XII intact

Labs

Na 133 mEq/L	Hgb 14.3 g/dL	Ca 8.4 mg/dL
K 3.8 mEq/L	Hct 44.6%	Mg 1.5 mEq/L
Cl 96 mEq/L	Plt 262 × $10^3/mm^3$	aPTT 48.1 sec
CO_2 24 mEq/L	WBC 18.1 × $10^3/mm^3$	PT 13.5 sec
BUN 25 mg/dL	Polys 89%	INR 1.2
SCr 2.1 mg/dL	Lymphs 9%	CPK 2171 IU/L
Glu 169 mg/dL	Monos 2%	CK-MB 196 IU/L
		LDH 281 IU/L

UA
Appearance: Yellow, hazy; SG 1.015; pH 7.5; protein 30 mg; glucose neg; ketones neg; Hgb 3+; WBC 2–5/hpf; RBC 5–10/hpf; epithelial cells occasional; bacteria 1+; leukocyte esterase neg; urobilinogen 0.2 EU/dL; bilirubin neg

ECG
Day 1: HR 94 bpm; NSR; acute anterior wall MI; anterolateral ST segment elevations; Q waves in V1 to V3 (see Figure 13–2).

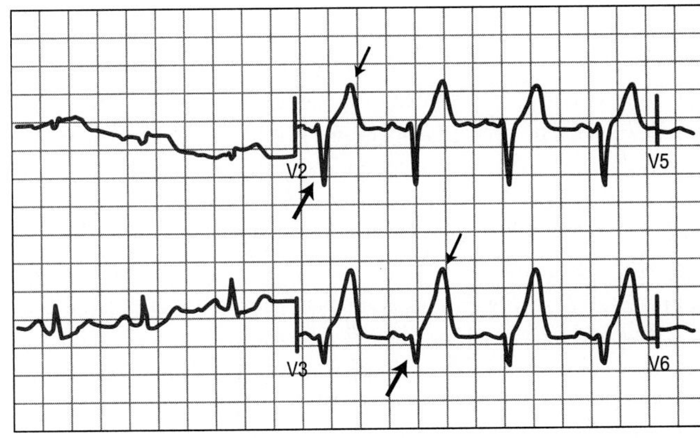

Figure 13–2. ECG leads V2 and V3 showing anterolateral ST segment elevations *(small arrows)* and Q waves *(large arrows)* that are consistent with anterior wall myocardial infarction.

▶ Clinical Course

During his hospitalization, he developed one episode of sustained asymptomatic VT with a BP of 70/40 mm Hg and HR of 105 bpm (see Figure 13–3). He also had multiple episodes of NSVT (8–10 beats) but still maintained his blood pressure and heart rate with no symptoms.

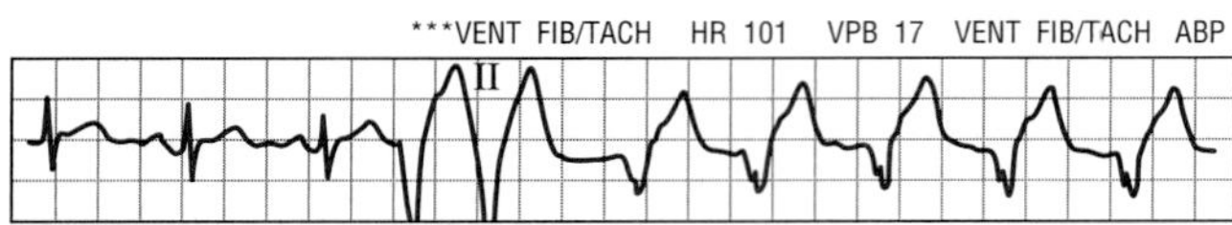

Figure 13–3. ECG (lead II) showing sustained ventricular tachycardia.

▶ Questions

Problem Identification

1. a. *What are the possible causes of sudden cardiac death and VT in this patient? What information presented in the case suggests these causes?*
   b. *How are VT and NSVT characterized on the ECG?*

Desired Outcome

2. *What are the goals of treatment for acute-onset VT?*

Therapeutic Alternatives

3. a. *What non-drug therapies may be useful for treating acute VT in this patient?*
   b. *What pharmacotherapeutic alternatives are available for the treatment of acute-onset VT?*

Optimal Plan

4. *What drug, dosage form, schedule, and duration of therapy are best for this patient for the treatment of acute-onset VT?*

Outcome Evaluation

5. *Which monitoring parameters are necessary to evaluate the therapy for achievement of the desired therapeutic outcome and to prevent toxicity?*

▶ Clinical Course

The patient received the treatment you recommended with no further episodes of VT. The abciximab infusion (0.125 mcg/kg/min) was subsequently discontinued. Other medications taken during the 3-day CCU hospitalization included heparin 500 units/hr by continuous IV infusion, nitroglycerin infusion 10 mcg/min, aspirin 325 mg po QD, clopidogrel 75 mg po QD, metoprolol 50 mg po BID, quinapril 20 mg po QD, and magnesium chloride 2 g IV × 1. The medication given for VT was discontinued after 2 days, and the patient was observed on telemetry. There was no recurrence of VT or NSVT after 3 days of telemetry observation, and the patient was then discharged on EC ASA 325 mg po QD, clopidogrel 75 mg po QD, metoprolol 50 mg po BID, and quinapril 20 mg po QD.

Patient Education

6. *What information should be provided to the patient to enhance patient understanding and compliance upon discharge?*

▶ Follow-Up Questions

1. *Create a list of the patient's drug therapy problems.*

▶ Self-Study Assignments

1. Patients with recurrent sustained VT after an acute MI (even after correction of precipitating factors) are at a high risk of sudden cardiac death. These patients are often taken to the electrophysiology lab and tested for inducibility of VT and are then given some form of preventative therapy (e.g., antiarrhythmics or implantable cardiac defibrillators). However, in patients who have asymptomatic NSVT, it is still not clear what treatment approach should be taken. The Multicenter Automatic Defibrillator Implantation Trial (MADIT) was conducted in patients with coronary artery disease and NSVT to determine whether all patients with asymptomatic NSVT require long-term preventative therapy.[6] Look up this article and write a one-page essay on your assessment of the study results.
2. The ACC/AHA guidelines[7] on management of acute MI suggest that all patients should receive ACE inhibitor therapy within the first 24 hours as long as there are no contraindications. Patients with asymptomatic or symptomatic LV dysfunction after an acute MI typically receive ACE inhibitors indefinitely because of decreased mortality (ISIS-4, GISSI-3, SOLVD trials). However, what is the duration of ACE inhibitor therapy in patients who do *not* develop asymptomatic or symptomatic LV dysfunction after an acute MI?

▶ Clinical Pearl

After an MI, β-blockers are the most effective prophylactic interventions against VT/VF for most patients. The role of amiodarone has expanded, and some patients at a higher risk of sudden cardiac death require an implantable defibrillator device or other antiarrhythmic therapy.

References

1. Hazinski MF, Cummins RO, eds. 2000 Handbook of Emergency Cardiac Care for Healthcare Providers. Dallas, American Heart Association, 2000.
2. Yusuf S, Peto R, Lewis J, et al. β-Blockade during and after myocardial infarction: An overview of the randomized trials. Prog Cardiovasc Dis 1985;27:335–371.
3. Joint National Committee on Prevention, Detection, Evaluation, and Treatment of High Blood Pressure. Sixth report. Arch Intern Med 1997;157:2413–2445.
4. MIAMI Trial Research Group. Metoprolol in acute myocardial infarction. Am J Cardiol 1985;56:1G–57G.

5. TIMI Study Group. Comparison of invasive and conservative strategies after treatment with intravenous tissue plasminogen activator in acute myocardial infarction: Results of the thrombolysis in myocardial infarction (TIMI) phase II trial. N Engl J Med 1989;320:618–627.
6. Moss AJ, Hall WJ, Cannon DS, et al. Improved survival with an implanted defibrillator in patients with coronary disease at high risk for ventricular arrhythmia. Multicenter Automatic Defibrillator Implantation Trial Investigators. N Engl J Med 1996;335:1933–1940.
7. Ryan TJ, Antman EM, Brooks NH, et al. 1999 update: ACC/AHA guidelines for the management of patients with acute myocardial infarction. A report of the American College of Cardiology/American Heart Association Task Force on Practice Guidelines (Committee on Management of Acute Myocardial Infarction). J Am Coll Cardiol 1999;34(3):890–911. Available at www.acc.org.

14 ATRIAL FIBRILLATION

▶ If It's Not Love, Head for the ER (Level II)

Bradley G. Phillips, PharmD

▶ After completing this case study, students should be able to:

- Determine therapeutic goals for patients presenting with new onset atrial fibrillation.
- Select appropriate pharmacotherapeutic regimens to achieve and maintain ventricular rate control in patients with atrial fibrillation.
- Recommend appropriate pharmacologic or other therapies to convert atrial fibrillation to normal sinus rhythm or maintain ventricular rate control.
- Recognize how treatment for lone atrial fibrillation differs from that associated with identifiable underlying causes.

PATIENT PRESENTATION

Chief Complaint

"I feel that my heart is beating too fast and I feel a bit dizzy."

HPI

Matthew Jacobson is a 63 yo man who presents to the ED with heart palpitations and dizziness. He first noticed the palpitations 3 hours ago while he was mowing his lawn. He describes the palpitations as a heavy fluttering sensation in his chest. The severity of his dizziness fluctuates; the dizziness was the worst when he was pushing his lawn mower. He has been seen in the medicine clinic for many years for his HTN and COPD and has a history of medication non-compliance.

PMH

HTN (uncontrolled because of non-compliance)
COPD × 15 years
BPH × 7 years

FH

Both parents had HTN; his mother died of a stroke at age 65, and his father died after suffering an AMI at the age of 62. He has one brother who is alive and well.

SH

Mr. Jacobson is retired and lives at home with his wife. He smoked 1 ppd for 20 years and quit 3 years ago. He drinks 1 to 2 beers every other week.

Meds

Terazosin 10 mg po once daily
Albuterol inhaler 2 puffs QID
Ipratropium bromide inhaler 2 puffs QID
Multivitamin 1 tablet po once daily

All

NKDA

ROS

No headache, blurred vision, chest pain, or fainting spells; complains of occasional wheezes, but has no cough or SOB; no present difficulty with urination.

PE

Gen

Cooperative overweight man in moderate distress

VS

BP 98/70 (supine), P 140 (irregular), RR 20, T 36.3°C; Ht 5′11″, Wt 93 kg

Skin

Cool to touch, normal turgor and color

HEENT

PERRLA, EOMI; funduscopic exam reveals mild arteriolar narrowing but no hemorrhages, exudates, or papilledema

Neck

Supple, no carotid bruits; no lymphadenopathy or thyromegaly

Pulm

Inspiratory and expiratory wheezes bilaterally without rales or rhonchi

CV

Tachycardia with irregular rate; varying S_1, S_2; no S_3 or S_4; no m/r/g

Abd

NT/ND, (+) BS; no organomegaly

Genit/Rect

Stool heme (–); prostate slightly enlarged and smooth

MS/Ext

Pulses 2+, full ROM, no CCE

Neuro

A & O × 3; CN II–XII intact. DTR 2+, negative Babinski

Labs (non-fasting)

Na 140 mEq/L
K 4.2 mEq/L
Cl 99 mEq/L
CO_2 24 mEq/L
BUN 23 mg/dL
SCr 1.5 mg/dL
Glu 125 mg/dL

Hgb 15.2 g/dL
Hct 48%
Plt $293 \times 10^3/mm^3$
WBC $12.1 \times 10^3/mm^3$
Polys 71%
Bands 2%
Lymphs 24%
Monos 3%

Ca 9.1 mg/dL
Mg 2.1 mEq/L

ECG

Atrial fibrillation, ventricular rate 144, no LVH

Chest X-Ray

No infiltrates, mild thoracic overinflation

Assessment

First episode of atrial fibrillation
Hypotension: Hold BP meds until rhythm disturbance is corrected and BP is stabilized
COPD: Continue current medications
BPH: Hold terazosin due to low BP and arrhythmia

▶ Questions

Problem Identification

1. a. *List and prioritize the patient's drug therapy problems.*
   b. *Does this patient have "lone" or "chronic" atrial fibrillation?*
   c. *Considering his presenting signs and symptoms, how would you characterize the severity of this patient's atrial fibrillation? State the rationale for your answer.*

Desired Outcome

2. *What are the acute goals for pharmacotherapy in this case?*

Therapeutic Alternatives

3. *Describe the benefits and risks of drugs that can be used to achieve and maintain acute ventricular rate control in patients with atrial fibrillation.*

Optimal Plan

4. *Which agent and dosage regimen would you recommend to achieve and maintain acute control of this patient's ventricular response rate?*

▶ Clinical Course

The drug regimen that you recommended to control the ventricular response was initiated. The rate prior to drug administration was 131 bpm with a BP of 101/71 mm Hg. The patient's baseline rhythm recorded just prior to drug therapy administration is shown in the top portion of Figure 14–1. The patient's rhythm and vital signs were monitored over the next 15 minutes. At 15 minutes, his rhythm showed atrial fibrillation with a ventricular response of 95 bpm and he had a BP of 108/83 mm Hg (see bottom portion of Figure 14–1). He stated that he felt better and did not notice the fluttering in his chest any longer. A continuous infusion of the same drug was initiated to maintain the patient's ventricular response rate. He also received heparin 5,000 units by IV bolus and was started on a heparin infusion of 1,000 U/hr. Shortly thereafter, the Cardiology Service arrived in the ED to evaluate the patient. The team decided to admit him to a telemetry bed for further evaluation with plans to perform cardioversion.

Outcome Evaluation

5. *How would you monitor and adjust the IV infusion to control his ventricular response rate?*

▶ Follow-Up Questions

1. *Is it possible that the drug therapy you recommended to control the ventricular response rate will also convert his atrial fibrillation to normal sinus rhythm?*
2. *If the cardiology team decides to chemically cardiovert the patient, why is it important to first control his ventricular rate?*

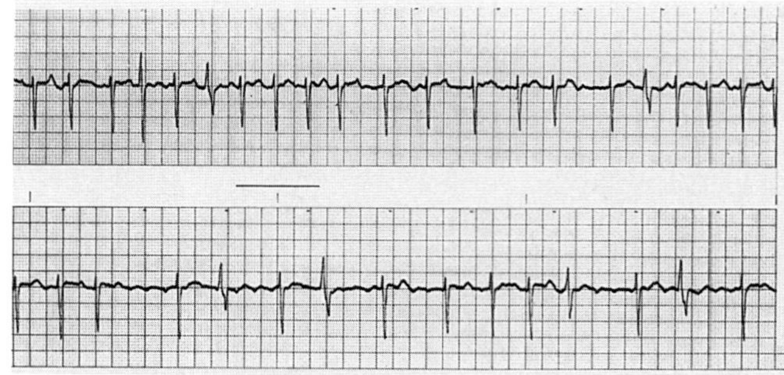

Figure 14–1. Rhythm recorded just prior to *(top)* and 15 minutes after *(bottom)* the administration of drug therapy. Top rhythm depicts atrial fibrillation with a ventricular response rate of 131 bpm. Bottom rhythm depicts atrial fibrillation with a rate of 95 bpm. Atrial fibrillation is characterized in each rhythm strip by the absence of atrial "p" waves and an irregular ventricular response (intervals between each QRS complex vary irregularly).

3. *Should this patient be continued in atrial fibrillation with ventricular rate control?*
4. *If the patient is successfully cardioverted, what drug therapy would you recommend long term?*

▶ Self-Study Assignments

1. Outline the antiarrhythmic drug regimen you would recommend to convert this patient's atrial fibrillation to normal sinus rhythm.
2. If this patient develops atrial fibrillation again, would you continue to control ventricular response rate or prescribe antiarrhythmic drug therapy to convert and maintain normal sinus rhythm chronically?
3. Give your recommendations for treating this patient's hypertension and the appropriateness of restarting terazosin for managing his BPH.

▶ Clinical Pearl

In atrial fibrillation, the ventricular rate must be controlled prior to chemical cardioversion so that paradoxical increases in ventricular response and subsequent hemodynamic instability do not occur.

References

1. Fuster V, Ryden LE, Asinger RW, et al. ACC/AHA/ESC Guidelines for the Management of Patients With Atrial Fibrillation: Executive Summary. A Report of the American College of Cardiology/American Heart Association Task Force on Practice Guidelines and the European Society of Cardiology Committee for Practice Guidelines and Policy Conferences (Committee to Develop Guidelines for the Management of Patients With Atrial Fibrillation). Developed in Collaboration With the North American Society of Pacing and Electrophysiology. Circulation 2001;104:2118–2150.
2. Snow V, Weiss KB, LeFevre M, et al. Management of newly detected atrial fibrillation: a clinical practice guideline from the American Academy of Family Physicians and the American College of Physicians. Ann Intern Med 2003;139:1009–1017.
3. Wyse DG, Waldo AL, DiMarco JP, et al. A comparison of rate control and rhythm control in patients with atrial fibrillation. N Engl J Med 2002;347:1825–1833.
4. Hagens VE, Ranchor AV, Van Sonderen E, et al. Effect of rate or rhythm control on quality of life in persistent atrial fibrillation. Results from the Rate Control Versus Electrical Cardioversion (RACE) Study. J Am Coll Cardiol 2004;43:241–247.
5. Carlsson J, Miketic S, Windeler J, et al. Randomized trial of rate-control versus rhythm-control in persistent atrial fibrillation: The Strategies of Treatment of Atrial Fibrillation (STAF) study. J Am Coll Cardiol 2003;41:1690–1696.
6. Hohnloser SH, Kuck KH, Lilienthal J. Rhythm or rate control in atrial fibrillation—Pharmacological Intervention in Atrial Fibrillation (PIAF): A randomised trial. Lancet 2000;356:1789–1794.
7. Phillips BG, Gandhi AJ, Sanoski CA, et al. Comparison of intravenous diltiazem and verapamil for the acute treatment of atrial fibrillation and atrial flutter. Pharmacotherapy 1997;17:1238–1245.
8. Roberts SA, Diaz C, Nolan PE, et al. Effectiveness and costs of digoxin treatment for atrial fibrillation and flutter. Am J Cardiol 1993;72:567–573.

15 HYPERTROPHIC CARDIOMYOPATHY

▶ The Air Force Recruit

William Linn, PharmD
Robert A. O'Rourke, MD

▶ After completing this case study, students should be able to:

- Describe the pathophysiology of hypertrophic cardiomyopathy (HCM).
- Recognize the most common clinical presentations of HCM and the typical physical findings.
- Risk-stratify patients with HCM and identify patients at highest risk of sudden cardiac death.
- Outline the various treatment options for patients with HCM.
- Differentiate the benefits and side effects of pharmacologic treatments for HCM.
- Advise and counsel patients on the appropriate use of medications used to treat HCM.
- Design monitoring parameters for achievement of the desired therapeutic outcomes while minimizing adverse effects of medications used to treat HCM.

PATIENT PRESENTATION

Chief Complaint

"I've been short of breath this week during training, and the drill instructor ordered me to report to sick call right away."

HPI

John Lawrence is an 18 yo recent high school graduate who presents to the general medical officer after referral by the corpsman. He was in a normal state of health for the past 18 years but has never been very physically active. John has recently reported for basic training at Lackland AFB after joining the Air Force. During his first week of training he complained of difficulty breathing when doing strenuous activity. The corpsman was called to assess John's condition after a near-syncopal episode on the obstacle course.

PMH

No known health problems. John had a viral-like URI at age 12 and right ear infections at ages 3 and 4.

FH

Father is alive and well at the age of 45. Mother has a heart murmur. Younger brother, age 15, is in good physical health. Older brother died suddenly at the age of 19 of unknown causes.

ROS

(+) for fatigue, palpitations with feelings of lightheadedness, dyspnea upon exertion.

Meds

No regular medications; occasional aspirin or ibuprofen use for headaches, aches, and pains.

All

NKDA

Physical Examination

Gen

John is a slightly anxious 18 yo male in no apparent distress.

VS

BP 116/84, P 80, RR 14, T 37.0°C; Wt 83.9 kg, Ht 6′2″

HEENT

PERRLA, EOMI, fundi benign, TMs intact

Neck

The carotid pulse is brisk and bifid with a "spike and dome" pattern. The JVP is normal.

Lungs

Clear to auscultation

CV

Loud S_1 with a physiologically split S_2; (+) S_4; there is a II/VI crescendo–decrescendo murmur heard best at the left sternal border which decreased in intensity with squatting.

Abd

Soft, NT/ND; normal and reactive bowel sounds

Ext

Radial pulses 4+ bilaterally; pedal pulses 3+ bilaterally.

Chest X-Ray

There is mild enlargement of the cardiac silhouette and the left ventricular contour is rounded.

ECG

Meets voltage criteria for left ventricular hypertrophy

24-Hour Holter Monitor

Multiple episodes of non-sustained ventricular tachycardia

Two-Dimensional Echocardiography

Diffuse hypertrophy of entire ventricular septum with a convex septal contour; there is dynamic left ventricular outflow obstruction associated with systolic anterior motion (SAM) of the mitral valve. There is extreme left ventricular hypertrophy with a wall thickness of 45 mm.

Doppler Echocardiography

There is a high velocity "dagger-shaped" signal on continuous wave doppler interrogation of the left ventricular outflow tract. The peak pressure velocity is 4 m/sec. Doppler color flow imaging revealed mild mitral regurgitation.

Assessment

18 year-old male with hypertrophic cardiomyopathy experiencing a near-syncopal episode during strenuous physical activity.

▶ Questions

Problem Identification

1. *What data are present to support the diagnosis of HCM in Mr. Lawrence? Is he a high-risk patient?*

Desired Outcome

2. *What are the goals of pharmacotherapy in this case?*

Therapeutic Alternatives

3. a. *What pharmacotherapeutic alternatives are available for the treatment of HCM?*
   b. *What other management options are available for patients with HCM?*

Optimal Plan

4. *What drug, dosage form, dose, schedule, and duration of therapy are best for this patient?*

Outcome Evaluation

5. *Which clinical and laboratory parameters are necessary to evaluate the therapy for achievement of the desired therapeutic outcome and to detect or prevent adverse effects?*

Patient Education

6. *What information should be provided to the patient to enhance compliance, ensure successful therapy, and minimize adverse effects?*

▶ Clinical Course

It has been 1 week since John's diagnosis, and he has responded well to his therapy with no complaints. His diary shows that his heart rate has been between 70 and 110 bpm this entire week with a normal blood pressure.

▶ Follow-Up Questions

1. *Are any adjustments in his medication dosage warranted at this time?*

▶ Self-Study Assignments

1. When a patient with HCM arrives at your pharmacy, what questions would you ask to assess his or her drug therapy?
2. Perform a literature search to determine when anticoagulation therapy should be initiated for HCM.
3. Perform a literature search on HCM using SumSearch (http://sumsearch.uthscsa.edu).

References

1. Maron BJ. Hypertrophic cardiomyopathy. In: Fuster V, Alexander RW, eds. Hurst's The Heart, 10th ed. New York, McGraw-Hill;2001:1967–1987.
2. Maron BJ. Hypertrophic cardiomyopathy: a systematic review. JAMA 2002;287: 1308–1320.
3. Spirito P, Seidman CE, McKenna WJ, et al. The management of hypertrophic cardiomyopathy. N Engl J Med 1997;336:775–785.
4. Watkins H. Sudden death in hypertrophic cardiomyopathy. N Engl J Med 2000;342:422–424.
5. Hess OM. Risk stratification in hypertrophic cardiomyopathy: fact or fiction? J Am Coll Cardiol 2003;42:880–881.
6. Monserrat L, Elliott PM, Gimeno JR, et al. Non-sustained ventricular tachycardia in hypertrophic cardiomyopathy: an independent marker of sudden death risk in young patients. J Am Coll Cardiol 2003;42:873–879.
7. Cannon RO 3rd. Assessing risk in hypertrophic cardiomyopathy. N Engl J Med 2003;349:1016–1018.
8. Maron BJ. Sudden death in young athletes. N Engl J Med 2003;349:1064–1075.
9. Maron BJ, Shen WK, Link MS, et al. Efficacy of implantable cardioverter-defibrillators for the prevention of sudden death in patients with hypertrophic cardiomyopathy. N Engl J Med 2000;342:365–373.
10. Kimmelstiel CD, Maron BJ. Role of Percutaneous Septal Ablation in Hypertrophic Obstructive Cardiomyopathy. Circulation 2004;109:452–455.

Acknowledgement: This case was modified from the case written for the fifth edition by Laura A. Bartels, PharmD.

16 DEEP VEIN THROMBOSIS

▶ Mrs. Houston, We Have a Problem (Level II)

Deanne L. Hall, PharmD
Meredith L. Rose, PharmD

▶ Upon completing this case study, students should be able to:

- Identify the signs and symptoms of deep-vein thrombosis (DVT) as well as associated risk factors for DVT.
- Compare the advantages and limitations of the therapeutic options for DVT in the outpatient setting.
- Develop an individualized therapeutic plan for a patient presenting with a DVT.
- Titrate warfarin doses in both the initiation and maintenance phases of therapy.
- Appropriately educate patients receiving anticoagulation therapy.

PATIENT PRESENTATION

Chief Complaint

"My calf started to swell last week. Now the pain is so bad that I'm having a hard time walking."

HPI

Mary Houston is a 47 yo woman who began to notice swelling of her right calf approximately 4 days ago. She reported to the ED of her local hospital 1 day after the onset of calf pain and swelling. Venous Dopplers were performed and the patient was told that she had a blood clot in her right leg. According to the patient, she was given a prescription for an injection and instructed to follow-up with her PCP within the next 1 to 2 days. She failed to have the prescription filled because her pharmacy did not have the drug in stock. Because of increasing pain and discomfort, Mrs. Houston was seen by her physician this morning who recommended hospitalization to initiate therapy for her blood clot.

PMH

Previous DVT at the age of 38; treated with warfarin for 3 months
TAH/BSO at the age of 38 secondary to endometriosis

FH

Father died at age 42 from MI; mother alive at 71 with breast cancer diagnosed 5 years ago, s/p radiation/chemotherapy; sister, alive and well. No family history of venous thromboembolic disease reported.

SH

Patient lives with her husband and 16 yo son; works in a department store as a cashier. 24 pack-year smoking history; currently smokes ½ to 1 ppd. (–) EtOH or IVDA.

Meds

Raloxifene 60 mg po once daily
Multiple vitamin 1 tablet po daily
Denies any herbal products

All

Codeine causes hives

ROS

(–) Fever, chills; (–) cough, shortness of breath, chest pain, diaphoresis or hemoptysis; (–) abdominal pain, N/V/D, constipation, or BRBPR; (–)

polyuria, dysuria, or hematuria; (+) acute pain and feeling of tightness in right lower leg, swelling of right calf to twice the normal size; (–) for swelling or pain in LLE

PE

Gen
This is a pleasant obese woman in NAD.

VS
BP 130/80, P 70, RR 16, T 36.6°C; Ht 5′2″; Wt 82 kg; O_2 sat 98% on RA

HEENT
PERRLA, EOMI, no icterus, mucous membranes pink and moist

Neck/LN
Supple; no thyromegaly, carotid bruits, JVD, or lymphadenopathy

Chest
CTA; no rales or rhonchi

Cardiac
RRR; no murmurs; no S_3 or S_4

Abd
Obese; soft, NT/ND; no masses, guarding, rebound or rigidity; no hepatosplenomegaly; normal BS

Genit/Rect
Normal; no rectal masses; heme-negative brown stool

Ext
No CCE; right calf swollen, erythematous, and warm to touch in posterior and anterior areas;(+) Homan's sign on right calf with no palpable cord; left calf non-tender, non-swollen, and without erythema.

Neuro
A & O × 3; no neurologic deficits noted

Labs

Na 139 mEq/L	Hgb 13.4 g/dL	AST 16 IU/L	aPTT 34.8 sec
K 3.6 mEq/L	Hct 39.5%	ALT 20 IU/L	PT 11.4 sec
Cl 103 mEq/L	WBC 9.4 × 10^3/mm^3	Alk Phos 67 IU/L	INR 1.0
CO_2 26 mEq/L	Plt 177 × 10^3/mm^3	GGT 20 IU/L	*Fasting Lipid Profile*
BUN 10 mg/dL		Ca 8.3 mg/dL	T. chol 250 mg/dL
SCr 0.7 mg/dL			LDL 169 mg/dL
Glu 119 mg/dL			HDL 43 mg/dL
			Trig 235 mg/dL

Hypercoagulability Profile

Factor V Leiden Mutation	Homozygous Positive
Factor II Prothrombin Gene Variant	Negative
Lupus Anticoagulant	Negative
Anticardiolipin Antibodies	Negative
Protein C Deficiency	Negative
Protein S Deficiency	Negative
Antithrombin III Deficiency	Negative
MTHFR Gene Variant	Negative

Chest X-Ray
No effusions or infiltrates present.

Spiral CT
Negative for pulmonary embolism.

Venous Compression Ultrasonography
RLE shows noncompressibility of the right posterior tibial vein with no color flow. There is normal compressibility and flow demonstrated within the right common femoral and iliac veins. LLE shows normal compressibility of the deep venous system from the level of the common femoral vein to the popliteal vein.

Assessment
DVT of the right posterior tibial vein requiring initiation of anticoagulation therapy. A venogram (see Figure 16–1) will not be necessary because of the positive ultrasound results.

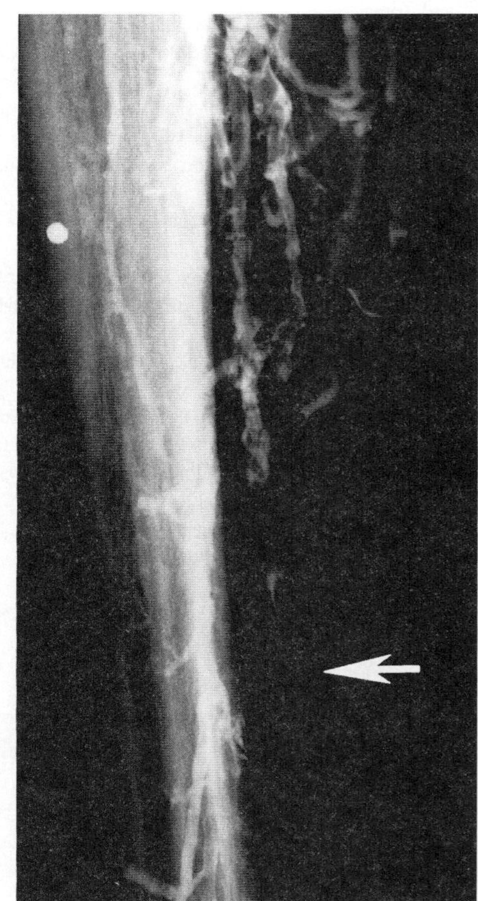

Figure 16–1. Venogram (not from this patient) documenting right posterior tibial vein thrombosis *(arrow)*. A venogram was not necessary in this patient because of the positive ultrasound results.

Questions

Problem Identification

1. a. *Create a problem list for this patient.*
   b. *What risk factors for DVT are present in this patient?*
   c. *What subjective and objective evidence is suggestive of a lower extremity DVT?*

Desired Outcome

2. *What are the acute and chronic goals of pharmacotherapy for this patient's DVT?*

Therapeutic Alternatives

3. a. *Discuss the available treatment options for initial anticoagulation in this patient.*
   b. *What alternatives are available if this patient has a history of heparin-induced thrombocytopenia (HIT)?*

Optimal Plan

4. *Design a treatment plan for the management of this patient's identified problems. Provide specific medication information including dosage form, dose, and schedule.*

Outcome Evaluation

5. *Which clinical and laboratory monitoring parameters should be assessed to ensure the efficacy and safety of anticoagulation therapy in this patient?*

Patient Education

6. *What information should be provided to the patient to enhance compliance, to minimize adverse effects, and to ensure successful therapy?*

Clinical Course

The patient was admitted and started on anticoagulation therapy (day 1). The following morning (day 2), a pharmacist-managed anticoagulation clinic was consulted to evaluate the patient for home low molecular weight heparin (LMWH) bridge therapy to warfarin. After careful evaluation, the pharmacist determined that the patient was an appropriate candidate for outpatient treatment of DVT. Additionally, the patient agreed with the treatment plan and had prescription drug coverage. Prior to discharge, the pharmacist educated the patient about her disease state and medication therapy with LMWH and warfarin. The pharmacist also taught the patient how to self-administer the LMWH and witnessed the patient's subcutaneous injection technique. The patient's prescriptions for both medications were filled and delivered to her before leaving the hospital. She was instructed to return to the clinic in 2 days for laboratory monitoring and evaluation of therapy. The patient's warfarin doses and laboratory values are listed in the following table.

Day	INR	Warfarin	Platelet Count	Comment
1	1.0	10 mg		Admitted to hospital
2	1.2	5 mg		Discharge to home
3		5 mg		
4	2.1	5 mg	$180 \times 10^3/mm^3$	Anticoag f/u visit
5		5 mg		
6	2.2			Anticoag f/u visit

Follow-Up Questions

1. *What day would you recommend to discontinue the LMWH?*
2. *What is your recommended treatment and monitoring plan based upon the patient visit on day 6?*
3. *What is the appropriate duration of warfarin therapy for this patient?*
4. *Three months later, the patient returns to the Anticoagulation Clinic for a 4-week follow-up assessment of her anticoagulation therapy. She has maintained a therapeutic INR on warfarin 5 mg daily for the past 2 months. Today her INR is measured at 5.6. What questions would you ask to assess this result?*
5. *Design a plan for the management and follow-up of this patient's supratherapeutic INR result.*

Self-Study Assignments

1. Discuss the issues surrounding therapeutic interchange of low-molecular-weight heparins.
2. In 2003, two randomized controlled trials evaluating long-term, low-intensity warfarin therapy for the prevention of recurrent VTE were published.[8,9] Based on your assessment of these studies, make a single conclusion that you would be able to share with your medical team. Your conclusion should be supported by your interpretation of the results of each study, identification of positive aspects of the studies, and any study design flaws or limitations.

Clinical Pearl

Unlike lepirudin, argatroban can result in prolongation of the INR. This INR elevation is linear with the argatroban dose administered. To assess warfarin's effect on the INR during concomitant therapy with argatroban, the argatroban infusion should be held for 4 to 6 hours prior to the INR measurement.[10]

References

1. Rosendaal FR, Koster T, Vandenbroucke JP, et al. High risk of thrombosis in patients homozygous for factor V Leiden (activated protein C resistance). Blood 1995;85:1504–1508.
2. Vandenbroucke JP, Koster T, Briet E, et al. Increased risk of venous thrombosis in oral-contraceptive users who are carriers of factor V Leiden mutation. Lancet 1994;344:1453–1457.

3. Tuprie AG, Chin BS, Lip GY. Venous thromboembolism: pathophysiology, clinical features, and prevention. BMJ 2002;325:887–890.
4. Buller HR, Davidson BL, Decousus H; Matisse Investigators. Subcutaneous fondaparinux versus intravenous unfractionated heparin in the initial treatment of pulmonary embolism. N Engl J Med 2003;349:1695–1702.
5. Eriksson H, Wahlander K, Gustafsson D, et al. A randomized, controlled, dose-guiding study of the oral direct thrombin inhibitor ximelagatran compared with standard therapy for the treatment of acute deep vein thrombosis: THRIVE I. J Thromb Haemost 2003;1:41–47.
6. Schiele F, Lindgaerde F, Eriksson H et al. Subcutaneous recombinant hirudin (HBW 023) versus intravenous sodium heparin in treatment of established acute deep vein thrombosis of the legs: a multicentre prospective dose-ranging randomized trial. International Multicentre Hirudin Study Group. Thromb Haemost 1997; 77:834–838.
7. Schulman S, Granqvist S, Holmstrom M, et al. The duration of oral anticoagulant therapy after a second episode of venous thromboembolism. The Duration of Anticoagulation Trial Study Group. N Engl J Med 1997;336:393–398.
8. Ridker PM, Goldhaber SZ, Danielson E, et al. Lon-term, low-intensity warfarin therapy for the prevention of recurrent venous thromboembolism. N Engl J Med 2003;348:1425–1434.
9. Kearon C, Ginsberg JS, Kovacs MJ, et al; Extended Low-Intensity Anticoagulation for Thrombo-Embolism Investigators. Comparison of low-intensity warfarin therapy with conventional-intensity warfarin for long-term prevention of recurrent venous thromboembolism. N Engl J Med 2003;349:631–639.
10. Dager WE, White RH. Treatment of heparin-induced thrombocytopenia. Ann Pharmacother 2002;136:489–503.

17 PULMONARY EMBOLISM

▶ The Clot Thickens (Level I)

Amy L. Seybert, PharmD
Ted L. Rice, MS, BCPS

▶ After completing this case study, students should be able to:

- Identify signs and symptoms of pulmonary embolism.
- Recognize risk factors predisposing a patient to pulmonary embolism.
- Design an appropriate pharmacotherapy regimen for the treatment of pulmonary embolism.
- Recommend patient education for anticoagulation therapy.

PATIENT PRESENTATION

Chief Complaint

"My chest hurts when I cough or take a deep breath."

HPI

Carol Pelungi is a 22 yo woman who presents to the ED following 12 days of illness. She states that approximately 2 weeks prior to admission she awoke with a sore throat, called her doctor, and received penicillin. The patient notes that in the morning of the second day of illness, she had acute onset of sharp, constant left-sided pleuritic chest pain and left-sided mid-back pain. The pain was made worse with lying flat, deep inspiration, and exercise. She became short of breath while talking. She also reports that pleuritic chest pain improves when seated. The patient has since had a mild cough productive of clear sputum tinged with bright red blood. Denies fever and chills. States the cough is worse in the morning and in the evening. Says she had been seen at an outside hospital and diagnosed with bronchitis and possible pericarditis. The penicillin was changed to ciprofloxacin and Percocet was added. She returned to the outside hospital as the pain persisted and prevented sleep. The ciprofloxacin dose was increased from 250 to 500 mg po BID. A review of records from the hospital reveal no ECG evidence of pericarditis. Chest x-ray performed 3 days prior to presentation here was read as normal by the radiologist. The patient presents complaining of continued pleuritic pain and cough.

PMH

Ovarian cyst that was drained 4 years ago

PSH

Tonsillectomy 2 years ago

SH

Denies tobacco, alcohol, or other drug use. She is a single student, living alone, no pets, and is sexually active.

ROS

No headache or blurred vision. No auditory complaints. No abdominal pain. No lightheadedness. No extremity or neurologic complaints. All other systems are negative, except for complaints noted in HPI.

Meds

Lo/Ovral × 3 years
Ciprofloxacin 500 mg po BID
Percocet 1 to 2 tabs po Q 6 H PRN

All

Sulfa → rash

PE

Gen

WDWN young woman who appears somewhat anxious.

VS

BP 110/64, HR 91, RR 24; T 37.9°C; Wt 63 kg; Ht 5′4″; O_2 sat 99% on room air

HEENT

Atraumatic; PERRLA; sclerae anicteric; TMs clear; oropharynx moist and pink, without erythema or exudate

Neck
No JVD; no lymphadenopathy; trachea midline; no thyromegaly

CV
RRR; no m/r/g

Lungs
There is some reproducible tenderness in the left lower costal margin; scattered inspiratory rales that clear with cough

Abd
Soft, NT/ND; normoactive bowel sounds

Rect
Normal sphincter tone; heme-negative stool

Ext
Well perfused, no CCE; normal distal pulses; negative Homan's sign; LE are without palpable cords, tenderness, and warmth; patient has a port wine stain on LLE

Neuro
A & O × 3; nonfocal exam; CN II–XII intact; DTRs 2+, Babinski ↓

Labs

Na 139 mEq/L	Hgb 11.5 g/dL	aPTT 24 sec
K 4.2 mEq/L	Hct 33.9%	PT 12.0 sec
Cl 103 mEq/L	Plt 284 × 10^3/mm^3	INR 0.9
CO_2 27 mEq/L	WBC 7.8 × 10^3/mm^3	Anticardiolipin IgG (–)
BUN 11 mg/dL	D-dimer 1500 ng/mL	Anticardiolipin IgM (–)
SCr 0.7 mg/dL		Factor V Leiden mutation: pending

PA Chest X-Ray
Demonstrates either a left lower lobe infiltrate notable at the costophrenic angle or perhaps a wedge infarct

ECG
Normal sinus rhythm at 91 bpm with a normal axis, normal intervals, and normal ST segments

Lower Extremity Venous Doppler Studies
Negative

Assessment
R/O PE vs. pneumonia

Plan
Initiate empiric treatment for both possible etiologies of the patient's complaints. Select and order either a helical computed tomography (CT) scan of the chest or a VQ scan with possible pulmonary angiogram.

▶ Questions

Problem Identification

1. a. *What risk factors for the development of a pulmonary embolus are present in this patient?*
   b. *What subjective and objective clinical evidence is suggestive of a pulmonary embolus in this patient? (See Figure 17–1).*

Desired Outcome

2. *What are the goals of therapy for this patient?*

Therapeutic Alternatives

3. a. *What nonpharmacologic therapeutic alternatives are available for the acute treatment of pulmonary embolism?*
   b. *What pharmacotherapeutic alternatives are available for the acute treatment of pulmonary embolism?*

Optimal Plan

4. a. *Design a pharmacotherapeutic plan for the empiric treatment of pulmonary embolism in this patient.*

▶ Clinical Course

In the ED, the patient was started on erythromycin for a possible pneumonia and the regimen that you recommended for empiric treatment of PE. She was then admitted for further work-up of possible PE.

V/Q scan report. Perfusion abnormality in the left base. There is a marked discrepancy between the perfusion defect and ventilation of the left lung, indicating an intermediate probability for pulmonary embolus (see *Figures 17–2* and *17–3*).

Pulmonary angiogram report. Consistent with pulmonary emboli in the left lower lobe pulmonary arteries (see *Figure 17–4*).

b. *Based on the new information, what additions or changes need to be made to the current therapy?*

Outcome Evaluation

5. a. *What monitoring parameters should be used to assess efficacy and toxicity of anticoagulation?*

▶ Clinical Course

Table 17–1 contains a summary of heparin/warfarin dosing (by the physician) in this patient.

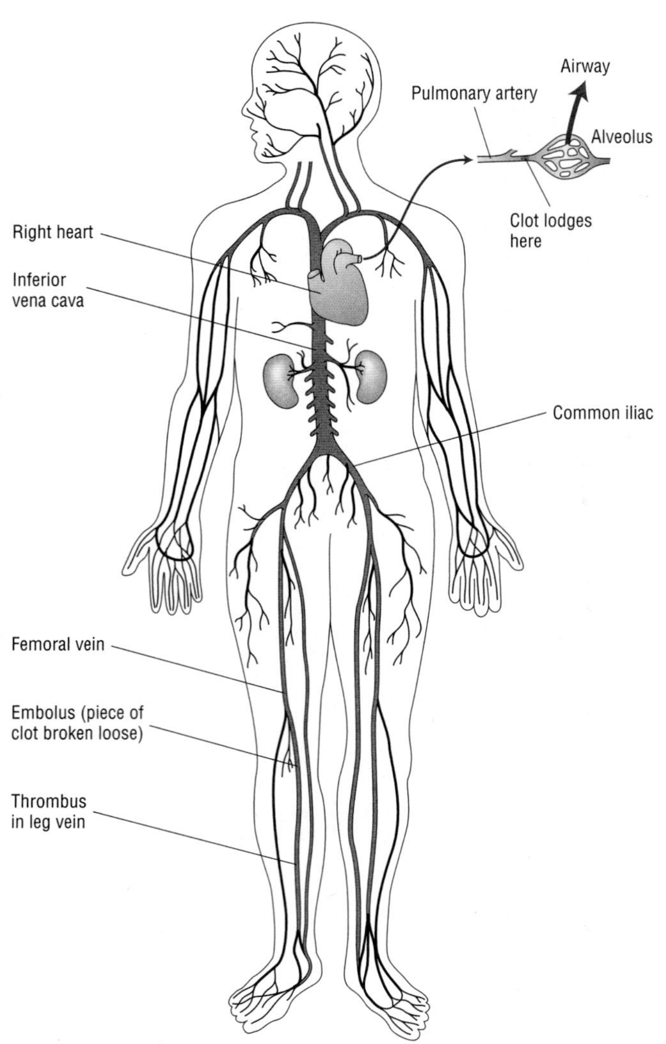

Figure 17–1. Development of pulmonary embolism. *(Reprinted with permission from Mulvihill ML. Human Diseases: A Systemic Approach, 4th ed. Norwalk, CT, Appleton & Lange, 1995:135.)*

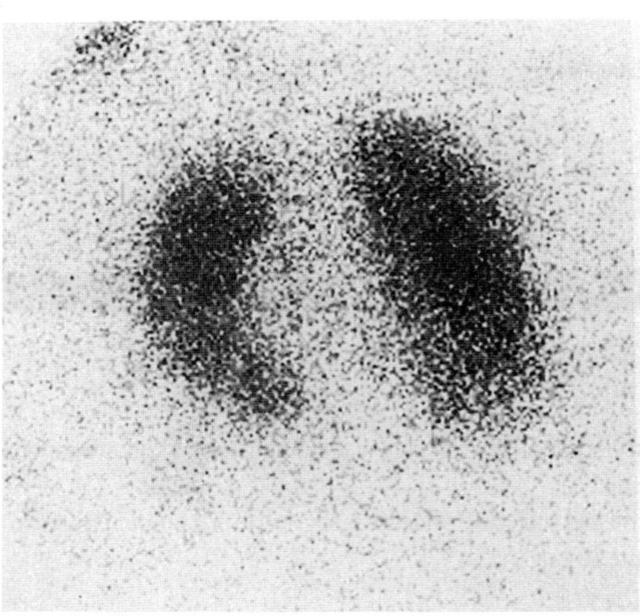

Figure 17–2. Xenon ventilation scan, posterior view. Asymmetry in ventilation due to elevation of diaphragm and decreased volume of the left hemithorax.

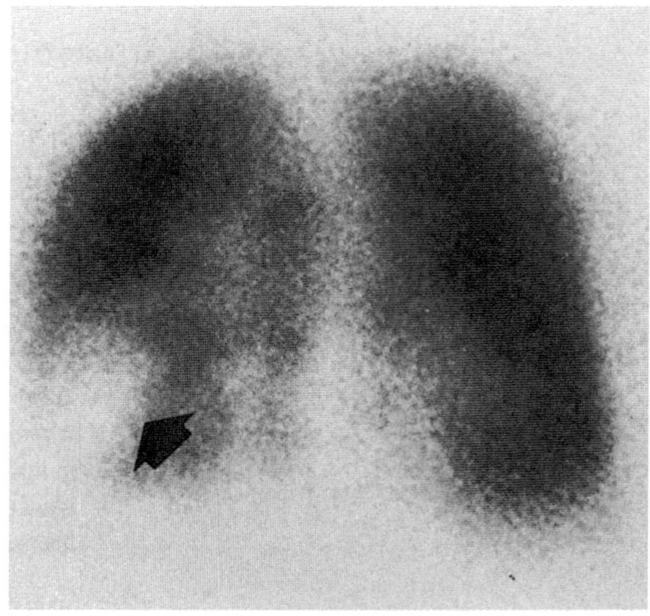

Figure 17–3. Perfusion lung scan, left posterior oblique view. Focal segmental perfusion defect at the left costophrenic angle, consistent with pulmonary embolism.

b. What is your assessment of the appropriateness of these interventions?

Patient Education

6. What medication information about warfarin should this patient receive at the time of hospital discharge?

► Self-Study Assignments

1. Prepare a written document that summarizes the primary literature on the use of thrombolytics in the treatment of pulmonary embolism.
2. Describe the alternative methods of birth control that could be used by this patient and provide patient education on these methods.

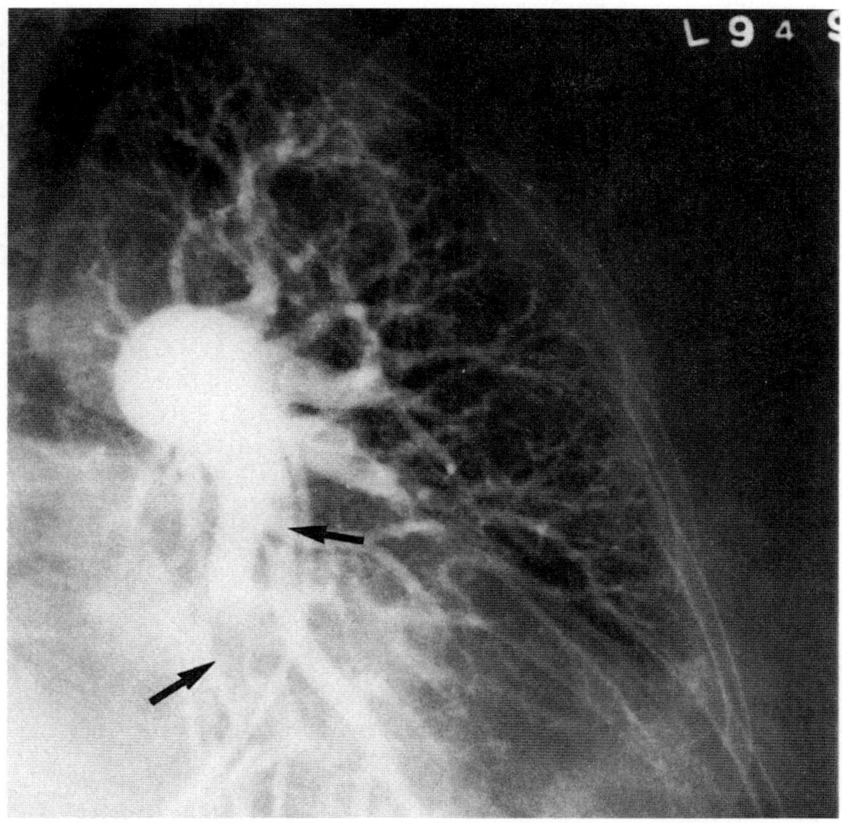

Figure 17–4. Anterior view of the left lung. Catheterization of the left pulmonary artery via the femoral vein and inferior vena cava. Emboli to basilar segments of the left lower lobe *(arrows)*.

▶ Clinical Pearl

Weight-based heparin dosing results in more rapid achievement of therapeutic aPTT than standard dosing and results in fewer recurrent episodes of venous thromboembolism.

References

1. Price H. Deaths from venous thromboembolism associated with combined oral contraceptives. Lancet 1997;350:450.
2. Rosing J, Tans G, Nicolaes GA, et al. Oral contraceptives and venous thrombosis: Different sensitivities to activated protein C in women using second- and third-generation oral contraceptives. Br J Haematol 1997;97:233–238.

TABLE 17–1. Heparin and Warfarin dosing as prescribed by the physician.

Hospital Day	Heparin Dose	Warfarin Dose	aPTT (sec)	PT (sec)/INR
1	5,000 units loading dose, then 1,100 units/h constant infusion	—	(6 h after starting heparin infusion) 32	12.1/1.0
2	1,500 units/h constant infusion, then rate decreased to 1,400 units/h constant infusion	5 mg	(6 h after change to 1,500 units/h) 90	Not done
			(6 h after change to 1,400 units/h) 76	Not done
3	1,300 units/h constant infusion	5 mg	(with AM labs) 70	14.4/1.2
4	1,300 units/h constant infusion	5 mg	(with AM labs) 68	19.0/1.7
5	Discontinued	5 mg	32	23.2/2.2

Reference ranges: aPTT 20–30 sec; PT 12 sec.

3. Goldhaber SZ, Grodstein F, Stampfer MJ, et al. A prospective study of risk factors for pulmonary embolism in women. JAMA 1997;277:642–645.
4. Fedullo PF, Tapson VF. The evaluation of suspected pulmonary embolism. N Engl J Med 2003;349:1247–1256.
5. Raschke RA, Reilly BM, Guidry JR, et al. The weight-based heparin dosing nomogram compared with a "standard care" nomogram. A randomized controlled trial. Ann Intern Med 1993;119:874–881.
6. Simonneau G, Sors H, Charbonnier B, et al. A comparison of low-molecular-weight heparin with unfractionated heparin for acute pulmonary embolism. N Engl J Med 1997;337:663–669.
7. Levine M, Gent M, Hirsh J, et al. A comparison of low-molecular-weight heparin administered primarily at home with unfractionated heparin administered in the hospital for proximal deep-vein thrombosis. N Engl J Med 1996;334:677–681.
8. Pinede L, Cucherat M, Duhaut P, et al. Optimal duration of anticoagulant therapy after an episode of venous thromboembolism. Blood Coagul Fibrinolysis 2000;11:701–707.
9. Hylek EM, Heiman H, Skates SJ, et al. Acetaminophen and other risk factors for excessive warfarin anticoagulation. JAMA 1998;279:657–662.

18 CHRONIC ANTICOAGULATION

▶ A Delicate Balance (Level II)

Beth Bryles Phillips, PharmD, BCPS

▶ After completing this case study, students should be able to:

- List the goals of oral anticoagulant therapy in preventing recurrent thromboembolism.
- Recognize common drug-drug interactions associated with warfarin therapy.
- Assess patients on chronic warfarin therapy.
- Appropriately educate patients about chronic warfarin therapy.

PATIENT PRESENTATION

Chief Complaint

"I'm here to get my blood drawn."

HPI

Nancy Hunt is an 84 yo woman with a history of recurrent DVT × 3, HTN, chronic venous stasis, and GERD who presents to the clinic for follow-up of her anticoagulant therapy. The most recent DVT occurred 3 years ago, at which time she was started on chronic warfarin therapy. She uses a pillbox to organize her warfarin tablets and states that she has not missed any doses in the last month. She reports having three nosebleeds over the past week, which is quite unusual for her. The nosebleeds lasted for about 5 minutes and the last one occurred 2 days ago. Otherwise, she denies any blood in the stool or urine, excessive bruising, severe headaches, abdominal pain, chest pain, shortness of breath, or pain in the lower extremities. She does not drink alcohol of any kind and she tries to avoid foods containing vitamin K. When asked if she has started any new medications, she reported that she has been taking cotrimoxazole DS (800/160 mg) BID for the past 6 days. She was seen in the ED last week for complaints of urinary frequency, urgency, and dysuria. She was diagnosed with a UTI and given a prescription for 7 days of cotrimoxazole. Except for the UTI, she denies being ill in the past month. She does report that her right leg sometimes aches and is swollen after standing on her feet all day. Her weight has been stable over the past year. Her use of OTC antacids (Pepcid AC) has increased over the last 3 weeks because of increasing heartburn. She states the heartburn has worsened despite wearing loose-fitting clothing, elevating the head of her bed, eating several small meals instead of three large meals, and avoiding chocolate, spicy, fatty, and caffeine-containing foods.

PMH

DVT × 3 (3, 15, and 40 years ago)
HTN
GERD
Chronic venous stasis of RLE
Obesity

FH

Mother died at age 75 due to CVA; father died at age 89 due to colon cancer; 2 children both living

SH

(–) EtOH; (–) Smoking

ROS

(+) For epistaxis and LE edema; (–) For CP, SOB, severe headaches, abdominal pain, leg pain, bruises, or change in color of stool or urine

Meds

Warfarin 5 mg po once daily
Hydrochlorothiazide 25 mg once daily
Calcium carbonate 500 mg 2 tablets po TID
Pepcid AC 10 mg po PRN

All

NKDA

PE

Gen

Pleasant obese woman in NAD

VS

BP 138/68, HR 72, RR 12, T 35.7°C; Wt 81.1 kg, Ht 5′5″

Skin

Normal turgor and color; warm; no rashes

HEENT

PERRLA, EOMI; disks flat; fundi with no hemorrhages or exudates

Neck/LN

No lymphadenopathy, thyromegaly, or carotid bruits

Lungs
CTA bilaterally

CV
RRR; normal S_1 and S_2; no S_3 or S_4; no m/r/g

Abd
Obese, non-tender, (+) BS

Genit/Rect
Deferred

Ext
1+ edema in right LE; no clubbing or cyanosis

Neuro
A & O × 3; CN II–XII intact; DTR 2+; Babinski negative

Labs

Date	PT/INR	Warfarin Dose
Today	56/5.4	5 mg daily
1 mo. ago	23/2.0	5 mg daily
2 mo. ago	26/2.3	5 mg daily
3 mo. ago	23/2.0	5 mg daily
4 mo. ago	22/2.0	5 mg daily
5 mo. ago	33/2.9	5 mg daily
6 mo. ago	28/2.5	5 mg daily

Assessment

Recurrent venous thromboembolism (VTE) requiring chronic anticoagulation with a target INR 2.5 (range, 2.0–3.0)
Supratherapeutic INR
GERD
Postphlebitic syndrome

▶ Questions

Problem Identification

1. a. *Identify this patient's drug therapy problems.*
   b. *Do any signs or symptoms indicate that this patient is over-anticoagulated?*
   c. *What questions would you ask this patient to assess her current warfarin therapy?*

Desired Outcome

2. *What are the goals of oral anticoagulant therapy in this patient?*

Therapeutic Alternatives

3. a. *What medications other than warfarin could be used to prevent recurrent thromboembolism in this patient?*
   b. *Because the patient is experiencing symptoms of GERD, the physician would like to prescribe a medication to relieve her symptoms. He would like to give her a prescription H_2-receptor antagonist (H_2RA) because she has had some relief with one on a PRN basis, but he is worried about drug interactions. What can you recommend that would be less likely to interact with her warfarin therapy?*

Optimal Plan

4. a. *Based on today's laboratory result, what is your recommendation for this patient's warfarin therapy?*
   b. *What can she do to help prevent supratherapeutic INRs in the future?*

Outcome Evaluation

5. *How will you monitor this patient's warfarin therapy?*

Patient Education

6. *What information should this patient know about her warfarin therapy?*

▶ Clinical Course

Upon return to clinic two days later, the patient reports she took her last dose of cotrimoxazole yesterday in the evening. Her PT and INR are 31 sec and 2.8, respectively. She reports no further episodes of epistaxis or any other symptoms of bleeding.

▶ Follow-Up Questions

1. *Based on this information, what are your recommendations for her warfarin therapy?*

▶ Self-Study Assignments

1. Vitamin K can be given to patients with excessive anticoagulation to lower INR values. When is it appropriate to consider vitamin K administration? Which route of administration (i.e., oral, intramuscular, or intravenous) would you recommend?
2. There are several mechanisms by which drugs may interact with warfarin. What are the major mechanisms of these interactions? Give examples of drugs that interact by each mechanism.
3. Anibiotics are a common cause of drug–drug interactions with warfarin. Which antibiotics are likely to interact with warfarin? Which antibiotics are reasonable alternatives to these drugs?

▶ Clinical Pearl

When assessing anticoagulant therapy in patients with a supratherapeutic INR, it is important to determine if the patient is experiencing any signs or symptoms of bleeding as this will guide therapeutic management.

References

1. Hirsh J, Dalen J, Anderson DR, et al. Oral anticoagulants: mechanism of action, clinical effectiveness, and optimal therapeutic range. Chest 2001;119(1 suppl): 8S–21S.
2. Ridker PM, Goldhaber SZ, Danielson E, et al; PREVENT Investigators. Long-term, low-intensity warfarin therapy for the prevention of recurrent venous thromboembolism. N Engl J Med 2003;348:1425–1434.
3. Kearon C, Ginsber JS, Kovacs MJ, et al; Extended Low-Intensity Anticoagulation for Thrombo-Embolism Investigators. Comparison of low-intensity warfarin therapy with conventional-intensity warfarin therapy for long-term prevention of recurrent venous thromboembolism. N Engl J Med 2003;349:631–9.
4. Hansten P, Wittkowsky. Warfarin drug interactions. In: Ansell JE, Wittkowsky AK, Oertel LB, eds. Managing Oral Anticoagulation Therapy: Clinical and Operational Guidelines. St. Louis, MO, Facts and Comparisons, 2003;35:1–35:14.
5. Cannegieter SC, Rosendaal FR, Wintzen AR, et al. Optimal oral anticoagulant therapy in patients with mechanical heart valves. N Engl J Med 1995;333:11–17.
6. The European Atrial Fibrillation Trial Study Group. Optimal oral anticoagulant therapy in patients with nonrheumatic atrial fibrillation and recent cerebral ischemia. N Engl J Med 1995;333:5–10.
7. Ansell J, Hirsh J, Dalen J, et al. Managing oral anticoagulant therapy. Chest 2001;119(1 suppl):22S–38S.

19 ISCHEMIC STROKE

► Brain Attack (Level II)

Susan R. Winkler, PharmD, BCPS

► After completing this case study, students should be able to:

- Identify and provide patient education on the risk factors for ischemic stroke.
- Discuss the various treatment options available for acute ischemic stroke.
- Develop an appropriate patient-specific therapeutic plan for the acute treatment of ischemic stroke.
- Develop an appropriate therapeutic plan for the outpatient management of a patient with ischemic stroke, including an appropriate agent to prevent stroke recurrence.

PATIENT PRESENTATION

Chief Complaint

"I can't move my right arm and leg."

HPI

John Gaines is a 76 yo man who was brought into the ED complaining of weakness in his right arm and leg and slurred speech. He stated that he awoke at 5:00 AM and went into the kitchen for a snack. He returned to bed but awoke at 6:00 AM and found he was unable to move his right arm and leg. This caused him to fall as he was trying to get out of bed. His daughter heard the "thump" and found him on the floor somewhat confused. She immediately called the paramedics. Approximately 2 weeks prior, he had had an episode in which he tried to speak but could not get the words out. This lasted about 2 minutes and did not recur.

PMH

Hypercholesterolemia
HTN
Seizure disorder (generalized tonic-clonic seizures of unknown etiology); last seizure 2 years ago

FH

Non-contributory

SH

Smokes 1 ppd × 54 years; h/o alcohol abuse

ROS

Slight headache; c/o double vision and slurred speech; no CP or SOB

Meds

Phenytoin 300 mg po at bedtime
Simvastatin 20 mg po at bedtime

All

NKDA

PE

Gen
WDWN right-handed, thin, African American man; appears slightly anxious

VS
BP 189/108, P 101, RR 22, T 37.2°C; Wt 76 kg, Ht 5′8″

Skin
Warm, dry

HEENT
PERRLA; no nystagmus; (+) diplopia; funduscopic exam reveals (+) arteriolar narrowing; no exudates, hemorrhages, or papilledema

Neck/LN
No carotid bruits; no lymphadenopathy; normal thyroid

Chest
Lungs clear

CV
RRR; S_1, S_2 normal, no S_3, (+) S_4

Abd
NT/ND; no HSM

Genit/Rect
Deferred

MS/Ext
Good pulses throughout; no CCE

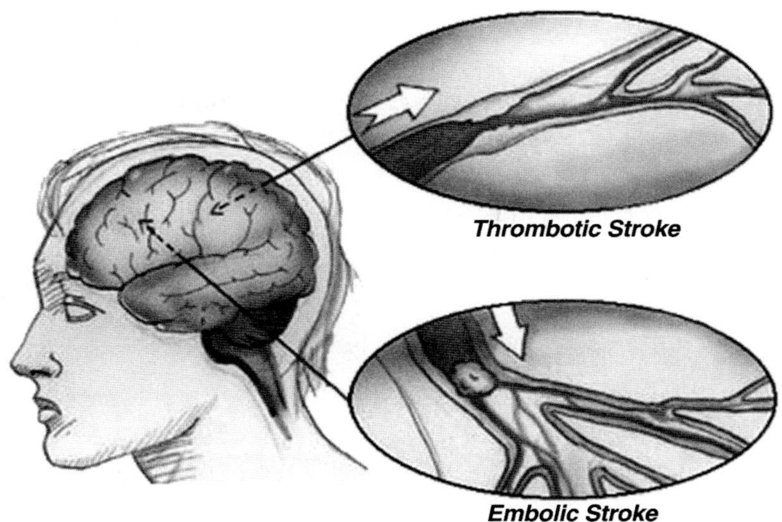

Figure 19–1. Ischemic strokes account for approximately 75% of all strokes. The cerebral infarction results either from a thrombus that forms in a blood vessel (thrombotic stroke) or an embolus that becomes lodged in a vessel (embolic stroke).

Neuro

A & O × 2, not oriented to time; (+) dysarthria; CN II–XII intact

Motor: RUE: 3/5 LUE: 5/5
RLE: 3/5 LLE: 5/5

Sensory: Normal pinprick and light touch

DTRs: 2+ throughout; Babinski normal

Labs

Na 143 mEq/L	Hgb 17.6 g/dL	Chol 333 mg/dL
K 4.2 mEq/L	Hct 51.5%	Phenytoin 18.6 mg/L
Cl 101 mEq/L	Plt 240 × 10^3/mm^3	
CO_2 21 mEq/L	WBC 6.7 × 10^3/mm^3	
BUN 23 mg/dL	PTT 22.0 sec	
SCr 1.2 mg/dL	PT 11.4 sec	
Glu 105 mg/dL		

ECG

Normal rhythm; tachycardia with a rate of 101 bpm

Brain CT Scan

Normal; no evidence of hemorrhage

Carotid Ultrasound

Normal flow

Assessment

Acute ischemic stroke (see Figure 19–1) in the left hemisphere in a 76 yo man with hypercholesterolemia, HTN, and seizure disorder

▶ Questions

Problem Identification

1. a. *Create a list of the patient's drug therapy problems.*
   b. *What non-modifiable and modifiable risk factors for acute ischemic stroke are present in this patient?*
   c. *Which signs and symptoms indicate the presence of an acute ischemic stroke?*

Desired Outcome

2. *What are the initial and long-term goals of pharmacotherapy in this case?*

Therapeutic Alternatives

3. a. *What nondrug therapies might be useful for this patient?*
   b. *What feasible pharmacotherapeutic alternatives are available for the treatment of acute ischemic stroke?*

Optimal Plan

4. *What initial therapy would you recommend for this patient?*

Outcome Evaluation

5. *What clinical and laboratory parameters are necessary to evaluate the chosen therapy for achievement of the desired effect and to detect or prevent adverse effects?*

► Clinical Course

The patient is now 5 days post-stroke and is ready for discharge from the hospital.

► Follow-Up Questions

1. *What nondrug therapies might be useful for preventing recurrent stroke in this patient?*
2. *a. What feasible pharmacotherapeutic alternatives are available for the primary prevention of acute ischemic stroke?*
   b. What feasible pharmacotherapeutic alternatives are available for the secondary prevention of acute ischemic stroke?
3. *What drug, dosage form, dose, schedule, and duration of therapy would you recommend for the secondary prevention of acute ischemic stroke in this patient?*
4. *How should the secondary prevention therapy you recommended be monitored?*
5. *In addition to the management of the ischemic stroke, what other therapeutic interventions should be undertaken for this patient?*

Patient Education

6. *What information should be provided to the patient about the secondary preventive therapy you recommended?*

► Self-Study Assignments

1. Perform a literature search and evaluate the role of ticlopidine, clopidogrel, and the combination of extended-release dipyridamole 200 mg plus immediate-release aspirin 25 mg (Aggrenox) in the secondary prevention of ischemic stroke.
2. Review the trials involving thrombolytics for acute stroke treatment. Pay particular attention to the inclusion and exclusion criteria used in each of the trials. Write a one-page essay summarizing your conclusions about the safety and efficacy of these agents for treatment of acute ischemic stroke.
3. Evaluate the role of statins for the primary and secondary prevention of acute ischemic stroke.

References

1. Camarata PJ, Heros RC, Latchaw RE. "Brain attack": The rationale for treating stroke as a medical emergency. Neurosurgery 1994;34:144–158.
2. National Institute of Neurological Disorders and Stroke rt-PA Stroke Study Group. Tissue plasminogen activator for acute ischemic stroke. N Engl J Med 1995;333:1581–1587.
3. Adams HP, Adams RJ, Brott T, et al. Guidelines for the early management of patients with ischemic stroke: A scientific statement from the Stroke Council of the American Stroke Association. Stroke 2003;34:1056–1083.
4. Furlan A, Higashida R, Wechsler L, et al. Intra-arterial prourokinase for acute ischemic stroke. The PROACT II study: A randomized controlled trial. Prolyse in acute cerebral thromboembolism. JAMA 1999;282:2003–2011.
5. Bath PM, Iddenden R, Bath FJ. Low-molecular-weight heparins and heparinoids in acute ischemic stroke: A meta-analysis of randomized controlled trials. Stroke 2000;31:1770–1778.
6. Sherman DG, Atkinson RP, Chippendale T, et al. Intravenous ancrod for treatment of acute ischemic stroke: the STAT study: A randomized controlled trial. Stroke Treatment with Ancrod Trial. JAMA 2000;283:2395–2403.
7. Straus SE, Majumdar SR, McAlister FA. New evidence for stroke prevention: Scientific review. JAMA 2002;288:1388–1395.
8. Chimowitz WI, Kokinos J, Strong J, et al. The warfarin–aspirin symptomatic intracranial disease study. Neurology 1995;45:1488–1493.
9. Diener HC, Cunha L, Forbes C, et al. European Stroke Prevention Study 2. Dipyridamole and acetylsalicylic acid in the secondary prevention of stroke. J Neurol Sci 1996;143:1–13.

20 HYPERLIPIDEMIA: PRIMARY PREVENTION

► Healthy as a Horse? (Level I)

Laurajo Ryan, PharmD, BCPS
Alicia M. Reese, PharmD, BCPS

► After completing this case study, students should be able to:

- Identify persons who should be screened for hyperlipidemia.
- Determine appropriate goal LDL, HDL, and total cholesterol concentrations for the primary prevention of coronary heart disease (CHD) in a patient with hyperlipidemia.
- Identify patients with hyperlipidemia who are candidates for therapeutic interventions.
- Outline a treatment regimen including both pharmacologic and lifestyle modifications for primary prevention of CHD in patients with hyperlipidemia.
- Design an appropriate monitoring plan for a patient receiving antihyperlipidemic therapy, including laboratory parameters and time intervals for follow-up.
- Educate patients on the goals, dosing, administration, adverse effects, and need for adherence to their treatment regimens.

PATIENT PRESENTATION

Chief Complaint

"My son had a heart attack and wants me to get checked."

HPI

Hillary Ingram-Banks is a 68 yo woman who has come to your clinic for a check-up and lipid profile. She had a cholesterol check performed 7 or 8 years ago, and she remembers that her total cholesterol then was around 225 mg/dL. At the time of her previous screening she was told to improve her diet and continue to exercise, but she was not given any specific instructions or follow-up plan. She has mild hypertension for which she takes a diuretic (when she remembers) and she swims for 2 hours every morning at the senior center. She does not smoke, and she tries to follow a "healthy diet."

PMH

HTN diagnosed 6 years ago
Hypothyroidism × 32 years

FH

Father died in MVA at age 54. Mother age 88, is alive with HTN and osteoporosis. She has three children, the eldest, age 47, was just released from the hospital following an acute MI. He had not been previously diagnosed with any health problems. Her daughters are twins aged 39 with no known health problems. The patient has a twin brother who is being treated for GERD. Her older brother is 71. He suffered a small stroke last year, and she knows that he has "stomach problems."

SH

She is very active, lives with her husband, and they do all of their own cooking, cleaning, and yard work. They are avid cooks and share a bottle of wine most evenings. She swims each morning before her volunteer session at the public library. She has never smoked cigarettes, although she does admit to experimenting with marijuana in the 1960's.

ROS

Patient states that she is "healthy as a horse" but does complain of occasional morning stiffness in her joints which is relieved by pain medicine she was given several years ago. She denies chest pain, SOB, melena, and recent changes in bowel or bladder habits. She is lactose intolerant; she experiences nausea, bloating and diarrhea after consuming dairy products. She went through menopause 25 years ago.

Meds

Chlorthalidone 12.5 mg po Q AM
Propoxyphene/acetaminophen 100/650mg 1–2 tabs Q 4–6 H PRN pain
MVI one tablet po daily

All

NKDA

PE

Gen
Patient is a well-groomed, thin, Caucasian woman in NAD

VS
BP 132/87, P 68, RR 13, T 37.2 °C, Ht 5′3″, Wt 116 lb.

Skin
Warm and dry, normal turgor, no lesions/tumors/moles

HEENT
PERRLA; EOMI; funduscopic exam deferred; TMs intact; oral mucosa clear

Neck/LN
Neck supple without lymphadenopathy; normal thyroid

Lungs/Thorax
CTA; no wheezes, crackles or rhonchi

CV
RRR, no murmurs, rubs, or gallops, normal S_1 and S_2; no S_3 or S_4

Abd
(+) BS, liver and spleen not palpable

Genit/Rect
Deferred

Ext
No pedal edema, pulses 2+ throughout

Neuro
No gross motor-sensory deficits present

Labs (fasting)

		Fasting Lipid Profile:
Na 141 mEq/L	Ca 9.6 mg/dL	TC 270 mg/dL
K 4.5 mEq/L	Mg 2.3 mEq/L	HDL 67 mg/dL
Cl 106 mEq/L	AST 35 U/L	LDL 172 mg/dL
CO_2 27 mEq/L	ALT 28 U/L	TG 150 mg/dL
BUN 15 mg/dL	T. bili 0.6 mg/dL	
SCr 0.9 mg/dL	T. prot 6.7 g/dL	
Glucose 88 mg/dL		

UA

Yellow, clear, SG 1.004, pH 5.4, (–) protein, (–) glucose, (–) ketones, (–) bilirubin, (–) blood, (–) nitrite, RBC 0/hpf, WBC 1/hpf, no bacteria, 1–5 epithelial cells

▶ Questions

Problem Identification

1. a. *Create a list of this patient's drug therapy problems.*
   b. *What signs, symptoms, and laboratory values indicate the presence and severity of hyperlipidemia in this patient?*
   c. *This patient has been diagnosed with hyperlipidemia. What are her risk factors (both modifiable and non-modifiable) for cardiovascular disease?*
   d. *Based on the data from the Framingham Heart Study, calculate this patient's 10-year cardiovascular risk.*
   e. *What are some potential sources of error in the measurement of the lipid profile?*

Desired Outcome

2. *List the goals of treatment for this patient.*

Therapeutic Alternatives

3. a. *What nonpharmacologic therapies are necessary for this patient to achieve and maintain adequate cholesterol control?*
   b. *What reasonable pharmacotherapeutic options are available for controlling this patient's hyperlipidemia?*

Optimal Plan

4. a. *Outline specific lifestyle modifications for this patient.*
   b. *Outline a specific and appropriate pharmacotherapeutic regimen for this patient, including drug, dose, dosage form, and schedule.*

Outcome Evaluation

5. *Based on your recommendations, what parameters should be monitored after initiating this regimen and throughout the treatment course? At what time intervals should these parameters be monitored?*

Patient Education

6. *Based on your recommendations, provide appropriate education for this patient.*

▶ Clinical Course

At Mrs. Banks' six-month follow-up appointment, she states that she has added kickboxing and weight training to her daily regimen. She has also decreased her daily intake of saturated fat and has been remembering to take her medications as prescribed. She states that she is experiencing mild, intermittent cramping in her calves. Her fasting lipid profile today is: TC 230 mg/dL, HDL 72 mg/dL, LDL 124 mg/dL, TG 170 mg/dL.

▶ Follow-Up Questions

1. *What instruction should you give the patient at this point in her therapy?*
2. *Suppose the patient now complains of intolerable adverse effects due to the current antihyperlipidemic drug therapy. Outline an appropriate change to her current therapy.*
3. *Suppose the patient is tolerating the current drug therapy but has not achieved the desired lipid control (TC 253 mg/dL, HDL 66 mg/dL, LDL 145 mg/dL, TG 210 mg/dL). Outline an appropriate change to her current therapy.*

▶ Self-Study Assignments

1. Outline the changes, if any, you would make to the pharmacotherapeutic regimen for this patient if she had presented at the initial visit with each of the following characteristics or history:
    - History of alcohol abuse
    - A younger pregnant woman
    - Diabetes mellitus
    - Chronic hepatitis C
    - End-stage renal disease, on hemodialysis three days per week
    - Low fixed income
2. Obtain product information and describe the proper use of a lipid profile monitor such as the Cholestech LDX monitor (Figure 20–1).

▶ Clinical Pearl

While using HMG-CoA reductase inhibitors, rare patients may experience symptoms of myopathy (weakness, soreness and cramping) without a rise in creatine kinase levels. In patients who experience these muscle symptoms despite dose reduction, therapy with an HMG-CoA reductase inhibitor should be discontinued.

References

1. Third Report of the National Cholesterol Education Program (NCEP) Expert Panel on Detection, Evaluation, and Treatment of High Blood Cholesterol in Adults (Adult Treatment Panel III) Executive Summary. National Institutes of Health NIH Publication No. 01–3670.
2. Pollare T, Lithell H, Berne C. A comparison of the effects of hydrochlorothiazide and captopril on glucose and lipid metabolism in patients with hypertension. N Engl J Med 1989;321:868–873.

A

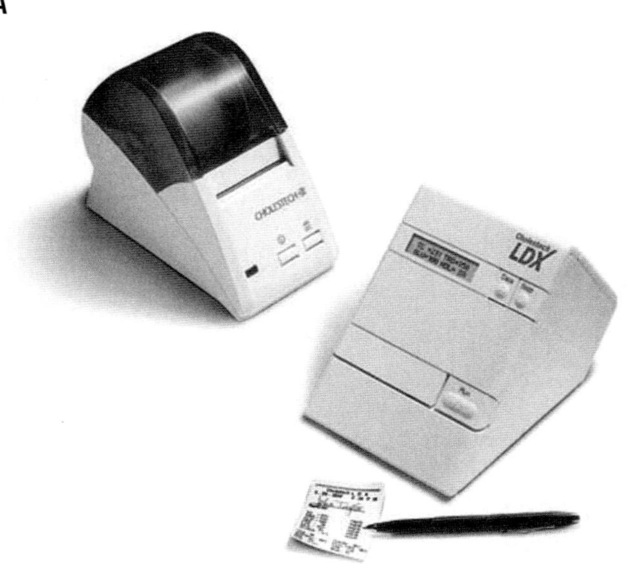

B

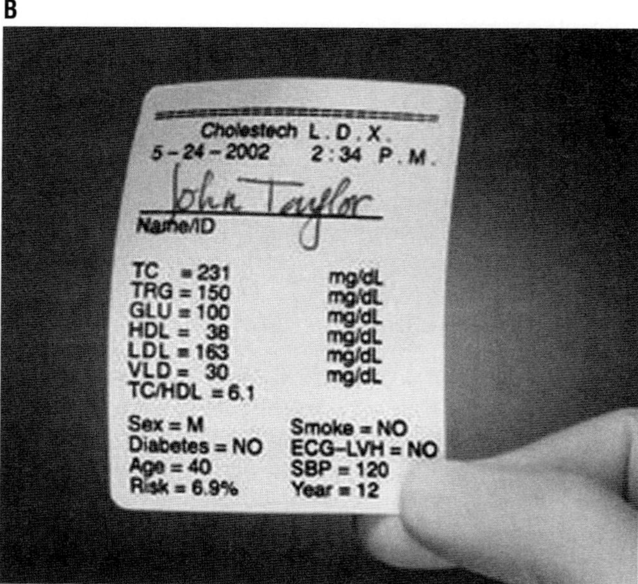

Figure 20–1. (A) The Cholestech LDX® analyzer. **(B)** Printout of sample lipid panel results from the LDX (not this patient). *(Cholestech LDX is a registered trademark of Cholestech Corporation.)*

3. Mosca L, Grundy SM, Judelson D, et al. Guide to preventive cardiology for women: AHA/ACC Scientific Statement: Consensus Panel Statement. Circulation 1999;99:2480–2484
4. Wong ND, Wilson PWF, Kannel WB. Serum cholesterol as a prognostic factor after myocardial infarction: the Framingham Study. Ann Intern Med 1991;115: 687–93.
5. Holme I. Cholesterol reduction and its impact on coronary artery disease and total mortality. Am J Cardiol 1995;76:10C–17C.
6. Hilleman DE, Wurdeman RL, Lenz TL. Therapeutic change of HMG-CoA reductase inhibitors in patients with coronary artery disease. Pharmacotherapy 2001;21:410–415.
7. Phillips PS, Haas RH, Bannykh S, et al. Statin-associated myopathy with normal creatine kinase levels. Ann Intern Med 2002;137:581–585.

21 HYPERLIPIDEMIA: SECONDARY PREVENTION

► A Sheltered Life (Level II)

Tina M. Hisel, PharmD, BCPS

► After completing this case study, students should be able to:

- Provide goal lipid levels for secondary prevention of cardiovascular events in patients with CHD.
- Choose appropriate antihyperlipidemic therapy for patients with CHD.
- Titrate drug doses based upon fasting lipid profiles to achieve appropriate goals.

PATIENT PRESENTATION

Chief Complaint

"I'm here to have my heart checked."

HPI

Michael Harper is a 54 yo male who was recently evaluated in the ED after experiencing chest pain while smoking a cigarette at home. He reports that he took a total of 3 sublingual nitroglycerin, separated by 5 minutes, with no relief. The pain was described as being substernal, heavy, and radiated to his neck and left arm. The chest pain was accompanied with diaphoresis and SOB. His ECG in the ED showed NSR and no acute ST segment changes from a previous ECG obtained 1 year earlier. Based on his significant cardiac history, the patient was admitted to the hospital for further evaluation. Three sets of biochemical cardiac markers were obtained and were WNL:

Date:	9/14	9/15	9/15
Time:	22:43	05:05	11:24
CK-MB	4.61	3.13	2.76
Troponin-I	<0.35	<0.35	<0.35

He remained asymptomatic during his admission and was discharged from the hospital the next day. He presents to the Family Practice clinic today for a 1-week F/U after his hospitalization. The patient has not been seen in the clinic for over 6 months as he did not appear for several scheduled appointments.

PMH

CHD; S/P MI and stent placement 7 years ago, S/P PTCA 1 year ago, and H/O multiple cardiac catheterizations
Chronic stable angina for the past 7 years, currently graded as Canadian CV Class II (angina with moderate exertion).
Dyslipidemia × 11 years
DM type 2 × ~11 years
HTN × 11 years
GERD
Obesity
Nicotine dependence × 30 years
H/O polysubstance abuse (cocaine, alcohol, marijuana, methamphetamine)

FH

Father died of lung CA in his 20's; Mother alive, with CHD and DM type 2. He is an only child.

SH

Continues cigarette smoking as described above. Denies current alcohol and illicit drug use. Unemployed for 4 months due to limitations in physical activity secondary to angina. Admits to lack of exercise and a sedentary lifestyle. He is not married and does not have any children. He currently lives at a homeless shelter. Based on his limited financial resources, he has been able to receive most of his medications at no cost from various pharmaceutical manufacturers. He states that he receives all of his meals from the homeless shelter and admits that he eats "whatever they have."

ROS

Positive for fatigue. All other systems negative except as described above.

Meds

EC aspirin 81 mg po daily
Lisinopril 10 mg po daily
Isosorbide mononitrate 60 mg po daily
Metoprolol XL 200 mg po daily
Simvastatin 40 mg po at bedtime
Nitroglycerin 0.4 mg SL PRN
Metformin XR 2,000 mg po Q PM
Glipizide XL 20 mg po Q AM
Esomeprazole 40 mg po daily

All

NKDA

PE

Gen

Patient is alert and oriented × 3 and in no distress.

VS
BP 143/93 mm Hg, P 68, RR 18, Wt 105 kg, Ht 70 inches, waist circumference 42 inches

Skin
Warm and moist with several tattoos throughout the body.

HEENT
Funduscopic exam reveals no hemorrhages or arterial narrowing.

Neck/LN
Neck is supple without lymphadenopathy or thyromegaly.

Lungs/Thorax
Clear to auscultation bilaterally without rales, rhonchi, or wheezes.

CV
Heart rate is regular with no appreciated murmurs or rubs; no S_3 or S_4.

Abd
Obese, soft, and nontender with normoactive bowel sounds and no organomegaly.

Ext
Free of cyanosis. There were no ulcerations or lesions on his feet.

Neuro
Cranial nerves II–XII were intact. Cerebellar exam was normal.

Labs
Labs drawn during his clinic visit today:

		Fasting Lipid Profile:
Na 144 mEq/L	AST 31 IU/L	T. chol 205 mg/dL
K 4.2 mEq/L	ALT 29 IU/L	HDL-C 29 mg/dL
Cl 101 mEq/L	Hgb A_{1c} 8.1%	LDL-C 121 mg/dL
CO_2 24 mEq/L	CRP <0.5 mg/L	Triglycerides 275 mg/dL
BUN 16 mg/dL		Non-HDL-C 176 mg/dL
SCr 0.8 mg/dL		
Glu 225 mg/dL		

UA
Urinary albumin-to-creatinine ratio: 58.4 mg/g

ECG
Evidence of an old anterior-lateral MI. No ST-segment changes evident

Assessment
Dyslipidemia
DM type 2 – uncontrolled
HTN – uncontrolled
Obesity
Tobacco abuse

Questions

Problem Identification

1. a. *Create a list of the patient's drug therapy problems.*
   b. *What signs, symptoms, or laboratory tests indicate the presence or severity of this individual's dyslipidemia?*
   c. *What additional information is needed to satisfactorily assess this patient?*

Desired Outcome

2. *What are the goals of pharmacotherapy in this case?*

Therapeutic Alternatives

3. a. *What nondrug therapies might be useful for this patient?*
   b. *What feasible pharmacotherapeutic alternatives are available for the treatment of this individual's dyslipidemia?*

Optimal Plan

4. *What drug, dose, schedule, and duration of therapy are best for the management of this patient's dyslipidemia?*

Outcome Evaluation

5. *Which parameters should be assessed to determine the effectiveness and adverse effects of the therapy you recommended?*

Patient Education

6. *What information should be provided to the patient to enhance compliance, ensure successful therapy, and minimize adverse effects?*

Clinical Course

The patient is initiated on the therapy you recommended and returns to the clinic in 4 weeks for a fasting lipid panel. The results are as follows: total cholesterol 179 mg/dL, TG 185 mg/dL, HDL-C 33 mg/dL, LDL-C 109 mg/dL, and non-HDL cholesterol 146 mg/dL.

Follow-Up Questions

1. *Based on this new information, what interventions, if any, should be made at this time?*
2. *Based on the patient's other comorbid conditions, what additional interventions should be made?*

Self-Study Assignments

1. Are elevations in triglycerides associated with adverse outcomes? What data support or refute these associations?
2. What role does C-reactive protein (CRP) play in cardiovascular risk assessment? Which patients are candidates for CRP measurements, and what is the significance of abnormal results?
3. Describe the educational information that you would provide to a patient who has been prescribed Pravigard® PAC (Figure 21–1).

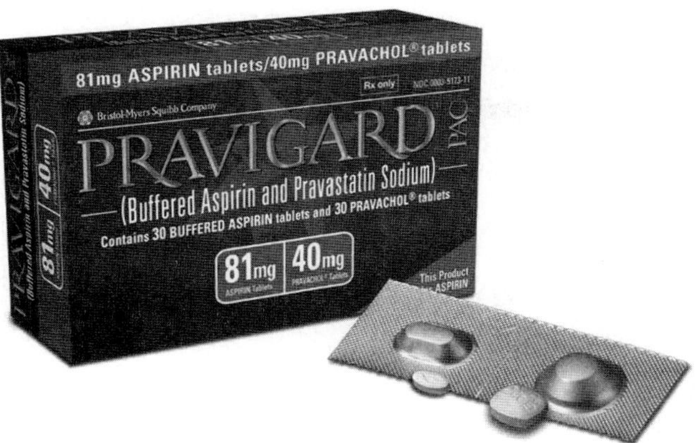

Figure 21–1. Pravigard PAC®, containing buffered aspirin 81 mg and pravastatin 40 mg per dose.

▶ Clinical Pearl

Each doubling of the dose of any HMG-CoA reductase inhibitor beyond the initial dose reduces LDL by an additional 6% from the results achieved with the starting dose. Therefore, subsequent dose increases can be estimated based on the patient's required LDL reduction.

References

1. Expert Panel on Detection, Evaluation, and Treatment of High Blood Cholesterol in Adults. Executive summary of the third report of the National Cholesterol Educational Program (NCEP) expert panel on detection, evaluation, and treatment of high blood cholesterol in adults (adult treatment panel III). JAMA 2001;285:2486–2497.
2. Jones P, Kafonek S, Laurora I, et al. Comparative dose efficacy study of atorvastatin versus simvastatin, pravastatin, lovastatin, and fluvastatin in patients with hypercholesterolemia (the CURVES study). Am J Cardiol 1998;81:582–587.
3. Scandinavian Simvastatin Survival Study Group. Randomised trial of cholesterol lowering in 4,444 patients with coronary heart disease: The Scandinavian Simvastatin Survival Study (4S). Lancet 1994;344:1383–1389.
4. Sacks FM, Pfeffer MA, Moye LA, et al. The effect of pravastatin on coronary events after myocardial infarction in patients with average cholesterol levels. Cholesterol and Recurrent Events Trial Investigators. N Engl J Med 1996;335:1001–1009.
5. The Long Term Intervention with Pravastatin in Ischemic Disease (LIPID) Study Group. Prevention of cardiovascular events and death with pravastatin in patients with coronary heart disease and a broad range of initial cholesterol levels. N Engl J Med 1999;339:1349–1357.
6. Coronary Drug Project Research Program. Clofibrate and niacin in coronary heart disease. JAMA 1975;231:360–381.

22 PERIPHERAL VASCULAR DISEASE

▶ The Colors of the Flag (Level III)

Susan D. Bear, BS, PharmD

▶ Upon completing this case study, the student should be able to:

- Describe the pathophysiology of Raynaud's phenomenon.
- Identify subjective and objective findings consistent with the diagnosis of Raynaud's phenomenon.
- Recommend appropriate nonpharmacologic strategies to minimize the frequency and severity of Raynaud's exacerbations.
- Select a pharmacotherapeutic regimen for the treatment of Raynaud's phenomenon.

PATIENT PRESENTATION

Chief Complaint

"I'm vomiting and I can't keep anything down. My joints hurt and I ache all over."

HPI

Jane Alexander is a 67 yo woman admitted with a 6-month history of weight loss, anorexia, fatigue, weakness, decreased appetite, intermittent diarrhea, GERD, and painful aching joints and fingers.

PMH

Type 2 DM × 4 years controlled with diet
Hypothyroidism
Chronic arthritis associated with systemic sclerosis
Hypercholesterolemia
HTN
S/P lumpectomy in 1988 for breast CA

FH

Mother died at age 98 from metastatic melanoma and father died at age 62 from an intracranial hemorrhage. Two sisters, both living, are hypothyroid. One brother who suffered from diabetes and PUD is deceased; another brother is living with heart disease.

SH

Widowed with one child; smoked 2 ppd × 52 years, (–) tobacco × 2 years; (–) alcohol

ROS

Positive for dry eyes, dry mouth, arthralgias of neck and hands, painful and swollen knees, headaches, reflux symptoms, diarrhea, vomiting, and fatigue. She notes numbness and pallor followed by cyanosis of fingers when exposed to cold and rubor and painful burning upon rewarming.

Meds

Synthroid 0.1 mg po once daily
Zocor 20 mg po once daily
Propranolol LA 60 mg po once daily
HCTZ 50 mg po once daily
Ibuprofen 200 mg po PRN (patient states 12–14 tablets per day in the last 10 to 14 days)

All

NKDA

PE

Gen
Awake, alert, tired-appearing female in NAD

VS
BP 150/95, HR 78, RR 18, T 36.6°C; Wt 57 kg, Ht 5′5″

Skin
Facial skin with diffuse tightening and absence of wrinkles, contracted oral orifice, smooth and shiny hidebound skin on fingers proximal to the MCP joint accompanied by decreased ROM, areas of ulceration on fingertips

HEENT
Dry mucous membranes; (–) JVD

Neck/LN
Neck painful to full ROM

Lungs/Thorax
CTA

Breasts
Atrophic; (–) lumps or masses; lumpectomy scar evident

CV
RRR with II/VI systolic murmur at the apex; (–) S_3, S_4 appreciated; carotids bilaterally palpable; (–) carotid bruit auscultated

Abd
Mild distention and epigastric tenderness; (+) bowel sounds

Genit/Rect
Hemoccult (+) × 3

Ext
(–) Rash, (+) limited ROM right shoulder, (+) swollen knees bilaterally

Neuro
Eye movements normal, facial muscle strength normal with normal facial symmetry, facial skin is taut, jaw opening and closing strength are normal, visual fields are full to confrontation. Skin on fingertips is quite taut and flexion is difficult; grip strength is adequate and finger abduction is fairly strong. Patient is able to ambulate slowly, but must use hands to push off to stand from a seated position.

Labs

Na 140 mEq/L	Hgb 9.2 g/dL	WBC 12.5 × 10^3/mm^3	CK 1530 IU/L	TSH 4.8 μIU/mL
K 4.1 mEq/L	Hct 29.1%	Neutros 84%	CK-MB 76 IU/L	Free T_4 0.7 ng/dL
Cl 100 mEq/L	Plt 585 × 10^3/mm^3	Lymphs 9%	% CK-MB 5%	B_{12} 144 pg/mL
CO_2 26 mEq/L	RBC 3.33 × 10^6/mm^3	Monos 7%	LDH 659 IU/L	Folate 2.5 ng/mL
BUN 55 mg/dL	MCV 87 μm^3	Eos 0%	Alb 2.8 g/dL	ESR 92 mm/hr
SCr 1.5 mg/dL	MCH 27.7 pg	Basos 0%	T. chol 150 mg/dL	RA 30 IU
Glu 139 mg/dL	MCHC 31.8 g/dL		Trig 140 mg/dL	ANA (+) speckled fluorescence
Ca 9.6 mg/dL			HbA_{1c} 6.2%	
Mg 1.8 mg/dL				
Phos 4.6 mg/dL				

HOSPITAL DAY 2 DIAGNOSTIC INFORMATION:

24-Hour Urine Collection
SCr 1.4 mg/dL, urine creatinine 45 mg/dL, total volume 1325 mL, CLcr 30 mL/min.

Other Tests
Urinalysis positive for 2+ protein; urine and stool cultures were negative.

Chest X-Ray
WNL

ECG
Sinus rhythm

Endoscopy
GE reflux with stricture, erosive esophagitis, diffuse gastritis, loss of mucosal folds, esophageal hypomotility

Colonoscopy
Diverticula noted in sigmoid and rectum; (–) internal hemorrhoids or polyps

EMG
Nerve conduction consistent with an active inflammatory process

Assessment
Systemic sclerosis
Raynaud's phenomenon
Renal insufficiency with proteinuria
GERD with stricture, erosive esophagitis, gastritis
Anemia with heme (–) stool
Malabsorption syndrome
Controlled hypercholesterolemia
Controlled primary hypothyroidism
Uncontrolled hypertension
Controlled type 2 DM

Questions

Problem Identification

1. a. *Create a list of this patient's drug therapy problems.*
   b. *What signs, symptoms, and laboratory values indicate the presence of Raynaud's phenomenon?*
   c. *Could any of the patient's peripheral vascular symptoms have been caused by drug therapy?*

Desired Outcome

2. *What are the goals of therapy for this patient's Raynaud's phenomenon?*

Therapeutic Alternatives

3. a. *What nondrug therapies could be useful for the treatment of the patient's painful symptoms associated with exacerbation of Raynaud's phenomenon?*
   b. *What pharmacotherapeutic alternatives are available for the treatment of Raynaud's phenomenon?*

Optimal Plan

4. a. *What drug, dose, and schedule would be most appropriate for treating this patient's Raynaud's phenomenon?*
   b. *In addition to initiating the new therapy that you suggested for control of the patient's peripheral vascular symptoms, what other adjustments would you make to her current drug regimen?*

Outcome Evaluation

5. *What clinical and laboratory parameters are needed to evaluate the patient's therapy for achievement of therapeutic goals and avoidance of adverse events?*

Patient Education

6. *What information should be provided to the patient to enhance compliance, ensure successful therapy, and minimize adverse events?*

Self-Study Assignments

1. Provide therapy recommendations for the treatment of chronic arthritis and the painful joint symptoms experienced by this patient with systemic sclerosis. Which drug classes should not be used? Why should they not be used?
2. Assume that the patient has used pseudoephedrine in the past for nasal congestion. If she requires a nasal decongestant in the future, should this drug be recommended?
3. Based on the NCEP III guidelines, how would this patient be risk stratified? What additional laboratory values would be needed to assist in the risk assessment and to determine if the patient is truly at goal LDL?

Clinical Pearl

An occupational therapist can be instrumental in instructing patients with Raynaud's phenomenon about lifestyle and occupational modifications to minimize trigger exposure and restrictions on activities of daily living.

References

1. Block JA, Sequeira W. Raynaud's Phenomenon. Lancet 2001;357:2042–2048.
2. Bolster MB, Maricq HR, Leff RL. Office evaluation and treatment of Raynaud's phenomenon. Cleve Clin J Med 1995;62:51–61.
3. Belch JJ, Ho M. Pharmacotherapy of Raynaud's phenomenon. Drugs 1996;52: 682–695.
4. Anderson ME, Moore TL, Hollis S, et al. Digital vascular response to topical glyceryl nitrate, as measured by laser Doppler imaging, in primary Raynaud's phenomenon and systemic sclerosis. Rheumatology 2002;41:324–328.
5. Dziadzio M, Denton CP, Smith R, et al. Losartan therapy for Raynaud's phenomenon and scleroderma: Clinical and biochemical findings in a fifteen-week, randomized, parallel-group, controlled trial. Arthritis Rheum 1999;42: 2646–2655.
6. Ferro CJ, Webb DJ. The clinical potential of endothelin receptor antagonists in cardiovascular medicine. Drugs 1996;51:12–27.
7. Belch JJ, Capell HA, Cooke ED, et al. Oral iloprost as a treatment for Raynaud's syndrome: A double blind multicentre placebo controlled study. Ann Rheum Dis 1995;54:197–200.
8. Coleiro B, Marshall SE, Denton CP, et al. Treatment of Raynaud's phenomenon with the selective serotonin reuptake inhibitor fluoxetine. Rheumatology 2001; 40:1038–1043.
9. Rey J, Cretel E, Jean R, et al. Serotonin reuptake inhibitors, Raynaud's phenomenon and erythromelalgia. Rheumatology 2003;42:601–602.
10. Dessein PH, Morrison RC, Lamparelli RD, et al. Triiodothyronine treatment for Raynaud's phenomenon: A controlled trial. J Rheumatol 1990;17:1025–1028.

23 HYPOVOLEMIC SHOCK

A Glass Half Full (Level II)

Brian L. Erstad, PharmD, FCCP, FCCM, FASHP

After completing this case study, students should be able to:

- Develop a plan for implementing fluid or medication therapies for treating a patient in the initial stages of shock.
- Outline the major parameters used to monitor hypovolemic shock and its treatment.
- List the major disadvantage of using isolated hemodynamic recordings, such as blood pressure measurements, for monitoring the progression of shock.
- Compare and contrast fluids and medications used for treating hypovolemic shock.

PATIENT PRESENTATION

Chief Complaint

Bill Hobbs is a 47 yo man admitted for fatigue and diarrhea.

HPI

Five days PTA, Mr. Hobbs had become nauseated and did not feel like eating. Although the nausea resolved after a couple of days, he began to have diarrhea, which led him to continue his avoidance of food intake. The diarrhea, in conjunction with increasing fatigue and lack of substantial fluid intake for 2 days, prompted his physician to hospitalize him for further evaluation and to temporarily stop his tacrolimus therapy (10 mg po BID); other medications were continued.

PMH

- S/P orthotopic liver transplantation 6 months PTA for sarcoidosis involving the liver; the transplant was complicated by an adrenal vein hemorrhage that required reoperation for ligation
- Diabetes mellitus posttransplant
- Moderate cellular rejection on recent biopsy

FH

Noncontributory

SH

Does not smoke, drink EtOH, or use illicit drugs

ROS

Patient has had a recent increase in weight over the past month (6 kg), although this has decreased by 2 kg in the past few days. Hearing is intact with no vertigo. No dizziness or fainting episodes. Colorless sputum. No chest pain or dyspnea, but heart has been "racing." Has had diarrhea for 3 days; no vomiting, abdominal pain, or cramping. No musculoskeletal pain or cramping.

Meds

- Prednisone 2.5 mg po every M, W, F
- Mycophenolate mofetil 250 mg po once daily
- Fluconazole 50 mg po every M, W, F
- Acyclovir 400 mg po BID
- Famotidine 20 mg po BID
- Spironolactone 200 mg po once daily

All

NKDA

PE

Gen

WDWN, but somewhat anxious man in mild distress

VS

BP 84/58 (baseline 135/85), but possible orthostatic changes not determined, HR 132 (baseline 80), RR 16, T 37°C; admission wt 78 kg

Skin

Pale color (including nail beds) and dry, but not cyanotic; no lesions

HEENT

Normal scalp/skull; conjunctiva pale and dry with clear sclerae; PERRLA, dry oral mucosa; remainder of ophthalmologic exam not performed

Neck/LN

Supple, no lymphadenopathy or thyromegaly

Lungs/Thorax

Decreased breath sounds since last exam

CV

RRR; S_1 and S_2 normal; apical pulse difficult to palpate; no m/r/g

Abd

Symmetrical with bulging flanks as a result of recent marked increase in ascites; palpable fluid wave; bowel sounds present; no tenderness or masses; scar from transplant evident

Genit/Rect

Normal male genitalia; prostate smooth, not enlarged; no hemorrhoids noted; stool heme (–)

MS/Ext

No deformities with normal ROM; 2–3+ leg edema; no ulcers or tenderness

Neuro

Mild muscular atrophy with weak grip strength; CN II–XII intact; 2+ reflexes throughout; Babinski downgoing

Labs

Na 118 mEq/L	Hgb 11.9 g/dL	Phos 6.3 mg/dL
K 4.3 mEq/L	Hct 34.3%	AST 86 IU/L
Cl 83 mEq/L	Plt $51 \times 10^3/mm^3$	ALT 59 IU/L
CO_2 25 mEq/L	WBC $6.3 \times 10^3/mm^3$	T. bili 1.6 mg/dL
BUN 66 mg/dL	PT 12.1 sec	Alk phos 83 IU/L
SCr 3.0 mg/dL	PTT 33 sec	
Glu 137 mg/dL		

Other Test Results

- I/O 1260/350 for first 14 hours of hospitalization
- Ultrasound of abdomen ordered with possible paracentesis planned
- Stool cultures negative for gastroenteric pathogens; O & P negative; negative *Clostridium difficile* titer
- Normal response to synthetic ACTH adrenal stimulation testing

Assessment

Volume depletion, possible nephrotoxicity from medications

Problem Identification

1. a. *Create a list of the patient's drug therapy problems.*
   b. *What information (signs, symptoms, laboratory values) indicates the presence or severity of hypovolemic shock?*

Desired Outcome

2. *What are the goals of pharmacotherapy in this case?*

Therapeutic Alternatives

3. a. *What nondrug therapies might be useful for this patient?*
   b. *What feasible pharmacotherapeutic alternatives are available for treatment of shock and the associated laboratory alterations?*

Optimal Plan

4. *What drug, dosage form, dose, schedule, and duration of therapy are best for this patient?*

Outcome Evaluation

5. *What clinical and laboratory parameters are necessary to evaluate the therapy for achievement of the desired therapeutic outcome and to detect or prevent adverse events?*

Patient Education

6. *What information should be provided to the patient to enhance compliance, ensure successful therapy, and minimize adverse effects?*

▶ Clinical Course

All cultures were negative and there was no other evidence of infection. However, the patient had a complicated clinical course since inadequate fluids were given because of concerns about fluid overload. Paracenteses were performed every few days to remove accumulated ascitic fluid; this led to further vascular depletion with decreased renal perfusion. After approximately 10 days, the patient had to be admitted to the ICU for renal failure precipitated by inadequate vascular expansion. However, there was no evidence of progressive organ rejection after resolution of the renal failure, and the tacrolimus was eventually restarted.

▶ Follow-Up Questions

1. *Why might this patient have changes in urine output, heart rate, and other parameters that are consistent with volume depletion even though he has edema on physical examination and his admission weight was indicative of volume overload?*

▶ Clinical Pearl

Although interstitial fluid accumulation in the lungs possibly leading to pulmonary edema is a concern, other sites of fluid accumulation such as the legs should not preclude adequate intravascular expansion, which is necessary to avoid organ hypoperfusion and subsequent dysfunction.

▶ Self-Study Assignments

1. Search the literature and be able to discuss the results of comparative trials involving crystalloids and colloids for plasma expansion.
2. Write a two-page report that compares the advantages and limitations of each type of fluid for the plasma expansion indication.

References

1. Fox DL, Vermeulen LC. UHC Technology Assessment: Albumin, Nonprotein Colloid, and Crystalloid Solutions. Oak Brook, IL, University HealthSystem Consortium, May 2000.
2. Choi PT, Yip G, Quinonez LG, et al. Crystalloids vs. colloids in fluid resuscitation: A systematic review. Crit Care Med 1999;27:200–210.
3. Finfer S, Bellomo R, Boyce N, et al; SAFE Study Investigators. A comparison of albumin and saline for fluid resuscitation in the intensive care unit. N Engl J Med 2004;350:2247–2256.

SECTION 3

Respiratory Disorders

24 ACUTE ASTHMA

▶ Attack of the Smokey Neighbor (Level I)

Tia D. Eddy, PharmD
Daniel T. Kennedy, PharmD, BCPS
Ralph E. Small, PharmD, FCCP, FASHP, FAPhA

▶ After completing this case study, students should be able to:

- Recognize the signs and symptoms of acute asthma.
- Describe pharmacologic and nonpharmacologic alternatives for the treatment of acute asthma according to patient signs and symptoms.
- Develop a pharmaceutical care plan for the treatment of acute asthma, including therapeutic endpoints, dosage regimens, monitoring parameters, and follow-up.
- Provide discharge education on the appropriate use of metered dose inhalers and peak flow meters as well as the role of different medications for the treatment of asthma.

PATIENT PRESENTATION

Chief Complaint

"Forty-five minutes ago, I started to get short of breath and my medicine doesn't help."

HPI

Jack Russell is a 56 yo man with a significant H/O HTN, asthma, and hyperlipidemia. He presents to the ED today with a H/O shortness of breath for 45 minutes and lower extremity muscle pain for 6 months. He reports that he was feeling well and in his usual state of health until about an hour ago, when he smelled something burning. Twenty minutes later, he began to feel short of breath and was wheezing. He tried using his albuterol inhaler without success, so he proceeded to the ED. When he arrived at the ED, he was tachycardic, tachypneic, wheezing, and hypertensive. His O_2 sats on RA were 87% to 88%. His last admission for an asthma attack was 2 months ago. He states that he has "felt better than he has in 10 years" with the addition of salmeterol to his asthma medications from that hospitalization. He denies recent cold or URI and says the albuterol usually helps him when he feels an attack coming on. When asked about triggers, he indicates that cigarette smoke, fireplace smoke, scented candles, and incense trigger his asthma. He suspects someone in his apartment building was burning something that triggered his asthma. In the ED, he was given 2 albuterol nebs (5 mg each, see Figure 24–1), and 125 mg IV Solu-Medrol. His chest x-ray was negative for any acute processes. He was noted to be hypoxic by measurements taken in the ED on 2L oxygen and had difficulty speaking in complete sentences. Patient was admitted to the hospital for further treatment.

PMH

Asthma; no previous intubations
GERD with Barrett's esophagus
Hyperlipidemia
Asthma
HTN
S/P Broken right forearm 2 years ago
S/P Renal stones 9 years ago
S/P ureteral stent placement then removal after shock wave lithotripsy

FH

Noncontributory

SH

Divorced with three children; lives alone in an apartment. Works as a carpenter. Denies current use or h/o tobacco, EtOH, IVDA, or crack/cocaine.

ROS

(+) chest tightness, labored breathing, increased heart rate and wheezing upon presentation to the ED. (+) leg muscle pain and weakness. No complaints of fatigue or fever.

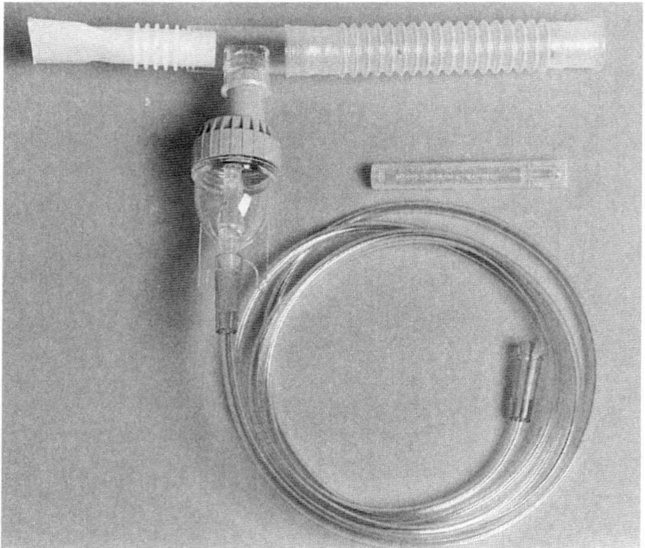

Figure 24–1. Nebulizer device used to administer inhaled β_2-agonist pharmacotherapy. The tubing is attached to an air compressor that takes air from the room and creates a high-pressure stream. An ultrasonic nebulizer uses sound vibrations instead of compressed air to create the aerosol. The liquid drug is placed into the plastic cup. Air from the compressor converts the drug into an aerosol mist that the patient inhales through the mouthpiece over 5 to 30 minutes until the liquid drug disappears. A mask can be worn by children or others who cannot hold the mouthpiece tightly in their lips.

Meds

- Albuterol MDI 2 puffs BID–QID PRN
- Salmeterol Diskus 1 inhalation QID
- Ipratropium bromide MDI 2 puffs QID
- Niacin 1500 mg po BID
- Nifedipine 60 mg SA po once daily
- Lovastatin 20 mg po at bedtime
- Aspirin 325 mg EC 1 po daily
- Lisinopril 10 mg po daily
- Lansoprazole 30 mg po BID

All

NKDA

PE

Gen

WDWN man in acute respiratory distress, labored breathing, using accessory muscles

VS

BP 155/92, P 112, T 37.8°C, R 24, pulsus paradoxus 14 mm Hg, Wt 68 kg, Ht 5′6″

HEENT

NC/AT, PEERLA, EOMI, hearing intact bilaterally, auditory canals without lesions or obstruction, septum midline, mucosa pink and moist, difficulty speaking

Neck

Trachea midline, neck supple, no JVD or lymphadenopathy

Respiratory

Expanded rib cage with accessory muscle use, decreased breath sounds bilaterally with high-pitched end-expiratory wheezes, tight air movement.

Cardiac

RRR, S_1 and S_2 WNL, no m/r/g. No bruits on examination.

Abdomen

Bowel sounds present, soft, non-tender, non-distended

Vascular

Pulses 2+ bilaterally in all extremities, no varicose veins noted.

Neuro

Alert and oriented × 3, CN II–XII grossly intact, DTRs 2+

Labs

Na 136.0 mEq/L	Hgb 14.5 g/dL	AST 26 IU/L	Ca 8.8 mg/dL
K 3.1 mEq/L	Hct 42.3%	ALT 24 IU/L	Mg 2.1 mg/dL
Cl 107 mEq/L	RBC 4.52 × 10^6/mm^3	Alk Phos 100 IU/L	Phos 2.9 mg/dL
CO_2 27 mEq/L	Plt 292 × 10^3/mm^3	T. bili 1.4 mg/dL	
BUN 12 mg/dL	WBC 8.9 × 10^3/mm^3	Alb 3.7 g/dL	
SCr 1.0 mg/dL	MCV 82.1 μm^3	INR 1.1	
Glu 114 mg/dL	MCH 27.6 pg		
	MCHC 33.7 g/dL		

Peak Flow

175 L/min (baseline at last office visit 480 L/min). Patient monitors peak flow once a week at home. One year ago: PFT = FEV_1 2.94 (85%), FEV_1/FVC 0.90.

ABG

pH 7.42, pCO_2 42 mm Hg, pO_2 88 mm Hg, HCO_3^- 23 mEq/L, O_2 sat 90% on 100% FIO_2

ECG

Sinus tachycardia

Chest X-Ray

No acute processes, no masses

Assessment

This is a 56 yo man admitted for an exacerbation of asthma probably secondary to exposure to smoke.

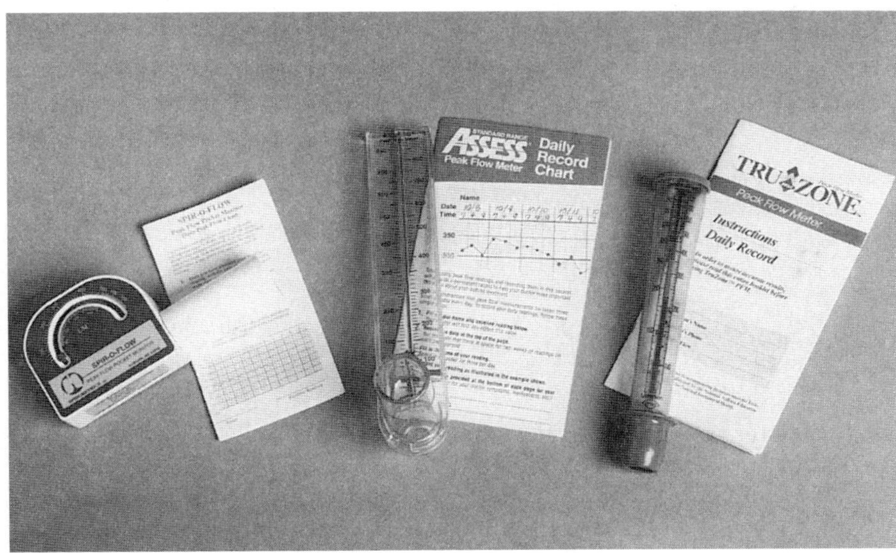

Figure 24–2. Examples of peak flow meters for assessing asthma control.

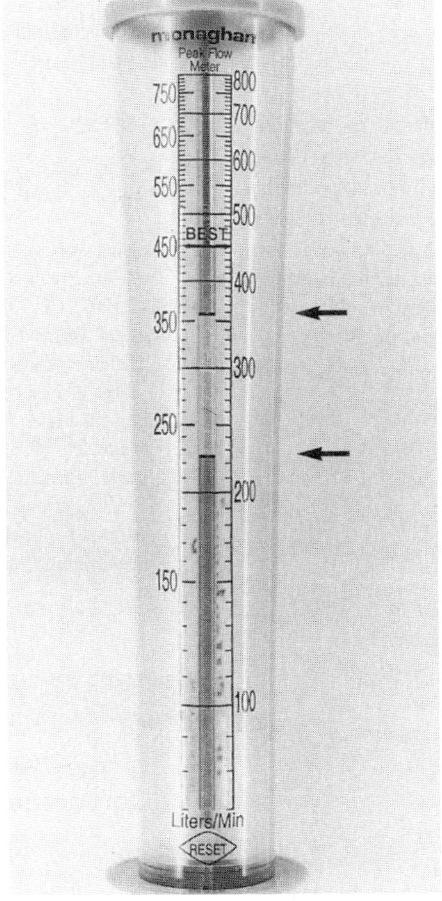

Figure 24–3. Scale of a peak flow meter. A reading in the green zone (above the top arrow) indicates that breathing is at least 80% of the patient's maximum flow rate (450 L/min). The yellow zone (between the arrows) indicates 50% to 79%, and the red zone (below the bottom arrow) indicates <50% of the patient's maximum flow rate.

Questions

Problem Identification

1. a. *Create a list of the patient's drug therapy problems.*
   b. *What information (signs, symptoms, laboratory values) indicates the severity of the acute asthma attack?*

Desired Outcome

2. *What are the acute goals of pharmacotherapy in this case?*

Therapeutic Alternatives

3. a. *What non-drug therapies might be useful for this patient?*
   b. *What feasible pharmacotherapeutic alternatives are available for the treatment of acute asthma?*

Optimal Plan

4. a. *What drug, dosage form, dose, schedule, and duration of therapy are best for this patient's acute asthma attack?*
   b. *What other pharmacotherapy would you recommend in the acute treatment of this patient?*

Clinical Course

Within 6 hours of admission, the patient had regained a normal breathing pattern. Upon further questioning, Mr. Russell reports poor sleep due to waking 1 to 3 times per night for SOB. He sleeps with his head elevated on two pillows to avoid SOB. He also reports sharing his bed with his 2 cats. The patient's PEF increased to >70% and was maintained for >24 hours with the plan you recommended. Only mild wheezing and minimal shortness of breath were reported, and the patient stated, "I feel much better." As treatment continued, the patient further improved and the decision was made to discharge the patient to home.

c. *What pharmacotherapy would you recommend for this patient upon discharge?*

Outcome Evaluation

a. *What are the long-term goals of asthma therapy for this patient?*
b. *What clinical parameters will you monitor to assess the efficacy of asthma pharmacotherapy in this patient?*
c. *What will you monitor to assess the side effects of drug therapy?*
d. *What laboratory tests or other objective measures are necessary to monitor therapy?*

Patient Education

6. a. *Describe the information that should be provided to this patient regarding inhaler technique, the differences between quick-relief and long-term-control medications, and avoiding triggers.*
   b. *Describe how you would explain to a patient how to use a peak flow meter (see Figures 24–2 and 24–3).*

Follow-Up Questions

1. *What preventive measures should be assessed to control the factors contributing to this patient's asthma severity?*

Self-Study Assignments

1. Discuss the mixed picture in respiratory disorders (i.e., COPD, asthma, chronic bronchitis) and how each component relates to the others.
2. Research the efficacy of peak flow-based action plans versus symptom-based action plans.
3. Conduct a literature search to determine the relationship between asthma and GERD.
4. Research the efficacy of albuterol via nebulization versus MDI in acute asthma.

Clinical Pearl

For proper treatment of an asthmatic patient, it is important to re-educate at every opportunity: (a) the role of each inhaler (rescue and scheduled) and when to use it, and (b) the proper technique for maximum efficacy.

References

1. Faulkner MA, Hilleman DE. Pharmacologic treatment of chronic obstructive pulmonary disease: past, present, and future. Pharmacotherapy 2003;23:1300–1315.
2. National Asthma Education and Prevention Program. Expert Panel Report: Guidelines for the Diagnosis and Management of Asthma Update on Selected Topics 2002. J Allergy Clin Immunol 2002;110(5 suppl):S141–S219.
3. National Asthma Education and Prevention Program. Expert Panel Report 2: Guidelines for the Diagnosis and Management of Asthma. Bethesda, MD, National Institutes of Health, 1997. www.nhlbi.nih.gov/guidelines/asthma/asthgdln.htm. Accessed March 14, 2003.
4. Williams DM. Clinical considerations in the use of inhaled corticosteroids for asthma. Pharmacotherapy 2001;21(suppl):38S–48S.
5. Mitchell C, Jenkins C, Scicchitano R, et al. Formoterol (Foradil) and medium-high doses of inhaled corticosteroids are more effective than high doses of corticosteroids in moderate-to-severe asthma. Pulm Pharmacol Ther 2003;16:229–306.

25 CHRONIC ASTHMA

A Tale of Cats, Colds, Compliance, and Corticosteroids (Level I)

Dennis M. Williams, PharmD, FASHP, FCCP, BCPS

After completing this case study, students should be able to:

- Recognize signs and symptoms of uncontrolled asthma.
- Identify potential causes of poorly controlled asthma.

- Describe a self-management plan and action plan for improving control of asthma.
- Recommend a rational, comprehensive approach to management of persistent asthma.

PATIENT PRESENTATION

Chief Complaint

"I am going to be kicked off my school's softball team because I have missed so much practice due to my asthma."

HPI

Randi Kerney is a 19 yo woman who presents to the student health service physician complaining of increased shortness of breath and wheezing. This episode began with a head cold about 4 days ago, and she has gotten progressively worse. When she first developed symptoms she began monitoring her peak flow rates twice daily and implemented an action plan that included frequent albuterol nebulizations. However, she has gotten progressively worse and has missed school and softball practice the last 2 days. Her peak flows for the past 4 days have ranged from 190 to 250 L/min and usually have been at the lower end of that range in the morning.

PMH

Moderate persistent asthma for 14 years; she has been hospitalized twice in the past 2 years for asthma exacerbations and has been to the ED 4 times in the past 7 months

Perennial allergic rhinitis

FH

Both parents living; mother 46 yo with HTN and a childhood history of asthma; father 52 yo with COPD (40 pack–year smoking history); one sibling age 24 in apparent good health except for seasonal allergies

SH

No alcohol or tobacco use; sexually active for 2 years with the same boyfriend. Patient is a college sophomore and chemistry major, and lives in a dormitory with her non-smoking roommate. Her boyfriend has a cat in his apartment.

Meds

Proventil HFA MDI 2 puffs PRN

Flovent MDI 220 mcg 2 puffs BID

Rhinocort aqua 1 spray each nostril once daily

Albuterol nebulization 2.5 mg in 3 mL NS PRN

Ortho Novum 7/7/7 one tablet po once daily

Compliance with above regimen is variable except for her OC, which she refills regularly on schedule. She indicates that she is typically a few weeks late on the steroid nasal and oral inhaler; patient obtains a Proventil HFA MDI approximately every 6 weeks. She frequently misses the evening dose of the steroid inhaler and experiences discomfort from the nasal spray.

All

Aspirin (urticaria and wheezing)

Cats (wheezing)

ROS

Unremarkable except for nasal stuffiness and heartburn. Patient also reports that she wakes up at least twice a week with shortness of breath and wheezing, and occasionally feels chest tightness in the morning.

PE

Gen

Anxious-appearing white woman in apparent distress with audible wheezing, unable to speak in complete sentences because of dyspnea. Suprasternal muscle retractions noted.

VS

BP 132/76, P 105, RR 28, T 38.2°C; Wt 58 kg

Skin

No rashes or bruises

HEENT

EOMI; PERLA; fundi benign, no hemorrhages or exudates; TMs intact; nasal mucosa boggy

Neck

Supple, no adenopathy or thyromegaly

Lungs

Diffuse wheezes bilaterally on exhalation and occasionally on inspiration

Breasts

Nontender without masses

CV

Tachycardia, regular rhythm; no murmurs, rubs, or gallops

Abd

Soft, NT/ND; bowel sounds active

Ext

Normal ROM; pulses 3+ throughout; no CCE

Neuro

Cranial nerves II–XII intact; no focal or sensory defects

Labs

Na 132 mEq/L	Hgb 12 g/dL	WBC $8.0 \times 10^3/mm^3$
K 4.4 mEq/L	Hct 36%	67% PMNs
Cl 102 mEq/L	Plt $180 \times 10^3/mm^3$	2% Bands
CO_2 26 mEq/L		20% Lymphs
BUN 22 mg/dL		8% Eos
SCr 0.9 mg/dL		3% Monos
Glu 104 mg/dL		Pulse ox 91% (on RA)

Nasal Smear

Numerous eosinophils

Chest X-Ray

Hyperinflated lungs; no infiltrates

Peak Flow

130 L/min (baseline 340 L/min)

Assessment

19 yo woman with moderate to severe exacerbation of asthma likely precipitated by viral upper respiratory infection and potential exposure to other triggers

▶ Clinical Course

The patient is admitted overnight for treatment with oxygen, inhaled bronchodilators, and oral prednisone (60 mg/day, given BID). She is discharged home with her previous regimen plus nebulized albuterol 2.5 mg TID for 5 days and a prednisone taper over 10 days starting at 60 mg daily. On follow-up at day 4 in the clinic, her lungs are clear without wheezing; her respiratory rate is 16 breaths/min; and her pulse oximetry is 97%. Her peak flow has improved to 270 L/min.

▶ Questions

Problem Identification

1. a. *Create a list of the patient's drug therapy problems.*
   b. *What information indicates the presence of uncontrolled chronic asthma and an acute asthma exacerbation?*
   c. *Could any of the patient's problems have been caused by drug therapy?*

Desired Outcome

2. *What are the goals of pharmacotherapy in this case?*

Therapeutic Alternatives

3. a. *What nondrug therapies might be useful for this patient?*
   b. *What feasible pharmacotherapeutic alternatives are available for treatment of this patient's chronic asthma?*

Optimal Plan

4. a. *Outline an optimal plan of treatment for this patient's chronic asthma.*
   b. *What alternatives would be appropriate if the initial therapy fails?*

Outcome Evaluation

5. *What clinical and laboratory parameters are necessary to evaluate the therapy for achievement of the desired therapeutic effect and to detect or prevent adverse effects?*

Patient Education

6. *What information should be provided to improve adherence, ensure successful therapy, and minimize adverse effects?*

▶ Clinical Course

With the institution of the changes you recommended, the patient's asthma is well controlled. She is questioned about her adherence to the medications and indicates that this has improved. Over the next several months, she notes only occasional nighttime symptoms that are responsive to albuterol. She needed to initiate her action plan (of increased β_2 agonist and inhaled corticosteroid use) only twice in the past 7 months.

▶ Self-Study Assignments

1. If this patient became pregnant, what impact would the pregnancy have on her asthma control and therapy?
2. If this patient continues to take inhaled corticosteroids when she is postmenopausal, can anything be done to minimize the problem of osteoporosis?
3. What recommendations can you make about stepping down her current regimen?
4. What ongoing monitoring is necessary as her medications are tapered or discontinued?
5. What role would immunotherapy play for her asthma and allergies?

▶ Clinical Pearl

All patients with persistent forms of asthma should receive the influenza vaccine annually. It is well established that viral respiratory infections, including influenza, are common triggers of asthma exacerbations in children and adults.

References

1. National Asthma Education and Prevention Program Expert Panel Report 2: Guidelines for the Diagnosis and Management of Asthma. Bethesda, MD, NIH, 1997: Pub. no. 97–4051. Also available on the Internet at www.nhlbi.nih.gov/guidelines/asthma/asthgdln.htm (accessed April 19, 2004).
2. National Asthma Education and Prevention Program Expert Panel Report 2: Guidelines for the Diagnosis and Management of Asthma. Update on Selected Topics 2002. Bethesda, MD, NIH, 2003: Pub. no. 02–5074. Also available on the Internet at: www.nhlbi.nih.gov/health/prof/lung/index.htm#asthma (accessed April 19, 2004).
3. Shrewsbury S, Pyke S, Britton M. Meta-analysis of increased dose of inhaled steroid or addition of salmeterol in symptomatic asthma (MIASMA). BMJ 2000;320:1368–1373.
4. Malmstrom K, Rodriguez-Gomez G, Guerra J, et al. Oral montelukast, inhaled beclomethasone, and placebo for chronic asthma: A randomized, controlled trial. Montelukast/Beclomethasone Study Group. Ann Intern Med 1999;130: 487–495.
5. Lofdahl CG, Reiss TF, Leff JA, et al. Randomized, placebo-controlled trial of effect of a leukotriene receptor antagonist, montelukast, on tapering inhaled corticosteroids in asthmatic patients. BMJ 1999;319:87–90.
6. Evans DJ, Taylor DA, Zetterstrom O, et al. A comparison of low-dose inhaled

budesonide plus theophylline and high-dose inhaled budesonide for moderate asthma. N Engl J Med 1997;337: 1412–1418.

7. Laviolette M, Malmstrom K, Lu S, et al. Montelukast added to inhaled beclomethasone in treatment of asthma. Montelukast/Beclomethasone Additivity Group. Am J Respir Crit Care Med 1999;160:1862–1868.

26 CHRONIC OBSTRUCTIVE LUNG DISEASE

▶ Waiting to Exhale (Level II)

Daren L. Knoell, PharmD

▶ After completing this case study, students should be able to:

- Differentiate the signs and symptoms of chronic bronchitis, emphysema, and mixed obstructive lung disease.
- Identify the importance of nonpharmacologic therapy in patients with COLD.
- Develop an appropriate medication regimen for a patient with COLD based on disease severity.
- Identify the association between cigarette smoking, lung disease, and the importance of smoking cessation strategies.
- Educate patients on the proper use of inhaled medications and determine which patients may benefit from spacers and/or holding chambers.
- Describe the relationship between α_1-antitrypsin deficiency and the development of emphysema.

PATIENT PRESENTATION

Chief Complaint

"I could barely breathe, and my cough was worse, so I went to the emergency room."

HPI

Johnny Carpenter is a 58 yo man with COLD who is admitted to the hospital after presenting to the ED with a 2-day history of progressive shortness of breath, cough, and increased production of sputum with fever and night sweats. He treated himself at home with Atrovent MDI but had increasing respiratory distress despite multiple puffs. Upon arrival to the ED, he was noted to have decreased breath sounds and was unable to speak full sentences. In the ED, he was placed on 4 L oxygen via face mask and given nebulized Atrovent and albuterol treatments. Solu-Medrol 60 mg IV and erythromycin 500 mg IV were given, and he was transferred to the floor.

PMH

COLD × 3 years
HTN × 20 years

His respiratory symptoms are often worse in the winter but usually respond to inhaled Atrovent. He states that he is compliant as long as his wife reminds him to take his medications. He admits that he does not like to use the Atrovent because it gives him blurred vision; he uses the open-mouth technique and does not currently use a spacer or holding chamber. The patient lacks coordination and demonstrates poor overall MDI technique. He last visited his PCP approximately 1 month ago, at which time his hypertension medication was changed from Dyazide to nadolol.

FH

Father died of lung cancer at age 75. Mother is alive and has HTN.

SH

Married × 35 years; wife is alive and in good health. Retired industrial contractor; primarily installed drywall. He does not drink except for an occasional beer. Has smoked cigarettes at least 1 ppd for more than 30 years. He has tried to cut back and is willing to consider smoking cessation because he understands that it is bad for his asthma and COPD. No history of IVDA.

ROS

(+) Shortness of breath with productive cough and purulent sputum; (+) weakness and myalgias. Denies chest pain; (+) fever.

Meds

Theo-Dur 100 mg po BID
Atrovent MDI 2 puffs BID
Nadolol 40 mg po once daily

All

Sulfa drugs; rash and hives

PE

Gen

Generally healthy appearing man, somewhat improved and now in moderate respiratory distress after receiving treatment in the ED

VS

BP 160/95, P 140, RR 34, T 37.9°C; pulsus paradoxus 12 mm Hg; Wt 80 kg, Ht 5′10″

Skin

Warm, dry

HEENT

PERRLA, EOMI; AV nicking on funduscopic exam; no hemorrhages or exudates; TMs intact; oropharynx clear

Neck/LN

(–) JVD, lymphadenopathy, or thyromegaly

Lungs

Diffuse inspiratory and expiratory wheezes bilaterally; no rales; (+) rhonchi

CV

RRR; normal S_1; accentuated S_2 sound, no S_3 or S_4

Abd
Soft, NT/ND; no organomegaly

Genit/Rect
Normal male genitalia; heme (–) stool

MS/Ext
Cyanotic nail beds; no clubbing or edema; pulses 2+ throughout

Neuro
A & O × 3; CN II–XII intact; DTRs 2+; Babinski downgoing

Labs

Na 130 mEq/L	Hgb 13.0 g/dL	AST 35 IU/L	*ABG on 6 L O_2 by NC*
K 3.7 mEq/L	Hct 39.5%	ALT 21 IU/L	pH 7.30
Cl 109 mEq/L	Plt 245 × 10^3/mm^3	T. bili 0.9 mg/dL	pO_2 100 mm Hg
BUN 14 mg/dL	WBC 8.0 × 10^3/mm^3	Alb 3.5 g/dL	pCO_2 55 mm Hg
SCr 0.9 mg/dL	PMNs 65%	Theoph 9.0 mg/L	HCO_3 25 mEq/L
Glu 110 mg/dL	Bands 3%		SaO_2 98%
	Lymphs 27%		
	Monos 5%		

Pulmonary Function Tests
Prebronchodilator FEV_1 = 2200 mL (Predicted is 3200 mL)
Prebronchodilator FVC = 3200 mL
Postbronchodilator FEV_1 = 2600 mL
Diffusion capacity (DL_{CO}) = 75% predicted (from tests performed 6 months ago)

Chest X-Ray
Flattened diaphragm; loss of peripheral vascular markings; no effusions or infiltrates noted

ECG
ST depression, flattened T-waves

Assessment
This is a normal appearing 58 yo man with acute respiratory insufficiency secondary to an acute exacerbation of COLD and suspected URI. He also has acute respiratory acidosis, and a history of HTN.

Meds Initiated After Transfer to Floor
Theo-Dur 100 mg po BID
Albuterol nebulized solution 1 mL of 0.5% solution (5 mg) in 3 mL NS Q 4 H
Atrovent MDI 4 puffs QID
Solu-Medrol 60 mg IV Q 6 H
Erythromycin 500 mg IV Q 6 H
Oxygen 2L via nasal cannula

▶ Questions

Problem Identification

1. a. *Create a list of this patient's drug therapy problems prior to treatment in the ED.*
   b. *What signs, symptoms, and laboratory data provide evidence that this patient is experiencing a COLD exacerbation? Based on the evidence, is his presentation more consistent with emphysema or chronic bronchitis?*
   c. *What additional information do you need to satisfactorily assess the adequacy of COLD treatment in this patient before he presented to the ED?*

Desired Outcome

2. *What are the desired goals for the treatment of this patient's COLD?*

Therapeutic Alternatives

3. a. *What non-drug therapies would be useful to improve this patient's COLD symptoms?*
   b. *What feasible pharmacotherapeutic alternatives are available for the treatment of COLD in this patient, particularly those that can be continued as an outpatient?*
   c. *Should home oxygen therapy be considered for the patient at this time?*
   d. *Is this patient a candidate for α_1-antitrypsin (Prolastin) therapy?*

Optimal Plan

4. *Develop a complete outpatient regimen for the treatment of COLD in this patient, including dose, route, frequency, and duration of therapy.*

Outcome Evaluation

5. *What clinical and laboratory parameters are necessary to evaluate the therapy for achievement of the desired therapeutic outcome and to detect or prevent adverse effects?*

Patient Education

6. *What information should be provided to the patient to enhance compliance, ensure successful therapy, and minimize adverse effects?*

▶ Self-Study Assignments

1. Describe and compare the expectations for deterioration in pulmonary function in normal healthy adults and smokers with emphysema. In particular, emphasis should be placed on expected patterns of change in DLco, FEV_1, and FVC, and general health over time in years.
2. Why would additional phenotyping be necessary if this patient were to have an abnormally low serum α_1-antitrypsin level? What are the

implications of the results if the patient were designated as homozygous ZZ, heterozygous MZ, or heterozygous SZ at the α_1-antitrypsin allele?

3. Search the Internet (see suggested site in references at end of chapter) for supplementary materials on smoking cessation guidelines for patients and health care providers. Study these materials and use them to work with an actual patient in the outpatient setting. Document your findings over time while working with this patient. The patient could be you.

▶ Clinical Pearl

Spacer devices and holding chambers are not interchangeable. Although both are designed to improve drug deposition in the airway, only the holding chamber avoids the need for the patient to coordinate actuation with inhalation. The Aerochamber and Inspirease are examples of holding chambers routinely used in practice.

References

1. Bach PB, Brown C, Gelfand SE, et al. Management of acute exacerbations of chronic obstructive pulmonary disease: a summary and appraisal of published evidence. Ann Intern Med 2001;134:600–620.
2. Snow V, Lascher S, Mottur-Pilson C. Evidence base for management of acute exacerbations of chronic obstructive pulmonary disease. Ann Intern Med 2001;134:595–599.
3. National Heart, Lung, and Blood Institute (NHLBI) Global Initiative for Chronic Obstructive Lung Disease. Available at www.goldcopd.com/docs.html. Accessed March 13, 2004.
4. MacDonald JL, Johnson CE. Pathophysiology and treatment of alpha 1-antitrypsin deficiency. Am J Health-Syst Pharm 1995;52:481–489.
5. Toogood JH. Helping your patients make better use of MDIs and spacers. J Resp Dis 1994;15:151–166.
6. American Thoracic Society. Standards for the diagnosis and care of patients with chronic obstructive pulmonary disease. Am J Resp Crit Care Med 1995;152:S77-S121.

Suggested Internet sites for smoking cessation information: Agency for Healthcare Research and Quality, www.ahrq.gov or The Virtual Office of the Surgeon General, www.surgeongeneral.gov/tobacco/. Both sites accessed March 13, 2004.

27 CYSTIC FIBROSIS

▶ Blood, Sweat, Lungs, and Gut (Level I)

Robert J. Kuhn, PharmD
Kimberly J. Novak, PharmD

▶ After completing this case study, students should be able to:

- Identify signs and symptoms of common problems in patients with cystic fibrosis (CF).
- Develop a monitoring plan for antimicrobial therapy in the treatment of acute pulmonary exacerbation in CF.
- Devise treatment strategies for common complications of drug therapy in patients with CF.
- Provide counseling on aerosolized medications in patients with CF, including appropriate instructions for dornase alfa and inhaled tobramycin.

PATIENT PRESENTATION

Chief Complaint

As reported by his mother: "Shortness of breath, increasing cough and sputum production, and decreased energy."

HPI

Eric Smith is a 9 yo male with a long history of CF; he was diagnosed with CF at 4 weeks of age. He had been doing well until 2 weeks ago when he developed shortness of breath, pulmonary congestion, and severe fatigue. Mother reported increasing cough productive of very-dark-colored sputum but no fever. The patient has had a decreased appetite and has lost 2 pounds. His oxygen saturation at home was 96% but is now 88% in clinic. Mother initially took him to clinic 5 days ago for the same symptoms and was given ciprofloxacin 500 mg po BID (~40 mg/kg/day). His prednisone was increased from 5 mg to 10 mg po once daily, and his mother was instructed to call or return if no improvement was seen. The patient now presents 5 days later with worsening respiratory symptoms.

PMH

Significant for 11 hospitalizations for acute pulmonary exacerbations of CF since his diagnosis.

H/O allergic bronchopulmonary aspergillosis, recently under control with corticosteroid treatment; last hospitalization was 8 weeks ago.

Pancreatic insufficiency requiring supplementation with 1,491 units/kg/meal of lipase to maintain weight gain.

Pulmonary changes c/w long-standing CF with bronchiectasis and two episodes of hemoptysis.

FH

Both parents are alive and well. Eric has one sister who had a recent cold and upper respiratory infection. Two maternal uncles died at ages 13 and 17 from CF.

SH

Eric attends third grade but has been homebound the last 2 months. Lives with his mother, father, and sister. They have city water and no pets; father smokes, but only outside of the home.

ROS

Patient complains of severe back pain, especially when coughing. Reduced ability to perform usual daily activities because of SOB. No current hemoptysis, vomiting, abdominal pain, or complaints of abnormal stool odor or character.

Meds

Aerosolized tobramycin 300 mg BID via nebulizer
Albuterol 0.083%, 3 mL (1 vial) TID via nebulizer
Pulmozyme 2.5 mg via nebulizer once daily
Flovent 110 mcg, 1 puff BID
Prednisone 10 mg po once daily
Azithromycin 250 mg po Q WMF
Creon 20, two caps with meals and one cap with snack
Ferrous sulfate 300 mg po once daily
ADEK one tablet po once daily

All

NKDA

PE

Gen

A pleasant, cooperative, 9-year-old boy who has shortness of breath with his oxygen cannula removed during the exam.

VS

BP 110/70, P 144, RR 44, T 36.9°C; Wt 59 lb.; Ht 50″
Oxygen saturation 95% with 1.5 L of oxygen; 88% on room air

HEENT

EOMI, PERRL; nares with dried mucus in both nostrils; no oral lesions, but secretions noted in the posterior pharynx

Neck/LN

Supple; no lymphadenopathy or thyromegaly

Lungs

Crackles heard bilaterally in the upper lobes greater than in the lower lobes

Heart

RRR without murmurs

Abd

Ticklish during exam; (+) bowel sounds; abdomen soft and supple. No steatorrhea noted

MS/Ext

Clubbing noted with no cyanosis; capillary refill < 2 seconds

Neuro

Eric is alert and awake; CNs intact; somewhat uncooperative with the full neurologic exam

Labs

Na 138 mEq/L	Hgb 15.4 g/dL	WBC $20.1 \times 10^3/mm^3$	AST 24 IU/L
K 4.5 mEq/L	Hct 45.2%	61% Segs	ALT 22 IU/L
Cl 102 mEq/L	MCV 91 μm^3	32% Bands	LDH 330 IU/L
CO_2 27 mEq/L	MCH 31.1 pg	6% Lymphs	GGT 42 IU/L
BUN 10 mg/dL	MCHC 34 g/dL	1% Monos	T. Prot 8.3 g/dL
SCr 0.7 mg/dL		Ca_i 4.6 mEq/L[a]	Alb 3.8 g/dL
Glu 188 mg/dL		Phos 4.6 mEq/L	

[a] Ca_i = ionized calcium

Urine Drug Screen

Negative

Sputum Culture Results

Organism A: *Pseudomonas aeruginosa*
Organism B: *Stenotrophomonas maltophilia*
Organism C: *Pseudomonas aeruginosa*—mucoid strain
Organism D: *Staphylococcus aureus*
Organism E: *Aspergillus* species

PFTs

FEV_1 56% of predicted; FVC_1 80% of predicted

Chest X-Ray

Bronchiectatic and interstitial fibrotic changes consistent with CF. No difference noted from previous exam 8 weeks ago.

▶ Questions

Problem Identification

1. a. *Identify this patient's drug therapy problems.*
   b. *What information indicates the disease severity and the need to treat his CF pharmacologically?*
   c. *Could any of his problems be caused by drug therapy?*

Desired Outcome

2. *What are the goals of pharmacotherapy in this case?*

Therapeutic Alternatives

3. a. *What nonpharmacologic therapies might be useful for this patient?*
   b. *What pharmacotherapeutic alternatives are available for treatment of this patient's acute pulmonary exacerbation?*

Optimal Plan

4. a. *What drugs, dosage forms, doses, schedules, and durations of therapy are best for this patient?*

▶ Clinical Course

Serum tobramycin concentrations drawn around the fourth dose of tobramycin 80 mg (3 mg/kg/dose) IV Q 8 H were as follows:
Peak: 5.9 mcg/mL collected 1 hour after the end of the 30 minute infusion
Trough: 0.4 mcg/mL collected just before the next dose

b. *Based on this new information, evaluate his drug therapy and if necessary, suggest modifications. Assume that the previous doses were administered on time.*

Outcome Evaluation

5. *What clinical and laboratory parameters are necessary to evaluate the therapy?*

Patient Education

6. *What information should you provide the patient regarding the administration of aerosolized drug therapy? The patient will be going home on aerosolized dornase alfa, tobramycin, and albuterol.*

▶ Self-Study Assignments

1. What potential problem is associated with the use of very-high-dose pancreatic enzymes in patients with CF? What dosage guidelines should be followed to minimize any potential risk?
2. What is the role of azithromycin in the chronic medical management of CF? What is/are the proposed mechanism(s) of action of azithromycin in CF management?
3. What are the recommendations for the administration of high-dose ibuprofen in patients with CF? When would you suggest that serum concentrations be drawn, and what levels are thought to be necessary to optimize therapy in a patient with CF?
4. What is the status of recommendations surrounding use of fluoroquinolones in children? What data support these recommendations?
5. Perform a literature search to determine the progress of gene therapy in CF.
6. What is the preferred treatment of acute bronchopulmonary aspergillosis in patients with CF? What long-term therapy is indicated?

▶ Clinical Pearl

Low doses of ibuprofen may increase the migration of neutrophils and inflammatory mediators in the lung and exacerbate the progression of lung disease. Care should be taken to evaluate the use of PRN ibuprofen in CF patients.

References

1. Konstan MW, Butler SM, Wohl ME, et al. Growth and nutritional indexes in early life predict pulmonary function in cystic fibrosis. J Pediatr 2003;142:624–630.
2. Yee CL, Duffy C, Gerbino PG, et al. Tendon or joint disorders in children after treatment with fluoroquinolones or azithromycin. Pediatr Infect Dis J 2002;21:525–529.
3. Saiman L, Campbell P, Burns J, et al. TOBI Consensus Conference. North American Cystic Fibrosis Conference, Nashville, TN, October 1997.
4. Saiman L, Marshall BC, Mayer-Hamblett N, et al. Azithromycin in patients with cystic fibrosis chronically infected with Pseudomonas aeruginosa: a randomized controlled trial. JAMA 2003;20:1749–1756.
5. Konstan MW, Byard PJ, Hoppel CL, et al. Effect of high-dose ibuprofen in patients with cystic fibrosis. N Engl J Med 1995;332:848–854.

SECTION 4

Gastrointestinal Disorders

28 GASTROESOPHAGEAL REFLUX DISEASE

► Banking on Relief (Level I)

Meredith L. Rose, PharmD

► After completing this case study, students should be able to:

- Identify the different clinical presentations of gastroesophageal reflux disease (GERD), including typical, atypical, and warning symptoms.
- Discuss available testing options for the diagnosis and evaluation of GERD.
- Define both nonpharmacologic and pharmacologic approaches to the treatment of GERD.
- Develop an individualized treatment plan for a patient with GERD, taking into consideration the efficacy, safety, and cost of available agents.
- Explain the role of maintenance therapy in the treatment of GERD.

PATIENT PRESENTATION

Chief Complaint

"I have been having a lot of heartburn and indigestion lately. I'm worried because I read in the newspaper that people who suffer from frequent heartburn are at risk for cancer."

HPI

Robert Wood is a 67 yo man who presents to his primary care doctor today for an evaluation of worsening gastroesophageal reflux symptoms. Over the past 3 months he has experienced increasing episodes of postprandial heartburn and regurgitation. Initially, he attempted to treat his symptoms with antacids and OTC H_2-receptor antagonists but experienced inadequate symptom relief. More recently, he completed the 14-day course of Prilosec OTC at the recommendation of his local pharmacist. He states that his symptoms were relieved by the Prilosec, but they returned within two weeks of stopping the therapy. The patient admits to frequent nocturnal awakenings secondary to epigastric discomfort but denies dysphagia or odynophagia. He is concerned because his symptoms are affecting his quality of life.

PMH

HTN × 20 years
CAD (s/p MI at 58)
Hyperlipidemia

FH

Father died at age 68 from CAD; mother died at age 77 from pneumonia; two siblings with "heart disease"

SH

Patient lives with his wife of 40 years. He is a retired investment banker and enjoys traveling with his wife. (+) social EtOH (1 to 2 martinis/week); 60 pack-year smoking history; currently smokes ½ ppd.

Meds

Aspirin 325 mg po daily
Atenolol 50 mg po daily
Hydrochlorothiazide 25 mg po daily
Simvastatin 20 mg po at bedtime

All

NKA

ROS

(–) HA, dizziness, visual changes, tinnitus or vertigo; (–) SOB, cough, hoarseness; (+) frequent episodes of non-radiating substernal CP, which he describes as burning in nature; (–) N/V/D, BRBPR, or dark/tarry stools; (–) urinary frequency, dysuria, nocturia; (+) recent 10-lb. weight loss (unintentional over 2 months)

PE

Gen

The patient is a well groomed Caucasian male who looks his stated age.

VS

BP 150/94; P 82—regular; RR 16; T 36.6°C; Ht 6′1″; Wt 85 kg

Skin

No rashes or lesions noted

HEENT

PERRLA, EOMI, no arterial narrowing or A–V nicking; pink, moist mucus membranes; gums without swelling or ulceration; tonsils absent; oropharynx clear

Neck

No thyromegaly, lymphadenopathy, or JVD

Lungs

CTA

CV

Regular rhythm, normal S_1 and S_2; no S_3 or S_4; II/VI SEM at the apex

Abd

Normoactive BS, soft, NT/ND; no HSM

Rect

No palpable rectal masses; brown stool without occult blood

Ext

No CCE

Neuro

A & O × 3, CN II–XII intact; 5/5 strength in upper and lower extremities bilaterally

Labs

Na 140 mEq/L	Ca 8.3 mg/dL	Hgb 13.5 g/dL
K 3.2 mEq/L	AST 20 IU/L	Hct 38.3%
Cl 95 mEq/L	ALT 32 IU/L	Plt 277 ×10^3/mm^3
CO_2 30 mEq/L	Alk Phos 67 IU/L	*Fasting Lipid Profile*
BUN 9 mg/dL	GGT 20 IU/L	T. chol 213 mg/dL
SCr 0.9 mg/dL		LDL 133 mg/dL
Glu 92 mg/dL		HDL 48 mg/dL
		Trig 144 mg/dL

Assessment

67 yo man who presents with worsening of symptoms of GERD over the past 3 months.

► Questions

Problem Identification

1. a. *Develop a list of this patient's drug therapy problems.*
   b. *What symptoms indicate the possible severity of the patient's GERD? Are the symptoms typical or atypical? Are any warning symptoms present?*
   c. *What factors may be contributing to the patient's symptoms of GERD? (Refer to Figure 28–1 for a depiction of possible causes of esophagitis.)*
   d. *What tests are used to evaluate a patient's symptoms and confirm the diagnosis of GERD?*

Desired Outcome

2. *What are the goals of pharmacotherapy for this patient's GERD?*

Therapeutic Alternatives

3. a. *What nonpharmacologic therapies or lifestyle modifications might be useful for managing this patient's GERD?*
   b. *What pharmacotherapeutic alternatives are available for treating this patient's GERD?*

Optimal Plan

4. *Based on the patient information provided, design an individualized pharmacotherapeutic plan for managing this patient's GERD.*

Outcome Evaluation

5. *What clinical and/or laboratory parameters should be evaluated at the patient's next follow-up appointment in order to assess for therapeutic response and to detect or prevent adverse effects?*

Patient Education

6. *How will you educate the patient about his GERD therapy in order to enhance compliance, minimize adverse effects, and promote successful therapeutic outcomes?*

► Clinical Course

Mr. Wood underwent an upper GI endoscopy that revealed multiple erosive lesions in the distal esophagus (see *Figure 28–2*). There was no evidence of ulceration, obstruction, or stricture. The patient was treated with an 8-week course of acid-suppressive therapy. Approximately 3 months after discontinuing acid suppressive therapy, the patient reported that his GERD

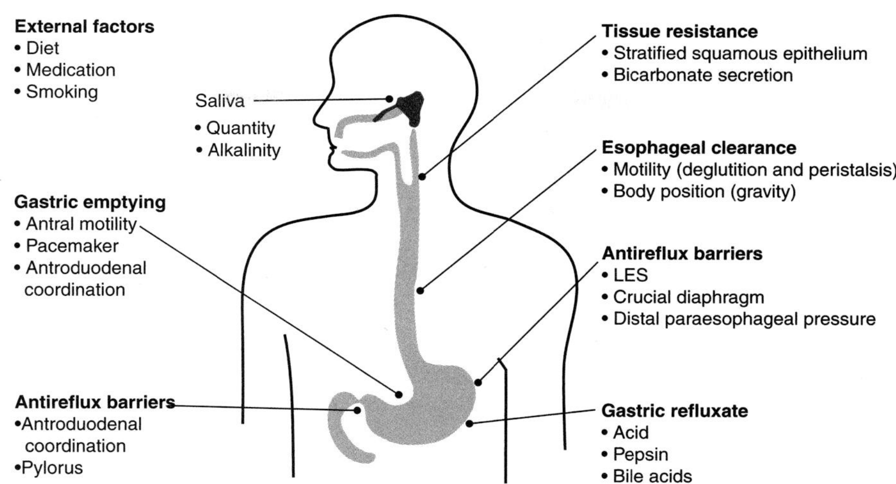

Figure 28–1. Factors involved in the pathogenesis of GERD. *(Reprinted with permission from Peterson WL. GERD: evidence-based therapeutic strategies. Bethesda, MD: American Gastroenterological Association; 2002.)*

symptoms had returned and that he was again suffering from frequent postprandial and nocturnal reflux episodes.

► Follow-Up Questions

1. *What is the role of maintenance therapy for controlling this patient's continued GERD symptoms?*
2. *What maintenance therapies could be recommended for the long-term management of GERD in this patient?*
3. *Should this patient be tested for H. Pylori? Please explain your answer.*

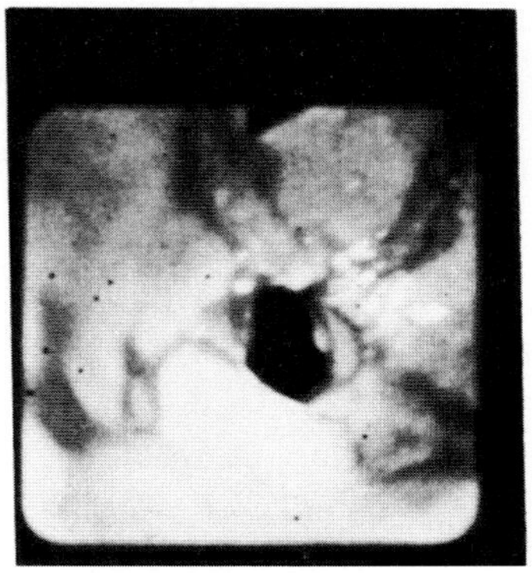

Figure 28–2. An endoscopic photograph of erosive esophagitis. The streaks are erosions, and the thick white material is exudate. *(Reprinted with permission from Gitnick G, ed. Principles and Practice of Gastroenterology and Hepatology, 2nd ed. Norwalk, CT, Appleton & Lange, 1994:46.)*

► Self-Study Assignments

1. Develop an algorithm for the diagnosis and treatment of GERD.
2. During an advanced practice experience rotation at a local pharmacy benefits management (PBM) organization, you are asked to evaluate the clinical impact of a formulary switch from omeprazole to lansoprazole. Conduct a literature search to identify at least two primary articles on formulary conversion of PPI agents. Provide a brief (2 to 3 paragraph) summary of each article highlighting the study population and methodology, pertinent results, and conclusions. Use this information to formulate a concise (1 to 2 paragraph) recommendation to the PBM regarding the clinical impact of the proposed switch.

► Clinical Pearl

Among the PPIs, rabeprazole is least affected by genotype differences in the CYP2C19 isoform since it is predominantly metabolized nonenzymatically.

References

1. Fass R, Fennerty MB, Vakil N. Non-erosive reflux disease (NERD)–current concepts and dilemmas. Am J Gastroenterol 2001;96:303–314.
2. Johnson DA, Fennerty MB. Heartburn severity underestimates erosive esophagitis severity in elderly patients with gastroesophageal reflux disease. Gastroenterology 2004;126:660–664.
3. Lagergren J, Bergstrom R, Lindgren A, et al. Symptomatic gastroesophageal reflux as a risk factor for esophageal adenocarcinoma. N Engl J Med 1999;340: 825–831.
4. DeVault KR, Castell DO. Updated guidelines for the diagnosis and treatment of gastroesophageal reflux disease. The Practice Parameters Committee of the American College of Gastroenterology. Am J Gastroenterol 1999;94:1434–1442.

5. Numans ME, Lau J, de Wit NJ, et al. Short-term treatment with proton-pump inhibitors as a test for gastroesophageal reflux disease: A meta-analysis of diagnostic test characteristics. Ann Intern Med 2004;140;518–527.
6. Provenzale D, Schmitt C, Wong JB. Barrett's esophagus: A new look at surveillance based on emerging estimates of cancer risk. Am J Gastroenterol 1999;94:2043–2053.
7. Kahrilas PJ, Quigley EM, Castell DO, et al. The effects of tegaserod (HTF 919) on oesophageal acid exposure in gastro-oesophageal reflux disease. Aliment Pharmacol Ther 2000;14:1503–1509.
8. Peterson WL. Improving the management of GERD: Evidence-based therapeutic strategies. Bethesda, MD: American Gastroenterological Association; 2002. Available on the Internet at www.gastro.org/edu/GERDmonograph.pdf. Accessed August 6, 2004.
9. Malfertheiner P, Megraud F, O'Morain C, et al. Current concepts in the management of *Helicobacter pylori* infection: The Maastricht 2–2000 Consensus Report. Aliment Pharmacol Ther 2002;16;167–180.

29 PEPTIC ULCER DISEASE

▶ Just a Gut Feeling (Level II)

Marie A. Chisholm, PharmD, FCCP
Mark W. Jackson, MD, FACG

▶ After completing this case study, students should be able to:

- Design a pharmaceutical care plan and evaluate pharmacotherapeutic outcomes for peptic ulcer disease (PUD) based on patient-specific information.
- Assess antiulcer regimens to detect and prevent adverse drug events.
- Understand the role of *Helicobacter pylori* in PUD and recommend appropriate regimens to eradicate this organism.
- Educate patients suffering from PUD on which medications to avoid.

PATIENT PRESENTATION

Chief Complaint
"My stomach has been hurting for over a month. I think something's wrong."

HPI
Margaret Fitzgerald is a 40 yo woman who presents to the clinic complaining of epigastric pain for more than 2 months and feeling weak for approximately 2 weeks. Her pain is non-radiating and occurs to the right of her epigastrium. This pain occurs daily, wavers in intensity, and increases at night and between meals. The patient states that ingesting food or antacids seems to decrease the severity of the pain. In addition to being constipated for more than 1 week, 5 days ago she noticed that she was having black, tarry bowel movements. She does not have any history of PUD or GI bleeding, and has not experienced anorexia, weight loss, nausea, or vomiting.

PMH
HTN × 6 years
Hypothyroidism × 8 years
Type 2 DM × 9 years
Occasional back pain

FH
Her father died at age 75 from colon cancer and her mother died at age 62 from an acute MI. She has two siblings who are alive and well.

SH
Presently employed as an elementary school teacher. She is married, and she and her husband Arnold have one daughter, who is 18 years old. She smokes approximately one pack of cigarettes per day and drinks two to three cans of beer per week.

Meds
Procardia XL 30 mg po once daily
Synthroid 100 mcg po once daily
DiaBeta 5 mg po once daily
Aspirin two tablets PRN back pain (she remembers taking at least 25 tablets over the last month)
Tums two tablets po PRN abdominal pain

All
NKDA

ROS
Unremarkable except for complaints noted above

PE

Gen
Well-nourished woman in slight distress

VS
BP 130/78 right arm, seated; P68; RR 14 reg; T 37.5°C; Ht 5′3,″ Wt 85 kg (80 kg 3 months ago)

Skin
Warm and dry

HEENT
PERRLA; EOMI; discs flat; no A-V nicking, hemorrhages, or exudates

Chest
Clear to A & P

CV
S_1 and S_2 normal; no m/r/g

Abd
Normal bowel sounds and mild epigastric tenderness; liver size normal; no splenomegaly or masses observed

GU

Pelvic exam normal and uterus is intact; LMP 2 weeks ago

Rect

Non-tender; melenic stool found in rectal vault; stool heme (+)

Ext

Normal ROM

Neuro

CN II–XII intact, DTRs 2+ throughout

Labs

Na 139 mEq/L	Hgb 10.2 g/dL	Ca 9.2 mg/dL
K 3.9 mEq/L	Hct 29%	Mg 2.0 mEq/L
Cl 98 mEq/L	Plt 230 × 10^3/mm^3	Phos 4.0 mg/dL
CO_2 26 mEq/L	WBC 6.5 × 10^3/mm^3	Alb 4.0 g/dL
BUN 10 mg/dL	MCV 74 μm^3	TSH 2.0 μIU/mL
SCr 1.0 mg/dL	Retic 0.3%	Total T_4 RIA 8.0 mcg/dL
FBG 89 mg/dL	Fe 49 mcg/dL	Free T_4 1.8 ng/dL

Peripheral Blood Smear

Positive for microcytic anemia

▶ Questions

Problem Identification

1. a. *Create a list of the patient's drug therapy problems.*
   b. *What information (signs, symptoms, tests, and laboratory values) indicates the presence of peptic ulcer disease?*

▶ Clinical Course (Part 1)

An EGD revealed a 7-mm ulcer in the roof of the duodenum (see Figure 29–1). The ulcer base is clear and without evidence of active bleeding. Inflammation of the antrum and the stomach was detected and biopsied. Refer to Figure 29–2 for common anatomic sites of peptic ulcerations.

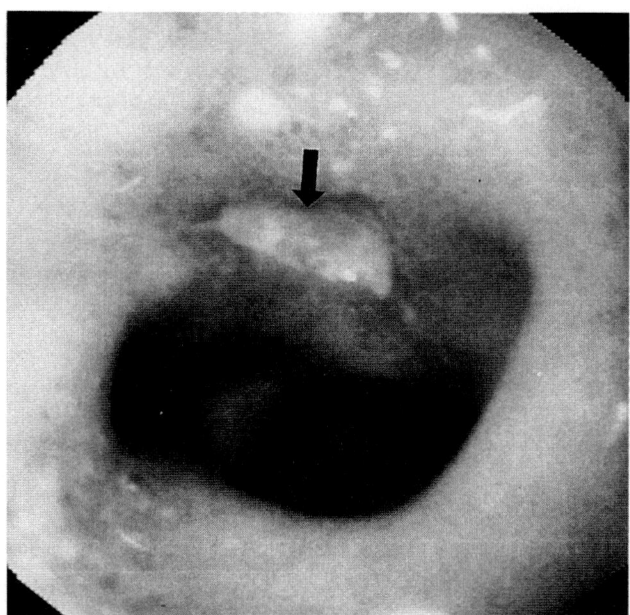

Figure 29–1. Endoscopy showing a 7-mm ulcer in the bulb of the duodenum *(arrow)*.

Desired Outcome

2. *What are the goals for treating this patient's PUD?*

Therapeutic Alternatives

3. a. *Considering this patient's presentation, what nonpharmacologic alternatives are available to treat her PUD?*
   b. *In the absence of information about the presence of Helicobacter pylori, what pharmacologic alternatives are available to treat duodenal ulcers?*

Optimal Plan

4. *Based on the patient's presentation and the current medical assessment, design a pharmacotherapeutic regimen to treat her duodenal ulcer and anemia.*

Outcome Evaluation

5. *Which clinical and laboratory parameters are necessary to evaluate therapy for achievement of the desired therapeutic outcomes and to detect or prevent adverse effects?*

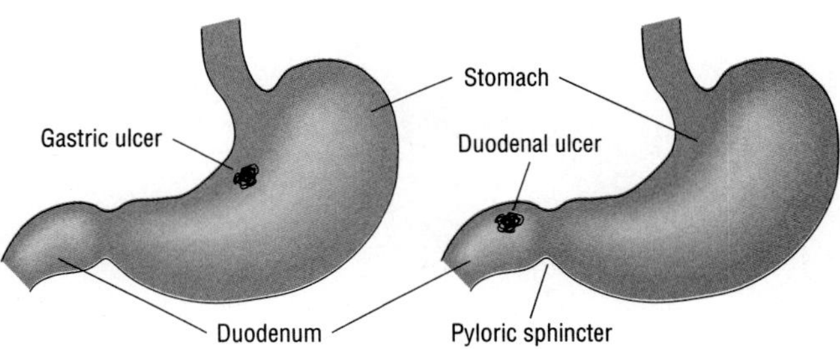

Figure 29–2. Common anatomic sites of peptic ulcers. *(Reprinted with permission from Mulvihill ML. Human Diseases: A Systemic Approach, 4th ed. Norwalk, CT, Appleton & Lange, 1995:174).*

Patient Education

6. *What information should be provided to the patient to ensure successful therapy, enhance compliance, and minimize adverse effects?*

▶ Clinical Course (Part 2)

At the time of endoscopy a biopsy of the gastric mucosa was taken and indicated the presence of inflammation and abundant *H. pylori*-like organisms (see Figure 29–3).

▶ Follow-Up Questions

1. *What is the significance of this new finding?*
2. *Based on this new information, how would you modify your goals for treating this patient's PUD?*
3. *What pharmacotherapeutic alternatives are available to achieve the new goals?*
4. *Design a pharmacotherapeutic regimen for this patient's ulcer that will accomplish the new treatment goals.*
5. *How should the PUD therapy you recommended be monitored for efficacy and adverse effects?*
6. *What information should be provided to the patient about her therapy?*

▶ Self-Study Assignments

1. Describe the advantages and limitations of diagnostic tests available to detect *H. pylori.*
2. After performing a literature search on *H. pylori* eradication therapy, compare the efficacy of proton pump inhibitors plus *H. pylori* antimicrobial therapy versus H_2-receptor antagonists plus *H. pylori* antimicrobial therapy.
3. Describe the role of pharmacists and nurse practitioners in treating peptic ulcer disease patients.

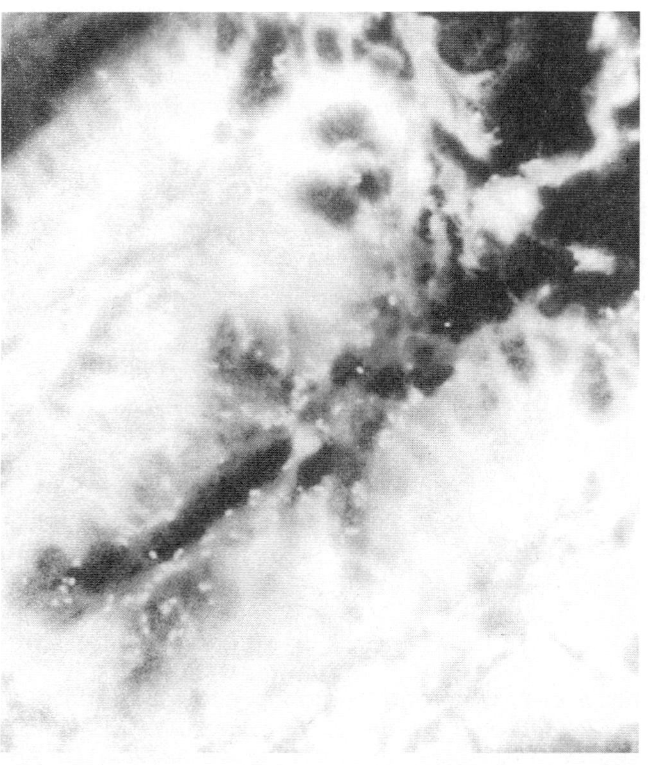

Figure 29–3. *Helicobacter pylori* organisms fluoresce above gastric epithelial cells.

▶ Clinical Pearl

Studies have indicated that the one-year recurrence rates of duodenal ulcer decreases from 70% to 90% with antisecretory agents to <15% after eradication of *H. pylori* infection.

References

1. Peterson WL. *Helicobacter pylori* and peptic ulcer disease. N Engl J Med 1991;324:1043–1048.
2. Graham DY. *Helicobacter pylori:* Its epidemiology and its role in duodenal ulcer disease. J Gastroenterol Hepatol 1991;6:105–113.
3. Soll AH. Consensus conference. Medical treatment of peptic ulcer disease. Practice guidelines. JAMA 1996;275:622–629.
4. ASHP Commission on Therapeutics. ASHP therapeutic position statement on the identification and treatment of *Helicobacter pylori*-associated peptic ulcer disease in adults. Am J Health-Syst Pharm 2001;58:331–337.
5. Chisholm MA, Jackson MW, Wade WE. Eradication of *Helicobacter pylori* in the management of uncomplicated peptic ulcer disease. Disease Management and Health Outcomes 1998;3(4):191–200.

30 NSAID-INDUCED ULCER DISEASE

▶ A Trip to Misadventure Land (Level II)

Cherokee Layson-Wolf, PharmD
Ralph E. Small, PharmD, FCCP, FASHP, FAPhA

▶ After completing this case study, students should be able to:

- Identify medications that may induce peptic ulcer disease (PUD).
- Identify the hallmark signs and symptoms of NSAID-induced PUD.
- Recommend appropriate therapy for the treatment of NSAID-induced PUD.
- Recommend alternative therapies for treatment of pain and inflammation in patients with PUD.
- Educate patients effectively on treatment options.

PATIENT PRESENTATION

Chief Complaint

"I have had some black stools and stomach pain in the past 2 weeks. I am worried that my ulcers have come back."

HPI

Jack Brown is a 76 yo man who presents to his PCP with complaints of black, tarry stools, and epigastric pain for 2 weeks. He stated he started taking TUMS for the stomach upset with little to no relief. These symptoms are consistent with those he experienced three times before when he was diagnosed with bleeding gastric ulcers.

PMH

- OA of the right hip and both knees × 15 years causing chronic pain and inability to exercise or perform daily activities such as mowing the lawn. Previous trials of Relafen, Lodine, and high-dose APAP were associated with eventual tolerance and return of pain; the pain has been controlled with ibuprofen for the past 6 months.
- H/O PUD × 3 episodes
- Hiatal hernia and GERD
- HTN
- Type 2 DM
- H/O BPH; S/P TURP 4 years ago
- S/P appendectomy after appendicitis in the 1970s
- CVA 4 years ago

FH

Father died of MI at age 70; mother died of cervical CA in her forties

SH

Retired tour guide from a large theme park; quit smoking cigars 12 years ago; denies EtOH; no regular exercise because of OA symptoms

Meds

- Clopidogrel 75 mg po QD
- Lisinopril 20 mg po QD
- Torsemide 20 mg, ½ tablet po Q AM
- Ibuprofen 600 mg po TID with food
- Glyburide 5 mg, ½ tablet po BID
- KCl 10 mEq po once daily
- TUMS 1 tablet po PRN stomach upset

All

Codeine, bee pollen, PCN: rash/hives

ROS

Denies headache or chest pain. Right-sided facial weakness with drooping. Occasionally experiences SOB. No heartburn, weakness, joint pain, polyphagia, polydipsia, or polyuria. Gait slow and shuffling but steady.

PE

Gen

The patient is a pleasant elderly man in mild distress.

VS

BP 130/60, P 80, RR 12, T 36.3°C, Ht 6′3″, Wt 84.8 kg

HEENT

PERRLA; funduscopic exam without hemorrhages, exudates, or papilledema; mild cataracts bilaterally

Neck/LN

Supple; no JVD or thyromegaly; no carotid bruits

Lungs

CTA

Cor

RRR, normal S_1, S_2

Abd

Normal BS, moderate epigastric pain on palpation

Genit/Rect

FOBT positive × 3

MS/Ext

No CCE; no skin breakdowns or ulcers, mild weakness of RUE

Neuro

A & O × 3; CN II–XII intact; negative Babinski

Labs

		Fasting Lipid Profile
Na 141 mEq/L	Hgb 7.2 g/dL	T. Chol 195 mg/dL
K 4.6 mEq/L	Hct 23%	LDL-C 125 mg/dL
Cl 107 mEq/L	Plt 390 × 10^3/mm^3	HDL-C 35 mg/dL
CO_2 27 mEq/L	WBC 7.0 × 10^3/mm^3	TG 175 mg/dL
BUN 21 mEq/L	Retic 1.8%	TSH 2.93 μIU/mL
SCr 1.1 mg/dL	HbA_{1c} 6.9%	
Glu 119 mg/dL		

Helicobacter pylori test

Positive as per FlexSure HP

UA

SG 1.005; straw-colored; pH 4.9; trace protein; glucose negative; ketones negative

EGD

Multiple gastric ulcers, none actively bleeding

▶ Questions

Problem Identification

1. a. *Create a list of the patient's drug therapy problems.*

   b. *What signs, symptoms, and laboratory values indicate the presence of PUD in this man?*

Desired Outcome

2. *What are the goals of pharmacotherapy in this case?*

Therapeutic Alternatives

3. a. *What pharmacologic alternatives are available for treating the gastric ulcers in this patient?*
   b. *What feasible pharmacotherapeutic options are available for preventing future gastric ulcers in this patient?*

Optimal Plan

4. a. *What is the optimal pharmacotherapeutic regimen for treating this patient's gastric ulcers?*
   b. *What pharmacotherapeutic regimen is best for treatment of this patient's osteoarthritis?*
   c. *Is this patient a candidate for prophylactic therapy against future NSAID-induced ulcers? If so, what drug and regimen would you recommend?*

Outcome Evaluation

5. *What measures would you implement for monitoring the efficacy and toxicity of the treatment regimen for gastric ulcers in this patient?*

Patient Education

6. *What information should be shared with this patient concerning the management of his gastric ulcers to enhance adherence, assure successful therapy, and minimize adverse effects?*

▶ Self-Study Assignments

1. Perform a literature search and assess current information on the efficacy of various agents in the secondary prevention of NSAID-induced ulcers.
2. Perform a literature search and assess current pharmacoeconomic data for the treatment of NSAID-induced peptic ulcer disease.
3. Perform a literature search and assess the cost effectiveness of *Helicobacter pylori* screening in patients on chronic NSAID therapy.

▶ Clinical Pearl

Risk factors for developing NSAID-induced ulcer disease include prior history of peptic ulcer disease, age > 60 years, prolonged use of NSAIDs, high NSAID doses, and concomitant use of anticoagulants, corticosteroids or other gastric irritants.

References

1. Lanza FL. A guideline for the treatment and prevention of NSAID-induced ulcers. Members of the Ad Hoc Committee on Practice Parameters of the American College of Gastroenterology. Am J Gastroenterol 1998;93:2037–2046.
2. Bannwarth B, Dorval E, Caekert A, et al. Influence of Helicobacter pylori eradication therapy on the occurrence of gastrointestinal events in patients treated with conventional nonsteroidal anti-inflammatory drugs combined with omeprazole. J Rheumatol 2002;29(9);1975–1980.
3. Lazzaroni M, Porro GB. Review article: Helicobacter pylori and NSAID gastropathy. Aliment Pharmacol Ther 2001;15 (Suppl 1):22–27.
4. Chan FK, To KF, Wu JC, et al. Eradication of Helicobacter pylori and risk of peptic ulcers in patients starting long-term treatment with non-steroidal anti-inflammatory drugs: A randomised trial. Lancet 2002;359:9–13.
5. Huang JQ, Sridhar S, Hunt RH. Role of Helicobacter pylori infection and non-steroidal anti-inflammatory drugs in peptic-ulcer disease: A meta-analysis. Lancet 2002; 359:14–22.
6. ASHP Commission on Therapeutics. ASHP Therapeutic position statement on the identification and treatment of Helicobacter pylori-associated peptic ulcer disease in adults. Am J Health Syst Pharm 2001:58; 331–337.
7. Hawkey CJ, Karrasch JA, Szczepanski L, et al. Omeprazole compared with misoprostol for ulcers associated with nonsteroidal anti-inflammatory drugs. N Engl J Med 1998;338: 727–734.
8. American College of Rheumatology Subcommittee on Osteoarthritis Guidelines. Recommendations for the medical management of osteoarthritis of the hip and knee: 2000 update. Arthritis Rheum 2000;43:1905–1915.
9. Cullen D, Bardhan KD, Eisner M, et al. Primary gastroduodenal prophylaxis with omeprazole for non-steroidal anti-inflammatory drug users. Aliment Pharmacol Ther 1998;12:135–140.
10. Graham DY, Agrawal NM, Campbell DR, et al; NSAID-Associated Gastric Ulcer Prevention Study Group. Ulcer prevention in long-term users of nonsteroidal anti-inflammatory drugs: results of a double-blind, randomized, multicenter, active- and placebo-controlled study of misoprostol vs. lansoprazole. Arch Intern Med 2002;162:169–175.
11. Scheiman JM, Yeomans, N, Hawkey CJ, et al. Esomeprazole reduces gastric and duodenal ulcer development among high risk NSAID users. Am J Gastroenterol. 2003; 98(9) Suppl:S52. Abstract.
12. Pavelka K, Gatterova J, Olejarova M, et al. Glucosamine sulfate use and delay of progression of knee osteoarthritis: a 3-year, randomized, placebo-controlled, double-blind study. Arch Intern Med 2002;162:2113–2123.
13. McAlindon TE, LaValley MP, Gulin JP, et al. Glucosamine and chondroitin for the treatment of osteoarthritis: a systematic quality assessment and meta-analysis. JAMA 2000;283:1469–1475.
14. Lichtenstein DR, Syngal S, Wolfe MM. Nonsteroidal anti-inflammatory drugs and the gastrointestinal tract: the double-edged sword. Arthritis Rheum 1995;38:5–18.
15. Rostom A, Dube C, Wells G, et al. Prevention of NSAID-induced gastroduodenal ulcers (Cochrane Review). In: The Cochrane Library, Issue 4, 2003. Chichester, UK: John Wiley & Sons, Ltd.

31 STRESS ULCER PROPHYLAXIS/UPPER GI HEMORRHAGE

▶ Prophylaxis Offers No Guarantee (Level I)

Kristie C. Reeves, PharmD, BCPS
Henry J. Mann, PharmD, FCCP, FCCM, FASHP

▶ After completing this case study, students should be able to:

- Identify risk factors associated with stress gastritis/ulceration and determine which critically ill patients should receive pharmacologic prophylaxis.
- Recommend appropriate pharmacologic alternatives including agent, route of administration, and dose for the prevention of stress-induced gastritis/ulceration.

- Identify and implement monitoring parameters for their recommended stress gastritis/ulceration prophylactic regimens.
- Discuss the pharmacologic approaches to the management of stress ulcer-induced bleeding.

PATIENT PRESENTATION

Chief Complaint

"Terrible pain everywhere around my stomach."

HPI

BJ is a 75 yo man who presents to the ED complaining of increasing abdominal pain over the last 24 hours. He noticed diffuse abdominal pain yesterday that was initially relieved by oxycodone 5 mg/acetaminophen 325 mg (Percocet) that he had left over from a previous prescription. This morning he rated his pain as a 10 on a 1 to 10 scale, with radiation to his back. He reports several vomiting episodes (yellow–green in color) in the last day, and that his last BM was about 48 hours ago.

PMH

HTN × approximately 20 years
CAD; S/P MI 8 years ago; s/p CABG × 3
CHF; EF 15% to 20% by transesophageal echocardiogram 4 years ago; currently experiences symptoms at rest
COPD
GI bleed secondary to NSAIDs eight months ago
OA
S/P cholecystectomy
S/P appendectomy

FH

Father died of "heart attack" at age of 55 and mother is in "good health."

SH

Patient is retired. He smokes cigarettes 1 ppd, which is down from a couple of years ago. He had previously smoked 2 ppd for 25 years.

ROS

Patient is nauseated with labored breathing; some confusion is noted when speaking with him. No complaints of chest pain, increased weakness, fatigue, or recent weight gain.

Meds

Furosemide 40 mg po BID
Digoxin 0.25 mg po once daily
Amlodipine 5 mg po once daily
Enalapril 10 mg po BID
Atrovent inhaler 2 puffs QID
Albuterol inhaler PRN
Colace 100 mg po BID
Celecoxib 200 mg once daily

All

PCN (hives)

PE

Gen

Elderly gentleman in obvious distress with difficulty breathing and significant abdominal pain.

VS

BP 105/65, P 120, RR 26, T 37.9°C; Ht 5′10″, Wt 71 kg

Skin

Warm, dry

Neck/LN

Supple; no JVD or bruits; no lymphadenopathy or thyromegaly

HEENT

PERRL, EOMI; fundi benign; nares patent; TMs intact

LUNG

Decreased breath sounds bilaterally with both inspiratory and expiratory wheezes bilaterally; no rales or rhonchi

CV

S_1, S_2 normal; sinus tachycardia with S_3, S_4

Abd

Firm, with diffuse tenderness to light palpation; no bowel sounds appreciated

Genit/Rect

Normal male genitalia; stool heme negative

Neuro

A & O × 2; somewhat confused

Labs

Na 138 mEq/L	Hgb 14.1 g/dL
K 3.8 mEq/L	Hct 40.8%
Cl 101 mEq/L	WBC 10.7 × 10^3/mm^3
CO_2 28 mEq/L	Plt 203 × 10^3/mm^3
BUN 21 mg/dL	Digoxin 0.5 ng/mL
SCr 1.6 mg/dL	
Glu 160 mg/dL	

ABG

pH 7.26, $PaCO_2$ 59 mm Hg, PaO_2 95 mm Hg

Abdominal X-Ray

Demonstrates free air

► Clinical Course

The patient was taken to the operating room for an exploratory laparotomy and was found to have a perforation of his cecum near the ileocecal valve. The surgeons noted minimal soilage, and the patient underwent a right hemicolectomy with a primary anastamosis. A central line was placed intraoperatively. He received 7 L of lactated Ringer's solution and 2 units of whole blood during the operation. He was taken to the surgical ICU postoperatively, mechanically ventilated and hemodynamically stable. He received antibiotic prophylaxis with clindamycin 900 mg IV Q 8 H plus aztreonam 1 g IV Q 8 H beginning before surgery and continuing for 24 hours after surgery to prevent surgical wound infection. Six hours postoperatively, his vital signs are BP 120/75, P 95, and CVP 14. Breath sounds are decreased bilaterally with bilateral rales now present. His urine output has been 60–80 mL/h for the past 6 hours. His blood glucose level is 160 mg/dL.

▶ Questions

Problem Identification

1. a. *As the pharmacist in the surgical ICU, you review the patient's chronic medications and recommend which medications should be restarted postoperatively and suggest any changes to these regimens during patient rounds. What are your recommendations for this patient's chronic medications and why?*

▶ Clinical Course

Two days postoperatively, the patient is improving but remains mechanically ventilated. Faint bowel sounds are now present but he is still NPO and requiring continuous NG suction. During rounds, the critical care team decides to stop continuous NG suction and initiate enteral feeds with Isosource VHN®, starting at 10 mL/hr, and advancing as tolerated by 20 mL/hr every 4 hours to a goal of 80 mL/hr. In addition to the medications restarted on your recommendation, he is also receiving lorazepam 1 mg IV Q 6 H, and morphine 2 mg/hr by continuous IV infusion. Recorded NG aspirate pH is 2.0.

b. *List all of the patient's drug therapy problems at this point in his hospital course (include both potential and actual drug therapy problems).*

c. *What are the risk factors for developing stress gastritis/ulceration in critically ill patients?*

d. *Do this patient's risk factors warrant prophylactic therapy to prevent stress ulceration?*

Desired Outcome

2. *What are the goals of pharmacotherapy for prevention of stress gastritis and ulceration?*

Therapeutic Alternatives

3. *Discuss the pharmacologic options available for the prophylaxis of stress ulceration in critically ill patients.*

Optimal Plan

4. *What would you recommend for stress ulcer prophylaxis in this patient?*

Outcome Evaluation

5. *What clinical parameters should be monitored to assess the effectiveness of this regimen?*

▶ Clinical Course

The surgical ICU team decides to use an H_2-receptor antagonist for prophylaxis. Morning labs: Na 141 mEq/L, K 4.3 mEq/L, BUN 29 mg/dL, SCr 1.9 mg/dL, Glu 180 mg/dL, WBC 11.2 × $10^3/mm^3$, Hgb 11.4 g/dL.

▶ Follow-Up Questions

1. *Based on your team's decision, what are the appropriate regimens for cimetidine, ranitidine, and famotidine in this patient?*

▶ Clinical Course

The following morning you note that the pH readings for the prior two nursing shifts (16 hours) have been 2.0 and 3.0, respectively, on the therapy you recommended. The nurse notes that the last measurement of NG residuals appeared to be blood-tinged and today's hemoglobin is 9.8 g/dL. You check the medication administration record and determine that all prescribed doses of therapy have been administered. Of note, the team thinks that he may be extubated later today with the possibility of moving him to the floor tomorrow.

2. *Based on the above information, what action should be taken to improve the patient's prophylaxis regimen?*

▶ Clinical Course

Later that day, a drop in BP to 90/50 mm Hg is noted by the nurse. His HR is 125 bpm, but he remains in NSR. Hgb is 8.5 g/dL. Two 500-mL saline flushes were given and resulted in an increase in his BP to 115/80 mm Hg. His HR decreased to 105 bpm. After he was determined to be hemodynamically stable, an EGD was performed. The gastroenterologist visualized multiple small gastric lesions that are oozing blood.

3. *What pharmacologic therapy would you suggest at this time?*

▶ Clinical Course

Three days later the NG aspirate has cleared of blood but remains guaiac positive. He has received a total of 2 units of PRBC and is hemodynamically stable and extubated. Bowel sounds are detected in all four quadrants, the NG tube is removed, and orders are written to initiate an oral diet, beginning with clear liquids and advancing as tolerated. Hgb 11.3 g/dL, BP 135/85 mm Hg, HR 85–90 bpm.

4. *What medication changes, if any, would you recommend at this time?*

▶ Self-Study Assignments

1. Describe how to mix and store omeprazole and lansoprazole suspensions.
2. Discuss how to mix, store, and administer IV pantoprazole.
3. Discuss the administration of sucralfate to renally-compromised patients who may be at risk for aluminum accumulation.
4. Identify potential drug interactions and adverse effects with antisecretory therapy (antacids, sucralfate, H_2-receptor antagonists, and proton pump inhibitors).
5. Discuss whether or not sucralfate use for stress ulcer prophylaxis decreases the incidence of nosocomial pneumonia in comparison to the use of H_2-receptor antagonists.
6. Discuss the prognostic significance of the appearance of an ulcer at the time of the initial endoscopy.

▶ Clinical Pearl

For agents administered through a nasogastric tube, check whether the patient is currently on active suction. If so, NG suction should be held for at least 30 to 60 minutes after the administration of any medication to prevent suctioning out significant amounts of the drug.

References

1. Bombardier C, Laine L, Reicin A, et al. Comparison of upper gastrointestinal toxicity of rofecoxib and naproxen in patients with rheumatoid arthritis. VIGOR Study Group. N Engl J Med 2000;343:1520–1528.
2. Pitt B, Zannad F, Remme WJ, et al. The effect of spironolactone on morbidity and mortality in patients with severe heart failure. Randomized Aldactone Evaluation Study Investigators. N Engl J Med 1999;341:709–717.
3. Cicoira M, Zanolla L, Rossi A, et al. Long-term, dose-dependent effects of spironolactone on left ventricular function and exercise tolerance in patients with chronic heart failure. J Am Coll Cardiol 2002;40:304–310.
4. MacLaren R, Jarvis CL, Fish DN. Use of enteral nutrition for stress ulcer prophylaxis. Ann Pharmacother 2001;35:1614–623.
5. van den Berghe G, Wouters P, Weekers F, et al. Intensive insulin therapy in critically ill patients. N Engl J Med 2001;345:1359–1367.
6. Tryba M, Cook D. Current guidelines on stress ulcer prophylaxis. Drugs 1997;54(4):581–596.
7. Cook DJ, Fuller HD, Guyatt GH, et al. Risk factors for gastrointestinal bleeding in critically ill patients. Canadian Critical Care Trials Group. N Engl J Med 1994;330:377–381.
8. Cook D, Heyland D, Griffith L, et al. Risk factors for clinically important upper gastrointestinal bleeding in patients requiring mechanical ventilation. Crit Care Med 1999;27:2812–2817.
9. American Society of Health-System Pharmacists. ASHP therapeutic guidelines on stress ulcer prophylaxis. Am J Health Syst Pharm 1999;56:347–379.
10. Levy MJ, Seelig CB, Robinson NJ, et al. Comparison of omeprazole and ranitidine for stress ulcer prophylaxis. Dig Dis Sci 1997;42:1255–1259.
11. Phillips JO, Metzler MH, Palmieri MT, et al. A prospective study of simplified omeprazole suspension for the prophylaxis of stress-related mucosal damage. Crit Care Med 1996;24:1793–1800.
12. Lasky MR, Metzler MH, Phillips, JO. A prospective study of omeprazole suspension to prevent clinically significant gastrointestinal bleeding from stress ulcers in mechanically ventilated trauma patients. J Trauma 1998;44:527–533.
13. Jung R, MacLaren R. Proton-pump inhibitors for stress ulcer prophylaxis in critically ill patients. Ann Pharmacother 2002;36:1929–1937.
14. Cook D, Guyatt G, Marshall J, et al. A comparison of sucralfate and ranitidine for the prevention of upper gastrointestinal bleeding in patients requiring mechanical ventilation. N Engl J Med 1998;338:791–797.
15. Mathot RA, Geus WP. Pharmacodynamic modeling of the acid inhibitory effect of ranitidine in patients in an intensive care unit during prolonged dosing: Characterization of tolerance. Clin Pharmacol Ther 1999;66:140–151.
16. Schupp KN, Schrand LM, Mutnick AH. A cost-effectiveness analysis of stress ulcer prophylaxis. Ann Pharmacother 2003;37:631–635.
17. Fennerty MB. Pathophysiology of the upper gastrointestinal tract in the critically ill patient: rationale for the therapeutic benefits of acid suppression. Crit Care Med 2002;30(6 Suppl):S351–S355.
18. Laterre PF, Horsmans Y. Intravenous omeprazole in critically ill patients: a randomized, crossover study comparing 40 with 80 mg plus 8 mg/hour on intragastric pH. Crit Care Med 2001;29:1931–1935.
19. Heiselman DE, Hulisz DT, Fricker R, et al. Randomized comparison of gastric pH control with intermittent and continuous intravenous infusion of famotidine in ICU patients. Am J Gastroenterol 1995;90:277–279.
20. Siepler JK, Trudeau W, Petty DE. Use of continuous infusion of histamine$_2$–receptor antagonists in critically ill patients. DICP 1989;23(10 Suppl): S40–S43.

32 CROHN'S DISEASE

▶ From Top to Bottom (Level II)

Kerry A. Cholka, PharmD

▶ **After completing this case study, students should be able to:**

- Identify the common signs and symptoms of Crohn's disease and classify the severity of the disease.
- Describe treatment options for a patient with chronic Crohn's disease and recommend a specific treatment plan that includes medication, dosing regimen, and monitoring parameters for efficacy and potential side effects.
- Educate a patient on the proper use of medications used to treat Crohn's disease.

PATIENT PRESENTATION

Chief Complaint

"I am doing okay, but my diarrhea continues to be a problem."

HPI

Diana Cummings is a 45 yo woman with a 30-year history of Crohn's disease. She was referred by her PCP to the GI Clinic. This is her initial GI Clinic visit. Her disease course has included stricturing small-bowel disease, multiple small-bowel resections in the past, and chronic steroid dependency with disease exacerbation when attempting to taper steroids. The patient had been on Azulfidine but stopped taking it and has not been treated with salicylates for many years. Because of the concerns about Ms. Cummings's current medical therapy for Crohn's disease, the PCP has sent the following tests results with the patient: (a) Cortrosyn stimulation test indicating adrenal insufficiency, and (b) DEXA scan measuring bone mineral density at 1.71 standard deviations below the young adult mean, which is diagnostic for osteopenia.

PSH

- Portion of jejunum resected in 1983 (Crohn's scarring/stricture leading to obstruction)
- Portion of small bowel resected in 1991 (stricture/acute inflammation)
- Portion of small bowel resected in 1996 (Crohn's stricture leading to obstruction) leaving 180 cm of small intestine beyond the Ligament of Treitz with an intact ileocecal valve and colon

PMH

- Crohn's diagnosed in 1973 (weight loss, diarrhea, vomiting, abdominal pain)
- HTN
- Depression with associated insomnia

FH

Remarkable for DM, HTN, and CAD in her mother; no family history of IBD

SH

Works as an assistant in a home for the mentally disabled; lives alone. Drinks alcohol socially; has a 23 pack-year history of smoking.

ROS

Up to 15 loose to semi-sold stools per day; no blood or mucus. Denies abdominal pain, cramps, fevers, or chills. Stable weight and good appetite. Denies headache, aphthous ulcers. Decreased visual acuity attributed to old corrective lenses. Lightheadedness upon rising; denies vertigo or tinnitus. Denies CP/SOB/cough, and denies joint pain or skin rashes. Some mild fatigue.

Meds

- Prednisone 10 mg po once daily
- Trazodone 100 mg po at bedtime for sleep
- Sertraline 100 mg po once daily
- Vitamin B_{12} 1000 mcg IM Q month
- Tramadol 50 mg po Q 6 H PRN
- Hydrochlorothiazide/triamterene 25 mg/37.5 mg 1 po daily (patient recently ran out)

All

NKDA

PE

Gen

Middle-aged African-American woman, somewhat anxious, in NAD, well developed, Cushingoid appearing.

VS

BP 146/92, P 72, RR 15, afebrile; Wt. 70 kg, Ht 5′2″

Skin

Warm and dry with flakiness

HEENT

PERRLA; EOMI; anicteric sclera, normal conjunctivae; mouth is moist and pink; pharynx is clear

Lungs

CTA and percussion bilaterally

CV

RRR with no murmurs

Abd

BS normally active, abdomen soft, NTND with no masses or organomegaly

Rectal

An external skin tag is present, but no other perianal lesions noted. No internal masses; stool is guaiac negative

MS/Ext

No CCE; 2+ dorsalis pedis and posterior tibial pulses bilaterally

Neuro

A & O × 3; CN II–XII intact; motor 5/5 upper and lower extremity bilaterally; sensation intact and reflexes symmetric with downgoing toes

Labs

Na 142 mEq/L	Hgb 13.9 g/dL	AST 18 IU/L	Ca 8.8 mg/dL
K 4.3 mEq/L	Hct 41.7%	ALT 19 IU/L	Mg 1.5 mEq/L
Cl 103 mEq/L	Plt 301 × 10^3/mm^3	Alk Phos 192 IU/L	Po_4 2.5 mg/dL
CO_2 25 mEq/L	WBC 9.3 × 10^3/mm^3	GGT 200 IU/L	PT 14.3 sec
BUN 6 mg/dL		T. bili 0.3 mg/dL	INR 1.2
SCr 0.7 mg/dL		T. prot 5.9 g/dL	
Glu 76 mg/dL		Alb 3.0 g/dL	

▶ Questions

Problem Identification

1. a. *Develop a drug therapy problem list for this patient.*
   b. *List the signs, symptoms, and laboratory values that indicate the presence of Crohn's disease in this patient.*
   c. *Based on the data presented, classify the severity of this patient's Crohn's disease. Explain the rationale for your decision and how it guides the approach to her treatment.*

Desired Outcomes

2. *What are the therapeutic goals for this patient?*

Therapeutic Alternatives

3. *What pharmacotherapeutic alternatives are available for the primary treatment of Crohn's disease?*

Optimal Plan

4. *What course of treatment (drug, dose, route, and schedule) would you recommend for this patient?*

Assessment Parameters

5. *What clinical and laboratory parameters can be used to evaluate the therapy for efficacy as well as adverse effects?*

Patient Education

6. *What information should be provided to the patient to help enhance adherence to the medications as well as prevent adverse events?*

▶ Clinical Course

Ms. Cummings receives the therapy that you recommended and was able to achieve remission of her Crohn's disease by her 4-week return visit. Eight months later, she returns to the GI clinic urgently, complaining of increased abdominal pain and diarrhea. Her abdominal pain is constant and is localized to the periumbilical region. She is again having up to 15 loose stools per day. She is tolerating oral nutrition, but her weight has dropped to 66 kg.

▶ Follow-Up Questions

1. *Considering this new information, what therapeutic intervention(s) are available for the secondary treatment of Crohn's disease?*
2. *What therapeutic regimen(s) would provide optimal therapy for the patient at this time?*

▶ Self-Study Assignments

1. Compare the prescription prices of the various mesalamine preparations and sulfasalazine in your geographic area.
2. Perform a literature search to learn about the use of infliximab in the treatment of Crohn's disease.
3. Create a dose equivalency table for the corticosteroids used in Crohn's disease.

▶ Clinical Pearl

Patients allergic to sulfas should not take sulfasalazine, and patients allergic to aspirin should not take sulfasalazine, olsalazine, or the mesalamine products.

References

1. Hanauer SB, Sandborn W; Practice Parameters Committee of the American College of Gastroenterology. Management of Crohn's disease in adults. Am J Gastroenterol 2001;96:635–643.
2. Pearson DC, May GR, Fick GH, et al. Azathioprine and 6-MP in Crohn's disease: a meta-analysis. Ann Intern Med 1995;122:132–142.
3. Feagan B, Rochon J, Fedorak RN. Methotrexate for the treatment of Crohn's disease. N Engl J Med 1995;332:292–297.
4. Ardizzone S, Porro GB. Inflammatory bowel disease: new insights into pathogenesis and treatment. J Intern Med 2002;252:475–496.
5. Garnett WR, Yunker N. Treatment of Crohn's disease with infliximab. Am J Health Syst Pharm 2001;58:307–316.
6. Kane SV, Schoenfeld P, Sandborn WJ, et al. The effectiveness of budesonide therapy for Crohn's disease. Aliment Pharmacol Ther 2002;16:1509–1517.

33 ULCERATIVE COLITIS

▶ The Schoolteacher's Lament (Level I)

Nancy S. Yunker, PharmD
Ralph E. Small, PharmD, FCCP, FASHP, FAPhA

▶ After completing this case study, students should be able to:

- Identify the common signs and symptoms of ulcerative colitis.
- Describe treatment options for an acute episode of ulcerative colitis and recommend a specific treatment plan for a patient that includes the medication, dosing regimen, potential side effects, and monitoring parameters.
- Develop a pharmacotherapeutic plan for an ulcerative colitis patient whose disease is in remission.
- Educate other health care professionals on recent advances in the pharmacotherapy of ulcerative colitis.

PATIENT PRESENTATION

Chief Complaint

"I've got blood in my stool and feel very weak."

HPI

John Frederickson is a 29 yo man who presents to the ED with the chief complaint of BRBPR and weakness. He was in his usual state of health until 4 days ago when he noticed BRBPR and an increased frequency of bowel movements (four to five each day). He describes bowel urgency and states that each bowel movement contains approximately 1 tablespoonful of blood; no bleeding is noted between bowel movements. He states that he has been weak for approximately 2 days. He has not traveled outside the city, been hospitalized, or received antibiotics recently.

PMH

HTN

FH

Father: history of ulcerative colitis, s/p colectomy 15 years ago

SH

Works as a schoolteacher; lives alone. No alcohol; quit smoking 1 year ago.

ROS

Negative for lightheadedness, previous episodes of rectal bleeding or spraying of toilet with blood, N/V, and muscle stiffness/soreness. Positive for occasional mild abdominal soreness.

Meds

Hydrochlorothiazide 25 mg po once daily × 3 years
Felodipine 5 mg po once daily × 6 months
Lactinex granules × 3 days

All

Sulfa drugs (rash/hives)

PE

Gen

A & O, pleasant, healthy-appearing white man in NAD; appears pale

VS

At 8 AM:

BP (lying down) 160/63 mm Hg, P 61 bpm
BP (standing) 157/65 mm Hg, P 89 bpm
RR 20 bpm, T 37.0°C, Pulse oximetry 96% on RA
Wt 81.2 kg (usual weight 83.0 kg), Ht 5′8″

Skin

No lesions; warm, adequate turgor

HEENT

PERRLA; EOMI; negative for iritis, uveitis, and conjunctivitis; funduscopic exam shows no AV nicking, hemorrhages, or exudates; moist mucous membranes; TMs intact

Lungs

CTA, no rales or rhonchi

CV

RRR, normal S_1 and S_2; no S_3, S_4

Abd

BS (+), soft, NTND, no palpable mass, no liver or spleen enlargement

Rectal

Somewhat tender; no hemorrhoids, fissures, or lesions by anoscopy; heme (+) stool

MS/Ext

No CCE; pulses 2+; normal ROM; normal strength bilaterally

Neuro

A & O × 3; CN II–XII intact; DTRs 2+

Labs

At 8:00 AM:

Na 139 mEq/L	Hgb 10.9 g/dL	WBC 6.8 × 10^3/mm^3	AST 32 IU/L
K 3.2 mEq/L	Hct 33.4%	PMNs 52%	ALT 30 IU/L
Cl 92 mEq/L	Plt 298 × 10^3/mm^3	Bands 5%	Alk phos 40 IU/L
CO_2 31 mEq/L	MCV 82 μm^3	Lymphs 36%	T. Bili 0.5 mg/dL
BUN 26 mg/dL	MCH 28 pg	Basos 1%	PT 12.0 sec
SCr 1.2 mg/dL	MCHC 32.6 g/dL	Monos 6%	INR 1.0
Glu 162 mg/dL			Ca 8.5 mg/dL
			PO_4 4.4 mg/dL

► Clinical Course

The patient received 1 L of 0.9% saline with KCl 30 mEq over 4 hours starting at 9:00 AM. Vital signs at 1:00 PM were as follows: BP (lying down) 155/82 mm Hg, P 62 bpm; BP (standing) 158/84 mm Hg, P 64 bpm. Repeat laboratory tests at 2:00 PM were as follows:

Na 137 mEq/L	Hgb 10.0 g/dL
K 3.5 mEq/L	Hct 31.3%
Cl 97 mEq/L	Plt 262 × 10^3/mm^3
CO_2 28 mEq/L	MCV 82 μm^3
BUN 11 mg/dL	MCH 26.2 pg
SCr 1.0 mg/dL	MCHC 32 g/dL
Glu 119 mg/dL	WBC 6.2 × 10^3/mm^3

ED assessment:

1. GI bleed; patient is stable after volume repletion
2. D/C to home with instructions to return to ED or PCP if symptoms return
3. Referral to GI clinic for colonoscopy

Follow-Up Evaluation

Colonoscopy (2 days after discharge from the ED): Adequate preparation. Diagnoses: (a) edema, erythema, crypt abscesses with mild oozing of blood; continuous from rectum to 1 cm below the splenic flexure, c/w moderate ulcerative colitis; (b) small internal hemorrhoids; (c) biopsy negative for cancer; (d) histology: distorted crypt architecture, mixed acute and chronic inflammation in the lamina propria, PMNs in the surface epithelium; no granulomas noted.

Assessment

Ulcerative colitis

Questions

Problem Identification

1. a. *List all of the patient's drug therapy problems, including those existing at his initial presentation to the ED.*
   b. *List the signs, symptoms, and laboratory values that indicate the presence and severity of ulcerative colitis; also include pertinent negative findings.*
   c. *Could the manifestations of the patient's ulcerative colitis have been precipitated by any event?*

Desired Outcome

2. *What are the short- and long-term pharmacotherapeutic goals for this patient?*

Therapeutic Alternatives

3. a. *What nondrug therapies might be useful for this patient?*
   b. *What feasible pharmacotherapeutic alternatives should be considered for the treatment of ulcerative colitis?*

Optimal Plan

4. a. *Based on your current assessment of the patient's disease severity, recommend an appropriate drug regimen.*
   b. *What alternatives should be considered if the patient fails to respond to initial therapy?*

Outcome Evaluation

5. *What clinical and laboratory parameters are necessary to evaluate the therapy for achievement of the desired therapeutic outcome and to detect or prevent adverse effects?*

Patient Education

6. *What information should be provided to the patient to enhance adherence, ensure successful therapy, and minimize adverse effects?*

Clinical Course

The patient successfully completed the initial course of therapy and returns to the physician 8 weeks later for follow-up. He states adherence with his therapeutic regimen, describes his bowel habits as normal, and has no complaints of weakness or abdominal/rectal tenderness. The repeat Hgb today is 13.1 g/dL.

Follow-Up Questions

1. *Considering this new information, what therapeutic intervention(s) do you recommend at this time?*
2. *What additional information should be provided to the patient?*

Self-Study Assignments

1. Review the literature comparing mesalamine, olsalazine, balsalazide, and sulfasalazine preparations regarding efficacy, adverse effects, and cost; include all currently available mesalamine dosage forms.
2. Perform a literature search to determine what new therapies are being evaluated for ulcerative colitis.
3. Review the literature regarding the currently proposed pathogenesis of ulcerative colitis, and relate your findings to the medications currently available and being investigated in clinical trials.
4. Conduct a literature search to determine how pharmacogenomics is affecting therapy of ulcerative colitis patients.

Clinical Pearl

Oral budesonide is a potent glucocorticoid with low systemic bioavailability used for Crohn's disease affecting the ileum and ascending colon. It has not been well studied for ulcerative colitis in the U. S. and is not an appropriate substitute for traditional oral glucocorticoid therapy in ulcerative colitis patients.

References

1. Chobanian AV, Bakris GL, Black HR, et al. The Seventh Report of the Joint National Committee on Prevention, Detection, Evaluation, and Treatment of High Blood Pressure: The JNC 7 report. JAMA 2003;289:2560–2572.
2. Sartor RB. Clinical applications of advances in the genetics of IBD. Rev Gastroenterol Disord 2003;3(Suppl 1):S9–S17.
3. Podolsky DK. Inflammatory bowel disease. N Engl J Med 2002; 347:417–429.
4. Motley RJ, Rhodes J, Ford GA, et al. Time relationships between cessation of smoking and onset of ulcerative colitis. Digestion 1987;37:125–127.
5. Sands BE. Therapy of inflammatory bowel disease. Gastroenterology 2000:118(2 Suppl 1):S68–S82.
6. Sutherland L, MacDonald JK. Oral 5-aminosalicylic acid for induction of remission in ulcerative colitis (Cochrane Review). In: *The Cochrane Library*, Issue 3, 2003. Oxford: Update Software.
7. Kornbluth A, Sachar DB. Ulcerative colitis practice guidelines in adults. American College of Gastroenterology, Practice Parameters Committee. Am J Gastroenterol 1997;92:204–211.
8. Hanauer SB, Present DH. The state of the art in the management of inflammatory bowel disease. Rev Gastroenterol Disord 2003;3:81–92.
9. Marshall JK, Irvine EJ. Putting rectal 5-aminosalicylic acid in its place: The role in distal ulcerative colitis. Am J Gastroenterol 2000;95:1628–1636.
10. Ardizzone S, Porro GB. A practical guide to the management of distal ulcerative colitis. Drugs 1998;55(4):519–542.
11. Sandborn WJ. Rational selection of oral 5-aminosalicylate formulations and prodrugs for the treatment of ulcerative colitis. Am J Gastroenterol 2002;97:2939–2941.
12. Sandborn WJ. Nicotine therapy for ulcerative colitis: A review of rationale, mechanisms, pharmacology, and clinical results. Am J Gastroenterol 1999;94:1161–1171.
13. Schultz M, Sartor RB. Probiotics and inflammatory bowel diseases. Am J Gastroenterol 2000;95(1 Suppl):S19–S21.
14. Cuffari C, Hunt S, Bayless T. Use of erythrocyte 6-thioguanine metabolite levels

to optimize azathioprine therapy in patients with inflammatory bowel disease. Gut 2001;48:642–646.

15. Sutherland L, Roth D, Beck P, et al. Oral 5-aminosalicylic acid for maintenance of remission in ulcerative colitis (Cochrane Review). In: *The Cochrane Library*, Issue 3, 2003. Oxford: Update Software.
16. Bernstein CN, Eaden J, Steinhart AH, et al. Cancer prevention in inflammatory bowel disease and chemoprophylactic potential of 5-aminosalicylic acid. Inflamm Bowel Dis 2002; 8:356–361.

34 NAUSEA AND VOMITING

▶ Family Ties (Level II)

Kelly K. Nystrom, PharmD, BCOP
Pamela A. Foral, PharmD, BCPS

▶ After completing this case study, students should be able to:

- Develop a regimen of prophylactic antiemetics based on the emetogenic risk associated with cancer chemotherapeutic agents to optimize the management of nausea and vomiting.
- Design an appropriate treatment regimen for anticipatory, breakthrough, and delayed nausea and vomiting.
- Design a monitoring plan to assess the effectiveness of an antiemetic regimen.
- Advise patients and caregivers on the reason for antiemetics, their appropriate use, and management of side effects.
- Recommend appropriate alternative antiemetic strategies based on patient-specific conditions such as response to the initial regimen and side effects.

PATIENT PRESENTATION

Chief Complaint

"I've been vomiting for 2 days."

HPI

Shelley Smith is a 35 yo woman who comes to the cancer center clinic 2 days after her first cycle of chemotherapy because of nausea and vomiting that started as she was leaving the clinic. She was diagnosed with Stage II epithelial ovarian cancer 1 month ago and underwent a unilateral salpingoophorectomy to preserve fertility. The current plan is for her to receive six cycles of carboplatin and paclitaxel therapy. Dosing consists of paclitaxel 175 mg/m^2 IV over 3 hours and carboplatin AUC 6 IV over 30 minutes, with both drugs repeated every 21 days for 6 cycles. Her antiemetics prior to her first cycle consisted of ondansetron 24 mg po and dexamethasone 12 mg po 30 minutes before her chemotherapy. She complained of nausea and vomiting as she was leaving the clinic, and the doctor ordered ondansetron 8 mg IV to be administered before she left. She was given prescriptions for prochlorperazine and lorazepam to be used for breakthrough nausea and vomiting and scheduled metoclopramide and dexamethasone to be started the following day to prevent delayed nausea and vomiting. The nausea and vomiting has persisted for 2 days, despite continued therapy.

PMH

Migraine headaches × 12 years
Severe motion sickness

FH

Maternal grandmother with ovarian cancer

SH

Married. One child, age 4. Works part-time as a teacher's aide. No alcohol or tobacco use. Physically very active and works out three to four times per week.

ROS

Complains of nausea, vomiting, epigastric discomfort, headache (migraine), fatigue. Denies fever, abdominal pain, diarrhea, change in stool color (i.e., melena), GU complaints, weakness, SOB, numbness or tingling in extremities.

Meds

Propranolol LA 80 mg po once daily
Midrin 2 po PRN migraine
Ortho-cyclen 1 po daily

All

No known allergies

PE

Gen

WDWN woman in moderate distress

VS

BP 115/75, P 97, RR 16, T 37°C; Wt 58 kg (60.5 kg 2 days ago), Ht 5′4″

Skin

Warm, dry, decreased turgor. No rashes or petechiae.

HEENT

PERRLA, EOMI, fundi benign, TMs intact, mucous membranes dry

Neck/LN

Thyroid NL. No adenopathy.

Lungs/Thorax
Lungs clear to auscultation

CV
RRR, no m/r/g

Abd
Soft, non-tender, well-healing abdominal incision

Genit/Rect
Genital exam not done. Rectal NL, stool guaiac negative

MS/Ext
No edema. Pulses 3+ throughout

Neuro
No visual abnormalities, cranial nerves intact, DTRs 2+

Labs

Na 140 mEq/L	Hgb 13.6 g/dL
K 3.0 mEq/L	Hct 43%
Cl 94 mEq/L	Plt 220 × 10^3/mm^3
CO_2 28 mEq/L	WBC 3.4 × 10^3/mm^3
BUN 30 mg/dL	48% PMNs
SCr 1.1 mg/dL	0% Bands
Glu 85 mg/dL	43% Lymphs
T. bili 0.7 mg/dL	6% Monos
	2% Eos
	1% Basos

Assessment
Dehydration and hypokalemia secondary to chemotherapy-induced emesis vs. migraine-associated nausea and vomiting

▶ Questions

Problem Identification

1. a. *Create a list of this patient's drug therapy problems.*
   b. *What are this patient's risk factors for nausea and vomiting?*

Desired Outcome

2. *What are the goals of therapy in this case?*

Therapeutic Alternatives

3. a. *What nondrug therapies may be useful to prevent nausea and vomiting?*
   b. *Why was the choice of antiemetic before she left the clinic inappropriate for the breakthrough nausea and vomiting episode?*
   c. *What pharmacologic alternatives may be helpful for the acute treatment of this patient?*
   d. *What therapeutic alternatives should be considered prior to her next cycle of chemotherapy to prevent future episodes of nausea and vomiting?*
   e. *If delayed nausea and vomiting is a concern, what measures can be implemented to prevent it?*

Optimal Plan

4. a. *Design a plan for the treatment of acute nausea and vomiting in this patient for subsequent cycles.*
   b. *Design a plan for the prevention of delayed nausea and vomiting in this patient for subsequent cycles.*
   c. *Design a regimen to treat breakthrough nausea and vomiting in this patient for subsequent cycles.*

Outcome Evaluation

5. a. *State how you will determine whether the antiemetic regimen you recommended for her acute treatment has been effective.*
   b. *Describe the information you will need to assess the efficacy and adverse effects of the prophylactic antiemetic regimen prior to each future course of chemotherapy.*

Patient Education

6. *How would you educate this patient on her antiemetic regimen?*

▶ Clinical Course

After treatment according to your recommendations, Mrs. Smith reports that she has not vomited for several hours and no longer feels nauseated. She will be coming back to the clinic in 3 weeks for her next course of carboplatin and paclitaxel, and she is fearful that she will again experience severe nausea and vomiting. In response to your education, she states that she feels less anxious. She agrees to take the medications you have recommended to her for her nausea and vomiting.

When she returns in 3 weeks, her physician follows your advice regarding antiemetics before and after her chemotherapy. Your follow-up phone call the next day confirms that she is taking her medications as instructed. She is experiencing no nausea or vomiting and no side effects of her antiemetics.

▶ Self-Study Assignments

1. Compare the indications, doses and costs of the 5-HT_3 antagonists dolasetron, ondansetron, granisetron, and palonosetron.
2. Perform a literature search on the use and efficacy of oral antiemetic regimens versus IV antiemetic regimens.
3. Discern in which patients it would be appropriate to use palonosetron or aprepitant, and the advantages and limitations of each drug.

▶ Clinical Pearl

Antiemetic regimens for the prevention and treatment of chemotherapy-induced nausea and vomiting should contain agents with different mechanisms of action to increase the effectiveness of the regimen.[3]

References

1. Siderov J, Zalcberg J, Chambers B, et al. Migraine following the use of a 5-hydroxytryptamine antagonist. Aust N Z J Med 1993;23:527–528.
2. Hesketh PJ, Kris MG, Grunberg SM, et al. Proposal for classifying the acute emetogenicity of cancer chemotherapy. J Clin Oncol 1997;15:103–109.
3. American Society of Health-System Pharmacists. ASHP therapeutic guidelines on the pharmacologic management of nausea and vomiting in adult and pediatric patients receiving chemotherapy or radiation therapy or undergoing surgery. Am J Health Syst Pharm 1999;56:729–764.
4. Osoba D, Zee B, Pater J, et al. Determinants of postchemotherapy nausea and vomiting in patients with cancer. Quality of Life and Symptom Control Committees of the National Cancer Institute of Canada Clinical Trials Group. J Clin Oncol 1997;15:116–123.
5. Inapsine® (droperidol). Product package insert. Shirley NY: American Regent Laboratories, Inc. Dec 2001.
6. Nolte MJ, Berkery R, Pizzo B, et al. Assuring the optimal use of serotonin antagonist antiemetics: The process for development and implementation of institutional antiemetic guidelines at Memorial Sloan-Kettering Cancer Center. J Clin Oncol 1998;16:771–778.
7. Emend® (aprepitant). Product package insert. Whitehouse Station NJ: Merck & Co, Inc, May 2003.
8. Aloxi® (palonosetron). Product package insert. Albuquerque NM: Cardinal Health, July 2003.

35 DIARRHEA

► Acute Diarrhea and Its Management (Level I)

Marie A. Abate, BS, PharmD
Charles D. Ponte, BS, PharmD, BCPS, CDE, FAPhA, FASHP, FCCP

► After completing this case study, students should be able to:

- Identify the common causes of acute diarrhea.
- Establish primary goals for the treatment of acute diarrhea.
- Recommend appropriate nondrug therapy for patients experiencing acute diarrhea.
- Explain the place of drug therapy in the treatment of acute diarrhea and recommend appropriate products.

PATIENT PRESENTATION

Chief Complaint

"I have diarrhea and I haven't been able to eat because I feel awful."

HPI

Tom Ellis is a 50 yo man who comes to the Internal Medicine Group Clinic with nausea, vomiting, cramping, and diarrhea. He had been well until two days ago, when he began to experience severe nausea that occurred about four hours after eating two chicken enchiladas with sour cream and cheese at the nearby Mexican restaurant. He chewed two Pepto-Bismol tablets at that time. The nausea persisted, and he subsequently vomited "several" times with some relief. As the evening progressed, he still felt "awful" and took Pepcid AC 2 tablets to settle his stomach. He began to feel achy and warm, and his temperature at the time was 38.2°C. He has continued to have nausea, vomiting, and a mild fever. He has not tolerated solid foods nor has he been able to keep down small amounts of fluid. Since yesterday, he has had six to eight liquid stools. He has not noticed any blood in the bowel movements. A friend brought him to the clinic because he was becoming weak and dizzy when he tried to stand up. He denies antibiotic use, laxative use, or excessive caffeine intake.

PMH

Hypertension × 6 years
Hyperlipidemia × 3 years

FH

Noncontributory

SH

No current tobacco use (5 pack–year history; quit 10 years ago); drinks wine or a mixed drink socially, usually not more than one glass per week; has about two cups of coffee daily. Works as an assistant manager in the finance department of a local health care organization. Married for 20 years.

ROS

Lightheadedness upon standing, denies sore throat, ear pain, or nasal discharge. Denies coughing or congestion. Frequent bouts of nausea. Frequent loose stools associated with significant cramping. Decreased urination; no pain upon urination. Complains of generalized fatigue, mild aching, feels like his heart is pounding.

Meds

HCTZ 25 mg one po daily × 6 years
Lipitor 10 mg po at bedtime × 3 years
One-A-Day po daily
Co-Q 10 (coenzyme Q-10) 100 mg BID (for HTN) × 2 weeks

All

Bactrim DS → itching, rash on legs 10 years ago
Pollen → sneezing, irritated eyes

PE

Gen

White male, appears ill, in moderate distress.

VS

BP 135/92, P 80 (supine); BP 110/70, P 100 (standing), RR 16, T 38°C; Ht 5′9″, Wt 75 kg

Skin

Slightly warm to touch, fair skin turgor

HEENT

Dry mucous membranes, non-erythematous TMs, PERRLA, some AV nicking, slight erythema in throat

Neck/LN
Without masses, lymphadenopathy, or thyromegaly

Chest
Clear to A & P

CV
RRR without m/r/g

Abd
Diffuse tenderness, no guarding or rebound, without organomegaly, non-distended, active bowel sounds

Genit/Rect
Heme (–) stool in the rectal vault; no gross blood, small internal hemorrhoids

MS/Ext
Normal muscle strength, no CCE

Neuro
A & O × 3; CN II–XII intact; normal reflexes, normal sensory and motor function

Labs

Na 138 mEq/L	Hgb 12.5 g/dL	AST 35 IU/L
K 3.5 mEq/L	Hct 35%	ALT 30 IU/L
Cl 100 mEq/L	Plt 350 × 10^3/mm^3	Total Chol 185 mg/dL
CO_2 25 mEq/L	WBC 12.0 × 10^3/mm^3	
BUN 20 mg/dL	50% PMNs	
SCr 1.1 mg/dL	48% Lymphs	
Glu 100 mg/dL	2% Monos	

UA
Clear, dark amber; SG 1.033; pH 6.0; protein (–); glucose (–); acetone (–), bilirubin (–), blood (–); microscopic: 0–2 WBC/hpf, 0–2 RBC/hpf, several hyaline casts

Assessment
Probable gastroenteritis; r/o acute infectious diarrhea
Hypertension
Hyperlipidemia

Plan
Admit to hospital for observation and acute therapy for diarrhea

---

▶ Questions

Problem Identification

1. a. *Create a list of the patient's drug therapy problems.*
   b. *What signs and symptoms does this man have that indicate the presence or severity of the diarrhea?*
   c. *What questions should you ask the patient or members of the medical team to obtain the additional information needed for a complete assessment of this patient?*
   d. *Could any of this patient's problems have been caused by drug therapy?*
   e. *What are other possible causes of this patient's diarrhea?*

Desired Outcome

2. *What are the goals of therapy for this patient?*

Therapeutic Alternatives

3. a. *What types of nondrug therapy should be considered for this patient?*
   b. *What feasible pharmacotherapeutic alternatives are available for treatment of diarrhea in this patient?*

Optimal Plan

4. *What nondrug interventions and specific pharmacotherapeutic regimens would you recommend for treating this patient's diarrhea?*

Outcome Evaluation

5. *What clinical and laboratory parameters are necessary to evaluate the diarrhea therapy for achievement of the desired outcome and to detect or prevent adverse effects?*

Patient Education

6. *What information should be provided to this patient to enhance adherence, ensure successful therapy, and minimize adverse effects?*

▶ Follow-Up Questions

1. *How should this patient's blood pressure be managed after he is rehydrated and leaves the hospital?*
2. *Does the patient need any changes with regard to his hyperlipidemia?*

▶ Clinical Course

The treatment and monitoring plan you recommended was initiated upon admission to the hospital. The patient's diarrhea had slowed by the evening of day 1. The patient had no further episodes of diarrhea or vomiting past midnight. On the morning of day 2, his orthostasis had resolved, his temperature was normal, the IV fluids were stopped, and he received clear liquids by mouth for breakfast and lunch. His stool cultures were negative. The patient was discharged during late afternoon.

▶ Self-Study Assignments

1. Identify the infectious causes of diarrhea. Design an effective pharmacotherapy treatment regimen for each cause.
2. Provide recommendations for the prevention of traveler's diarrhea.
3. Describe whether or not antidiarrheal products can be safely recommended for use in very young children (< 3 yo) and if so, the specific products that could be used.
4. Describe when oral rehydration products should be used, and recommend a specific product and dosage for young or older patients who present with mild to moderate diarrhea and minimal dehydration.

▶ Clinical Pearl

Dehydration and electrolyte imbalances are major concerns with diarrhea, particularly when accompanied by nausea and vomiting; repletion and maintenance of body water and electrolytes are primary treatment goals.

References

1. Ilnyckyj A. Clinical evaluation and management of acute infectious diarrhea in adults. Gastroenterol Clin N Am 2001;30(3):599–609.
2. Aranda-Michel J, Giannella RA. Acute diarrhea: A practical review. Am J Med 1999;106:670–676.
3. Ramzan NN. Traveler's diarrhea. Gastroenterol Clin N Am 2001;30(3):665–678.
4. Coenzyme Q-10. Natural Medicines Comprehensive Database. Stockton:CA; 2003. Available at www.naturalmedicinesdatabase.com (Accessed June 1, 2004).
5. Manatsathit S, Dupont HL, Farthing M, et al. Guideline for the management of acute diarrhea in adults. J Gastroenterol Hepatol 2002;17(Suppl 1):S54–S71.
6. Wingate D, Phillips SF, Lewis SJ, et al. Guidelines for adults on self-medication for the treatment of acute diarrhoea. Aliment Pharmacol Ther 2001;15:773–782.

36 IRRITABLE BOWEL SYNDROME

▶ It's A Strain (Level II)

Nancy S. Yunker, PharmD
William R. Garnett, PharmD, FCCP

▶ After completing this case study, students should be able to:

- Identify the signs and symptoms of irritable bowel syndrome (IBS) associated with abdominal discomfort, bloating, and constipation.
- Devise patient management strategies for patients with IBS including pharmacologic and nonpharmacologic options.
- Outline parameters for monitoring the safety and efficacy of therapy used in patients with IBS associated with abdominal discomfort, bloating, and constipation.
- Identify treatment options for IBS associated with abdominal discomfort, fecal urgency, and diarrhea.
- Evaluate the efficacy of treatment options for patients with IBS.

PATIENT PRESENTATION

Chief Complaint

"My colon feels all stopped up and I feel really bloated. Can you prescribe something to help me?"

HPI

Sarah Smith is a 34 yo woman who presents to her PCP with the chief complaint of a 4-month history of hard pellet-like stools and difficulty when passing stools. She states that she constantly feels bloated and has taken to wearing loose-fitting clothing as she can not tolerate anything tight around her abdomen. She states that she was diagnosed with "spastic colon" in college but was able to tolerate the symptoms until about 6 months ago when she began to notice some bloating and a decrease in the number of bowel movements per week. She attributes the worsening symptoms to increased stress at work and her recent enrollment in an evening MBA program. Prior to 6 months ago, she states that she averaged about 5 stools a week. She estimates that she has had 1 or 2 bowel movements a week for the past month. She complains of straining to pass her stools and states that she has to get up 30 minutes earlier in the morning to allow for an attempt to pass a stool. She also states that the abdominal pain is not limited to when she passes a stool. She complains of abdominal pain and bloating almost continuously throughout the day for the past 2 months, although her symptoms are somewhat alleviated by passing a "good stool." She also states that the symptoms are worse when she has midterms or finals or when she needs to complete a major college writing assignment. She resumed taking psyllium powder 3 months ago but could not stand the taste and has switched to Metamucil wafers.

PMH

Seasonal allergies
Tension headaches
Anxiety

PSH

Cholecystectomy 2 years ago

FH

Separated from husband for 6 months – question of abuse; divorce is pending. Her 11 yo son lives with her. Mother is alive with HTN and her father is alive with hypercholesterolemia. No siblings.

SH

Social alcohol use; No smoking. Recently promoted to assistant bank manager after working as a teller for 7 years. Has been told that when she finishes her MBA she will be candidate for a branch manager position. She states that the additional money will help her to support her son.

ROS

Occasional headaches, usually associated with stress or allergy symptoms; occasional nausea, no vomiting; (–) blood in the stool or tarry stools; (+) flatulence & bloating. States that the abdominal symptoms may improve at night before bedtime especially if she uses a heating pad; she is not awakened at night with abdominal pain.

Meds

Diphenhydramine 25 mg po Q 6 H PRN allergy symptoms
Ibuprofen 200 mg, 2 tabs po Q 4–6 H PRN headaches, menstrual cramps
Metamucil wafers (cinnamon), 2 wafers po TID with water
Lo-Ovral (discontinued 5 months ago)

All

NKDA

PE

Gen

A & O, WDWN, pleasant white female currently appearing slightly anxious

VS

BP 126/85, P 72, RR 18, T 37.1°C; Ht 5′4″ Wt 59 kg

Skin

Dry skin on lower extremities, no rashes noted

HEENT

PERRLA, EOMI, moist mucus membranes, TMs intact

Neck/LN

No thyromegaly, lymphadenopathy, or JVD

Lungs

CTA; no rales or rhonchi

Breasts

Symmetrical; no lumps or masses detected; nipples without discharge

CV

RRR, normal S_1 and S_2; no S_3 or S_4

Abd

(+) BS, slightly tender in LLQ, no HSM

Genit/Rect

Vulva normal; no palpable rectal masses; brown stool with no occult blood; no hemorrhoids

MS/Ext

No CCE, pulses 2+, normal ROM, normal strength bilaterally

Labs

Na 139 mEq/L	WBC 6.2×10^3/mm^3
K 4.2 mEq/L	Hgb 14.2 g/dL
Cl 103 mEq/L	Hct 32.5%
CO_2 28 mEq/L	
BUN 15 mg/dL	
SCr 1.1 mg/dL	
Glu 120 mg/dL	

Stool: Negative for blood
Serum Pregnancy Test: Negative

Assessment:

Irritable bowel syndrome associated with abdominal discomfort, bloating, and constipation.

▶ Questions

Problem Identification

1. a. *Create a list of the patient's drug therapy problems.*
   b. *List the signs, symptoms, and laboratory values that indicate the presence and severity of abdominal discomfort, bloating, and constipation associated IBS; also include pertinent negative findings.*
   c. *Could any of the patient's problems have been caused by drug therapy?*
   d. *Are any of the patient's problems amenable to pharmacotherapy?*
   e. *What additional information is needed to satisfactorily assess this patient?*

Desired Outcome

2. *Differentiate the patient's goals of therapy from those of her health care providers.*

Therapeutic Alternatives

3. a. *What nondrug therapies might be useful for this patient?*
   b. *What feasible pharmacotherapeutic alternatives are available for the treatment of the IBS associated with abdominal discomfort, bloating, and constipation?*
   c. *What pharmacotherapeutic alternatives are available for the treatment of IBS associated with abdominal discomfort, fecal urgency, and diarrhea?*
   d. *What psychosocial considerations are applicable to this patient?*

Optimal Plan

4. a. *What drug, dosage form, dose, schedule, and duration of therapy are best for this patient?*
   b. *What alternatives would be appropriate if the initial therapy fails or cannot be used?*

Outcome Evaluation

5. *What clinical and laboratory parameters are necessary to evaluate the therapy for achievement of the desired therapeutic outcome and to detect or prevent adverse effects?*

Patient Education

6. *What information should be provided to the patient to enhance compliance, ensure successful therapy, and minimize adverse effects?*

► Clinical Course

The patient returns to the physician 2 months later and reports that her symptoms are much improved and the abdominal pain has resolved. She is happy with her medication regimen, but her friends have suggested that peppermint oil or herbal medications may be just as effective. She would like more information about the use of these products for IBS.

► Follow-Up Questions

1. *What therapeutic regimen would you recommend for this patient at this time?*
2. *What information would you provide regarding the addition or substitution of alternative medications (e.g., dietary supplements) to this patient's regimen?*

► Self-Study Assignments

1. Conduct a literature search to determine what types of alternative therapies have been tried for IBS. Include an evaluation of the scientific rigor of these studies.
2. Conduct a search for IBS patient information available on the Internet. Select two sites and compare their scientific rigor and the usefulness of the information provided to the patient.
3. Conduct an informal survey among friends, family members, coworkers and fellow students about the incidence of IBS and what therapeutic options they would recommend to a person suffering from IBS.

► Clinical Pearl

Probiotics are living organisms that are thought to exert health benefits beyond general nutrition after ingestion. A few small studies have examined the effect of probiotics, especially *Lactobacillus spp*., in IBS patients. It has been suggested that probiotics may offer some benefit to IBS patients, particularly those with pain and flatulence.[12] However, more rigorous trials are needed before definitive recommendations can be made on the use of probiotics in IBS patients.

References

1. Drossman DA, Camilleri M, Mayer EA, et al. AGA technical review on irritable bowel syndrome. Gastroenterology 2002;123:2108–2131.
2. American Gastroenterological Association Clinical Practice Committee. American Gastroenterological Association medical position statement: irritable bowel syndrome. Gastroenterology 2002; 123:2105–2107.
3. Miller S, Heck A. Irritable bowel syndrome. US Pharmacist 2000;Nov (Suppl): 3–13.
4. American College of Gastroenterology Functional Gastrointestinal Disorders Task Force. Evidenced-based position statement on the management of irritable bowel syndrome in North America. Am J Gastroenterol 2002;97(11 Suppl):S1-S5.
5. Fass R, Longstreth GF, Pimentel M, et al. Evidence- and consensus-based practice guidelines for the diagnosis of irritable bowel syndrome. Arch Intern Med 2001;161:2081–2088.
6. Brandt LJ, Bjorkman D, Fennerty MB, et al. Systematic Review on the management of irritable bowel syndrome in North America. Am J Gastroenterol 2002;97(11 Suppl):S7–26.
7. FDA talk paper. FDA updates Zelnorm labeling with new risk information. www.fda.gov/bbs/topics/answers/2004/ans01285.html (accessed June 2, 2004).
8. Jailwala J, Imperiale TF, Kroenke K. Pharmacologic treatment of the irritable bowel syndrome: A systematic review of randomized, controlled trials. Ann Intern Med 2000;133:136–147.
9. Tougas G, Snape WJ, Otten MH, et al. Long-term safety of tegaserod in patients with constipation-predominant irritable bowel syndrome. Aliment Pharmacol Ther 2002;16:1701–1708.
10. Bensoussan A, Talley NJ, Hing M, et al. Treatment of irritable bowel syndrome with Chinese herbal medicine: A randomized controlled trial. JAMA 1998;280: 1585–1589.
11. Pittler MH, Ernst E. Peppermint oil for irritable bowel syndrome: A critical review and metaanalysis. Am J Gastroenterol 1998;93:1131–1135.
12. Spanier JA, Howden CW, Jones MP. A systematic review of alternative therapies in the irritable bowel syndrome. Arch Intern Med 2003;163:265–274.

37 PEDIATRIC GASTROENTERITIS

► Dihydrogen Monoxide and Other Critical Elements (Level II)

William McGhee, PharmD
Basil J. Zitelli, MD, FAAP

► After completing this case study, students should be able to:

- Recognize the signs and symptoms of diarrhea with dehydration and be able to assess the severity of the problem.
- Recommend appropriate oral rehydration therapy (ORT) products and treatment regimens for varying degrees of dehydration severity.
- Understand the limited role of antidiarrheal products for the treatment of acute diarrhea in children and be able to educate parents on their appropriate use.
- Properly assess the effectiveness of ORT using both clinical and laboratory parameters.
- Identify the signs and symptoms indicating severe dehydration that requires referral to an ED for immediate IV volume replacement.

PATIENT PRESENTATION

Chief Complaint

James Robinson is a 5-month-old infant who presented to the ED with a 5-day history of fever, vomiting, and diarrhea.

HPI

The patient was in good health when, 5 days prior to presentation, he felt warm to his mother and did not eat as well as usual. He normally takes between 6 and 8 ounces of Similac with iron formula every 4 to 6 hours. The mother introduced rice cereal into his diet 2 weeks prior to the onset of symptoms. The mother did not take the child's temperature but gave acetaminophen, one dropperful every 6 hours, when he felt warm.

In the evening of the first day of illness, James vomited shortly after feeding. The emesis was non-bloody and non-bilious. He continued to vomit after each feeding for the next three meals and was more irritable than usual. Four days prior to presentation, James developed loose, watery stools after each attempt at feeding and several times between feeds. The stools did not appear to contain blood or mucus.

Vomiting and diarrhea continued, and 3 days prior to presentation the mother called her pediatrician, who recommended 12 hours of clear liquids given in frequent but small amounts. The mother gave a variety of clear liquids, including water, Pedialyte, Jell-O water, and flat Coca-Cola. The vomiting stopped, but the diarrhea continued despite these measures. Fever was intermittent, and the child became more lethargic. The mother continued the clear fluids that her doctor had recommended.

On the day of presentation, the mother stated that James was irritable, sleepy, and had a decreased number of wet diapers. She noted that his lips appeared dry. James is in day care, and other day care mates have had similar illnesses recently. At a recent doctor's appointment 7 days prior to presentation, his weight was 7.1 kg.

PMH

Born at 37 weeks' gestation; uncomplicated labor, pregnancy, and delivery; hospitalized at 2 months of age for fever and possible sepsis.

ROS

Small patches of eczema over the nape of his neck. History of a heart murmur heard at 2 months of age (mother didn't know what the doctors meant when they called it "innocent"). Immunizations are up-to-date, including hepatitis B vaccine. Development is age-appropriate.

All

No known allergies

FH

Mother is 24 yo, in good health; Father is 26 yo, in good health. A 2 yo sibling recently had diarrhea that lasted for 3 days but had no vomiting or fever.

SH

James lives with his parents and sibling; they have one dog and use a city water supply. He attends day care regularly.

PE

Gen

Patient is ill appearing, lying limply in his mother's lap; sleepy, but arousable.

VS

BP 90/58, P 140, RR 45, T 38.8°C; Wt 6.5 kg

Skin

Pink, decreased skin turgor, capillary refill 2 to 3 seconds

HEENT

TMs gray and translucent; nose with crusted secretions; lips dry and cracked; tongue dry; anterior fontanelle and eyes sunken

Neck/LN

Normal

Lungs/Thorax

Tachypneic and hyperpneic; no retractions; no crackles or wheezes

Heart

Tachycardia; no murmur noted; pulses were normal; capillary refill was 2 to 3 seconds

Abd

Scaphoid; active bowel sounds; soft, nontender; no masses or organomegaly

Genit/Rect

Normal circumcised male; testes descended; greenish, watery stool in the diaper

MS/Ext

Normal

Neuro

Sleepy but arousable; irritable when awake; no focal deficits noted

Labs

Na 138 mEq/L	Hgb 13.6 g/dL
K 4.6 mEq/L	Hct 42%
Cl 110 mEq/L	WBC $13.0 \times 10^3/mm^3$
CO_2 13 mEq/L	49% Polys
BUN 24 mg/dL	5% Bands
SCr 0.5 mg/dL	27% Lymphs
Glu 84 mg/dL	17% Monos
	2% Basos

UA

Normal except for specific gravity of 1.028; ketones 2+

Assessment

1. Typical viral gastroenteritis, probably rotavirus infection
2. Dehydration with metabolic acidosis

▶ Questions

Problem Identification

1. a. *Create a list of the patient's drug therapy problems.*
   b. *What information (signs, symptoms, laboratory values) indicates the presence or severity of gastroenteritis?*

Desired Outcome

2. *What are the goals of pharmacotherapy in this case?*

Therapeutic Alternatives

3. a. *What nondrug therapies might be useful for this patient?*
   b. *What feasible pharmacotherapeutic alternatives are available for treatment of this patient's diarrhea?*

Optimal Plan

4. *What drug(s), dosage forms, schedule, and duration of therapy are best for this patient?*

Outcome Evaluation

5. *What clinical and laboratory parameters should be monitored to evaluate therapy for achievement of the desired therapeutic outcome?*

Patient Education

6. *What information should be provided to the child's parents to enhance compliance, ensure successful therapy, and minimize adverse effects?*

▶ Self-Study Assignments

1. In what circumstances would antimicrobial therapy be considered for children with diarrhea and dehydration?
2. What is the role of drug therapy in the prevention of diarrhea when traveling to some foreign countries?
3. What barriers exist to the widespread implementation of ORT, including parents and physicians? How can these barriers be overcome? (Hint: Explore the advantages of ORT versus IV rehydration therapy, including ease of care at home versus hospitalization, insurance issues, and physician reluctance).
4. Write a two-page essay describing the role of the community-based pharmacy practitioner in the care of patients with pediatric gastroenteritis and dehydration.

▶ Clinical Pearl

Oral rehydration therapy is equivalent to IV therapy in rehydrating children with gastroenteritis and diarrhea with mild to moderate dehydration. Oral rehydration therapy is the standard of care in the treatment of these patients, and antidiarrheal, antiemetic, and antimicrobial therapies are rarely necessary. IV rehydration is necessary only in patients with severe dehydration.

References

1. Glass RI, Lew JF, Gangarosa RE, et al. Estimates of morbidity and mortality rates for diarrheal diseases in American children. J Pediatr 1991;118(4 [Pt 2]):S27–S33.
2. Duggan C, Santosham M, Glass RI. The management of acute diarrhea in children: Oral rehydration, maintenance, and nutritional therapy. MMWR Morb Mortal Wkly Rep 1992;41(RR-16):1–20.
3. Provisional Committee on Quality Improvement, Subcommittee on Acute Gastroenteritis. Practice parameter: The management of acute gastroenteritis in young children. Pediatrics 1996;97:424–435.
4. Snyder J. The continuing evolution of oral therapy for diarrhea. Semin Pediatr Infect Dis 1994;5:231–235.
5. Santosham M. Oral rehydration therapy: Reverse transfer of technology. Arch Pediatric Adolesc Med 2002;156:1177–1179. Editorial.
6. Costa-Ribeiro H, Ribeiro TC, Mattos AP, et al. Limitations of probiotic therapy in acute, severe dehydrating diarrhea. J Pediatr Gastroenterol Nutr 2003; 36:112–115
7. McClung HJ, Murray RD, Heitlinger LA. The Internet as a source for current patient information. Pediatrics 1998;101:1065. Abstract.
8. Centers for Disease Control and Prevention. Managing acute gastroenteritis among children: Oral rehydration, maintenance, and nutritional therapy. MMWR Morb Mortal Wkly Rep 2003;52 (RR-16):1–16.

38 CONSTIPATION

▶ Bound to Be Slow (Level I)

Beth Bryles Phillips, PharmD, BCPS

▶ After completing this case study, students should be able to:

- Identify medications that can exacerbate constipation.
- Describe the advantages and disadvantages of each class of laxatives and discuss the appropriate use of each class.
- Recommend an appropriate plan for the treatment of constipation, including lifestyle modifications and drug therapy.
- Educate patients regarding laxative therapy.

PATIENT PRESENTATION

Chief Complaint

"I've been having some difficulties going to the bathroom lately."

HPI

Evelyn Purnham is a 69 yo woman who presents to the general medicine clinic for an initial visit. She complains of feeling bloated and constipated lately, sometimes going an entire week with only one bowel movement. She reports straining the majority of the time, although she denies pain during these straining episodes. A recent colonoscopy was unremarkable. She has not attempted medications to provide relief of her constipation.

In addition, she reports frequent heartburn, most often occurring in the late evening when she goes to bed. Upon a friend's advice, she purchased some Amphojel (aluminum hydroxide) over-the-counter to try to help alleviate the heartburn. She has had some success with this. Around the same time the heartburn started, she began having trouble sleeping. She was given a prescription for amitriptyline and reports this has helped her insomnia. She reports using Advil 2 tablets, one to two times weekly for arthritic pain in her hands and knees. She states that her hands and knees are painful and tender. She has stopped her regular walks in the park due to the worsening pain in her knees.

PMH

HTN
Osteoarthritis
GERD
S/P TAH 15 years ago
S/P CVA 1 year ago; no residual deficits

FH

Father and mother both died of heart disease in their 80s.

SH

(–) Alcohol or tobacco use; (+) caffeine use, 1 cup of coffee each AM; widowed × 1 year, has 2 daughters, both healthy

ROS

(+) For constipation, lower abdominal fullness, heartburn, occasional arthritic pain in hands and knees with movement, and infrequent headache.

Meds

Verapamil SR 240 mg po once daily
Tylenol 650 mg po QID
Amitriptyline 75 mg po at bedtime
Amphojel® 600 mg po PC (sometimes at bedtime)
Advil 1–2 tabs PRN arthritic pain/HA

All

NKDA

PE

Gen
Patient is a pleasant woman in NAD

VS
BP 135/85, P 78, RR 19, T 37.7°C; Ht 5′2″, Wt 63.5 kg

Skin
Normal skin turgor and color

HEENT
PERRLA and EOM full without nystagmus, sclerae clear, fundi show flat disks with no hemorrhages or exudates; external auricular canal clear; TMs normal; oropharynx well hydrated

Neck/LN
Supple, no lymphadenopathy or JVD; no thyromegaly or bruits

CV
Regular rate and rhythm

Lungs
CTA

Abd
No hepatomegaly, splenomegaly, or masses; no tenderness or guarding; (+) slight distention; normoactive bowel sounds

Rectal
No fissures, hemorrhoids, or strictures; no evidence of rectal bleeding; large amount of stool in rectal vault

MS/Ext
(+) Tenderness in hands bilaterally, no clubbing, peripheral pulses intact, decreased strength and limited ROM in both LE

Neuro
Alert and oriented × 3, CN II–XII symmetric and intact, DTRs 2+

Labs

Na 142 mEq/L	Glu 123mg/dL
K 4.3 mEq/L	Ca 8.9 mg/dL
Cl 105 mEq/L	TSH 2.70 (IU/mL
CO_2 26 mEq/L	Free T_4 1.2 ng/dL
BUN 14 mg/dL	
SCr 1.2 mg/dL	

Questions

Problem Identification

1. a. *Develop a list of the potential drug therapy problems in this patient other than those related to her constipation.*
   b. *What signs or symptoms are indicative of constipation in this patient?*
   c. *What are some of the possible nonpharmacologic contributors to her constipation?*
   d. *What are some of the possible pharmacologic contributors to constipation in this patient?*
   e. *What information might you want to obtain from a patient who presents with a chief complaint of constipation?*

Desired Outcome

2. *What are the goals of pharmacotherapy in treating constipation?*

Therapeutic Alternatives

3. a. *What are some nonpharmacologic steps that might be useful in treating constipation?*
   b. *What are the pharmacologic options for the treatment of constipation?*
   c. *Is this patient's current regimen for reflux appropriate? If not, what recommendations can you make to optimize this regimen?*

Optimal Plan

4. *After nonpharmacologic measures have been attempted, what would be the most appropriate choice of drug therapy for her, including dose and schedule? Provide the rationale for your answer.*

Outcome Evaluation

5. *How would you monitor this patient to ensure that your pharmacotherapeutic goals have been achieved? What would be an appropriate follow-up measure?*

Patient Education

6. *When educating this patient on using a bulk-forming laxative, what information should you convey to her to ensure appropriate use of this product?*

► Clinical Course

One month later, Ms. Purnham returns to the clinic. The interventions you made were put into place. She reports that she has been using the drug therapy you recommended and has had some relief but still is constipated. She asks if there is something else she can take.

► Follow-Up Questions

1. *What agent would you recommend in a patient who reports only partial relief of constipation with a bulk-forming laxative?*

► Self-Study Assignments

1. Suggest pharmacotherapeutic plans for the drug therapy problems you identified in questions 1.a. and 1.d.
2. List some of the drug classes that commonly cause constipation. For agents in these classes, discuss what the non-constipating alternatives might be. For example, should an agent in another class be chosen instead, or could a dose reduction be attempted?

► Clinical Pearl

Constipation is often a sign of an underlying problem, such as an adverse reaction to a medication or a symptom of a disease; these possibilities should always be considered when evaluating a patient complaining of constipation.

References

1. Lembo A, Camilleri M. Chronic constipation. N Engl J Med 2003;349:1360–1368.
2. Xing JH, Soffer EE. Adverse effects of laxatives. Dis Colon Rectum 2001;44:1201–1209.

39 ASCITES MANAGEMENT IN PORTAL HYPERTENSION AND CIRRHOSIS

► A Pint Is a Pound (Level I)

Joette M. Meyer, PharmD

► After completing this case study, students should be able to:

- Identify signs and symptoms of cirrhosis and its complications.
- Develop a diuretic regimen for patients with ascites.
- Recommend appropriate monitoring for the diuretic regimen.
- Educate patients on pharmacologic and nonpharmacologic therapy to control ascites and prevent further decompensation of their liver disease.
- Recommend pharmacologic therapy to treat or prevent complications of ascites and portal hypertension (i.e., prophylaxis of spontaneous bacterial peritonitis, variceal bleeding, and hepatic encephalopathy).

PATIENT PRESENTATION

Chief Complaint

"My belly is swelling up."

HPI

Hector Quintana is a 47 yo Hispanic man with a history of hepatitis C and alcoholic cirrhosis admitted to the hospital from the outpatient clinic with abdominal swelling, 6.8-kg weight gain over the past 2 weeks, diffuse abdominal pain, fatigue, lethargy, and mild confusion. He has been approved for liver transplantation and is on the waiting list.

PMH

Cirrhosis secondary to alcohol and hepatitis C diagnosed 5 years ago by liver biopsy
H/O of multiple upper GI bleeds secondary to esophageal varices
H/O ascites with moderate accumulation of fluid
H/O spontaneous bacterial peritonitis (SBP) 1 year ago
Type 2 DM

FH

No liver disease; otherwise non-contributory

SH

Recently divorced, living with his teen-age daughter and girlfriend. Unemployed for the past 7 years; previously worked in a liquor store. Receives Medicaid and SSI. History of ethanol abuse, quit 5 years ago. Previously drank three 6-packs of beer/day × 18 years. History of IVDA (heroin); quit 5 years ago.

Meds

Human 70/30 Insulin 44 units subQ Q AM and 20 units subQ Q PM
Lactulose 15 mL po once daily
H/O interferon alfa-2b 3 million units subQ 3 times/week plus ribavirin 400 mg po Q AM and 600 mg po Q PM × 6 months

All

None

ROS

Increasing abdominal girth and weight gain; vague abdominal pain. No fever, chills, nausea, vomiting, cough, chest pain, or shortness of breath.

PE

Gen

Alert and oriented man in NAD; slow to answer questions, poor historian

VS

BP 118/56, P 85, R 20, T 36.2°C; current weight is 61.7 kg, Ht 5′6″

Skin

(+) Spider angiomata on chest; no apparent jaundice

HEENT

Icteric sclera, PERRL, EOMI, TMs intact; O/P moist, no erythema, no lesions

Neck/LN

Supple, (–) JVD; thyroid palpable, no nodules

Chest

CTA bilaterally, good air exchange bilaterally, (+) gynecomastia

CV

RRR, normal S_1 and S_2, no S_3, S_4, or murmurs

Abd

Distended, firm, slightly tender; (+) shifting dullness; hepatomegaly; spleen not palpated; bowel sounds present; no guarding or rebound tenderness

Genit/Rect

Heme-negative stool, external genitalia normal

MS/Ext

Slight asterixis, no lesions or edema, no palmar erythema, no deficit in extremities

Neuro

A & O × 2, slow to answer questions, normal tone and reflexes, CNs grossly intact

Labs

Na 137 mEq/L	Hgb 13.5 g/dL	AST 105 IU/L	T. prot 5.6 g/dL
K 4.4 mEq/L	Hct 39.1%	ALT 87 IU/L	Alb 2.5 g/dL
Cl 108 mEq/L	Plt 83 × 10^3/mm^3	Alk Phos 224 IU/L	Ca 8.7 mg/dL
CO_2 23 mEq/L	WBC 4.5 × 10^3/mm^3	LDH 169 IU/L	Mg 1.7 mg/dL
BUN 7 mg/dL	PT 15.6 sec	T. bili 2.7 mg/dL	Phos 2.4 mg/dL
SCr 0.5 mg/dL	PTT 45.4 sec	D. bili 0.9 mg/dL	HCV PCR 9597 copies/mL
Glu 241 mg/dL		HIV negative	AFP 9.8 IU/mL

Child–Pugh Score

11, "C" classification

Diet

Patient has been instructed to follow a 2-g sodium diet, unrestricted protein

Assessment

End-stage liver disease with cirrhosis due to alcohol and hepatitis C complicated by a history of variceal bleeding, ascites, and SBP. Now presenting with worsening ascites and encephalopathy. R/O recurrent SBP.

▶ Clinical Course

A large volume paracentesis was performed and 5 L of fluid was removed. Cell count: 200 WBC with 13% neutrophils; albumin < 1.0 g/dL; protein < 3.0 g/dL; no growth on culture. A 24-hour urine collection was completed that showed sodium excretion of 102 mEq/day.

▶ Questions

Problem Identification

1. a. Create a list of the patient's drug therapy problems.
b. What information (signs, symptoms, laboratory values) indicates the presence or severity of ascites secondary to liver cirrhosis? (See Figure 39–1.)

Desired Outcome

2. What are the goals of pharmacotherapy for the management of ascites in this case?

Therapeutic Alternatives

3. a. What nondrug therapies might be useful for this patient?
b. What feasible pharmacotherapeutic alternatives are available for treatment of cirrhotic ascites?

Optimal Plan

4. a. What drug, dosage form, dose, schedule, and duration of therapy are best for this patient?
b. What pharmacologic alternatives would be appropriate if the initial therapy fails or cannot be used?

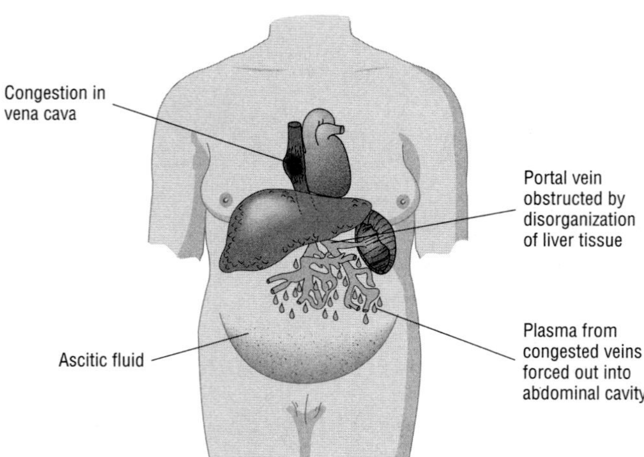

Figure 39–1. Development of ascites with portal hypertension due to cirrhosis. *(Reprinted with permission from Mulvihill ML. Human Diseases: A Systemic Approach, 4th ed. Norwalk, CT, Appleton & Lange, 1995:203)*

Outcome Evaluation

5. *What clinical and laboratory parameters are necessary to evaluate the therapy for achievement of the desired therapeutic outcome and to detect or prevent adverse effects?*

Patient Education

6. *What information should be provided to the patient to enhance adherence to drug therapy, ensure successful therapy, and minimize adverse effects?*

Additional Case Questions

1. *How serious a condition is SBP, and what pharmacologic alternatives are available for secondary prevention in a patient with a prior episode of SBP?*
2. *What pharmacologic alternatives are available for the secondary prevention of variceal bleeding?*
3. *How can pharmacologic therapy be optimized to control hepatic encephalopathy in this patient?*

► Self-Study Assignments

1. Compare the pharmacokinetics and pharmacodynamics of the diuretics used in the treatment of cirrhotic ascites. Explain the rationale for using furosemide and spironolactone in combination.
2. Discuss the pros and cons of using antibiotics as prophylaxis against recurrent SBP, and identify high-risk patients who would benefit from this therapy.

► Clinical Course

Sodium restriction alone reduces ascites in approximately 10% of patients. The combination of sodium restriction and oral spironolactone plus furosemide improves ascites in 90% of patients.

References

1. Rimola A, Garcia-Tsao G, Navasa M, et al. Diagnosis, treatment, and prophylaxis of spontaneous bacterial peritonitis: A consensus document. J Hepatol 2000;32:142–153.
2. Runyon BA. Management of adult patients with ascites caused by cirrhosis. Hepatology 1998;27:264–72.
3. Rossle M, Ochs A, Gulberg V, et al. A comparison of paracentesis and transjugular intrahepatic portosystemic shunting in patients with ascites. N Engl J Med 2000;342:1701–1707.
4. Bhuva M, Granger D, Jensen D. Spontaneous bacterial peritonitis: An update on evaluation, management, and prevention. Am J Med 1994;97:169–175.
5. Tito L, Rimola A, Gines P, et al. Recurrence of spontaneous bacterial peritonitis in cirrhosis: frequency and predictive factors. Hepatology 1988;8:27–31.
6. Such J, Runyon BA. Spontaneous bacterial peritonitis. Clin Infect Dis 1998;27:669–76.
7. Soares-Weiser K, Brezis M, Tur-Kaspa R, et al. Antibiotic prophylaxis of bacterial infections in cirrhotic inpatients: a meta-analysis of randomized controlled trials. Scand J Gastroenterol 2003;38:193–200.
8. Garcia-Tsao G. Current management of the complications of cirrhosis and portal hypertension: Variceal hemorrhage, ascites, and spontaneous bacterial peritonitis. Gastroenterology 2001;120:726–748.
9. Bernard B, Lebrec D, Mathurin P, et al. Beta-adrenergic antagonists in the prevention of gastrointestinal rebleeding in patients with cirrhosis: A meta-analysis. Hepatology 1997;25:63–70.
10. Gournay J, Masliah C, Martin T, et al. Isosorbide mononitrate and propranolol compared with propranolol alone for the prevention of variceal rebleeding. Hepatology 2000;31:1239–1245.

This case presentation contains the professional views of the author and does not necessarily represent the official position of the FDA.

40 ESOPHAGEAL VARICES

► It's All About Making the Gradient (Level I)

Cesar Alaniz, PharmD

► After completing this case study, students should be able to:

- List nonpharmacologic options for the management of patients with bleeding esophageal varices.
- Recommend appropriate pharmacologic therapy for the control of bleeding esophageal varices.
- Provide appropriate patient education for patients receiving therapy for portal hypertension.

PATIENT PRESENTATION

Chief Complaint

Bloody stools

HPI

Dirk Grady is a 48 yo man with a history of alcoholic cirrhosis with grade 1 varices who was admitted to the hospital approximately 1 month ago for a

GI bleed. Endoscopy at that time revealed grade 1 esophageal varices that were too small to band. He was subsequently discharged on nadolol for management of portal hypertension. Today he presents to the ED reporting a 2-day history of feeling "out of sorts". This morning he was feeling bloated and then had two bowel movements consisting of tarry stools. He describes lightheadedness and weakness without CP, SOB, hematuria, or hematemesis. He has had decreased oral intake.

PMH
Alcoholic cirrhosis
Esophageal varices (grade 1)

FH
Father had diabetes

SH
He smokes about 1 ppd and has for many years. He has a 20-year history of alcohol consumption but hasn't had any in 3 years. He does not use any illicit drugs.

ROS
Negative except for complaints noted above

Meds
Nadolol 20 mg po once daily
Furosemide 40 mg po once daily
KCl 20 mEq once daily

All
NKDA

PE

Gen
Ill-appearing male in NAD

VS
BP 98/70, P 96, RR 18, T 37.0°C, sitting; not orthostatic but increase in HR to 120s on standing

Skin
Pale, normal turgor, no palmar erythema

HEENT
PERRLA, anicteric sclera, oropharynx clear without erythema or exudate

Neck/LN
Neck supple, no masses

Lungs/Thorax
Clear to auscultation

CV
Reg S_1, S_2; no S_3; no MR appreciated

Abd
Soft, mild distention with minimal diffuse tenderness with no rebound or guarding. No palpable or pulsatile masses. No fluid wave, with liver edge non-palpable; spleen not palpable.

Rect
Heme positive

Ext
Warm, trace edema; symmetric pulses

Neuro
A & O × 3, CN II–XII intact, no asterixis

Labs (on admission)

Na 141 mEq/L	Hgb 7.1 g/dL	AST 113 IU/L	Protein 7.4 g/dL
K 4.6 mEq/L	Hct 24.3%	ALT 91 IU/L	Alb 2.6 g/dL
Cl 111 mEq/L	WBC 9.2 × 10^3/mm^3	Alk phos 143 IU/L	Ca 8.1 mg/dL
CO_2 24 mEq/L	Plt 75 × 10^3/mm^3	LDH 232 IU/L	Phos 2.7 mg/dL
BUN 19 mg/dL	aPTT 28.6 sec	T. bili 1.8 mg/dL	
SCr 0.8 mg/dL	PT 12.9 sec		
Glu 116 mg/dL	INR 1.2		

ECG
NSR; no ST changes; no Q waves

Assessment
48 yo man with history of chronic alcohol use and cirrhosis who presents with a probable upper GI bleed that is likely variceal in origin. Plan to perform emergent endoscopy.

▶ Clinical Course

The patient underwent emergent endoscopy, which confirmed presence of bleeding esophageal varices.

▶ Questions

Problem Identification (see Figure 40–1)

1. a. *Create a list of the patient's drug therapy problems.*
   b. *What information supports the diagnosis of bleeding esophageal varices, and what indicates the relative severity of disease?*

Desired Outcome

2. *What are the goals for managing this patient's clinical condition?*

Therapeutic Alternatives

3. a. *What nonpharmacologic interventions should be considered for this patient?*
   b. *What pharmacologic interventions should be considered for this patient's current condition?*

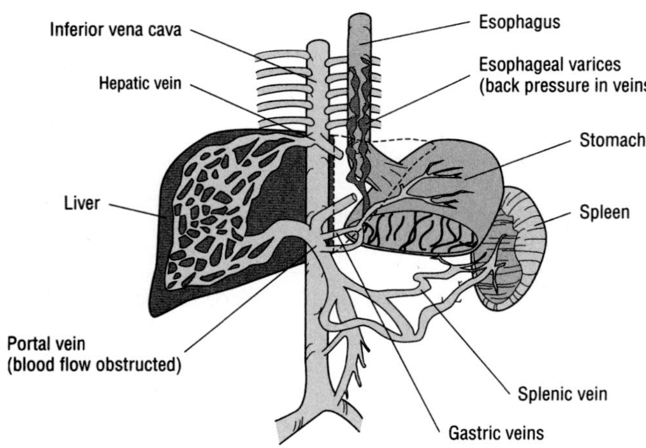

Figure 40–1. Anatomic relationships among intestinal veins affected by alcoholic cirrhosis. *(Reprinted with permission from Mulvihill ML. Human Diseases: A Systemic Approach,4th ed. Norwalk, CT, Appleton & Lange, 1995; 202).*

Optimal Plan

4. *What pharmacotherapeutic plan should be outlined for managing the patient's current problems?*

Outcome Evaluation

5. *What clinical and laboratory parameters should be followed to evaluate therapeutic interventions and to minimize the risk of adverse effects?*

Patient Education

6. *What information should be provided to the patient about his medication therapy?*

▶ Clinical Pearl

Although octreotide is generally well tolerated, its use should be monitored carefully. Octreotide may cause hyperglycemia, which may increase morbidity or mortality. Prolonged infusions (i.e., longer than 5 days) should be avoided.

▶ Self-Study Assignments

1. Compare the efficacy of pharmacologic vs. nonpharmacologic therapy for preventing repeat episodes of variceal bleeding.
2. Describe the benefits and limitations of using hepatic venous pressure gradient (HVPG) measurements for guiding pharmacologic therapy of portal hypertension.
3. Describe the role of transjugular intrahepatic portosystemic shunt (TIPS) in the management of bleeding esophageal varices.

References

1. de Franchis R. Updating consensus in portal hypertension: Report of the Baveno III Consensus Workshop on definitions, methodology and therapeutic strategies in portal hypertension. J Hepatol 2000;33:846–852.
2. Villanueva C, Ortiz J, Minana, et al. Somatostatin treatment and risk stratification by continuous portal pressure monitoring during acute variceal bleeding. Gastroenterology 2001;121:110–117.
3. Escorsell A, Bandi JC, Andreu V, et al. Desensitization to the effects of intravenous octreotide in cirrhotic patients with portal hypertension. Gastroenterology 2001;120:161–169.
4. Bosch J, Abraldes JG, Groszmann R. Current management of portal hypertension. J Hepatol 2003;38(Suppl 1):S54–S68.

41 HEPATIC ENCEPHALOPATHY

▶ State of Confusion (Level I)

Carrie Sincak, PharmD

▶ After completing this case study, students should be able to:

- Identify and correct the precipitating factors associated with the development of hepatic encephalopathy in a cirrhotic patient.
- Recommend appropriate nonpharmacologic and pharmacologic intervention for a cirrhotic patient who develops hepatic encephalopathy.
- Design a plan for monitoring the efficacy and adverse effects of recommended treatments for hepatic encephalopathy.
- Provide patient education for those receiving treatment for hepatic encephalopathy.

PATIENT PRESENTATION

Chief Complaint (from husband)

"She is acting strange and seems very confused."

HPI

Helen Markey is a 58 yo woman who was brought to the ED by her husband because of hallucinations and disorientation. He states that she was well until about 3 days ago when she started becoming confused and very slow to respond. At that time, she also complained of abdominal pain and lack of bowel movements. Since then, she has imagined bugs crawling all over the room and cannot orient herself to time or place. This morning, she could not recognize him and has become increasingly short-tempered.

PMH

Liver cirrhosis diagnosed 3 years ago secondary to heavy alcohol use. She was admitted multiple times for alcohol-related problems, uncontrolled ascites, and bleeding esophageal varices.

FH

Father died at age 42 in MVA; mother died at age 60 of heart disease. She has two brothers who are both living; the older brother lives out of state and is a recovering alcoholic. One sister died at age 38 of ALS.

SH

Unemployed. History of alcoholism, quit 3 years ago when liver cirrhosis was diagnosed. Lives alone with husband; they have a grown daughter and son.

ROS

Confused; some abdominal discomfort.

Meds

Spironolactone 100 mg po once daily
Furosemide 40 mg po once daily
MVI 1 tablet po once daily
Thiamine 100 mg po once daily
Folic Acid 1 mg po once daily
Propranolol 20 mg po BID
Lactulose 30 mL po BID
Patient has a history of noncompliance with her diet and medications.

All

No known drug or food allergies

PE

Gen

Dehydrated and jaundiced woman who is disoriented to time, place, and people

VS

BP 114/60, P 62 (supine); BP 90/60, P 83 (standing); RR 20, T 36.5°C; Ht 5′1″, Wt 68 kg (per patient's husband)

Skin

Decreased skin turgor; dry; jaundiced; spider angiomata on chest; (+) palmar erythema

HEENT

PERRLA; TMs intact; EOMI; fundi benign; dry mucous membranes; icteric sclerae

Lungs

Few rales bilaterally

CV

RRR; S_1 and S_2 normal; no S_3 or S_4

Abd

Mild tenderness; distended abdomen; (+) shifting dullness but fluid wave difficult to ascertain; prominent veins observed on abdomen; liver palpable 9 cm below the right costal margin; spleen is palpable. Bowel sounds normal.

Rect

Heme (–) stool

Ext

2+ pedal edema

Neuro

Confused; not oriented to time, place, and people; (+) asterixis; CN II–XII intact; DTRs 2+

Labs

Na 134 mEq/L	Hgb 11.4 g/dL	WBC 6.9×10^3/mm^3	AST 57 IU/L	Ca 7.4 mg/dL
K 3.2 mEq/L	Hct 32%	48% PMNs	ALT 69 IU/L	Mg 1.2 mg/dL
Cl 107 mEq/L	MCV 76 μm^3	2% Bands	ALK 154 IU/L	Phos 4.5 mg/dL
CO_2 27 mEq/L	MCHC 30 g/dL	3% Eos	T. bili 3.4 mg/dL	PT 17.9 sec
BUN 40 mg/dL	Retic 0.3%	38% Lymphs	D. bili 0.6 mg/dL	aPTT 40.2 sec
SCr 1.5 mg/dL	Plt 98×10^3/mm^3	9% Monos	Alb 2.1 g/dL	
Glu 82 mg/dL				

Assessment

Hepatic encephalopathy

Questions

Problem Identification

1. a. *Create a list of the patient's drug therapy problems.*
   b. *What information indicates the presence of hepatic encephalopathy in this patient?*
   c. *What precipitating factors in this patient could potentially cause hepatic encephalopathy?*
   d. *What additional information is needed to satisfactorily assess the hepatic encephalopathy of this patient?*

Desired Outcome

2. *What are the general principles for the management of hepatic encephalopathy and desired therapeutic outcomes?*

Therapeutic Alternatives

3. a. *What nondrug interventions are important before initiating pharmacotherapeutic agents for the treatment of hepatic encephalopathy?*
   b. *What pharmacotherapeutic alternatives are available for the treatment of hepatic encephalopathy? Include the mechanism of action of each drug in your answer.*

Optimal Plan

4. *Outline a pharmacotherapeutic plan that is most suitable for this patient. Include the drug, dosage form, dose, schedule, and duration of treatment.*

Outcome Evaluation

5. *How would you monitor the efficacy and adverse effects of the treatment you recommended? (See Figure 41–1.)*

Number Connection Test 1.

Patient's Name	
Date	
Completion Time (seconds)	
Tester's Initials	
PT. Chart No.	
Patient's Signature	

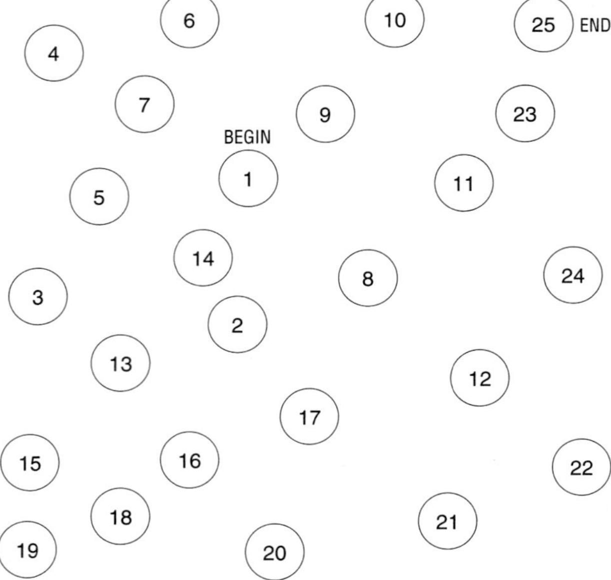

Figure 41–1. Number Connection Test part A (NCT-A), which measures cognitive motor abilities. Subjects have to connect the numbers printed on paper consecutively from 1 to 25, as quickly as possible. Errors are not counted, but patients are instructed to return to the preceding correct number and then carry on. The test score is the time the patient needs to perform the test, including the time needed to correct all errors. A low score represents a good performance. *(Reprinted with permission from reference 5.)*

▶ Clinical Course

Five days after beginning treatment with the regimen you recommended, the patient is responding positively, and the dose has been titrated appropriately. She is oriented to time, place, and people, and only slight asterixis is detected. The plan is to discharge the patient home tomorrow.

Patient Education

6. *What medication-related information should be provided to the patient about her therapy upon discharge?*

▶ Self-Study Assignments

1. Perform a literature search to assess the efficacy and the potential role of flumazenil and bromocriptine in the treatment of hepatic encephalopathy.
2. List the amino acid contents in the commercially available oral and parenteral formulations of branched-chain amino acid products; determine the cost of these products in your area.
3. List the potential advantages and disadvantages of using antibiotics for the treatment of hepatic encephalopathy.

▶ Clinical Pearl

All patients with chronic liver disease should be evaluated for signs and symptoms of acute hepatic encephalopathy. Aggressive treatment is required and precipitating factors controlled. Patients may have clinical conditions that increase their risk for developing encephalopathy (e.g., bleeding esophageal varices).

References

1. Blei AT and Cordoba J; Practice Parameters Committee of the American College of Gastroenterology. Hepatic encephalopathy. Am J Gastroenterol 2001;96:1968–1976.
2. Blei AT. Diagnosis and treatment of hepatic encephalopathy. Baillieres Best Pract Res Clin Gastroenterol 2000;14(6):959–974.
3. Gerber T, Schomerus H. Hepatic encephalopathy in liver cirrhosis: Pathogenesis, diagnosis and management. Drugs 2000;60(6):1353–1370.
4. Alexander T, Thomas K, Cherian AM, et al. Effect of three antibacterial drugs in lowering blood & stool ammonia production in hepatic encephalopathy. Indian J Med Res 1992;96:292–296.
5. Quero JC, Schalm SW. Subclinical hepatic encephalopathy. Semin Liver Dis 1996;16:321–328.

42 ACUTE PANCREATITIS

▶ Cuts Like a Knife (Level II)

Charles W. Fetrow, PharmD
Maria Yaramus, PharmD

▶ After completing this case study, students should be able to:

- Recognize signs, symptoms, and laboratory abnormalities commonly associated with acute pancreatitis.
- Describe potential systemic complications associated with acute pancreatitis.
- Recommend appropriate analgesic, nutritional, and enzyme therapy for patients with acute pancreatitis.
- Outline monitoring parameters to assist in realization of desired pharmacotherapeutic outcomes.

PATIENT PRESENTATION

Chief Complaint

"It feels like I've got a knife through my stomach."

HPI

Gerald Sherman is a 59 yo man who presents to the ED because of intense mid-epigastric pain radiating to the back. He states that he has had sharp, intermittent epigastric/abdominal pain for 3 to 4 weeks, which has been increasing in severity and duration over the last 3 days.

PMH

- Pneumonia 4 years ago that resolved with appropriate antimicrobial therapy
- S/P open-reduction internal fixation of left femur secondary to MVA 18 years ago

FH

Father died at age of 75 from complications related to CVA; mother approximately 70 years of age, alive and well. One brother, also alive and without significant illness

SH

Married with 2 children. Employed as an electrician. Denies any smoking or alcohol consumption

Meds

- Multiple vitamin 1 po daily
- Extra-strength Tylenol several doses per day started recently PRN pain

All

NKDA

ROS

States that he has been feeling "overheated" and has experienced periodic bouts of nausea and vomiting for the past 3 to 4 days. Also describes an approximate 6.8-kg weight loss over the past 2 months secondary to anorexia and intense postprandial pain. He has noted a reduction in the frequency of bowel movements. No complaints of diarrhea or blood in the stool; no knowledge of any prior history of uncontrolled blood sugars

PE

Gen

The patient seems restless and in moderate distress but otherwise is a well-appearing, well-nourished male who looks his stated age.

VS

BP 100/68, P 118, RR 30, T 38.5°C; Wt 68 kg, Ht 5′8″

HEENT

PEERLA; EOMI; oropharynx pink and clear; oral mucosa dry

Skin

Dry with poor skin turgor; some skin tenting noted

Neck/LN

Supple; no bruits, lymphadenopathy, or thyromegaly

Cor

Sinus tachycardia; no m/r/g

Lungs

Bilateral basilar rales

Abd

Moderately distended with active but diminished bowel sounds; (+) guarding; pain is elicited on light palpation of left upper and mid-epigastric region. No rebound tenderness, masses, or HSM

Ext

Extremities are warm and well perfused. Good pulses present in all extremities

Rect

Normal sphincter tone; no bright red blood or masses visible; stool is guaiac negative; prostate may be slightly enlarged

Neuro

Patient is A & O × 3; neuro exam essentially benign; CN II–XII intact; strength is equal bilaterally in all extremities

Labs

Na 130 mEq/L	Hgb 18 g/dL	AST 349 IU/L	Ca 8.0 mg/dL
K 3.9 mEq/L	Hct 52%	ALT 154 IU/L	Mg 1.8 mEq/L
Cl 95 mEq/L	WBC 16.2 × 10^3/mm^3	Alk phos 275 IU/L	Phos 2.3 mg/dL
CO_2 23 mEq/L	Neutros 70%	LDH 225 IU/L	Trig 1182 mg/dL
BUN 32 mg/dL	Bands 5%	T. bili 0.7 mg/dL	Repeat Trig 1021 mg/dL
SCr 1.4 mg/dL	Eos 1%	Alb 3.3 g/dL	
Glu 399 mg/dL	Basos 1%	Prealb 19 mg/dL	
	Lymphs 21%	Amylase 2244 IU/L	
	Monos 2%	Lipase 1548 IU/L	

UA

Color yellow; turbidity clear; SG 1.010; pH 7.0; glucose > 1,000 mg/dL; bilirubin (–); ketones (–); Hgb (–); protein (–); nitrite (–); crystals (–); casts (–); mucous (–); bacteria (–); urobilinogen: 0.2 EU/dL; WBC 0–5/hpf; RBC 0/hpf; epithelial cells: 0–10/hpf

Chest X-Ray

AP view of chest shows the heart to be normal in size. The lungs are clear without any infiltrates, masses, effusions, or atelectasis

Abd Ultrasound

Non-specific gas pattern; no dilated bowel. Questionable opacity/abnormality of common bile duct. Cannot rule out gallstone/obstruction

ECG

Sinus tachycardia; rate 140 bpm

Assessment

- Acute pancreatitis precipitating hyperglycemia
- R/O choledocholithiasis

▶ Questions

Problem Identification (see Figure 42–1)

1. *a. What signs, symptoms, and laboratory tests are consistent with the diagnosis of acute pancreatitis?*
   b. What are the likely etiologies that may explain the development of acute pancreatitis in this case?
   c. Construct a drug therapy problem list for this patient.

Desired Outcome

2. *What are the desired goals of therapy for this patient?*

Therapeutic Alternatives

3. *What therapies may be instituted to achieve the goals outlined above? Provide a rationale for each therapy.*

Optimal Plan

4. *Develop a pharmacotherapeutic care plan for this patient.*

Outcome Evaluation

5. *Outline monitoring parameters for efficacy and adverse effects of therapy for pain management.*

▶ Clinical Course

TPN is instituted after 24 hours. After several days of improvement in the hospital, the patient develops a WBC count of $20.4 \times 10^3/mm^3$ with neutrophils 77%, bands 11%, eosinophils 1%, basophils 0%, lymphocytes 7%, and monocytes 4%. He has a temperature of 39.8°C and is noted to be orthostatic (BP 128/76 sitting, 98/60 standing) with a glucose of 675 mg/dL. He has also experienced several episodes of diarrhea and steatorrhea.

Because of these setbacks in the patient's progress, a contrast-enhanced CT scan is obtained. The results demonstrate peri-pancreatic and retroperitoneal edema. The pancreas itself appears relatively normal with the exception of small non-enhancing areas around the neck of the pancreas, which are suggestive of necrosis.

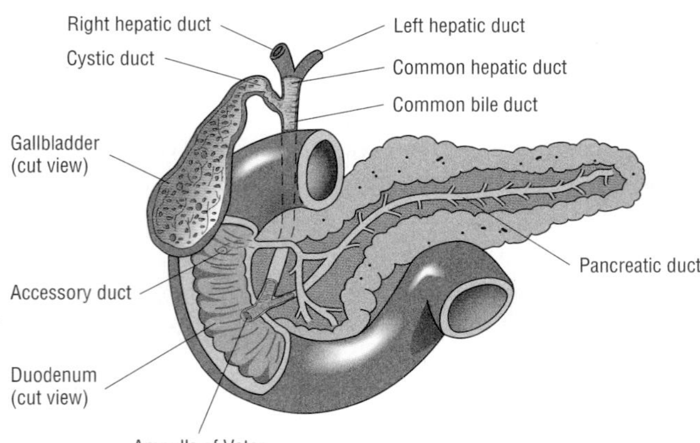

Figure 42–1. Anatomic relationship between the pancreas and other digestive organs.
(Reprinted with permission from Mulvihill ML. Human Diseases: A Systemic Approach, 4th ed. Norwalk, CT, Appleton & Lange, 1995:209)

▶ Follow-Up Questions

a. What potential etiologies might explain this patient's fever and relapsing acute pancreatitis?
b. What are the new treatment goals for this patient?
c. Given this new information, what therapeutic interventions should be considered for this patient?
d. How should these new therapies be monitored for efficacy and adverse effects?
e. Which medications have been associated with the development of drug-induced acute pancreatitis?

Patient Education

6. *The patient is being discharged today after a prolonged hospital course. The attending physician would like you to talk with the patient about his discharge medications. What information should be provided?*

▶ Self-Study Assignments

1. Describe the pathophysiology through which autodigestion of the pancreas occurs.
2. Investigate the experimental use of CCK-receptor blockers, octreotide, and cytokine antagonists for their potential to improve outcomes related to acute pancreatitis.
3. Compose a list of drugs thought to aggravate or give rise to drug-induced pancreatitis.
4. Review information published regarding opiate effects on the sphincter of Oddi. Specifically review the article by Isenhower and Mueller.[3]

▶ Clinical Pearl

More expensive microencapsulated pancreatic enzyme products have not consistently been shown to be superior to standard therapeutic doses of the less expensive, non-enteric coated dosage forms.[3]

References

1. Steinberg W, Tenner S. Acute pancreatitis. N Engl J Med 1994;330:1198–1210.
2. Mitchell RM, Byrne MF, Baillie J. Pancreatitis. Lancet 2003;361:1447–1455.
3. Isenhower HL, Mueller BA. Selection of narcotic analgesics for pain associated with pancreatitis. Am J Health Syst Pharm 1998;55:480–486.
4. Balthazar EJ, Ranson JH, Naidich DP, et al. Acute pancreatitis: Prognostic value of CT. Radiology 1985;156:767–772.
5. Rattner DW, Legermate DA, Lee MJ, et al. Early surgical debridement of symptomatic pancreatic necrosis is beneficial irrespective of infection. Am J Surg 1992;163:105–109.
6. Beger HG, Bittner R, Block S, et al. Bacterial contamination of pancreatic necrosis. A prospective clinical study. Gastroenterology 1986;91:433–438.

7. Bassi C. Infected pancreatic necrosis. Int J Pancreatol 1994;16:1–10.
8. Pederzoli P, Bassi C, Vesentini S, et al. A randomized multicenter clinical trial of antibiotic prophylaxis of septic complications in acute necrotizing pancreatitis with imipenem. Surg Gynecol Obstet 1993;176:480–483.
9. Manes G, Rabitti PG, Menchise A, et al. Prophylaxis with meropenem of septic complications in acute pancreatitis: A randomized, controlled trial versus imipenem. Pancreas 2003 Nov;27(4):e79–e83.
10. DiMagno EP, Go VL, Summerskill WH. Relations between pancreatic enzyme outputs and malabsorption in severe pancreatic insufficiency. N Engl J Med 1973;288:813–815.
11. Lankisch PG. Enzyme treatment of exocrine pancreatic insufficiency in chronic pancreatitis. Digestion 1993;54(Suppl 2):21–29.
12. Tenner S, Levine RS, Steinberg WM. Drug treatment of acute and chronic pancreatitis. In: Lewis JH, ed. A Pharmacologic Approach to Gastrointestinal Disorders. Baltimore, Williams & Wilkins, 1994:311–340.

43 CHRONIC PANCREATITIS

► Uneasy Rider (Level II)

Susan D. Bear, BS, PharmD
Donna S. Wall, PharmD

► After completing this case study, students should be able to:

- Identify subjective and objective findings consistent with chronic pancreatitis and acute exacerbation of chronic pancreatitis.
- Evaluate patient-specific data and develop a problem list for the patient with acute exacerbation of chronic pancreatitis.
- Understand the rationale for "pancreatic rest" in the resolution of pain and symptoms of an acute exacerbation.
- Discuss therapeutic alternatives and outline a patient-specific plan for pain management during an acute exacerbation.
- Recommend appropriate enzyme replacement therapy for management of steatorrhea in a patient with chronic pancreatitis.

PATIENT PRESENTATION

Chief Complaint

"I'm having terrible pain in my stomach with vomiting and diarrhea."

HPI

Harold Bertoli is a 46 yo man who presents to the ED with complaints of sharp epigastric pain that radiates up into the chest, down to the scrotum, and around to the back. He states that he has had nausea and vomiting for 6 days with an unintentional 6.8-kg weight loss over the last 4 weeks. Upon further questioning, he relates that he has had a fever and malodorous watery green stools for 3 days.

PMH

The patient reports being hospitalized 3 times in the last year for similar episodes. His last admission was 3 months ago. He left AMA after 3 days because "that doctor wouldn't do anything for my pain. I know my own body better than anyone." He describes what appears to be a celiac block procedure that was done 6 months ago. He has had several episodes of gastritis over the last several years, but no episodes in the last 6 months. Old medical records are unavailable for review.

FH

Father died at age 62 of COPD. Mother is still alive and in relatively good health. The patient is an only child.

SH

He is unmarried and currently employed in a tool and die shop. He reports a 20-year history of ethanol abuse, "probably 3 cases of beer a week." He smoked 2 packs of cigarettes per day × 15 years. He states that he has had no alcohol or cigarettes since a motorcycle accident 3 years ago.

ROS

No hematemesis; no complaints other than those above

Meds

Propoxyphene 65 mg po PRN (he reports up to 10 capsules per day for the last week with little to no pain relief)

All

NKDA

PE

Gen

Thin, ill-appearing white male in obvious distress

VS

BP 130/90, HR 75, RR 23, T 37.5°C; Wt 63.5 kg, Ht 5′11″

Skin

No abdominal bruising or ecchymosis, no spider angiomata, poor skin turgor

HEENT

PERRLA; EOMI; oropharynx clear; mucous membranes dry

Neck/LN

Supple, (–) JVD, thyromegaly, lymphadenopathy, or bruits

Lungs/Thorax

Prolonged expiratory phase, mild scattered expiratory wheeze

CV

RRR without m/r/g

Abd

Decreased bowel sounds; no distention; some voluntary guarding, worse near the RUQ; no rebound

Genit/Rect

Normal sphincter tone, no masses, guaiac (–)

Ext

(–) Clubbing, cyanosis, or edema

Neuro

A & O × 3, CN II–XII intact

Labs

Na 132 mEq/L	Hgb 14.3 g/dL	Ca 9.8 mg/dL	Lipase 120 IU/L
K 3.2 mEq/L	Hct 32.3%	Mg 2.0 mEq/L	Amylase 283 IU/L
Cl 97 mEq/L	WBC 11.3 × $10^3/mm^3$	Phos 3.6 mg/dL	
CO_2 23 mEq/L	T. Bili 0.4 mg/dL		
BUN 8 mg/dL	Alk Phos 113 IU/L		
SCr 1.0 mg/dL	Alb 2.9 g/dL		
FBG 240 mg/dL	Prealb 20 mg/dL		

KUB

Unremarkable

Upright Abdominal X-Ray

Consistent with pancreatic calcification

ERCP

Changes consistent with chronic pancreatitis, including dilation of the main pancreatic duct

Assessment

Acute exacerbation of chronic pancreatitis

▶ Questions

Problem Identification

1. a. *Create a list of this patient's drug therapy problems.*
   b. *What subjective and objective information is consistent with the diagnosis of chronic pancreatitis?*
   c. *Which signs, symptoms, and test results indicate that the patient is experiencing an acute exacerbation of chronic pancreatitis?*
   d. *Are any of the patient's problems amenable to drug therapy?*
   e. *What additional information is needed to satisfactorily assess this patient?*

Desired Outcome

2. *What are the goals of pharmacotherapy in this case?*

Therapeutic Alternatives

3. a. *What non-drug therapies could be useful in this patient?*
   b. *What feasible pharmacotherapeutic alternatives are available for treatment of this acute exacerbation of chronic pancreatitis?*

Optimal Plan

4. *What drug, dosage form, and duration of therapy are best for this patient?*

Outcome Evaluation

5. *Which clinical and laboratory parameters are necessary to evaluate the therapy for achievement of the desired therapeutic outcome and to detect or prevent adverse events?*

▶ Clinical Course

After 2 weeks of appropriate management, Mr. Bertoli's pain has resolved. A low-fat oral diet has been initiated, but nursing documentation indicates that the patient is having two to three malodorous stools each day. The assessment is that the patient has steatorrhea.

▶ Follow-Up Questions

Problem Identification

1. *What is the nature of this problem, and what pharmacotherapeutic intervention should be initiated to correct it?*

Desired Outcome

2. *What are the goals of pharmacotherapy for this condition?*

Therapeutic Alternatives

3. *What feasible pharmacotherapeutic alternatives are available for treatment of this condition?*

Optimal Plan

4. *What drug, dosage form, dose, schedule, and duration of therapy are optimal for this patient?*

Assessment Parameters

5. *Which clinical and laboratory parameters are necessary to evaluate the therapy for achievement of the desired therapeutic outcome and to detect or prevent adverse effects?*

Patient Education

6. *After 5 additional days of the therapy that you recommended, the patient is ready for discharge. What information should be provided to enhance compliance, ensure successful therapy, and minimize adverse events?*

▶ Self-Study Assignments

1. Obtain information on the diagnostic test referred to as "ERCP" and describe its role in the diagnosis of chronic pancreatitis.
2. Review the pathway of pancreatic pain fibers.
3. What role do elevated triglycerides play in acute exacerbation of chronic pancreatitis? Is it a cause or an effect?
4. This patient later develops erosive gastritis requiring treatment with an H_2-receptor antagonist. What effect will this intervention have on his enzyme replacement therapy?

▶ Clinical Pearl

When seeking treatment for acute exacerbation, patients with long-standing pancreatitis may not present with extreme elevations in amylase and lipase levels. The diseased organ lacks the functional capacity to produce large amounts of enzyme. This limits the use of enzyme elevation to evaluate severity of exacerbation.

References

1. Owyang C, Levitt M. Chronic pancreatitis. In: Yamada T, ed. Textbook of Gastroenterology. Philadelphia, Lippincott-Raven, 1995:2091–2112.
2. Lankisch PG, Burchard-Reckert S, Lehnick D. Underestimation of acute pancreatitis: Patients with only a small increase in amylase/lipase levels can also have or develop severe acute pancreatitis. Gut 1999;44:542–544.
3. Beckingham IJ, Bornman PC. ABC of diseases of liver, pancreas and biliary system. BMJ 2001;322:595–598.
4. Schmid SW, Uhl W, Friss H, et al. The role of infection in acute pancreatitis. Gut 1999;45:311–316.
5. Principles of Analgesic Use in the Treatment of Acute Pain and Cancer Pain, 4th ed. Glenview, IL: American Pain Society, 1999.
6. Apte MV, Keogh GW, Wilson JS. Chronic pancreatitis: Complications and management. J Clin Gastroenterol 1999;29:225–240.

44 VIRAL HEPATITIS A VACCINATION

▶ Taking a Shot (Level I)

Juliana Chan, PharmD

▶ After completing this case study, students should be able to:

- Determine which patient populations are at greatest risk for contracting hepatitis A.
- Recommend hepatitis A immunization for appropriate individuals based on current guidelines of the Centers for Disease Control and Prevention (CDC).
- Assess the efficacy and adverse effects of hepatitis A vaccines.
- Educate eligible patients on the benefits of hepatitis A vaccination and the possible adverse effects associated with its use.

PATIENT PRESENTATION

Chief Complaint

"I'm feeling well today. I just came to clinic for my annual physical, and now they say I might need some kind of shot."

HPI

Edgar Zeller is a 57 yo man who presented to medicine clinic earlier today for a routine annual physical exam. During the medical history, the patient reported that he will be leaving for China in 3 months for a 4-week vacation. He has been referred to this travel clinic today for further evaluation and possible hepatitis A vaccination.

PMH

Gout × 25 years
Glaucoma × 18 years
H/O Kidney stones in 1987
Hepatitis B carrier

PSH

Trabeculectomy in right eye 2 years ago
Cataract removal in right eye 1 year ago

FH

Mother died in her thirties, father died of pancreatic cancer at age 51; four brothers all with a history of gout; one sister died of heart failure and a second sister is alive and well.

SH

Married for 29 years and lives with his wife and daughter. Does not smoke or drink. Retired greenskeeper at the local country club.

ROS

The patient is quite active. He denies any angina, dyspnea on exertion, palpitations, fainting, cough, sputum, wheezing, abdominal pain, change in bowel habits, melena, hematochezia, urinary urgency or frequency, or sexual dysfunction.

Meds

Allopurinol 300 mg po once daily
Pred Forte eye drops; 1 gtt in right eye BID

All

None

PE

Gen
The patient is a healthy Caucasian man in no apparent distress

VS
BP 104/60, P 62, RR 20, T 36.9°C; Wt 75 kg; Ht 5′8″

Skin
Warm and dry

HEENT
PERRLA, EOMI; fundi normal; TMs clear

Neck/LN
No adenopathy or goiter

Chest
Clear without wheezes, rhonchi, or rales

CV
RRR, S_1, S_2 normal; no S_3 or S_4

Abd
(+) Bowel sounds, no mass, non-tender

Genit/Rect
Testes normal with no masses; prostate soft and non-tender without nodules; no rectal masses

MS/Ext
Normal range of motion throughout; no CCE

Neuro
A & O × 3; CN II–XII intact; no focal deficits

Labs

Na 139 mEq/L	Hgb 15.1 g/dL	AST 38 IU/L	T. chol 198 mg/dL
K 4.1 mEq/L	Hct 43.3%	ALT 39 IU/L	Trig 341 mg/dL
Cl 107 mEq/L	WBC 5.6 × 10^3/mm^3	Alk phos 85 IU/L	HDL 39 mg/dL
CO_2 26 mEq/L	Plt 181 × 10^3/mm^3	T. bili 0.6 mg/dL	anti-HA (–)
BUN 17 mg/dL		LDH 167 IU/L	HbsAg (+)
SCr 0.8 mg/dL		PT 13.7 sec	Urate 4.9 mg/dL
Glu (non-fasting) 102 mg/dL		Alb 4.5 g/dL	PSA 0.9 ng/mL

ECG
Sinus bradycardia without arrhythmia or infarction

Assessment
The patient is healthy with no complaints. He is here to be evaluated for hepatitis A vaccination.

Questions

Problem Identification

1. a. *What patient factors make this patient a candidate for hepatitis A vaccination?*
   b. *What other patient populations or environments present an increased risk for infection with hepatitis A?*

Desired Outcome

2. *What are the goals of hepatitis A vaccination?*

Therapeutic Alternatives

3. a. *What nonpharmacologic recommendations should be made to this patient to minimize his risk of developing hepatitis A infection while in China?*
   b. *What commercial products are available for vaccination against hepatitis A, and how effective are they in providing protective efficacy?*

Optimal Plan

4. *Outline a treatment regimen that includes dose, dosage, route of administration, and the number of doses required for this patient.*

Outcome Evaluation

5. a. *How should the therapy you recommended be monitored for efficacy?*
   b. *What adverse effects may be experienced with the therapy you recommended, and how may these events be treated?*

Patient Education

6. *What information should be provided to the patient about the hepatitis A vaccine?*

▶ Clinical Course

Two weeks prior to Mr. Zeller's departure for vacation, his daughter, Lilly, and wife, Helen, decide to go with him to China. Lilly is anti-HAV-negative, is not a carrier of hepatitis B, and is otherwise healthy. Helen's anti-HAV status is unknown, but she recalls receiving one dose of a hepatitis A vaccine about 13 months ago and is immunized against hepatitis B.

▶ Follow-Up Question

1. *What preventive measures do you recommend for Lilly and Helen, who will leave this country within 2 weeks and travel to an area that is endemic for hepatitis A?*

▶ Self-Study Assignments

1. Compare and contrast the mechanism of action, immunogenicity rate, and adverse effects of the two commercially available hepatitis A vaccines.
2. Determine what other vaccines can be given simultaneously with the hepatitis A vaccine.
3. Compare the cost of administering the Havrix and Energix-B vaccines separately versus the combination product Twinrix for an adult.

Clinical Pearl

According to the CDC, vaccination of children living in states and communities with consistently elevated rates of hepatitis A will provide protection from disease and is expected to reduce the overall incidence of hepatitis A.[1]

References

1. Centers for Disease Control and Prevention. Prevention of hepatitis A through active or passive immunization: Recommendations of the Advisory Committee on Immunization Practices (ACIP). MMWR Morb Mortal Wkly Rep 1999;48(RR12): 1–37.
2. Kemmer NM, Miskovsky EP. Hepatitis A. Infect Dis Clin North Am 2000;14(3): 605–615.
3. Twinrix Prescribing Information. GlaxoSmithKline. Research Triangle Park, NC; August 2003.

45 VIRAL HEPATITIS B

▶ The Infected Family (Level II)

Juliana Chan, PharmD

▶ After completing this case study, students should be able to:

- Outline a pharmacologic and nonpharmacologic regimen for patients with chronic hepatitis B.
- Determine clinical and laboratory endpoints for treatment of chronic hepatitis B.
- Assess the efficacy and adverse effects of chronic hepatitis B treatment with interferon, lamivudine, and adefovir dipivoxil.
- Recommend hepatitis B immunization for appropriate individuals based on current guidelines of the Centers for Disease Control and Prevention (CDC).
- Provide patient education on lamivudine and adefovir dipivoxil treatment.

PATIENT PRESENTATION

Chief Complaint

"My family doctor sent me here for evaluation of my liver problem. I think I have hepatitis B."

HPI

Steven Sung is a 45 yo Chinese man with no significant past medical history except for HTN. According to the patient, he had blood tests done as part of a routine physical exam required for his new job 1 year ago. At that time, he was told that his liver enzymes were elevated, and he was advised to see his family doctor for further assessment. Because he did not feel ill, he did not follow this advice. At a visit to his family doctor 3 weeks ago for assessment of his HTN, he was again told that his liver enzymes were abnormal and that additional tests suggested hepatitis B. He was referred to the liver clinic today for further evaluation and possible treatment.

PMH

HTN

FH

Father died of lung cancer at age 65; mother died of hepatitis at age 62; three siblings are alive and well.

SH

Married for 10 years and lives with his wife and their two 5-year-old twins. His wife is 7 months pregnant with their third child and is HbsAg (+). The twins are positive for anti-HBs. He smokes 1 ppd and drinks one can of beer with meals daily. Employed as a machinist.

Meds

Hydrochlorothiazide 25 mg, 1 tablet by mouth daily

All

Penicillin ("rash all over the body")

ROS

Denies any symptoms except increased tiredness (which he attributes to lack of sleep) and weight loss. No changes in urine or stool color and no history of icteric sclerae.

PE

Gen

The patient is a cachectic, lethargic man.

VS

BP 139/90, P 64, RR 16, T 37.1°C; Wt 84 kg; Ht 6′0″

Skin

Warm and dry; no obvious icterus; no spider nevi or palmar erythema

HEENT

PERRLA, EOMI, sclerae anicteric; funduscopic exam normal; TMs intact

Cor

RRR, S_1, S_2 normal; no S_3 or S_4

Lungs

Clear to P & A

Abd

Soft, non-tender; liver span 10 cm; no evidence of ascites; spleen is not palpable

Rect

Guaiac negative

MS/Ext

Normal range of motion throughout; no C/C/E

Neuro

CN II–XII intact; DTRs 2+ throughout; negative Babinski

Labs (today)

Na 142 mEq/L	Hgb 13.5 g/dL	HIV negative
K 4.0 mEq/L	Hct 43%	HCV negative
Cl 102 mEq/L	Plt 175 × 10^3/mm^3	
CO_2 23 mEq/L	WBC 7.5 × 10^3/mm^3	
BUN 13 mg/dL	65% PMNs	
SCr 1.3 mg/dL	2% Bands	
Glu (non-fasting) 113 mg/dL	25% Lymphs	
	8% Monos	

Liver function tests and hepatitis screen values were compared with those obtained on his initial evaluation 1 year ago:

Test	12 Months Ago	3 Weeks Ago
AST	142 IU/L	130 IU/L
ALT	120 IU/L	110 IU/L
Alk phos	84 IU/L	81 IU/L
T. bili	1.0 mg/dL	0.9 mg/dL
PT	13.2 sec	13.5 sec
Alb	3.0 g/dL	2.9 g/dL
HbsAg	(+)	(+)
Anti-HBs	Not done	(–)
HBeAg	Not done	(+)
HBV DNA	Not done	2,562,035 copies/mL
Anti-HCV	(–)	(–)
HIV	(–)	(–)

Assessment

Because of the persistent elevations in hepatic enzymes, a liver biopsy was performed. The results revealed features consistent with chronic active hepatitis without cirrhosis.

▶ Questions

Problem Identification

1. a. *Create a list of this patient's drug therapy problems.*
   b. *In addition to the liver biopsy results, which clinical findings, laboratory values, and items in the medical history suggest the presence of chronic hepatitis B virus (HBV) infection?*

Desired Outcome

2. *What are the goals of treatment for chronic active HBV infection?*

Therapeutic Alternatives

3. a. *What nonpharmacologic measures should be considered for this patient?*
   b. *What pharmacotherapeutic alternatives are available for treatment of this patient?*

Optimal Plan

4. *What drug, dose, dosage form, schedule, and duration of therapy should be recommended?*

Outcome Evaluation

5. a. *How should the therapy you recommended be monitored for efficacy and adverse effects?*
   b. *Which baseline parameters suggest that this patient may have a favorable response to treatment (i.e., sustained loss of HBeAg and HBV DNA)?*

Patient Education

6. *What information should be provided to this patient regarding the treatment?*

▶ Follow-Up Questions

1. *For the hepatitis B vaccines currently available, outline treatment regimens for each age category (including Steven's newborn baby at birth) that include number of doses, dosage schedule, and dose in micrograms.*
2. *What preventive measures will you recommend for each member of the patient's family?*

▶ Clinical Course

The patient tolerated the initial therapy very well. After 12 months of treatment, his physician had stopped his therapy. However, at month 13, serum HBV DNA was detectable. His lab results for the last few months of treatment were as follows:

	ALT (IU/L)	Hepatitis B DNA (pg/mL)	Hepatitis B Serologies
Month 13	23	0	HbeAb (+)
Month 15	70	0.58	HbeAg (+)

His physician decides to reinitiate therapy for an additional year. These are his laboratory values for the second year of therapy:

	ALT (IU/L)	Hepatitis B DNA (pg/mL)	Hepatitis B Serologies
Month 17	83	2,325.62	HbeAg (+)
Month 19	89	2,413.34	HbeAg (+)
Month 22	98	2,424.98	HbeAg (+)
Month 25	103	2,550.67	HbeAg (+)

In addition, Steven started to develop more fatigue and edema in his legs in the past 6 months.

3. *What is your assessment of these laboratory results?*
4. *Based on these results, what changes in therapy would you recommend? Include the drug name, dose, dosage form, schedule, and duration of therapy.*
5. *What adverse effects might occur with this new therapy? How would you monitor for them?*
6. *What information should be provided to this patient about the new treatment?*

▶ Self-Study Assignments

1. Describe the ideal hepatitis B candidate to respond to lamivudine therapy and what you would monitor for therapeutic efficacy and adverse effects.
2. Compare and contrast the mechanism of action, immunogenicity rate, and adverse effects of the two commercially available hepatitis B vaccines.
3. Survey several pharmacies to estimate the approximate retail cost of adefovir dipivoxil, lamivudine, and interferon therapy for the treatment of hepatitis B.
4. Review the time course of serologic markers after acute hepatitis B virus infection and explain their significance to one of your peers (see Figure 45–1).

▶ Clinical Pearl

To eliminate HBV transmission that occurs during infancy and childhood, the Immunization Practice Advisory Committee of the Centers of Disease Control recommends that all newborn infants be vaccinated regardless of the hepatitis B status of the mothers.[3,4,9,10]

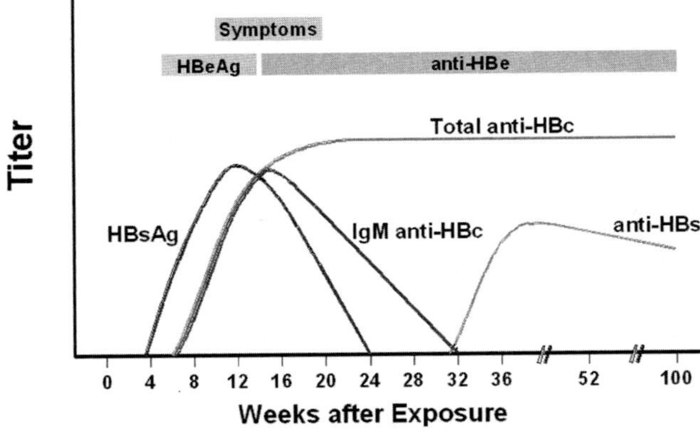

Figure 45–1. Typical Serologic Course of Acute Hepatitis B Virus Infection with Recovery. Note: Serologic markers of infection vary depending on whether the infection is acute or chronic. *(Source: National Center for Infectious Diseases: Hepatitis B Virus. http://www.cdc.gov/ncidod/diseases/hepatitis/slideset/hep_b/slide_3.htm (accessed June 7, 2004).)*

References

1. Lok AS, McMahon BJ; Practice Guidelines Committee, American Association for the Study of Liver Diseases. Chronic hepatitis B. Hepatology 2001;34:1225–1241.
2. Conjeevaram HS, Lok ASF. Management of chronic hepatitis B. J Hepatol 2003;38(Suppl 1):S90–S103.
3. Centers for Disease Control and Prevention. Hepatitis B virus: A comprehensive strategy for eliminating transmission in the United States through universal childhood vaccination. Recommendations of the Immunization Practices Advisory Committee (ACIP) MMWR Morb Mortal Wkly Rep 1991; 40(RR13):1–19.
4. Notice to readers update: Recommendations to prevent hepatitis B virus transmission—United States. MMWR Morb Mortal Wkly Rep 1995;44(30):574–575.
5. Marcellin P, Chang TT, Lim SG, et al. Adefovir dipivoxil for the treatment of hepatitis B e antigen-positive chronic hepatitis B. N Engl J Med 2003;348:808–816.
6. EASL Jury. EASL International Consensus Conference on Hepatitis B. 13–14 September, 2002: Geneva, Switzerland. Consensus statement (short version). J Hepatol 2003;38:533–540.
7. Lai CL, Chien RN, Leung NW, et al. A one-year trial of lamivudine for chronic hepatitis B. Asia Hepatitis Lamivudine Study Group. N Engl J Med 1998;339:61–68.
8. Most recently published hepatitis B postexposure prophylaxis recommendations. MMWR Morb Mortal Wkly Rep 1997;46(RR18):22–23.
9. Notice to readers: Alternate two-dose hepatitis B vaccination schedule for adolescents aged 11–15 years. MMWR Morb Mortal Wkly Rep 2000;49(12):261.

46 VIRAL HEPATITIS C

▶ Interfering with the Bridge from Fibrosis to Cirrhosis (Level I)

Cesar Alaniz, PharmD
Nancy P. Lam, PharmD, BCPS

▶ After completing this case study, students should be able to:

- Develop a treatment plan for patients with chronic hepatitis.
- Evaluate the clinical and laboratory endpoints for treatment of chronic hepatitis C.
- Develop a plan for monitoring efficacy and adverse effects of pharmacologic management of chronic hepatitis C.
- Provide education for patients with chronic hepatitis C regarding their medications.

PATIENT PRESENTATION

Chief Complaint

"I was told that my liver tests are abnormal."

HPI

Gina Starring is a 42 yo woman who has been referred by her family doctor to the liver clinic for assessment of her abnormal liver enzymes. She reports remote use of recreational drugs in high school, including IV cocaine. She drinks alcohol occassionally (1 to 2 glasses of wine per week). She states that she feels fine with periodic fatigue. She has no past history of liver problems.

PMH
IV drug abuse in high school

FH
No known family history of liver disease. Both parents are alive and well.

SH
Married for 10 years; no children. Non-smoker; denies illicit drug or inhalant use; drinks about one to two glasses of wine per week.

ROS
Denies any signs or symptoms of liver diseases except for occasional fatigue. No changes in urine color. Recalls having icteric sclerae briefly in high school.

Meds
MVI 1 tablet po daily
Calcium carbonate 1250 mg daily

All
No known drug or food allergies

PE

Gen
Well nourished woman in NAD

VS
BP 108/76, P 74, RR 16, T 37.0°C; Wt 75 kg; Ht 5′5″

Skin
No jaundice; no spider angiomata or palmar erythema

HEENT
PERRLA; EOMI; sclerae anicteric; funduscopic exam normal; TMs intact

Neck/LN
Neck supple; no lymphadenopathy or thyromegaly; no carotid bruits

Lungs
Normal breath sounds

CV
RRR, S_1, S_2 normal; no S_3 or S_4

Abd
Liver span 10 cm; spleen not palpable; no evidence of ascites

MS/Ext
No CCE; peripheral pulses 2+ throughout; normal ROM

Neuro
A & O × 3; CN II–XII intact; DTRs 2+

Labs
Obtained 2 weeks ago from patient's family physician:

Na 141 mEq/L	Hgb 14.2 g/dL	AST 117 IU/L	HbsAg (–)
K 4.2 mEq/L	Hct 40.2%	ALT 137 IU/L	Anti-HAV(–)
Cl 107 mEq/L	Plt 245 × 10^3/mm^3	Alk phos 96 IU/L	Anti-HCV (+)
CO_2 23 mEq/L	WBC 7.2 × 10^3/mm^3	T. bili 1.6 mg/dL	HCV RNA (bDNA assay)
BUN 11 mg/dL	65% PMNs	Alb 3.2 g/dL	3.4 million copies/mL
SCr 1.2 mg/L	2% Bands	PT 12.3 sec	HIV-negative (non-fasting)
Glu 118 mg/dL	25% Lymphs	ANA (–)	
	8% Monos		

Liver Biopsy (performed after liver clinic visit)
Moderate degree of fibrosis and inflammation consistent with chronic hepatitis

Assessment
Chronic hepatitis C

▶ Questions

Problem Identification

1. a. *Create a list of patient's drug-related problems.*
   b. *What physical findings, laboratory values, or medical history information suggests the presence of chronic hepatitis C virus (HCV) infection?*

Desired Outcome

2. *What are the goals of treatment of chronic HCV infection?*

Therapeutic Alternatives

3. a. *What nonpharmacologic measures should be considered for this patient?*
   b. *What pharmacotherapeutic alternatives are available for treatment of this patient?*
   c. *Does this patient have any concurrent medical conditions that are considered contraindications to receiving the treatments discussed in the previous question?*

Optimal Plan

4. *Design a pharmacotherapeutic plan for this patient. Include the drug, dose, schedule, and duration of therapy.*

Outcome Evaluation

5. a. *How should the therapy you recommended be monitored for efficacy and adverse effects?*
   b. *Which baseline parameters of this patient have been suggested as predictors of poor response to the treatment you recommended?*

c. *What actions can be taken if the patient develops intolerable adverse effects to the treatment you recommended?*

Patient Education

6. *What information should be provided to this patient regarding her treatment?*

▶ Clinical Course

Ms. Starring has been on the treatment you recommended for 24 weeks. Overall, she tolerates the treatment well without any significant adverse effects. The laboratory tests from the week 24 visit revealed the following: AST 90 IU/L, ALT 100 IU/L, and qualitative HCV RNA test (+).

▶ Follow-Up Questions

1. a. *Based on this new information, what changes, if any, would you recommend for the treatment of chronic hepatitis C for this patient?*
   b. *Outline a plan for vaccination of this patient against other forms of viral hepatitis.*

▶ Self-Study Assignments

1. Estimate the cost of a 12-month course of interferon and ribavirin treatment for chronic hepatitis C. Include the cost of syringes and needles, monthly clinic visits, and laboratory tests.
2. Perform a literature search to compare the differences in the pharmacokinetic properties of interferon and peginterferon.
3. Perform a literature search on efforts to develop a vaccine for hepatitis C.

▶ Clinical Pearl

The course of chronic hepatitis C infection and treatment response can be adversely affected by alcohol consumption. Patients should be advised to stop all alcohol consumption.

References

1. Manns MP, McHutchinson JG, Gordon SC, et al. Peginterferon alfa-2b plus ribavirin compared with interferon alfa-2b plus ribavirin for initial treatment of chronic hepatitis C: A randomised trial. Lancet 2001;358:958–965.
2. Fried MW, Shiffman ML, Reddy KR, et al. Peginterferon alfa-2a plus ribavirin for chronic hepatitis C virus infection. N Engl J Med 2002;347:975–982.
3. Pawlotsky JM, Bouvier-Alias M, Hezode C, et al. Standardization of hepatitis C virus RNA quantification. Hepatology. 2000;32:654–659.
4. National Institutes of Health Consensus Development Conference Statement: Management of hepatitis C: 2002 – June 10–12, 2002. Hepatology 2002;36(5 Suppl 1):S3–S20.

SECTION 5

Renal Disorders

47 DRUG-INDUCED ACUTE RENAL FAILURE

► Unintended Consequences (Level II)

Mary K. Stamatakis, PharmD

► After completing this case study, students should be able to:

- Evaluate common clinical and laboratory findings in a patient with acute renal failure.
- Develop a pharmacologic plan for the treatment of complications associated with acute renal failure.
- Assess appropriateness of serum aminoglycoside concentrations in relation to efficacy and toxicity.
- Provide recommendations to prevent development of drug-induced acute renal failure.
- Adjust drug dosages, as needed, based on a patient's creatinine clearance.
- Recommend pharmacologic alternatives that do not adversely affect kidney function.

PATIENT PRESENTATION

Chief Complaint
Not available

HPI
The renal consult team has been asked to see James Edwards, a 71 yo man who originally presented to the hospital with symptoms of CHF that necessitated aortic and mitral valve replacement surgery. His surgery was complicated by a 1-hour hypotensive episode, with BP as low as 70/50. Three days postoperation, the patient was found to have purulent drainage from the surgical site and was diagnosed with mediastinitis. At this time, the patient was also found to have a *Serratia* bacteremia (blood cultures × 4 positive for *Serratia marcescens,* sensitive to gentamicin, piperacillin, and ciprofloxacin) and was started on gentamicin and piperacillin. He has currently completed day 25 of a 6-week course of antibiotics. An increase in BUN and creatinine from baseline and volume overload have been noted over the past week. He is now 28 days postsurgery.

PMH
Type 2 DM
Gout
Osteoarthritis
HTN
Atrial fibrillation

FH
Father with type 2 DM

SH
(–) Smoking; occasional EtOH; retired coal miner (9 years ago)

ROS
Currently complains of cough, trouble breathing, and pain in joints in hands. No fever or chills

Meds
Gentamicin IVPB × 25 days (see table for dosages)
Piperacillin 3 g IVPB Q 4 H × 25 days
Colace 100 mg po BID
Prazosin 2 mg po TID
Furosemide 40 mg IV Q 12 H × 2 days
Digoxin 0.25 mg po once daily
Allopurinol 100 mg po once daily
Ranitidine 150 mg po Q 12 H
Meperidine 25 mg IM Q 4–6 H PRN pain
Sliding scale insulin

Celecoxib 200 mg po once daily (started today for symptoms related to arthritis)

All

NKDA

PE

Gen

A & O × 3

VS

BP 154/70, P 80, RR 26, T 37.7°C; Current Wt 84 kg (baseline Wt 78 kg), Ht 5′9″

HEENT

PERRLA, EOMI, poor dentition

Neck/LN

(–) JVD

Chest

Basilar crackles, inspiratory wheezes

CV

S_1, S_2 normal, no S_3, irregular rhythm

Abd

Soft, non-tender, (+) BS, (–) HSM

Genit/Rect

(–) Masses

MS/Ext

2+ Ankle/sacral edema

Neuro

Grossly intact, no focal deficits noted

Labs (Current)

Na 138 mEq/L	Hgb 9.0 g/dL	Ca 8.5 mg/dL
K 3.8 mEq/L	Hct 27.5%	Mg 2.0 mg/dL
Cl 104 mEq/L	Plt 263 × 10³/mm³	Phos 4.7 mg/dL
CO_2 25 mEq/L	WBC 9.9 × 10³/mm³	
BUN 52 mg/dL	(BUN 15 mg/dL on admission)	
SCr 3.2 mg/dL	(SCr 1.3 mg/dL on admission)	
Glu 146 mg/dL		

UA

Color, yellow; character, hazy; glucose (–); ketones (–); SG 1.020; pH 5.0; protein 30 mg/dL; coarse granular casts 5–10/lpf; WBC 5–10/hpf; RBC 2–5/hpf; no bacteria; nitrite (–); blood small; osmolality 325 mOsm; urinary sodium 77 mEq/L; creatinine 63 mg/dL

Renal Function and Serum Gentamicin Concentrations During Hospitalization

Postop Day	SCr (mg/dL)	BUN (mg/dL)	Gentamicin Conc. (mcg/mL) Peak[a]	Trough[b]	Gentamicin Dosages
3	1.4	15			160 mg × 1, then 120 mg Q 12 H
5	1.2	22	4.5	1.2	Change to 160 mg Q 12 H
7	1.4	21			
10	1.4	22	8.1	2.1	Change to 240 mg Q 24 H
14	1.2	21			
17	1.4	26	9.6	1.0	Change to 180 mg Q 24 H
21	1.7	27			
24	2.4	38	7.4	2.6	Change to 180 mg Q 48 H
26	2.9	44			
28	3.2	52			

[a] Levels drawn 30 minutes after a 30-minute infusion.
[b] Levels drawn immediately before the next dose.

I/O and Daily Weights

Day	I/O	Wt (kg)
3 days ago	3,100 mL/1100 mL	N/A
2 days ago	3,250 mL/1050 mL	83
Yesterday	2,850 mL/1250 mL	N/A
Today	N/A	84

Assessment

Acute renal failure and extracellular fluid expansion

Plan

Monitor creatinine daily to assess change in renal function. Fluid restriction and maximize IV diuretics to put him in negative fluid balance. He needs to lose 6 to 7 kg body water to return to his usual weight of 78 kg.

▶ Questions

Problem Identification

1. a. *Create a list of the patient's drug therapy problems.*
   b. *What information (signs, symptoms, laboratory values) indicates the presence or severity of each problem?*
   c. *What additional laboratory information would assist in the assessment of this patient?*
   d. *Could any of the patient's problems be caused by drug therapy?*
   e. *What risk factors did the patient have for gentamicin-induced acute renal failure?*

Desired Outcome

2. *What are the goals of pharmacotherapy in this case?*

Therapeutic Alternatives

3. a. *What non-drug therapies might be useful for this patient?*
   b. *What pharmacotherapeutic alternatives are available for treatment of acute renal failure in this patient?*

Optimal Plan

4. *What drug recommendations are optimal at this point?*

Outcome Evaluation

5. *What clinical and laboratory parameters are necessary to evaluate therapy for achievement of the desired therapeutic outcomes and to detect or prevent adverse effects?*

Patient Education

6. *What information should be provided to the patient to enhance compliance, ensure successful therapy, and minimize adverse effects?*

Additional Case Questions

1. *Based on the patient's creatinine clearance of 21 mL/min, do any of his medications require dosage adjustment?*
2. *What therapeutic interventions can decrease the likelihood of developing gentamicin-induced nephrotoxicity?*
3. *When assessing fractional excretion of sodium (FE_{NA}), what influence do previous dosages of furosemide have on interpretation of the results?*

▶ Self-Study Assignments

1. Based on the original set of gentamicin plasma concentrations obtained (peak 4.5 mcg/mL drawn 30 minutes after a 30 minute infusion, trough 1.2 mcg/mL drawn immediately before the next dose) on the dosing regimen of gentamicin 120 mg IVPB Q 12 H, calculate Mr. Edwards's pharmacokinetic parameters and determine an appropriate dosage regimen for him that would have avoided elevated trough concentrations.
2. Review the literature to determine whether once-daily dosing of aminoglycosides (i.e., large dose–extended interval dosing method) has been shown to decrease the incidence of nephrotoxicity, and if this approach should have been initially recommended in this patient.
3. Recommend an appropriate dosage of digoxin for this patient given a trough digoxin concentration of 2.7 ng/mL.
4. Estimate the patient's original creatinine clearance using the MDRD Study equation, which can be accessed at www.nephron.com.

▶ Clinical Pearl

There is a strong correlation between aminoglycoside clearance and creatinine clearance. If a patient's renal function deteriorates, a similar decline will be seen in aminoglycoside clearance.

References

1. Triggs E, Charles B. Pharmacokinetics and therapeutic drug monitoring of gentamicin in the elderly. Clin Pharmacokinet 1999;37:331–341.
2. Brater DC. Pharmacology of diuretics. Am J Med Sci 2000;319:38–50.
3. Bellomo R, Chapman M, Finfer S, et al. Low-dose dopamine in patients with early renal dysfunction: A placebo-controlled randomised trial. Australian and New Zealand Intensive Care Society (ANZICS) Clinical Trials Group. Lancet 2000;356:2139–2143.
4. Kellum JA, Decker JM. Use of dopamine in acute renal failure: A meta-analysis. Crit Care Med 2001;29:1526–1531.
5. Lam YW, Banerji S, Hatfield C, et al. Principles of drug administration in renal insufficiency. Clin Pharmacokinet 1997;32:30–57.

48 ACUTE RENAL FAILURE

▶ It Happened in the OR (Level II)

Reina Bendayan, PharmD
Michelle D. Furler, BSc Pharm

▶ After completing this case study, students should be able to:

- Recognize the clinical and laboratory manifestations of acute renal failure (ARF).
- Understand the pathogenesis of prerenal, intrinsic, and postrenal failure.
- Discuss the efficacy of adjunctive agents, including diuretics, dopamine, and enteral and parenteral nutritional support in ARF.
- Compare the use of conventional versus continuous hemodialysis methods in patients with ARF.

PATIENT PRESENTATION

Chief Complaint

"Weakness, dizziness."

HPI

Zhi Chiu is a 78 yo man who was admitted to the hospital with an acute GI bleed with BRBPR that started 1 hour before admission. Upon admission, the patient is pale and sweaty. His blood pressure is 96/48 mm Hg.

PMH

HTN × 25 years
CHF × 8 years
No known renal disease

FH

Father died of an acute MI; mother was diabetic.

SH

Retired and living at home with his wife. Before retirement, the patient was employed as an accountant. No alcohol, no tobacco use.

ROS

Not done, patient is acutely ill.

Meds

Digoxin 0.125 mg po once daily
Furosemide 40 mg po once daily
Enalapril 20 mg po once daily
Famotidine 20 mg po BID

All

NKA

PE

Gen

A pale and diaphoretic elderly Chinese male in acute distress

VS

BP 96/48, P 120, RR 24, T 37.1°C; Wt 66 kg, Ht 5′6″

Skin

Pale and moist

HEENT

Fundi normal, conjunctiva pale, ears normal, tongue dry

Neck/LN

No JVD or HJR; no lymphadenopathy or thyromegaly

CV

Normal S_1, S_2; no S_3; faint S_4, no murmurs

Lungs

No rales

Abd

Soft, NT; No HSM

Rect

No lesion palpable but (+) BRBPR; no prostate enlargement

MS/Ext

Normal; no peripheral edema

Neuro

A & O; CNs intact; Motor—no focal weakness; DTRs symmetric; toes downgoing; sensation—normal coordination, gait normal

Labs

Na 136 mEq/L
K 5.3 mEq/L
Cl 103 mEq/L
CO_2 24 mEq/L
BUN 46.6 mg/dL
SCr 2.4 mg/dL
Glu 214 mg/dL

Hgb 9.0 g/dL
Hct 30%
Ca 8.6 mg/dL
Phos 3.9 mg/dL

Hospital Course

Upon admission, the patient was resuscitated with O_2 therapy, aggressive IV hydration (1 L of normal saline, over the first hour) and multiple transfusions (4 units of PRBC). The furosemide dose was withheld. His BP stabilized and he underwent a colonoscopy, which showed multiple diverticula in the ascending and descending colon that were the presumed sources of bleeding. He continued to bleed in-hospital and received 4 more units of PRBC. Because of this, the patient was taken to the OR for a partial colectomy. He was hypotensive in the OR (BP 70 mm Hg systolic) and postoperatively his urine output was very low (hourly: 0, 0, 0, 0, 0, 5 mL, 20 mL, 20 mL, 15 mL, 15 mL, 7 mL, 15 mL). He was aggressively hydrated with normal saline but his urine output remained low and his serum creatinine began to rise. Urinalysis at that time showed heme granular casts, protein 1+, WBC 2+, glucose1+, and RBC 2+; a diagnosis of ATN was made. A renal dose of dopamine (3 mcg/kg/min) and furosemide 80 mg IV Q 8 H were administered. Two days postoperatively, his CXR showed CHF. A femoral vein catheter was inserted and he underwent continuous venovenous hemodiafiltration (CVVHD) for 3 days. Serum chemistry values during this period were as follows:

Parameter	Immediately Postoperatively	One Week Postoperatively
Na (mEq/L)	137	133
K (mEq/L)	4.2	3.6
Cl (mEq/L)	104	94
CO_2 (mEq/L)	22	30
BUN (mg/dL)	42	29
SCr (mg/dL)	3.7	3.9
Glu (mg/dL)	176	148
Hgb (g/dL)	9.5	10.5
Hct (%)	30	35
Ca (mg/dL)	7.8	7.7
Phos (mg/dL)	5.8	3.9
T. prot (g/dL)	4.3	4.1
Alb (g/dL)	2.4	1.8

The heart failure resolved and the catheter was removed. His subsequent hospital course was uneventful. Upon discharge, his outpatient medications were restarted.

Discharge Assessment

Acute GI bleed due to multiple diverticula; partial colectomy performed. Complications included: (a) ARF as a result of severe hypotension and hypovolemia, and (b) CHF as a result of fluid overload.

▶ Questions

Problem Identification

1. a. *Create a list of the patient's drug therapy problems during this hospital admission.*
   b. *What information (signs, symptoms, laboratory values) indicates the presence or severity of GI bleed, severe hypotension on admission, and acute renal failure?*

Desired Outcome

2. *What are the goals of pharmacotherapy in this patient upon admission, during surgery, and postoperatively?*

Therapeutic Alternatives

3. a. *Were the nondrug therapies that were administered to this patient upon admission and postoperatively appropriate?*
   b. *Were the pharmacotherapeutic measures that were instituted during the patient's episode of acute renal failure appropriate? Provide the rationale for your answer.*

Optimal Plan

4. *Design an optimal therapeutic plan for the management of this patient's postoperative episode of acute renal failure.*

Outcome Evaluation

5. *Outline the clinical and laboratory parameters necessary to evaluate your treatment regimen for the patient's episode of ARF.*

Patient Education

6. *What information should be provided to the patient to ensure successful therapy of CHF when he leaves the hospital?*

▶ Self-Study Assignments

1. Review the drugs that can induce acute renal failure by causing: (a) glomerulonephritis; (b) acute tubular necrosis; (c) acute interstitial nephritis; (d) nephrolithiasis; and (e) hemodynamic changes.
2. Discuss the use of experimental therapies such as growth factors and atrial natriuretic peptide (ANF) in acute renal failure.

▶ Clinical Pearl

The presence of heme granular casts in the urine of a hypotensive oliguric patient is indicative of ATN.

References

1. Dubose TD Jr, Warnock DG, Mehta RL, et al. Acute renal failure in the 21st century: Recommendations for management and outcomes assessment. Am J Kidney Dis 1997;29:793–799.
2. Palevsky PM. Acute renal failure. J Am Soc Nephrol 2003;2:41–76.
3. Denton MD, Chertow GM, Brady HR. "Renal dose" dopamine for the treatment of acute renal failure: scientific rationale, experimental studies and clinical trials. Kidney Int 1996;50:4–14.
4. Burton CJ, Tomson CR. Can the use of low dose dopamine for treatment of acute renal failure be justified? Postgrad Med J 1999;75:269–274.
5. Kellum JA. Decker J. Use of dopamine in acute renal failure: A meta-analysis. Crit Care Med 2001;29:1526–1531.
6. Shilliday IR, Quinn KJ, Allison ME. Loop diuretics in the management of acute renal failure: A prospective, double-blind, placebo-controlled, randomized study. Nephrol Dial Transplant 1997;12:2592–2596.

49 PROGRESSIVE RENAL DISEASE

▶ Don't Fail Me Now (Level III)

Reina Bendayan, PharmD
Michelle D. Furler, BSc Pharm

▶ After completing this case study, students should be able to:

- Differentiate acute renal failure from chronic renal failure.
- Identify risk factors for progression of renal disease.
- Recognize potential comorbid or pathologic conditions that are frequently associated with chronic renal insufficiency.
- Recommend nonpharmacologic and pharmacologic interventions to alter the rate of progression of renal disease.
- Educate patients on the common medications prescribed for chronic renal insufficiency.

PATIENT PRESENTATION

Chief Complaint

"I'm here to check the results of my urine test."

HPI

Rob Brandon is a 52 yo man with diabetes mellitus who visited his PCP 2 weeks ago for a routine examination. His laboratory tests revealed a serum creatinine of 1.6 mg/dL, which was elevated over his baseline of 1.3 mg/dL 1 year ago. A 24-hour urine collection was performed last week and he was scheduled to return to clinic today for further evaluation of his kidney function. He states that he has not been checking his blood glucose at home because his machine is not working. However, he asserts that he has been taking his medications faithfully.

PMH

Type 2 DM × 16 years (failed glyburide, currently on insulin)
HTN × 2 years
Hypercholesterolemia × 5 years (noncompliant with diet)

FH

His father had DM and died in an MVA 3 years ago; his mother had HTN and died at the age of 50 secondary to MI.

SH

A high school teacher, married with 1 child (24 yo). No tobacco use but occasional alcohol (2 or 3 beers on weekends). Usual diet includes eggs and sausages for breakfast, turkey sandwiches for lunch, and pasta and salad for dinner.

ROS

Occasional headaches; no c/o polyuria, polydipsia, polyphagia, sensory loss, or visual changes. No dysuria, flank pain, hematuria, pedal edema, CP, or SOB

Meds

Humulin N 35 units SubQ Q AM, 20 units SubQ Q PM (for 5 years)
Humulin R 12 units SubQ Q AM, 8 units SubQ Q PM
Hydrochlorothiazide 25 mg po once daily (× 2 years)
Pravastatin 40 mg po once daily (× 5 years; on current dose for 1 year)
Acetaminophen 650 mg po Q 6 H PRN headaches

All

Sulfa (anaphylaxis)

PE

Gen

The patient is a moderately obese African-American man in NAD

VS

BP 150/95 sitting and standing in both arms, HR 76, RR 16, T 37.2°C; Wt 88.5 kg, Ht 5′8″

Skin

Warm, dry

HEENT

PERRLA, EOMI, fundi revealed microaneurysms consistent with diabetic retinopathy; no retinal edema or vitreous hemorrhage. TMs intact. Oral mucosa moist with no lesions.

Neck/LN

Supple; no cervical adenopathy or thyromegaly

Lungs/Thorax

CTA

CV

Heart sounds are normal

Abd

NT; no masses or organs palpable. No abdominal bruits

Gent/Rect

Normal rectal exam; prostate benign; heme (–) stool

MS/Ext

No CCE

Neuro

A & O × 3; CNs intact; normal DTRs

Labs (2 weeks ago, fasting)

		Fasting Lipid Profile
Na 140 mEq/L	Hgb 12.2 g/dL	T. chol 225 mg/dL
K 4.8 mEq/L	Hct 36.5%	Trig 135 mg/dL
Cl 108 mEq/L	WBC 10.8 × 10^3/mm^3	LDL 152 mg/dL
CO_2 26 mEq/L	Plt 148 × 10^3/mm^3	HDL 46 mg/dL
BUN 27 mg/dL	Ca 9.3 mg/dL	
SCr 1.6 mg/dL	Phos 2.5 mg/dL	
Glu 194 mg/dL	Uric acid 6.9 mg/dL	
HbA_{1c} 9%	Alb 3.2 g/dL	

UA (1 week ago)

1+ glucose, (–) ketones, >3+ protein, (–) leukocyte esterase & nitrite; (–) RBC; 2–5 WBC/hpf

24-Hour Urine Collection

Total urine volume 2.1 L, urine creatinine 60 mg/dL, urine albumin 680 mg/24hr

Assessment

52-year-old man newly diagnosed with diabetic nephropathy

▶ Questions

Problem Identification

1. a. *Create a list of the patient's drug therapy problems*
   b. *What are the signs and symptoms of diabetic nephropathy, diabetes mellitus, hypertension, and hypercholesterolemia in this patient?*
   c. *Calculate this patient's creatinine clearance (CLcr in mL/min) using the following data: (i) baseline CLcr from 1 year ago; (ii) current CLcr using the SCr from 2 weeks ago; (iii) current CLcr using the data from the 24-hour urine collection. Discuss whether (ii) and (iii) provide good estimates of the patient's GFR.*
   d. *Briefly discuss the advantages and limitations of estimating glomerular filtration rate (GFR) using the Modification of Diet in Renal Disease (MDRD) equation, and calculate this patient's current GFR using the equation.*

e. *What degree of renal failure is shown by this patient? Compare the definition, classification, and prognosis of chronic renal failure to acute renal failure.*

Desired Outcome

2. *What are the goals of pharmacotherapy for the management of the patient's renal insufficiency, diabetes, hypertension, and hypercholesterolemia?*

Therapeutic Alternatives

3. a. *What nonpharmacologic therapies might be useful to control this patient's medical conditions?*
   b. *What are the pharmacotherapeutic alternatives for the prevention of renal disease progression and the management of diabetes mellitus, hypertension, and hyperlipidemia in this patient?*

Optimal Plan

4. *What drug regimens would provide optimal therapy for this patient's current medical problems?*

Outcome Evaluation

5. *Outline the clinical and laboratory parameters necessary to evaluate the efficacy and safety of the recommended regimens for the patient's nephropathy, diabetes mellitus, hypertension, and hypercholesterolemia.*

Patient Education

6. *What information should be provided to the patient to ensure successful therapy and minimize adverse effects of the antihypertensive and insulin therapy?*

▶ Clinical Course

The plan you recommended is implemented, and the patient returns to his PCP one month later. His blood pressure is 145/90 mm Hg (sitting and standing) and HR is 90 bpm. He has no new complaints and reports tolerating his new medications well. He also states that he has been watching his diet and has been using Cardia Salt (46% NaCl, 54% K/Mg salt) in his meals for the last 5 days. His laboratory results are BUN 30 mg/dL, SCr 1.6 mg/dL, Na 142 mEq/L, K 5.4 mEq/L, Cl 110 mEq/L, CO_2 28 mEq/L, Glu 135 mg/dL.

▶ Follow-Up Questions

1. *What new or persistent drug therapy problems does this patient have?*
2. *What changes, if any, would you recommend in the patient's drug regimen?*

▶ Self-Study Assignments

1. Discuss the role of diuretic therapy in patients with normal renal function compared to those with creatinine clearance values < 20 mL/min.
2. Review and compare the effects of antihypertensive agents on renal blood flow and glomerular filtration rate in patients with hypertension and diabetic nephropathy.

▶ Clinical Pearl

Normotensive patients with type 2 diabetes and persistent microalbuminuria should be treated with an ACE inhibitor to slow the progression of diabetic nephropathy.

References

1. National Kidney Foundation. K/DOQI clinical practice guidelines for chronic kidney disease: Evaluation, classification, and stratification. Am J Kidney Dis, 2002;39(2 Suppl 1):S1-S266.
2. Walser M. Assessing renal function from creatinine measurements in adults with chronic renal failure. Am J Kidney Dis 1998;32:23–31.
3. National Kidney Foundation. Clinical practice guidelines for managing dyslipidemias in chronic kidney disease. Am J Kidney Dis 2003;41(4 Suppl 3):S1–S91. Available online at: www.kidney.org/professionals/kdoqi/guidelines_lipids/index.htm (accessed April 19, 2004).
4. Pedrini MT, Levey AS, Lau J, et al. The effect of dietary protein restriction on the progression of diabetic and nondiabetic renal diseases: A meta-analysis. Ann Intern Med 1996;124:627–632.
5. Kasiske BL, Lakatua JD, Ma JZ, et al. A meta-analysis of the effects of dietary protein restriction on the rate of decline in renal function. Am J Kidney Dis 1998;31:954–961.
6. Kopple JD. National Kidney Foundation-K/DOQI clinical practice guidelines for nutrition in chronic renal failure. Am J Kidney Dis 2001;37(1 Suppl 2):S66–S70.
7. Midgley JP, Matthew AG, Greenwood CM, et al. Effect of reduced dietary sodium on blood pressure: A meta-analysis of randomized controlled trials. JAMA 1996;275:1590–1597.
8. Joint National Committee on Prevention, Detection, Evaluation, and Treatment of High Blood Pressure. The sixth report of the Joint National Committee on Prevention, Detection, Evaluation, and Treatment of High Blood Pressure. Arch Intern Med 1997;157:2413–2446.
9. Stefanick ML, Mackey S, Sheehan M, et al. Effects of diet and exercise in men and postmenopausal women with low levels of HDL cholesterol and high levels of LDL cholesterol. N Engl J Med 1998;339:12–20.
10. ALLHAT Officers and Coordinators for the ALLHAT Collaborative Research Group. The Antihypertensive and Lipid-Lowering Treatment to Prevent Heart Attack Trial. Major outcomes in high-risk hypertensive patients randomized to angiotensin-converting enzyme inhibitor or calcium channel blocker vs diuretic: The Antihypertensive and Lipid-Lowering Treatment to Prevent Heart Attack Trial (ALLHAT). JAMA. 2002;288:2981–2997.

Note: All NKF K/DOQI Clinical Practice Guidelines are available online at www.kidney.org/professionals/kdoqi/guidelines.cfm

50 END-STAGE RENAL DISEASE

▶ A Return to the Machine (Level II)

James D. Coyle, PharmD

▶ Upon completing this case study, students should be able to:

- Assess all available information to identify medication-related problems in an end-stage renal disease patient on hemodialysis.

- State the desired therapeutic outcomes of each problem.
- List therapeutic alternatives for managing each problem.
- Develop a plan for managing each problem that includes plans for monitoring patient response to interventions.
- Outline a plan for helping the patient understand and effectively implement medication-related interventions.

PATIENT PRESENTATION

Chief Complaint

"My kidney doesn't work anymore."

HPI

John Brooks is a 64 yo man who presented to the outpatient dialysis center for staff-assisted hemodialysis. His ESRD is secondary to a congenital kidney defect and long-standing HTN. He received a cadaveric renal transplant approximately 15 years ago, but the transplant was recently rejected. He had an AV Gore-Tex graft placed in his left forearm 17 days prior to this first dialysis session.

PMH

Congenital kidney defect diagnosed at age 19 as a result of a HTN work-up. He was dialyzed for 3 years prior to his transplant 15 years ago.

FH

Mother died of cancer at age 93. Status of father unknown. Two brothers in good health. Three daughters in good health.

SH

Lives by himself. Employed full-time doing light maintenance work (currently on sick leave). He relates that his daughters "care about me, but don't do enough to help me out." Occasional social alcohol use. Minimal caffeine consumption. No tobacco use.

ROS

Negative except for dry, itchy skin; feeling tired and weak over the past several weeks; loss of appetite, with frequent N & V over the past week; constipation; and swelling in feet and lower legs. No other complaints related to central or peripheral nervous system or cardiovascular system. Wears glasses for reading and driving.

Meds

Atenolol 50 mg po at bedtime
Paxil 10 mg ½ tab po once daily
Restoril 30 mg po at bedtime

All

PCN (upper body rash after oral PCN approximately 10 years ago)

PE

Gen

The patient is a WDWN African-American man in NAD who appears his stated age.

VS

BP 170/100, P 82, RR 16, T 36.8°C; Wt 72.5 kg, Ht 5′10″

Skin

Dry, scaly arms and legs are noted.

Ext

Mild bilateral foot/ankle edema.
The remainder of the PE was WNL.

Labs

Na 142 mEq/L	Hgb 9.3 g/dL	AST 16 IU/L	T. chol 228 mg/dL	Iron 90 μg/dL
K 5.3 mEq/L	Hct 27.9%	ALT 21 IU/L	HDL 33 mg/dL	TIBC 275 μg/dL
Cl 110 mEq/L	RBC $3.41 \times 10^6/mm^3$	LDH 371 IU/L	LDL 149 mg/dL	T. sat 33%
CO_2 20 mEq/L	MCV 81.7 μm^3	Alk phos 124 IU/L	Chol/HDL 6.9	Ferritin 349 ng/mL
Anion gap 18	MCHC 33.4 g/dL	T. bili 0.5 mg/dL	Trig 229 mg/dL	Aluminum 14 μg/L
BUN 120 mg/dL	WBC $6.9 \times 10^3/mm^3$	D. bili 0.3 mg/dL	Ca 8.6 mg/dL	PTH 1835 pg/mL
SCr 9.2 mg/dL		T. prot 6.1 g/dL	Phos 7.4 mg/dL	Osm 308 mOsm/kg
Glu 85 mg/dL		Alb 3.6 g/dL	Urate 5.5 mg/dL	

Mr. Brooks's nephrologist provided the following dialysis prescription:

Dialyze 3.5 hours per session, 3 times per week
Dry weight: 67.5 kg
Dialyzer: Fresenius F80
Blood flow rate: 400 mL/min
Dialysate flow rate: 500 mL/min
Dialysate: Bicarbonate
Na 145 mEq/L, K 2.0 mEq/L, Ca 2.5 mEq/L, HCO_3^- 35 mEq/L
Heparin: 2,000 unit bolus, then 500 units/hr until 1 hour before termination

▶ Questions

Problem Identification

1. a. *Create a list of this patient's drug therapy problems.*
   b. *Which information (signs, symptoms, laboratory values) indicates the severity of this patient's end-stage renal disease?*

Desired Outcome

2. *State the goal of pharmacotherapy with respect to each problem identified.*

Therapeutic Alternatives

3. *What therapeutic options are available for each of this patient's medication-related problems? Indicate the advantages and disadvantages of each option.*

Optimal Plan

4. *Which of the available therapeutic options identified in question 3 would you recommend for this patient? Provide a rationale for each recommendation. Include the name, dosage form, dose, schedule, and duration of therapy for any drugs recommended.*

Outcome Evaluation

5. *What clinical and/or laboratory parameters would you recommend to evaluate the desired and undesired consequences of each of your recommended interventions?*

Patient Education

6. *What information should be provided to the patient to enhance compliance, ensure successful therapy, and minimize adverse effects?*

▶ Self-Study Assignments

1. Assume that Mr. Brooks presents as above except that his serum iron is 45 mcg/dL, serum ferritin is 72 ng/mL, MCV is 70 μm^3, and MCHC is 27 g/dL. Develop a therapeutic plan, including a monitoring plan, to treat his anemia under this scenario.
2. Compare the content and cost of a variety of water-soluble vitamin supplements appropriate for use by ESRD patients. Select the product that you would recommend for use by your patients.
3. Assume that Mr. Brooks develops an infection that requires tobramycin. Develop a therapeutic plan for the use of tobramycin in this patient, including a monitoring plan.

▶ Clinical Pearl

Epoetin is an important but not sufficient requirement for normal red blood cell production—ya gotta have iron, too!

References

1. National Kidney Foundation. K/DOQI clinical practice guidelines for anemia of chronic kidney disease: Update 2000. Am J Kidney Dis 2001;37(Suppl 1): S182–S238.
2. National Kidney Foundation. K/DOQI clinical practice guidelines for bone metabolism and disease in chronic kidney disease. Am J Kidney Dis 2003;42(4 Suppl 3):S1–S202.
3. Gennari FJ, Rimmer JM. Acid–base disorders in end-stage renal disease. Semin Dial 1990;3:81–85.
4. Zoccali C and Dunea G. Hypertension. In: Daugirdas JT, Blake PG, Ings TS, eds. Handbook of Dialysis, 3rd ed. Philadelphia, Lippincott Williams & Wilkins, 2001:466–476.
5. Chobanian AV, Bakris GL, Black HR, et al. Seventh Report of the Joint National Committee on Prevention, Detection, Evaluation, and Treatment of High Blood Pressure. Hypertension 2003;42:1206–1252.
6. Executive summary of the third report of The National Cholesterol Education Program (NCEP) Expert Panel on Detection, Evaluation, and Treatment of High Blood Cholesterol in Adults (Adult Treatment Panel III). JAMA 2001;285: 2486–2497.
7. National Kidney Foundation. Clinical practice guidelines for managing dyslipidemias in chronic kidney disease. Am J Kidney Dis 2003;41(4 Suppl 3):S1–S91.
8. Aranesp® (darbepoetin alfa) package insert. Amgen Inc, 2002.
9. Fishbane S. Safety in iron management. Am J Kidney Dis 2003;41(5 Suppl):S18–S26.
10. Felsenfeld AJ. Considerations for the treatment of secondary hyperparathyroidism in renal failure. J Am Soc Nephrol 1997;8:993–1004.
11. National Kidney Foundation. K/DOQI clinical practice guidelines for nutrition in chronic renal failure. Am J Kidney Dis 2000;35(6 Suppl 2):S1–S140.
12. Robertson KE, Mueller BA. Uremic pruritus. Am J Health Syst Pharm 1996;53:2159–2170.

51 CHRONIC GLOMERULONEPHRITIS

▶ An Ongoing Battle With Lupus (Level III)

Melanie S. Joy, PharmD

▶ After completing this case study, students should be able to:

- Identify the risk factors for kidney disease progression in a patient with lupus-induced glomerulonephritis.
- Recognize laboratory and urinalysis abnormalities associated with lupus nephritis.
- Identify treatment options that are available for lupus-induced diffuse proliferative glomerulonephritis.
- Recognize the clinical significance of glucocorticoid-induced complications and recommend appropriate treatment options.
- Provide patient education regarding drug therapy for lupus nephritis and its complications.

PATIENT PRESENTATION

Chief Complaint

"I have pain in my hips and lower back and fatigue."

HPI

The patient is a 23 yo African-American woman with a history of diffuse proliferative glomerulonephritis (DPGN) as a consequence of SLE, which decreased in activity after two courses of IV cyclophosphamide (10 and 6 years ago). Past treatment with azathioprine therapy was unsuccessful. During recent follow-up nephrology clinic appointments, urinalyses demonstrated increased disease activity.

PMH

- Lupus-induced DPGN × 10 years
- History of oligomenorrhea
- HTN
- Hypercholesterolemia
- Recent DEXA scan revealed decreased bone mineral density of the spine and hip
- S/P tonsillectomy as a child

SH

The patient works as an executive assistant. She drinks alcohol socially. There is no history of tobacco or illicit drug use.

FH

Paternal grandmother and two aunts also have SLE. No family history of DM, HTN, CVA, or MI.

ROS

Complains of arthralgias and pain around the hip and lower back. Denies rash, fever, chills, nausea, vomiting, symptoms of Raynaud's phenomenon, pleuritic chest pain, or shortness of breath.

Meds

- Prednisone 15 mg po daily (with fluctuating doses over the past 10 years)
- Atenolol 25 mg po daily
- Clonidine patch 0.2 mg weekly

All

Gemfibrozil (rash) and cefadroxil ("swelling")

PE

Gen

WDWN white woman in NAD

VS

BP 160/115, P 64, RR 18, T 36.5°C; Wt 49 kg

Skin

Small papules over the PIPs and MCPs of first and second digits bilaterally. No alopecia

HEENT

NC/AT; clear sclerae, fundi show copper wiring alone; oropharynx is clear without exudates; no oral or nasal ulcers

Neck/LN

No cervical, supraclavicular, or axillary adenopathy; normal thyroid

Lungs

CTA bilaterally

CV

RRR; normal S_1, S_2; no m/r/g

Abd

Soft, non-tender, without hepatosplenomegaly

MS/Ext

No synovitis; pulses are 2+ and equal without bruits; no clubbing or cyanosis; 2+ edema of the lower extremities; (+) pain during hip extension and flexion

Neuro

A & O × 3; CN II–XII are grossly intact; strength is 5/5 in all four extremities; 2+ DTRs in all four extremities

Labs

Na 144 mEq/L	Hgb 10.4 g/dL	AST 25 IU/L	Chol 400 mg/dL
K 4.2 mEq/L	Hct 31.7%	ALT 23 IU/L	LDL 204 mg/dL
Cl 110 mEq/L	Plt 318 × 10^3/mm^3	Alk phos 54 IU/L	HDL 34 mg/dL
CO_2 26 mEq/L	WBC 8.9 × 10^3/mm^3	GGT 27 IU/L	C3 75 mg/dL
BUN 45 mg/dL	Ca 7.8 mg/dL	T. Bili 0.2 mg/dL	C4 22 mg/dL
SCr 2.2 mg/dL	Mg 2.1 mg/dL	Alb 2.5 g/dL	DS DNA Ab (+)
Glu 71 mg/dL	Phos 5.1 mg/dL	Ferritin 200 ng/mL	EPO < 2 mIU/mL
		T. Sat 45%	

UA

Dipstick demonstrates: pH 5, 3+ Hgb, 3+ protein, > 250 RBCs. Microscopic examination reveals 10 RBC/hpf, some are dysmorphic; two waxy casts and three finely granular casts, oval fat bodies, and RBC casts (see Figure 51–1).

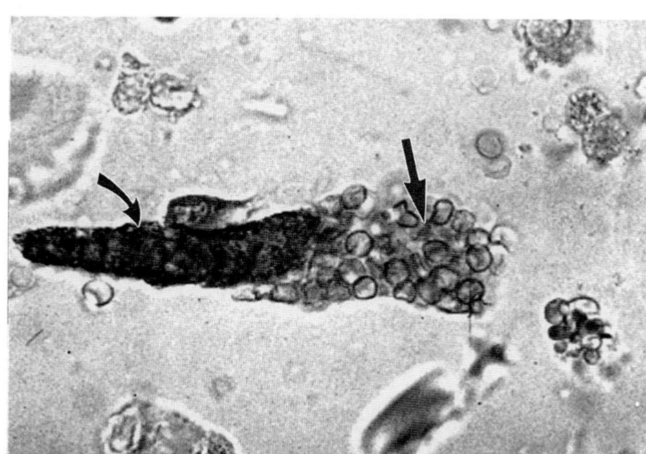

Figure 51–1. Photomicrograph of a nephritic urine sediment with a cast that is a red blood cell cast at one end *(straight arrow)* and a pigmented cast at the other end *(curved arrow)*. (Phase contrast × **750.**) *(Photo courtesy of J. Charles Jennette, MD.)*

24-Hour Urine Collection

Urine protein 603 mg/dL, urine creatinine 54.5 mg/dL, volume 2151 mL. Results 6 months ago were urine creatinine 81 mg/dL, volume 1200 mL, with SCr 1.2 mg/dL.

Renal Biopsy

Features of lupus-induced DPGN are present, with an increased chronicity score and a decreased activity score. There is persistent hypercellularity in > 50% of the glomeruli; 50% of the glomeruli are globally sclerotic, and there is advanced tubular atrophy and interstitial fibrosis.

DEXA Scan

BMD of the spine (L1–L2) measured 0.763 g/cm^2 (T score 2.58 SD below the mean). Total BMD of the proximal right femur measured 0.719 g/cm^2 (T score 2.14 SD below the mean).

Assessment

1. Active lupus-induced DPGN with nephrotic syndrome
2. Anemia
3. HTN (uncontrolled)
4. Corticosteroid-induced osteoporosis
5. Hypercholesterolemia

▶ Questions

Problem Identification

1. a. *Create a list of this patient's drug therapy problems.*
   b. *Which information obtained from the medical history, physical examination, and laboratory analysis indicates the presence of glomerulonephritis?*
   c. *Which information indicates complications from the disease itself or long-term treatment?*
   d. *Calculate the patient's measured creatinine clearance (CLcr)/glomerular filtration rate (GFR) from the present 24-hour urine collection and the MDRD equation and compare these to the measured CLcr 6 months ago to assess the rate of progression of chronic kidney disease.*
   e. *What other risk factors for renal disease progression does this patient have?*
   f. *Describe the possible glomerular lesions attributable to SLE in this patient.*
   g. *What is the typical clinical presentation of SLE, and which attributes are present in this patient?*

Desired Outcome

2. *What are the pharmacotherapy goals for this patient's lupus nephritis?*

Therapeutic Alternatives

3. *What treatment alternatives are available for achieving the goals related to lupus nephritis and its complications?*

Optimal Plan

4. *Based on the available therapeutic options, design a pharmacotherapeutic plan for the management of lupus nephritis and its complications.*

Outcome Evaluation

5. *Outline a clinical and laboratory monitoring plan for each of the patient's drug therapy problems.*

Patient Education

6. *What should the patient be told regarding the drug therapy she is to receive to treat her condition and its complications?*

▶ Clinical Course

At the 3-month visit, the patient complained of nausea and vomiting. Labs: SCr 1.2 mg/dL, BUN 25 mg/dL, Albumin 3.0 g/dL, AST 17 IU/L, ALT 11 IU/L, Alk phos 41 IU/L, GGT 19 IU/L, amylase 182 IU/L, lipase 253 IU/L. Urinalysis results: Ucr 65 mg/dL, urinary protein 458 mg/dL, volume 1,510 mL; CLcr 57 mL/min. A mild pancreatitis, possibly caused by mycophenolate mofetil, was suspected because of the elevated amylase and lipase values and concurrent symptoms of nausea and vomiting. The dose of mycophenolate was decreased from 1000 mg po BID to 500 mg po BID.

▶ Self-Study Assignments

1. What effects on the immune system do each of the various therapies for lupus-induced DPGN have?
2. What is the role of hyperlipidemia in progression of renal disease, and what therapies may be effective?
3. What are the current recommendations regarding prevention of corticosteroid-induced osteoporosis?
4. What alternatives to mycophenolate mofetil exist if intolerable GI side effects continue and/or hepatic function worsens in this patient?

▶ Clinical Pearl

Severe forms of glomerular disease are manifest clinically as nephrotic range proteinuria, declining creatinine clearance, hematuria with dysmorphic red blood cells, presence of urinary casts, hypertension, edema, anemia, and hypercholesterolemia.

References

1. Levey AS, Bosch JP, Lewis JB, et al. A more accurate method to estimate glomerular filtration rate from serum creatinine: A new prediction equation. Modification of Diet in Renal Disease Study Group. Ann Intern Med 1999;130: 461–470.

2. Austin HA, Balow JE. Treatment of lupus nephritis. Semin Nephrol 2000;20: 265–276.
3. Cameron JS. Lupus nephritis. J Am Soc Nephrol 1999;10:413–424.
4. Korbet SM, Lewis EJ, Schwartz MM, et al. Factors predictive of outcome in severe lupus nephritis. Lupus Nephritis Collaborative Study Group. Am J Kidney Dis 2000;35:904–914.
5. Mok CC, Lai KN. Mycophenolate mofetil in lupus glomerulonephritis. Am J Kidney Dis 2002;40:447–457.
6. Chan TM, Li FK, Tang CS, et al. Efficacy of mycophenolate mofetil in patients with diffuse proliferative lupus nephritis. Hong Kong-Guangzhou Nephrology Study Group. N Engl J Med 2000;343:1156–1162.
7. Kingdon EJ, McLean AG, Psimenou E, et al. The safety and efficacy of MMF in lupus nephritis: A pilot study. Lupus 2001;10:606–611.
8. Remuzzi G, Tognoni G, for the GISEN Group. Randomised placebo-controlled trial of effect of ramipril on decline in glomerular filtration rate and risk of terminal renal failure in proteinuric, non-diabetic nephropathy. Lancet 1997;349: 1857–1863.
9. Wierzbicki AS. Lipids, cardiovascular disease and atherosclerosis in systemic lupus erythematosus. Lupus 2000;9:194–201.
10. Recommendations for the prevention and treatment of glucocorticoid-induced osteoporosis. American College of Rheumatology Task Force on Osteoporosis Guidelines. Arthritis Rheum 1996;39:1791–1801.
11. National Kidney Foundation. K/DOQI clinical practice guidelines for bone metabolism and disease in chronic kidney disease. Am J Kidney Dis 2003;42:Suppl 3:S1–S202.

52 SYNDROME OF INAPPROPRIATE ANTIDIURETIC HORMONE RELEASE

▶ An Out-of-Body Experience (Level I)

Rex W. Force, PharmD, FCCP, BCPS

▶ After completing this case study, students should be able to:

- Identify the etiologies of hyponatremia and specifically the syndrome of inappropriate antidiuretic hormone (SIADH) release.
- Recognize risk factors for the development of hyponatremia and SIADH.
- Understand the importance of assessing osmotic and fluid status in patients with hyponatremia.
- Recommend and monitor appropriate therapy and alternative treatments for SIADH.
- Educate patients on treatment options, proper administration of selected treatments, and observed side effects.

PATIENT PRESENTATION

Chief Complaint

"Where am I!?! What's going on?!?!"

HPI

Jane Hokanson is a 63 yo woman who presents to the ED after suffering what, according to her husband, sounds like a seizure at home. She began to develop nausea, body aches, confusion, and weakness about 12 hours PTA. She is accompanied by her husband, who stated that she had become progressively more confused and disoriented prior to her seizure. The patient stated that she has never felt this way before. Shortly after presentation to the ED she experienced another generalized tonic-clonic seizure that lasted approximately 1 minute. She was given 1 g of phenytoin IV. Postictally, she immediately became combative and agitated. She was given 5 mg of diazepam IV every 5 minutes × 4 (total of 20 mg) with no resolution of agitation. At that time, chlorpromazine 75 mg IM was administered, which resulted in rapid sedation.

PMH

Headaches
Major depression
Seasonal allergies
S/P total abdominal hysterectomy

FH

Mother died at 81 and had no chronic medical problems. Father is living with diabetes at age 89; he had a small MI 2 years ago.

SH

Married with no children. Denies smoking or alcohol consumption. Employment history is unknown.

ROS

Difficult to obtain because of decreased mental status. Husband states that she is healthy except for her headaches, depression, and occasional allergy symptoms.

Meds

Multivitamins
Sertraline 100 mg daily
Black cohosh, licorice, grapeseed extract, and other herbal products (husband can't recall all the names)

All

NKDA

PE

Gen

Preictal: A & O × 3 but disoriented about recent events. Patient appears her stated age and is of ideal body weight. Postictally she was agitated and then somnolent and disoriented.

VS

BP 152/92, P 108, RR 56, T 35.8°C

Skin

Diaphoretic centrally and very warm; no lesions or rashes noted

HEENT

NC/AT; EOMI; pupils equal at 4 mm with decreased response to light; no strabismus, nystagmus, or conjunctivitis; TMs WNL bilaterally

Neck/LN
Supple without lymphadenopathy, masses, goiter, or bruits

Lungs/Chest
Clear to A & P bilaterally with decreased inspiratory effort

CV
RRR; no m/r/g

Abd
Soft, NT/ND w/o masses or organomegaly; decreased bowel sounds in all four quadrants

Genit/Rect
Deferred

MS/Ext
Normal ROM; muscle strength 5/5 and equal bilaterally; pulses 2+ throughout; no CCE; capillary refill < 2 sec

Neuro
CN II–XI intact; no focal or lateralizing signs; DTRs 2/4 and equal bilaterally; sensory intact; negative Babinski

Labs (fasting)

Na 117 mEq/L	Ca 9.2 mg/dL	T. chol 177 mg/dL	Cl 81 mEq/L	Uric acid 3.2 mg/dL	HDL 55 mg/dL
K 3.1 mEq/L	Phos 2.3 mg/dL	TG 72 mg/dL	CO_2 28 mEq/L	AST 87 IU/L	LDL 108 mg/dL
			BUN 16 mg/dL	ALT 59 IU/L	VLDL 38 mg/dL
			SCr 1.0 mg/dL	T. bili 0.7 mg/dL	T4 6.9 mcg/dL
			Glu 116 mg/dL	LDH 256 IU/L	Serum osm 238 mOsm/kg

UA
SG 1.008, pH 6.8, leukocyte esterase (–), nitrite (–), protein (–), ketones (–), urobilinogen nl, bilirubin (–), blood (–), glucose 80 mg/dL, spot urine sodium 112 mEq/L, osmolality 321 mOsm/kg

ECG
Sinus tachycardia

CT Head
Subtle low density in the left operculum at the gray-white matter junction; very likely an artifact, but subtle changes secondary to old ischemic disease, tumor, or old contusion are possible; no acute hemorrhage is present

Chest X-Ray
Normal except for old compression fracture noted at T7

Assessment
SIADH, electrolyte disturbances, and seizure in an otherwise healthy woman

▶ Questions

Problem Identification

1. a. *Create a list of the patient's drug therapy problems.*
   b. *What information (signs, symptoms, laboratory values) indicates the presence or severity of SIADH as the cause of her hyponatremia?*
   c. *Could any of the patient's problems have been caused by drug therapy?*

Desired Outcome

2. *What are the goals of pharmacotherapy in this case?*

Therapeutic Alternatives

3. a. *What nondrug therapies might be useful for this patient?*
   b. *What pharmacotherapeutic alternatives are available for the treatment of hyponatremia?*

Optimal Plan

4. *What drug dosage form, dose, schedule, and duration of therapy are most appropriate for initial treatment of this patient?*

Outcome Evaluation

5. *What clinical parameters are necessary to evaluate the therapy for achievement of the desired therapeutic outcome and to detect or prevent adverse effects?*

Patient Education

6. *What information should be provided to the patient to enhance compliance, ensure successful therapy, and minimize adverse effects?*

▶ Clinical Course

The patient received treatment you recommended, and her serum electrolytes normalized over the next 48 hours. At that time, the patient admitted to taking one of her husband's metolazone 5-mg tablets for what she called "fluid retention" on the day prior to her initial presentation.

▶ Follow-Up Questions

1. *Does this information alter your assessment of the patient's drug therapy problems?*

▶ Self-Study Assignments

1. What is the formula for calculating serum osmolality? Based on that formula, what is this patient's calculated serum osmolality?
2. Are phenothiazines appropriate for the treatment of agitated postictal patients?
3. Perform a literature or Internet search to determine the possible medicinal benefits of black cohosh, grapeseed extract, and herbal licorice.
4. What are the risk factors for selective serotonin reuptake inhibitors to cause hyponatremia?

▶ Clinical Pearl

Excessive serum concentrations of osmotically active substances such as glucose may cause hyponatremia as a consequence of movement of water from the intracellular compartment to extracellular spaces in an attempt to normalize osmolality. For each 100 mg/dL increase in serum glucose concentration, sodium will decrease by approximately 1.6–2.4 mEq/L.

References

1. Sterns RH. Severe symptomatic hyponatremia: Treatment and outcome. A study of 64 cases. Ann Intern Med 1987;107:656–664.
2. Adrogue HJ, Madias NE. Hyponatremia. N Engl J Med 2000;342:1581–1589.
3. Hillier TA, Abbott RD, Barrett EJ. Hyponatremia: Evaluating the correction factor for hyperglycemia. Am J Med 1999;106:399–403.
4. Fried LF, Palevsky PM. Hyponatremia and hypernatremia. Med Clin North Am 1997;81: 585–609.
5. Laureno R, Karp BI. Myelinolysis after correction of hyponatremia. Ann Intern Med 1997;126: 57–62.
6. Milionis HJ, Liamis GL, Elisaf MS. The hyponatremic patient: A systematic approach to laboratory diagnosis. CMAJ 2002;166:1056–1062.
7. Kirby D, Ames D. Hyponatraemia and selective serotonin re-uptake inhibitors in elderly patients. Int J Geriatr Psychiatry 2001;16:484–493.
8. Mulloy AL, Caruana RJ. Hyponatremic emergencies. Med Clin North Am 1995;79:155–168.

53 HYPERKALEMIA, HYPERPHOSPHATEMIA, AND HYPERCALCEMIA

▶ A Lesson in Homeostasis (Level II)

Mary K. Stamatakis, PharmD

▶ After completing this case study, students should be able to:

- Interpret clinical and biochemical findings which support the diagnosis of hyperkalemia, hyperphosphatemia, and hypercalcemia.
- Recommend a patient-specific therapeutic plan for the treatment of hyperkalemia, hyperphosphatemia, and hypercalcemia.
- Monitor the effectiveness of the pharmacotherapeutic plan.
- Educate patients with kidney disease on over-the-counter medications that can worsen hyperkalemia and hyperphosphatemia.

PATIENT PRESENTATION

Chief Complaint

"I'm not feeling too good."

HPI

Terry James is a 34 yo man with IDDM, HTN, and stage 5 chronic kidney disease (end-stage renal disease). He receives hemodialysis 3 times a week with a high-flux hemodialysis membrane (see Figure 53–1). Two days prior to admission, he developed fever, chills, general malaise, and SOB. On the day of admission, he complains of nausea and vomiting. He admits to missing his HD session yesterday.

PMH

IDDM since age 18
HTN × 12 years
Stage 5 chronic kidney disease on HD for the past 3 years, receives HD with a high-flux cellulose triacetate membrane (no residual renal function)
Left arm AV graft thrombus formation with thrombectomy last month
AV graft infected with MRSA 2 months ago
Hyperlipidemia

FH

Father with CAD; no family history of DM, HTN, CA

SH

Retired from a glass factory; on disability; past history of smoking, quit 3 years ago; (–) EtOH for the past 7 years; H/O IVDA, quit 7 years ago

ROS

Decreased appetite, intermittent headache, and left arm pain

Meds

Warfarin 2.5 mg po daily
Ranitidine 150 mg po daily
Calcium acetate 667 mg, 2 po TID
Nephrocaps, 1 po daily
Clonidine patch, TTS-2, 1 patch Q week
Procardia XL 60 mg po daily
Lipitor 10 mg po daily
NPH insulin 30 units SQ Q AM and 15 units SQ Q PM
Epogen 6,000 IU IV 3 times a week with HD
Calcijex 2 mcg IV 3 times a week with HD
Ensure nutritional supplement, 1 can (240 mL) po TID

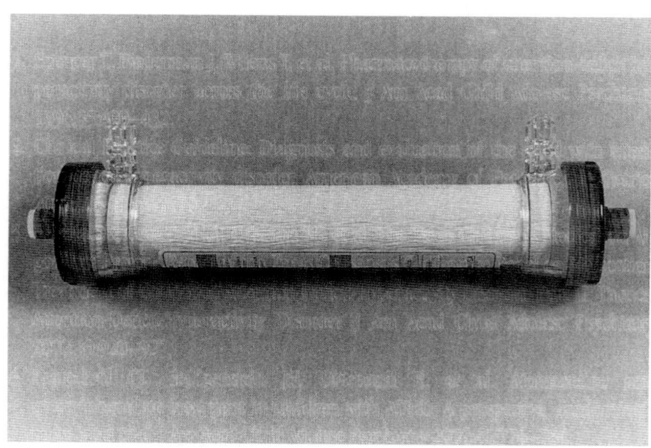

Figure 53–1. Example of a high-flux hemodialysis membrane.

All
NKDA

PE

Gen
Patient appears to be in mild to moderate distress

VS
BP 172/86, P 122, RR 18, T 39.0°C; dry body weight 72 kg, Ht 5′11″

Skin
Erythematous left arm AV graft site with marked tenderness, warm to the touch

HEENT
NC/AT, PERRLA, EOMI, funduscopy WNL, oral pharyngeal mucosa clear

Neck/LN
No JVD or lymphadenopathy, normal thyroid

Lungs
CTA bilaterally

CV
Tachycardia; normal S_1 and S_2; no S_3 or S_4; II/VI SEM at apex radiating to LSB

Abd
Soft, NT/ND, no HSM

Genit/Rect
Normal prostate, guaiac negative stool

MS/Ext
Trace bilateral pedal edema, no clubbing or cyanosis

Neuro
A & O × 3, CN II–XII intact, normal DTRs bilaterally

Labs

Na 135 mEq/L	Hgb 9.3 g/dL	Ca 10.6 mg/dL
K 5.8 mEq/L	Hct 28.5%	Mg 1.9 mg/dL
Cl 97 mEq/L	Plt 192 × 10^3/mm^3	Phos 7.4 mg/dL
CO_2 22 mEq/L	WBC 14.4 × 10^3/mm^3	AST 35 IU/L
BUN 71 mg/dL		ALT 29 IU/L
SCr 8.8 mg/dL		T. Bili 0.9 mg/dL
Glu 200 mg/dL		Alk Phos 87 IU/L
		Alb 3.0 g/dL
		Intact PTH 110 pg/mL (last month 125 pg/mL)

Chest X-Ray
No infiltrates or effusions

ECG
Sinus tachycardia

Bacteriology
Blood culture from AV graft positive for coagulase-positive cocci

Assessment
34 yo man with IDDM, ESRD on HD with infected AV graft site, hyperkalemia, hyperphosphatemia, and anemia

Plan
1. Start vancomycin for probable MRSA-infected dialysis graft.
2. Patient missed HD session yesterday. Will dialyze now to correct some of the electrolyte abnormalities.

▶ Questions

Problem Identification

1. a. *Create a list of the patient's drug therapy problems.*

Problem 1: Hyperkalemia

b. *What information (signs, symptoms, laboratory values) indicates the presence or severity of hyperkalemia?*

c. *Could anything the patient is taking be contributing to his hyperkalemia?*

d. *What is the pathophysiology of the patient's hyperkalemia?*

e. *What are the clinical consequences of hyperkalemia?*

Desired Outcome

2. *What are the goals for treating this patient's hyperkalemia?*

Therapeutic Alternatives

3. a. *What nondrug therapies are available for the treatment of hyperkalemia?*

b. *What feasible pharmacotherapeutic alternatives are available for treatment of hyperkalemia?*

Optimal Plan

4. *What pharmacotherapeutic recommendations are optimal for treatment of this patient's hyperkalemia?*

Outcome Evaluation

5. *Which clinical and laboratory parameters are necessary to evaluate the therapy for achievement of the desired therapeutic outcomes and to detect or prevent adverse effects?*

Patient Education

6. *What information should be provided to the patient regarding OTC medications that should be avoided to reduce the risk of hyperkalemia?*

Problem 2: Hyperphosphatemia and Hypercalcemia

1. a. *What information (signs, symptoms, laboratory values) indicates the presence or severity of hyperphosphatemia and hypercalcemia?*
   b. *Could any of the patient's medications be contributing to his hyperphosphatemia and hypercalcemia?*
   c. *What is the pathophysiology of the patient's hyperphosphatemia and hypercalcemia?*
   d. *What are the clinical consequences of hyperphosphatemia and hypercalcemia?*

Desired Outcome

2. *What are the goals of pharmacotherapy for treating this patient's hyperphosphatemia and hypercalcemia?*

Therapeutic Alternatives

3. a. *What nondrug therapies are available for the treatment of hyperphosphatemia?*
   b. *What feasible pharmacotherapeutic alternatives are available for the treatment of hyperphosphatemia when dietary phosphorus restriction is inadequate to control hyperphosphatemia?*
   c. *What pharmacotherapeutic options are available for the treatment of hypercalcemia?*

Optimal Plan

4. *What drug recommendations are optimal for treatment of this patient's hyperphosphatemia and hypercalcemia?*

Outcome Evaluation

5. *How should laboratory parameters be monitored to assess the effectiveness of the therapy for hyperphosphatemia and hypercalcemia?*

Patient Education

6. *What information should be provided to the patient to help ensure successful therapy and prevent future complications?*

▶ Follow-Up Questions

1. *What is an appropriate dosage of vancomycin for treatment of presumed MRSA bacteremia in this patient who receives dialysis with a cellulose triacetate (high-flux) dialyzer?*
2. *What additional information do you need to assess this patient's anemia of chronic kidney disease?*

▶ Clinical Pearl

Electrolyte disorders, such as hyperkalemia and hypercalcemia, can be prevented in dialysis patients by lowering dialysate potassium or calcium concentrations.

▶ Self-Study Assignments

1. The following laboratory values and erythropoietin dosages were available from the outpatient hemodialysis unit. Formulate a treatment plan to correct the patient's anemia of chronic kidney disease.

Time	Hgb (g/dL)	Ferritin (ng/mL)	% Transferrin Saturation	Erythropoietin Dosage
2 weeks ago	9.3	85	16	6,000 IU IV 3 ×/week
1 month ago	9.5	—	—	6,000 IU IV 3 ×/week

2. Compare the cost of a 1-month supply of calcium carbonate, calcium acetate, and sevelamer HCl using usual doses for treatment of hyperphosphatemia.

References

1. Ahmed J, Weisberg LS. Hyperkalemia in dialysis patients. Semin Dial 2001;14:348–56.
2. Block GA, Hulbert-Shearon TE, Levin NW, et al. Association of serum phosphorus and calcium × phosphate product with mortality risk in chronic hemodialysis patients: A national study. Am J Kidney Dis 1998;31:607–617.
3. Goodman WG, Goldin J, Kuizon BD, et al. Coronary-artery calcification in young adults with end-stage renal disease who are undergoing dialysis. N Engl J Med 2000;342:1478–1483.
4. The NKF-Kidney Disease Outcomes Quality Initiative (K/DOQI) clinical practice guidelines: Bone metabolism and disease in chronic kidney disease. Am J Kidney Dis 2003;42 (4 Suppl 3):S1–S201.

54 HYPERCALCEMIA OF MALIGNANCY

▶ Too Much of a Good Thing (Level I)

Laura L. Jung, PharmD
Rowena N. Schwartz, PharmD, BCOP

▶ After completing this case study, students should be able to:

- Recognize the signs and symptoms of hypercalcemia.
- Evaluate laboratory data and clinical symptoms for assessment and monitoring of hypercalcemia, hypercalcemia treatment, and complications of hypercalcemia.
- Recommend a pharmacotherapeutic plan for the initial treatment of cancer-related hypercalcemia.
- Recognize and develop management strategies for toxicities associated with treatment options for hypercalcemia.

PATIENT PRESENTATION

Chief Complaint

"I'm really tired and I feel as if I'm acting funny."

HPI

Tom Jones is a 43 yo man who presented to his oncologist's office today with a 2-day history of fatigue, somnolence, lethargy, and constipation. He states he has not felt like himself for the past 2 days. His wife states that since yesterday he has not complained of pain, and he has not used any immediate-release morphine sulfate for breakthrough pain. She states that his dose of sustained-released morphine was increased 1 week ago from 60 mg BID to 90 mg BID, and she attributes this to the changes in her husband's actions. She feels he is acting "doped up"; she thinks that he is now overmedicated. She reports that his last bowel movement was 5 days ago despite increased use of milk of magnesia, and she attributes the constipation to his increase in pain medication.

PMH

Renal cell carcinoma of the left kidney diagnosed 3 years ago. S/P left nephrectomy. Diagnosed with metastatic recurrence 1 year ago with metastases to the lung. S/P high-dose aldesleukin × 3 cycles, last cycle 4 months ago. Therapy was discontinued secondary to progressive disease in the lung. New disease in the inguinal lymph nodes and metastatic disease to the left femur diagnosed 2 months ago. He is currently being evaluated for a clinical trial.

Hypertension × 8 years

Tonsillectomy 1968

FH

Mother alive and healthy; father died of MI 5 years ago; brother killed in MVA 2 years ago; no history of cancer in other family members.

SH

No tobacco, EtOH, or recreational drug use. Former airline pilot for 15 years. Forced to retire early secondary to renal cell carcinoma. Lives at home with wife of 18 years.

ROS

States that he is nauseated and feels very tired. However, his wife has noted that he is more tired, has constipation, and is nauseated, which she believes has affected his appetite and contributed to an unintentional weight loss of 20 pounds over the past 6 months. Mr. Jones has no other complaints except a history of sharp aching pain in his left lower back with numbness and shooting pain down his left leg that began 3 months ago. Currently, Mr. Jones is not complaining of pain.

Medications

- Morphine sulfate sustained-release 90 mg po Q 12 H (increased 1 week ago)
- Morphine sulfate immediate-release 15 mg po Q 2 H PRN pain (estimated use 8 ×/24 hours prior to dose increase of morphine sulfate sustained-release)
- Gabapentin 300 mg po Q 8 H
- Hydrochlorothiazide 25 mg po Q AM
- Docusate sodium 200 mg po at bedtime
- MOM 30 mL po daily PRN constipation; increased to Q 6 H three days ago

All

NKDA

PE

Gen

Patient is cachectic; does not appear to be in any discomfort

VS

BP 100/68, P 110, RR 20, T 37.3°C; Wt 63 kg; Ht 6′1″

Skin

Dry with tenting on the dorsal surfaces of both hands; slow capillary refill bilaterally. Nephrectomy scar present on left lower backside extending around to left lower abdomen

HEENT

PERRLA, EOMI, fundi benign; TMs intact; oropharynx clear; mucus membranes dry

Neck/LN

Palpable inguinal lymph nodes

Cor

RRR, S_1, S_2 normal; no m/r/g

Lungs

CTA bilaterally with normal respirations, no crackles

Abd

Firm, distended, nontender; high-pitched BS; no abdominal masses

Genit/Rect

Normal male genitalia; normal rectal tone; stool heme (–)

MS/Ext

Pronounced muscle wasting in left leg compared to right

Neuro

Lethargic, oriented × 3 (self, location, and year). Speech is clear but slow. Language normal. Follows simple commands. Answers questions with prompting from wife. Cranial nerves grossly intact; moves all extremities, but LLE weakness compared to RLE

Labs

Na 144 mEq/L	Hgb 12.1 g/dL	AST 32 IU/L	Ca 12.1 mg/dL
K 3.6 mEq/L	Hct 36.3%	ALT 25 IU/L	Mg 1.5 mEq/L
Cl 101 mEq/L	Plt 110 × 10^3/mm^3	Alk phos 150 IU/L	Phos 3.5 mEq/L
CO_2 28 mEq/L	WBC 6.5 × 10^3/mm^3	LDH 200 IU/L	
BUN 38 mg/dL	45% PMNs	T. bili 1.2 mg/dL	
SCr 1.5 mg/dL	2% bands	D. bili 0.5 mg/dL	
Glu 95 mg/dL	32% lymphs	T. prot 5.6 g/dL	
	12% monos	Alb 2.0 g/dL	
	4% eos		
	5% basos		

Assessment/Plan

1. 43 yo man with metastatic renal cell carcinoma presenting with first episode of documented tumor-induced hypercalcemia and associated complications
2. Somnolence and lethargy: R/O infection, brain metastases
3. Admit to inpatient oncology service for further management of hypercalcemia and related complications

▶ Questions

Problem Identification

1. a. *Create a list of this patient's drug therapy problems.*
   b. *What information (signs, symptoms, laboratory values) indicates the presence or severity of hypercalcemia?*
   c. *What is Mr. Jones' corrected serum calcium level based on his serum albumin level?*
   d. *Could any of the patient's problems have been exacerbated by his current drug therapy?*
   e. *What are the possible etiologies of hypercalcemia in this patient?*
   f. *What additional information is needed to satisfactorily assess this patient?*

Desired Outcome

2. *What are the goals of pharmacotherapy in this case?*

Therapeutic Alternatives

3. *What are the available therapeutic options for the acute and chronic treatment of hypercalcemia?*

Optimal Plan

4. *Outline an optimal treatment regimen for hypercalcemia in this patient. Include drug(s), dose, schedule, and duration.*

Outcome Evaluation

5. *How would you monitor the therapy you recommended for efficacy and adverse effects?*

Patient Education

6. *What information would you provide Mr. Jones and his family about the treatment regimen you recommended for his hypercalcemia?*

▶ Follow-Up Questions

1. *Mr. Jones' wife is unfamiliar with the neurologic side effects of hypercalcemia and thinks her husband is "dopey" from pain medications. She requests that you stop all pain medications because he has no pain at this time. Outline a plan to manage Mr. Jones' pain until his hypercalcemia resolves.*

▶ Clinical Course

Mr. Jones completed his initial treatment for hypercalcemia without any problems, except that new renal cell carcinoma metastases were found in his right femur. He was discharged on the same pain regimen he was taking prior to admission. One week after discharge, Mr. Jones began complaining of increased left leg and hip pain. His pain was controlled with increases in sustained-release morphine sulfate to 120 mg po Q 12 H, immediate-release morphine sulfate to 30 mg po Q 2 H PRN pain, and gabapentin to 300 mg po Q 6 H. Six weeks after his initial treatment for hypercalcemia, Mr. Jones' wife noticed that her husband was again becoming confused and lethargic. His use of immediate-release morphine dropped from four times a day to zero over a period of 3 days. Upon presentation at his oncologist's office, Mr. Jones is found to have a serum calcium level of 13.0 mg/dL with an albumin of 2.2 g/dL and is oriented × 1 to self only. Normal saline at 150 cc/hr is initiated and he is admitted to the inpatient oncology service for further management.

▶ Follow-Up Questions

2. *What is Mr. Jones' corrected serum calcium level based on his serum albumin level, and what is your assessment of this value?*
3. *What pharmacotherapeutic regimen would you recommend for Mr. Jones now? State the rationale for your answer.*

▶ Clinical Course

Mr. Jones's hypercalcemia resolves with treatment and he reports that his pain is well controlled. He is discharged from the hospital on the same pain regimen he was taking prior to admission. Over the next 2 months, Mr. Jones experiences episodes of hypercalcemia with increasing frequency. The last two episodes were separated by 2 weeks, and both were treated by his outpatient oncologist with normal saline rehydration and zoledronic acid. One week after his last treatment with zoledronic acid, Mr. Jones reports to his outpatient oncologist's office with complaints of nausea, disorientation, and dehydration.

Labs

Na 142 mEq/L	Hgb 10.9 g/dL	AST 34 IU/L
K 3.7 mEq/L	Hct 33%	ALT 30 IU/L
Cl 105 mEq/L	Plt 150 × 10^3/mm^3	Alk phos 300 IU/L
CO_2 28 mEq/L	WBC 4.5 × 10^3/mm^3	T. bili 1.1 mg/dL
BUN 30 mg/dL	50% PMNs	D. bili 0.2 mg/dL
SCr 1.2 mg/dL	4% bands	Alb 2.1 g/dL
Glu 110 mg/dL	28% lymphs	Ca 12.5 mg/dL
	10% monos	Mg 1.8 mEq/L
	3% eos	Phos 4.0 mEq/L
	5% basos	

▶ Follow-Up Questions

4. *What treatment option might be considered for Mr. Jones at this time and why?*
5. *How would you monitor the therapy you have recommended for efficacy and adverse effects?*

▶ Self-Study Assignments

1. What are the roles of oral bisphosphonates and intranasal calcitonin in the treatment of hypercalcemia?
2. What nonmalignant disease states can induce hypercalcemia?
3. What treatment(s) can decrease the risk of developing hypercalcemia in patients receiving calcitriol for anticancer therapy?

▶ Clinical Pearl

When evaluating a patient for hypercalcemia, a corrected calcium must be used to account for the patient's albumin level.

References

1. Chisholm MA, Mulloy AL, Taylor AT. Acute management of cancer-related hypercalcemia. Ann Pharmacother 1996;30:507–513.
2. National Cancer Institute. Hypercalcemia (PDQ() supportive care—Health professionals. Available at: http://cancer.gov/cancerinfo/pdq (accessed April 19, 2004).
3. Leyland-Jones B. Treatment of cancer-related hypercalcemia: The role of gallium nitrate. Semin Oncol 2003(2 Suppl 5);30:13–19.
4. Payne RB, Carver ME, Morgan DB. Interpretation of serum total calcium: Effects of adjustments for albumin concentration on frequency of abnormal values and on detection of change in the individual. J Clin Pathol 1979;32:56–60.
5. Berenson JR. Treatment of hypercalcemia of malignancy with bisphosphonates. Semin Oncol 2002(6 Suppl 21);29:12–18.
6. Body JJ, Bartl R, Burckhardt P, et al. Current use of bisphosphonates in oncology. International Bone and Cancer Study Group. J Clin Oncol 1998;16:3890–3899.
7. Zojer N, Keck AV, Pecherstorfer M. Comparative tolerability of drug therapies for hypercalcaemia of malignancy. Drug Saf 1999;21:389–406.
8. Major P, Lortholary A, Hon J, et al. Zoledronic acid is superior to pamidronate in the treatment of hypercalcemia of malignancy: A pooled analysis of two randomized, controlled clinical trials. J Clin Oncol 2001;19:558–567.

55 HYPOKALEMIA AND HYPOMAGNESEMIA

▶ Double Trouble (Level II)

Denise R. Sokos, PharmD, BCPS
W. Greg Leader, PharmD

▶ After completing this case study, students should be able to:

- Identify potential causes of electrolyte disorders given a patient case history.
- Select the appropriate route of administration and dose of electrolyte replacement therapy specific for a patient.
- Monitor patients receiving electrolyte replacement therapy for efficacy and toxicity.

PATIENT PRESENTATION

Chief Complaint

"I've had belly pain for three days."

HPI

Elizabeth Farrs is a 35 yo woman who was evaluated in the ED five days ago because of emesis and diarrhea. Tonight, she presents with intermittent diffuse abdominal pain, 3 days in duration. She rates the pain as 7 on a 10-point scale. States the pain is unlike the pancreatitis pain that she has had previously. For the past week, she admits to excessive EtOH intake and decreased appetite. She also complains of weakness, a chronic cough with whitish sputum, and intermittent diarrhea for 4 months. She has lost 125 pounds in the last 8 months after gastric bypass surgery.

PMH

Gastric bypass surgery
Chronic pancreatitis
Alcoholic hepatitis
Type 2 DM
Depression/Anxiety
Pneumonia 1 month ago (hospitalized)
Cholecystectomy

FH

Mother ↑ diabetes; Father ↓ 68 years old from "heart attack"; 2 brothers, both ↑ diabetes

SH

Lives with her husband. She had one son who was murdered 2 months ago. Reports drinking 1 pint of whiskey every day for the last week (abstinent × 3 years until 2 months ago); denies IVDA.

ROS

Denies fever, chills, headache, chest pain, or respiratory difficulties (dyspnea, PND, orthopnea). No hematemesis or melena. Reports intermittent polyuria and polydipsia, but denies dysuria or incontinence. Occasional nausea. States that she has had some generalized muscle weakness for the last few days and reports lightheadedness upon standing. Has feelings of sadness and anxiety.

Meds

Glimeperide 2 mg po daily
Citalopram 10 mg po daily – started one month ago
Pancrelipase 2 po QID with meals
MVI with minerals 1 po TID AC
Ferrous Sulfate 325 mg po daily
Immunization History: "Tetanus shot" 5 years ago

All

Codeine – nausea and hives

PE

Gen

The patient is A & O × 2; mild confusion, cooperative. Flat affect.

VS

Supine BP 130/90, P 90; Upright BP 108/69, P 110; RR 18, T 37.1°C; Ht 5′4″, Wt 70 kg

Skin

Skin warm, dry, no abnormal nevi, no spider angiomata

HEENT

NC/AT; PERRLA; EOM intact; no nystagmus. Disc demarcation clear; no A-V nicking, exudates, or papilledema. Throat not erythematous. Dry mucous membranes. TMs intact.

Neck/LN

Jugular vein flat; no lymphadenopathy; thyroid smooth and not enlarged

Lungs

Clear to auscultation bilaterally; a few crackles at the base of the right lung

CV

RRR; normal S_1 and S_2; no murmurs, rubs, or gallops; apical pulse at 4th intercostal space

Abd

Soft, not distended, moderate epigastric tenderness; no fluid wave or shifting dullness; no rebound or guarding; liver palpable 4 cm below the RCM. Spleen not palpable. BS present in all four quadrants.

Genit/Rect

GU deferred. Rect: heme (–) stool; (+) hemorrhoids

Ext

No C/C/E or tenderness. Pulses palpable bilaterally. Full ROM in all extremities.

Back

No CVA tenderness

Neuro

CN II–XII intact. Muscle strength 4/5 in upper and lower extremities. DTR 2+ throughout. Plantars downgoing.

Labs

Na 138 mEq/L	Hgb 11.6 g/dL	Ca 8.0 mg/dL	Alk Phos 184 IU/L
K 2.6 mEq/L	Hct 34.5%	Mg 0.9 mEq/L	GGT 268 IU/L
Cl 111 mEq/L	WBC 6.1 × 10^3/mm^3	Phos 3.3 mEq/L	Alb 2.8 g/dL
CO_2 21 mEq/L	Plt 239 × 10^3/mm^3	AST 226 IU/L	Amylase116 IU/L
BUN 7 mg/dL		ALT 100 IU/L	Lipase 200 IU/L
SCr 0.5 mg/dL		T. bili 0.3 mg/dL	
Glu 290 mg/dL			

ABG

pH 7.39, $PaCO_2$ 37 mm Hg, PaO_2 79 mm Hg, bicarbonate 22 mEq/L on room air

Abd Ultrasound

Slightly enlarged, fatty infiltrated liver with mild intra- and extrahepatic biliary ductal dilatation, post cholecystectomy. Normal pancreas.

ECG

NSR, no ischemic changes

Assessment

Admit as observation to inpatient bed.

1. Electrolyte abnormalities
2. Abdominal pain
3. EtOH abuse
4. Depression/anxiety
5. Type 2 DM
6. Chronic intermittent diarrhea

▶ Questions

Problem Identification

1. a. *Create a list of the patient's drug therapy problems.*
   b. *What information (signs, symptoms, laboratory values) indicates the presence and severity of the electrolyte abnormalities?*
   c. *What are the potential causes of the electrolyte disorders in this patient?*
   d. *What additional information is needed to satisfactorily assess this patient?*

Desired Outcome

2. *What are the goals of pharmacotherapy in this patient?*

Therapeutic Alternatives

3. *What feasible pharmacotherapeutic alternatives are available for treatment of dehydration, hypokalemia, and hypomagnesemia?*

Optimal Plan

4. *Given the therapeutic alternatives outlined above, what therapy would be the most appropriate?*

Outcome Evaluation

5. *Which clinical and laboratory parameters are necessary to evaluate the therapy for the desired therapeutic outcome and prevention of adverse effects?*

Patient Education

6. *When the patient is to be discharged on oral potassium and magnesium supplementation, what information should be provided to her to ensure successful therapy and minimize adverse effects?*

▶ Follow-Up Questions

1. *What medical options are available for the treatment of this patient's chronic pancreatitis?*
2. *What changes should be made in the therapy for the patient's other medical conditions?*
3. *What vaccinations should this patient receive?*

▶ Self-Study Assignments

1. Outline a therapeutic plan for the treatment of chronic pain in this patient.
2. Search the literature for information on the treatment or prevention of withdrawal symptoms in hospitalized alcoholics. What drug therapy would you recommend? Defend your choice.
3. Describe how a patient's acid–base status can affect serum electrolyte concentrations.

▶ Clinical Pearl

The addition of small amounts of potassium (20–30 mEq/L) to dextrose solutions for replacement may lead to a transient decrease in serum potassium. The glucose solution may stimulate insulin secretion causing an intracellular shift of potassium.

References

1. Dyckner T, Wester PO. Ventricular extrasystoles and intracellular electrolytes in hypokalemic patients before and after correction of the hypokalemia. Acta Med Scand 1978;204:375–379.
2. Hamill-Ruth RJ, McGory R. Magnesium repletion and its effects on potassium homeostasis in critically ill adults: Results of a double-blind, randomized, controlled trial. Crit Care Med 1996;24:38–45.
3. Kruse JA, Carlson RW. Rapid correction of hypokalemia using concentrated intravenous potassium chloride infusions. Arch Intern Med 1990;150:613–617.
4. Hamill RJ, Robinson LM, Wexler HR, et al. Efficacy and safety of potassium infusion therapy in hypokalemic critically ill patients. Crit Care Med 1991;19:694–699.

56 METABOLIC ACIDOSIS

▶ Of Proximal Tubules, Normal Anion Gaps, and RTA (Level II)

Kimberly A. Dornbrook-Lavender, PharmD, BCPS
Melanie S. Joy, PharmD

▶ After completing this case study, students should be able to:

- Recognize the clinical and laboratory manifestations of metabolic acidosis.
- Differentiate between the types of renal tubular acidosis.
- Develop a patient-specific pharmacotherapeutic plan for the treatment of chronic metabolic acidosis.
- Provide medication education for patients with chronic metabolic acidosis.

PATIENT PRESENTATION

Chief Complaint

"I just feel so weak all the time."

HPI

The patient is a 27 yo woman who was referred to the nephrology clinic for the management of fatigue, dyspnea, somnolence, lethargy, and increased proximal muscle weakness, particularly with hip extension. She requires the use of her upper extremities to arise from a seated position. In addition, she also notes increasing pain in the left shoulder and hips, as well as discomfort in the quadriceps region. There is no history of diarrhea.

PMH

Four pregnancies with normal uncomplicated vaginal deliveries

SH

She has been divorced from her husband for 8 years and currently lives with her four children. There is no history of tobacco habituation or recreational drug use.

FH

History of unspecified arthritis and cancer, and a questionable history of renal disease in the patient's mother.

ROS

As per HPI

Meds

None

All

NKDA

PE

Gen

Pleasant African-American woman in NAD

VS

BP 124/80, P 80, RR 22, T 37.2°C; Wt 75 kg, Ht 5′7″

HEENT

No hemorrhages or exudates on funduscopic examination

Neck/LN

JVP was 5 cm; carotid pulses were 2+ bilaterally; no thyromegaly or lymphadenopathy

Lungs

CTA & P

CV

Unable to palpate PMI; regular rate and rhythm; normal S_1 and S_2; no murmurs

Abd

Obese, soft, non-tender, normoactive bowel sounds, no organomegaly

MS/Ext

Minimal sternal and quadriceps tenderness

Neuro

No focal cranial nerve deficits, weakness in hip flexion and extension with strength graded at 3/5. DTRs are 1+ brachioradialis, 2+ biceps, 2+ quadriceps, 1+ ankle jerks, toes downgoing bilaterally

Labs

Na 143 mEq/L	Hgb 15 g/dL	AST 13 IU/L	1, 25-OH-D_3 32 pg/mL
K 3.2 mEq/L	Hct 45%	ALT 7 IU/L	25-OH D_3 10 ng/mL
Cl 119 mEq/L	Plt 225 × $10^3/mm^3$	Alk phos 113 IU/L	T4 5.8 mcg/dL
CO_2 12 mEq/L	WBC 7.6 × $10^3/mm^3$	GGT 14 IU/L	TSH 4.5 (IU/mL
BUN 15 mg/dL	Ca 7.4 mg/dL	T. bili 0.4 mg/dL	
SCr 1.2 mg/dL	Mg 2.2 mg/dL	Alb 4.6 g/dL	
Glu 75 mg/dL	Phos 1.0 mg/dL		

ABG on RA

pH 7.27, pCO_2 27 mm Hg, pO_2 106 mm Hg, bicarbonate 12.1 mEq/L

UA

SG 1.010; pH 5.0. Fractional excretion of bicarbonate (following bicarbonate infusion to increase serum level to 25 mEq/L) > 25%

KUB

No nephrocalcinosis

Radiology

Bilateral femur and tibia films demonstrated pseudofracture or stress response to the right proximal femur; cortical reabsorption in the left proximal femur

Assessment

1. Acidosis
2. Hypocalcemia
3. Hypokalemia
4. Hypophosphatemia
5. Osteomalacia

▶ Questions

Problem Identification

1. a. *Identify the type of acidosis (metabolic versus respiratory) this patient exhibits, calculate the anion gap, and identify the potential causes.*
   b. *What medical conditions present in this patient are either untreated or inadequately treated?*
   c. *Which information obtained from the patient's symptoms, physical examination, and laboratory analysis indicates the presence of a chronic metabolic acidosis with a renal tubular acidosis component or one of its complications?*
   d. *What are the different types of renal tubular acidosis (RTA), and how do they differ with respect to etiology, mechanisms, and clinical/laboratory findings?*
   e. *Which type of RTA is most likely present in this patient?*

Desired Outcome

2. *What are the pharmacotherapy goals for this patient?*

Therapeutic Alternatives

3. *What treatment alternatives are available to achieve the desired therapeutic outcomes?*

Optimal Plan

4. *Design a pharmacotherapeutic plan for the management of metabolic acidosis and its complications in this patient.*

Outcome Evaluation

5. *Outline a clinical and laboratory monitoring plan to assess the patient's response to the pharmacotherapeutic regimen you recommended.*

Patient Education

6. *How should the patient be educated about the drug therapy to treat chronic metabolic acidosis and renal tubular acidosis?*

▶ Clinical Course

At the patient's 6-month clinic visit, 2+ pedal edema and symptoms of depression are noted. During the patient interview, she suggests that she has not been compliant with medications because of depressive symptoms.

Labs

Na 139 mEq/L	Ca 7.1 mg/dL
K 3.3 mEq/L	Mg 1.9 mg/dL
Cl 114 mEq/L	Phos 0.9 mg/dL
CO_2 14 mEq/L	Alb 4.6 g/dL
BUN 12 mg/dL	UA: Trace glucose
SCr 0.9 mg/dL	
Glu 99 mg/dL	

Furosemide 40 mg po daily, Neutra-Phos 3 packets po TID, and amitriptyline 25 mg po at bedtime were added to the medication regimen. In addition, the patient was advised to take an extra 80 mEq potassium over the ensuing 24 hours.

▶ Self-Study Assignments

1. Differentiate between the bone disease of metabolic acidosis versus that associated with chronic renal failure and osteoporosis.
2. Discuss the basis for the diagnosis of the various forms of RTA by evaluating the urinalysis and serum chemistries.

▶ Clinical Pearl

When differentiating between the various types of RTA, consider the urine pH, fractional excretion of bicarbonate, serum potassium, presence or absence of nephrocalcinosis and bone disease, and dose of bicarbonate needed to normalize plasma bicarbonate (Table 1).

TABLE 1. Differential diagnosis of various types of RTA.

	Proximal RTA (Type 2)	Distal RTA (Type 1)	Hyperkalemic RTA (Type 4)
Serum potassium[a]	↔ or ↓	↔ or ↓	↑
Urinary anion gap (UAG)	Negative	Positive	Positive
Urine pH	< 5.5	> 5.5	< 5.5
Ammonium excretion	↔	↓	↓
Fractional bicarbonate excretion[b]	> 10–15%	< 5%	> 5–10%
Nephrocalcinosis/lithiasis[c]	–	++	–
Bone involvement[c]	++	+	–

[a] ↓,decreased; ↑, increased; ↔, normal or no change
[b] After alkali loading with a bicarbonate infusion
[c] –, absent; +, rarely present; ++, often present

References

1. Rodriguez Soriano J. Renal tubular acidosis: The clinical entity. J Am Soc Nephrol 2002;13:2160–2170.
2. Gregory MJ, Schwartz GJ. Diagnosis and treatment of renal tubular disorders. Semin Nephrol 1998;18(3):317–329.
3. Unwin RJ, Capasso G. The renal tubular acidoses. J R Soc Med 2001;94:221–225.
4. Gluck SL. Acid–base. Lancet 1998;352:474–479.
5. Penney MD, Oleesky DA. Renal tubular acidosis. Ann Clin Biochem 1999;36(pt 4):408–422.
6. Bushinsky DA, Frick KK. The effects of acid on bone. Curr Opin Nephrol Hypertens 2000;9:369–379.
7. Bushinsky DA. Acid-base imbalance and the skeleton. Eur J Nutr 2001;40:238–244.
8. Rastegar A, Soleimani M. Hypokalemia and hyperkalemia. Postgrad Med J 2001;77:759–764.

57 METABOLIC ALKALOSIS

▶ The Carpenter's Mixed Bag (Level I)

Thomas D. Nolin, PharmD, PhD

▶ After completing this case study, students should be able to:

- Determine the type of acid–base disorder a patient is experiencing when given patient history and pertinent laboratory values.
- Describe patient-specific factors that contribute to the development of metabolic disorders.
- Recommend appropriate therapeutic alternatives for the treatment of metabolic alkalosis.
- Formulate a patient-specific pharmacotherapeutic plan for the treatment and monitoring of metabolic alkalosis.

PATIENT PRESENTATION

Chief Complaint

"I can't catch my breath."

HPI

Henry Alstoff is a 62 yo man who presents to the ED with complaints of shortness of breath and generalized pain. He was discharged 2 days ago from a hospital near his home where he had been admitted with symptoms consistent with CHF. During that hospitalization he was treated with furosemide and supplemental oxygen. He was breathing comfortably on discharge. The patient also reports worsening shortness of breath and increased weakness over the past 24 hours.

PMH

Hx CHF
Hypertension
Hyperlipidemia
CABG 4 years ago
Chronic kidney disease (SCr 2.2 mg/dL 6 months ago)
Insulin-dependent diabetes mellitus × 25 years

FH

Not available

SH

Significant history of alcohol consumption but has not had an alcoholic beverage for 8 years. There is no history of tobacco or illicit drug use. He is a carpenter and lives at home with his wife.

ROS

The patient denies recent weight gain or loss, loss of appetite, nausea, or vomiting. Also denies fever, chills, or night sweats. Does admit to a nonproductive cough. No reported chest pain, palpitations, or diaphoresis. Denies diarrhea, constipation, change in bowel habits, or color of stool. Urine output has decreased over the past 24 hours.

Meds

Furosemide 80 mg po daily (increased from 20 mg po daily 2 days ago upon discharge from the hospital)
KCl 10 mEq po daily
Calcium carbonate 500 mg po BID × 8 months
Atorvastatin 10 mg po daily
Humulin-N insulin 24 units SQ Q AM, 18 units SQ Q PM; last dosage change 1 month ago
Lisinopril 40 mg po daily × 1 year

All

NKDA

PE

Gen

The patient appears to be uncomfortable. Breathing is labored.

VS
BP 132/78, HR 76, RR 26, T 37.4°C; Wt 111 kg; Ht 5′10″; O_2 sat 89% on RA

Skin
Soft, intact, warm and dry.

HEENT
NC/AT, EOMI, PERRLA, sclerae anicteric. Funduscopic exam is normal. No sinus tenderness. Moist mucous membranes. No oral lesions or exudates.

Neck/LN
No JVD or bruits. No lymphadenopathy or thyromegaly.

Chest
Scattered rhonchi at bases

CV
RRR, normal S_1, S_2, no S_3 or S_4, no murmurs

Abd
Soft, NT/ND; old surgical scars evident; (+) bowel sounds

GU
Noncontributory

Ext
Distal pulses trace bilaterally. Femoral pulses 1+ bilaterally.

Neuro
A & O × 3. DTR 1+ and symmetrical bilaterally. UE/LE strength 4/5. CN II–XII intact. Babinski negative bilaterally.

Labs

Na 137 mEq/L	Hgb 12.0 g/dL	AST 13 IU/L
K 5.5 mEq/L	Hct 37.1%	ALT 23 IU/L
Cl 90 mEq/L	Plt 361 × 10^3/mm^3	GGT 30 IU/L
CO_2 36 mEq/L	WBC 7.4 × 10^3/mm^3	T. bili 0.4 mg/dL
BUN 49 mg/dL	Mg 2.5 mEq/L	PT 12.1 sec
SCr 2.9 mg/dL	Phos 2.7 mg/dL	PTT 21.9 sec
Glu 305 mg/dL		

ABG
pH 7.46, pCO_2 52 mm Hg, pO_2 83 mm Hg on RA

UA
Urine sodium 14 mEq/L, potassium 10 mEq/L, chloride 18 mEq/L

Chest X-Ray
Interstitial pulmonary edema and cardiomegaly (see Figure 57–1)

ECG
Normal

Assessment
Admit patient for uncontrolled congestive heart failure, worsening renal function, and electrolyte abnormalities

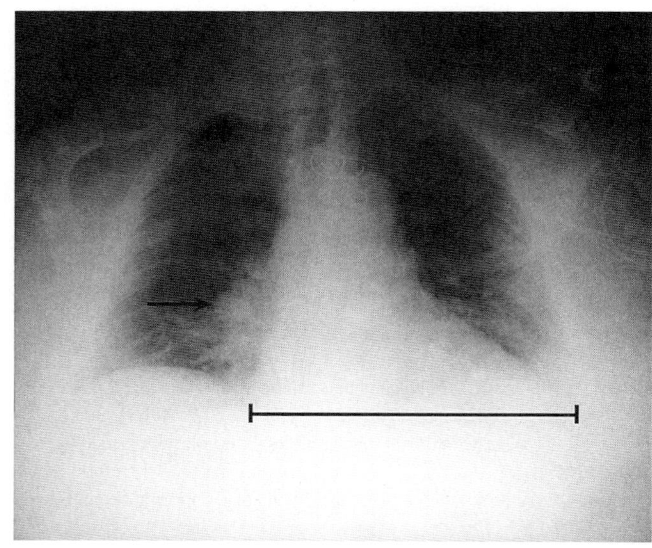

Figure 57–1. Chest x-ray showing findings compatible with interstitial pulmonary edema *(small arrow)* and cardiomegaly *(horizontal line).* Sternal wires and mediastinal clips are also noted.

▶ Questions

Problem Identification

1. a. *Identify the type of acid–base disturbance present in this patient. Explain how the patient's arterial blood gas results and medical history support your response.*
   b. *Create a list of this patient's drug therapy problems.*
   c. *Describe the clinical findings that are consistent with metabolic alkalosis and those that are inconsistent with this acid–base disorder.*
   d. *Explain how diuretics such as furosemide can result in metabolic alkalosis.*

Desired Outcome

2. *What are the desired therapeutic outcomes for this patient?*

Therapeutic Alternatives

3. *What pharmacologic and nonpharmacologic alternatives should be considered for the treatment of metabolic alkalosis in this patient?*

Optimal Plan

4. a. *What drug, dosage form, dose, schedule, and duration of therapy are best for this patient?*
   b. *What other modifications to the patient's current drug regimen are warranted? Include your rationale.*

Outcome Evaluation

5. a. *What clinical and laboratory parameters are necessary to evaluate the therapy for achievement of the desired outcome and prevention of adverse effects?*

▶ Clinical Course

The patient was started on IV fluids for metabolic alkalosis. Urine output improved from 15 mL/hr during the first 2 hours after admission to 40 mL/hr. Total fluid intake was 4.2 L and urine output was 1.2 L for the first 24 hours. The next morning, a chest X-ray showed a small increase in the degree of pulmonary edema. Laboratory values 24 hours after the initiation of therapy are as follows:

Na 142 mEq/L	BUN 40 mg/dL	ABG
K 4.8 mEq/L	SCr 2.6 mg/dL	pH 7.46
Cl 99 mEq/L	Mg 2.3 mEq/L	pCO_2 48 mm Hg
CO_2 33 mEq/L		pO_2 90 mm Hg

For the treatment of congestive heart failure, the patient's lisinopril was discontinued and isosorbide dinitrate 20 mg po TID and hydralazine 25 mg Q 8 H were initiated.

b. *What is your assessment of the patient's response to the IV fluid therapy initiated for treatment of metabolic alkalosis? Is a modification of therapy warranted?*

Patient Education

6. *What information should be provided to the patient regarding the isosorbide dinitrate and hydralazine started for the treatment of CHF?*

▶ Self-Study Assignments

1. Discuss the use of hydrochloric acid in the treatment of metabolic alkalosis and include indications, dosing, infusion preparation, and safe administration technique in your discussion.
2. Discuss how urine electrolytes play a role in the diagnosis and treatment of metabolic alkalosis.

▶ Clinical Pearl

It is important to identify the cause of metabolic alkalosis and correct it. However, correcting the underlying cause does not always reverse the alkalosis, and additional therapy will be required.

References

1. Galla JH. Metabolic alkalosis. J Am Soc Nephrol 2000;11:369–375.
2. Mazur JE, Devlin JW, Peters MJ, et al. Single versus multiple doses of acetazolamide for metabolic alkalosis in critically ill medical patients: A randomized double-blind trial. Crit Care Med 1999;27:1257–1261.
3. Brimioulle S, Berre J, Dufaye P, et al. Hydrochloric acid infusion for treatment of metabolic alkalosis associated with respiratory acidosis. Crit Care Med 1989;17:232–236.
4. Cochran EB, Kamper CA, Phelps SJ, et al. Parenteral nutrition in the critically ill patient. Clin Pharm 1989;8:783–799.

Editor's Note: This case was modified from the case written for the fifth edition by Jennifer Stoffel, PharmD, BCPS.

SECTION 6

Neurologic Disorders

58 MULTIPLE SCLEROSIS

▶ White Dots and Black Holes (Level I)

Jacquelyn L. Bainbridge, BS Pharm, PharmD, FCCP
John R. Corboy, MD

▶ After completing this case study, students should be able to:

- Describe the signs and symptoms of multiple sclerosis (MS) that often mimic those of other neurologic diseases.
- Design a pharmacotherapeutic regimen for treatment of an acute exacerbation of MS.
- Identify patients for whom disease-modifying therapy would be appropriate and recommend the most appropriate alternative for an individual patient.
- Educate a patient on the proper dosing, self-administration, adverse effects, and storage of interferon beta-1a, interferon beta-1b, and glatiramer acetate.

PATIENT PRESENTATION

Chief Complaint

"My left foot is numb, and I'm having trouble walking."

HPI

Cathy Olson is a 24 yo woman who was in excellent health until 10 months ago when she developed progressive sensory loss on her right face, distorted hearing in the right ear, and intense vertigo. These symptoms intensified over 10 days, at which time she was hospitalized. A brain MRI showed an enhancing lesion in her right pons and a total of six other lesions, three of which are periventricular. CSF evaluation revealed elevated IgG Index and oligoclonal bands. She presents to clinic today indicating that she has had progressive left-sided sensory loss resulting in difficulty ambulating that began about a week ago when she had a mild URI and was experiencing increased stress at work.

PMH

Frequent migraine headaches since adolescence that have been difficult to control despite therapy with ibuprofen and sumatriptan

Mild recurrent bouts of depression that have not been treated pharmacologically

FH

The patient is of Norwegian descent. She was born and raised in Wisconsin. She has no siblings, and both parents are alive and well. There is no family history of neurologic disease.

SH

The patient is single and is employed as an accountant. She has not smoked for 3 years; prior to that she smoked 1 ppd. Her use of alcohol is limited to an occasional glass of wine or beer on weekends.

Meds

Ibuprofen 400 mg po PRN headache

All

NKDA

ROS

Unremarkable except that she reports feeling run-down and tired. Also reports past difficulty with urinary control (incontinence) and a subjective feeling of weakness in hot weather. No previous history of visual disturbance (e.g., pain, blurred or double vision) or motor disturbance.

PE

Gen
The patient is a white woman who appears to be slightly anxious but is otherwise in NAD.

VS
BP 106/60, P 72 and regular, RR 12, T 36.2°C Wt 55 kg, Ht 5′5″

Skin
Normal turgor; no obvious lesions, tumors, or moles

HEENT
NC/AT, TMs clear

Neck/LN
Supple, without lymphadenopathy or thyromegaly

Cor
RRR; S_1, S_2 normal; no m/r/g

Lungs
Clear to A&P

Abd
NT/ND

Genit/Rect
Deferred

MS/Ext
Normal ROM; pulses 2+ throughout

Neuro
The patient is alert, oriented, and cooperative.

CN II– XII: Mild subjective sense of auditory distortion and tinnitus right ear despite intact auditory acuity. PERRLA; visual acuity is 20/20 both eyes. Funduscopic exam is normal. EOMs are full in extent. Slight nystagmus present.

Motor tone and strength are normal throughout. DTRs are hyperactive throughout. Sensory exam reveals moderate diminution in the subjective intensity of light touch and pinprick on the left, with maximal deficits noted in the left foot. Coordination testing is normal except for modest unsteadiness on performing tandem walking. Romberg maneuver is positive.

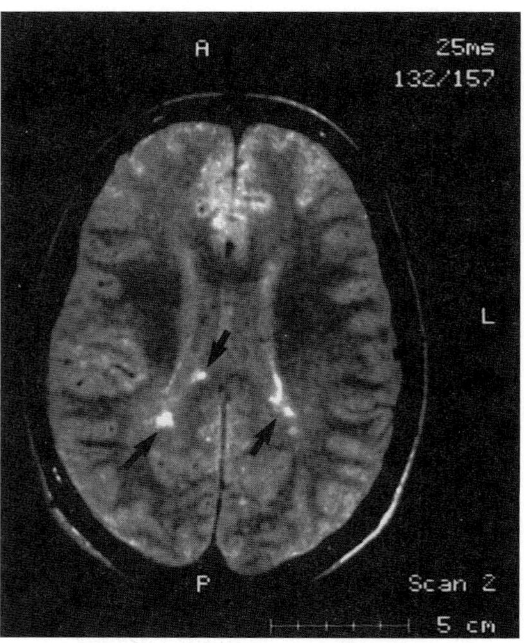

Figure 58–1. Brain MRI scan. Arrows highlight typical periventricular white matter lesions seen in multiple sclerosis.

Labs

Na 140 mEq/L	AST 12 IU/L
K 4.1 mEq/L	ALT 40 IU/L
Cl 99 mEq/L	GGT 33 IU/L
CO_2 23 mEq/L	Wintrobe ESR 20 mm/hr
BUN 11 mg/dL	TSH 2.0 mIU/L
SCr 0.9 mg/dL	ANA negative
Glu 109 mg/dL	CRP 1.0 mg/dL
	Lyme serology negative

Brain MRI

Multiple areas of increased periventricular white matter signal (plaque); see Figure 58–1.

▶ Questions

Problem Identification

1. a. *Which clinical information (patient demographics, signs, symptoms, lab values) suggests the diagnosis of multiple sclerosis in this patient?*
   b. *What additional information (laboratory tests, diagnostic procedures) may be useful in assessing this patient?*

Desired Outcome

2. *What are the goals of therapy for this patient?*

Therapeutic Alternatives

3. a. *What pharmacotherapeutic options are available to treat this patient's acute exacerbation, and which one would you recommend?*
   b. *What adjunctive treatments may be indicated for this patient?*
   c. *What adverse effects might be anticipated for both first-line and adjunctive treatments?*

▶ Clinical Course

The patient was treated with the regimen you recommended with gradual resolution of her symptoms. Six months after the initial presentation, she returns to clinic with complaints of increased difficulty walking and some blurring of her vision. Her muscle strength is intact in the upper extremities, but there is marked weakness in the lower extremities, especially the left side. DTRs are hyperactive in the lower extremities, and tone is slightly spastic. The patient's gait is slow, but she is able to walk without assistance. Her affect is sad, and she is tearful during the examination. She states that she is concerned about the progression of her disease.

d. What therapeutic options are available to modify this patient's disease course?

Optimal Plan

4. Design an optimal pharmacotherapeutic plan for reducing the frequency of MS exacerbations in this patient.

Outcome Evaluation

5. Which clinical and laboratory parameters are necessary for assessment of both efficacy and toxicity?

Patient Education

6. What information would you provide to this patient about her long-term MS therapy?

▶ Self-Study Assignments

1. Identify recent clinical trials assessing the efficacy and toxicity of mitoxantrone or IV immune globulin (IVIG) for MS. Considering the data available, define the potential role(s) of these agents for patients with MS.
2. Review the clinical studies evaluating glatiramer acetate for MS. How does this agent compare to interferon beta-1b and interferon beta-1a in terms of both efficacy and toxicity?
3. Outline a plan for providing patient education on the dosing, administration, and storage of interferon beta-1b, interferon beta-1a, and glatiramer acetate.
4. Obtain relevant information and formulate an opinion on the role of plasmapheresis in the treatment of MS.

▶ Clinical Pearl

Many patients do not feel better with interferon therapy and may experience unpleasant adverse effects. It is important to re-enforce that the ABC-R (Avonex, Betaseron, Copaxone, Rebif) medications do not alter ongoing symptoms of the disease but will reduce attacks and progression of disability over time. Adequate education about the potential benefits and expected side effects is essential to ensuring adherence to the therapy.

References

1. Schapiro RT. Symptom management in multiple sclerosis. Ann Neurol 1994;36(Suppl):S123–S129.
2. The INFB Multiple Sclerosis Study Group and the British Columbia MS/MRI Analysis Group. Interferon beta-1b in the treatment of multiple sclerosis. Final outcome of the randomized controlled trial. Neurology 1995;45:1277–1285.
3. Jacobs LD, Cookfair DL, Rudick RA, et al. Intramuscular interferon beta-1a for disease progression in relapsing multiple sclerosis. The Multiple Sclerosis Collaborative Research Group. Ann Neurol 1996;39:285–294.
4. Jacobs LD, Beck RW, Simon JH, et al. Intramuscular interferon beta-1a therapy initiated during a first demyelinating event in multiple sclerosis. CHAMPS Study Group. N Engl J Med 2000;343:898–904.
5. Corboy JR, Goodin DS, Frohman EM. Disease-modifying therapies for multiple sclerosis. Curr Treat Options Neurol 2003;5:35–54.
6. Johnson KP, Brooks BR, Cohen JA, et al. Extended use of glatiramer acetate (Copaxone) is well tolerated and maintains its clinical effect on multiple sclerosis relapse rate and degree of disability. Copolymer 1 Multiple Sclerosis Study Group. Neurology 1998;50:701–708.
7. PRISMS (Prevention of Relapses and Disability by Interferon beta-1a Subcutaneously in Multiple Sclerosis) Study Group and the University of British Columbia MS/MRI Analysis Group. PRISMS-4: Long-term efficacy of interferon-beta-1a in relapsing MS. Neurology 2001;56:1628–1636.
8. Goodin DS, Frohman EM, Garmany GP, et al. Disease modifying therapies in multiple sclerosis. Report of the therapeutics and technology assessment subcommittee of the American Academy of Neurology and the MS Council for Clinical Practice Guidelines. Neurology 2002;58:169–178.

59 COMPLEX PARTIAL SEIZURES

▶ A Lifelong Pattern (Level I)

James W. McAuley, RPh, PhD

▶ After completing this case study, students should be able to:

- Identify necessary patient- and disease-specific data to collect for patients with complex partial seizures.
- Define potential drug-related problems for established and new antiepileptic drugs.
- List desired therapeutic outcomes for patients with complex partial seizures.
- Based on patient characteristics, choose appropriate pharmacotherapy for treatment of partial seizures and develop a suitable care plan.

PATIENT PRESENTATION

Chief Complaint

"My regular doctor told me I should see a neurologist about my seizures."

HPI

Peggy Livingston is a 60 yo woman referred to the epilepsy clinic by her PCP for evaluation of anticonvulsant therapy. She continues to have seizures, with the last seizure occurring 1 week ago, which resulted in a fall down a flight of stairs. Her seizures started at a very early age. She remembers initially having them in first grade and being confused a lot throughout her schooling. She was briefly tried on phenobarbital but has been on phenytoin most of her life. She has poor seizure control with no extended seizure-free periods. She has not seen a neurologist for years, if ever. She has not had any neuroimaging studies and provides no previous EEG results.

Most of her seizures are complex partial seizures where she "blacks out" and loses sense of time. Occasionally, she has secondarily generalized tonic-clonic convulsions. She is more likely to have a seizure if she gets "overtired" or stressed. She has no significant risk factors for seizures. She states that at some time in her past, she "felt terrible" on higher doses of phenytoin. She confirms that she is very compliant, although she has run out of her medications more than once. Because she is having seizures, she does not drive and therefore must rely on others for transportation.

Data gathered from reviewing her seizure calendar with her and her husband suggest that she is experiencing approximately two "small" seizures per week (complex partial seizures with no secondary generalization) and one "big" seizure per month (a secondarily generalized tonic-clonic seizure). Her interview details and her overall score on her responses to the Quality of Life in Epilepsy questionnaire (QOLIE-89) show a significant impact of her seizures on her quality of life. Her scores on the energy/fatigue, pain, and social support domains are especially low in comparison to a cohort of other patients with epilepsy.

PMH
S/P hysterectomy at age 44

FH
Both parents deceased, one younger brother in good health. No seizure disorder, cancer, or cardiovascular disease.

SH
Married; retired from a local seamstress shop; denies tobacco and alcohol use; finished high school.

ROS
Tires easily, but no problem with balance

Meds
Phenytoin 100 mg po TID

All
NKDA

PE

Gen
Pleasant woman in NAD

VS
BP 126/73, P 63, RR 17, T 36.2°C; Ht 5′11″, Wt 50.8 kg

Skin
Normal color, hydration, and temperature

HEENT
Mild hirsutism, (+) gingival hyperplasia, (+) cataract left eye

Neck/LN
(–) JVD, (–) lymphadenopathy

Lungs/Thorax
CTA

Breasts
Deferred

CV
Normal S_1 and S_2, RRR, NSR, normal peripheral pulses

Abd
NTND, (+) BS, no HSM

Genit/Rect
Deferred

MS/Ext
Significant burn on right hand from seizure while cooking

Neuro
CN II–XII intact, slight lateral gaze nystagmus noted. Motor: 4/5 muscle strength on left side, 5/5 on right side. DTRs: 2+ RUE, 1+ LUE, 0 RLE, 0 LLE. Sensory: normal light touch and pin prick. Station: nl

Labs

Na 137 mEq/L	Hgb 14.5 g/dL	AST 31 IU/L
K 4.1 mEq/L	Hct 41.7%	ALT 22 IU/L
Cl 100 mEq/L	RBC 4.71 × 10^6/mm^3	Alk phos 187 IU/L
CO_2 29 mEq/L	MCV 88.6 μm^3	GGT 45 IU/L
BUN 9 mg/dL	MCHC 34.7 g/dL	Ca 7.3 mg/dL
SCr 0.6 mg/dL	Plt 212 × 10^3/mm^3	Alb 3.9 g/dL
Glu 107 mg/dL	WBC 5.4 × 10^3/mm^3	

EEG
Abnormal for bitemporal slowing, which is more significant in the left temporal region as characterized with polymorphic and epileptiform discharges consistent with a history of seizure disorder

Assessment
Uncontrolled complex partial seizures, with occasional secondary generalization

▶ Questions

Problem Identification

1. a. *Create a list of the patient's drug therapy problems.*
   b. *Which information (signs, symptoms, laboratory values) indicates the presence or severity of complex partial seizures?*

Desired Outcome

2. *What are the goals of pharmacotherapy in this case?*

Therapeutic Alternatives

3. a. *What non-drug therapies might be useful for this patient?*
   b. *What feasible pharmacotherapeutic alternatives are available for treatment of complex partial seizures in this patient?*

Optimal Plan

4. *What drug, dosage form, dose, schedule, and duration of therapy are best for this patient?*

Outcome Evaluation

5. *Which clinical and laboratory parameters are necessary to evaluate the therapy for achievement of the desired therapeutic outcome and to detect or prevent adverse effects?*

Patient Education

6. *What information should be provided to the patient to enhance adherence, ensure successful therapy, and minimize adverse effects?*

▶ Clinical Course

A collective decision was made among the health care practitioners, the patient, and her husband to add one of the new antiepileptic drugs to her current drug regimen and to see her back in two months. She was given written and verbal information on this new drug and instructed to call with any questions, problems, or concerns. She verbalized understanding. At her next visit, the patient reported that there had been an initial response to the addition of the new antiepileptic drug (i.e., fewer seizures), but then a return to two "small" seizures per week and one "big" seizure per month. There are no recent laboratory data. Her neurologic exam is unchanged.

▶ Follow-Up Questions

1. *Other than non-adherence, what are the potential explanations for this situation?*

▶ Clinical Course

Upon further questioning about adherence, the patient reports that she has not been taking her new antiepileptic drug for the last month. This was a result of having no prescription insurance coverage and financial problems at home. She was able to continue her phenytoin as directed. She is offered enrollment forms for a patient assistance program in order to obtain her medications at a reduced cost, and the need to be compliant with her medications was reemphasized. She then stated that 1 month ago she fell and broke her hip. It has healed well, but she is now more concerned about her "brittle bones."

▶ Self-Study Assignments

1. Outline a plan for assessing this patient's compliance with her medication regimen.
2. What risk factors does this patient have for osteoporosis? What interventions should be made?
3. Would switching this patient from phenytoin to carbamazepine be an appropriate alternative? If so, would Tegretol XR or Carbatrol be an appropriate dosage form?

▶ Clinical Pearl

Although epilepsy affects men and women equally, there are many women's health issues in epilepsy, including menstrual cycle influences on seizure activity, contraceptive–antiepileptic drug interactions, teratogenicity of antiepileptic drugs, and influence of treatment in postmenopausal women with epilepsy.

References

1. Wiebe S, Eliasziw M, Matijevic S. Changes in quality of life in epilepsy: How large must they be to be real? Epilepsia 2001;42:113–118.
2. Mohanraj R, Brodie MJ. Measuring the efficacy of antiepileptic drugs. Seizure 2003;12:413–443.
3. Cramer JA, Fisher R, Ben-Menachem E, et al. New antiepileptic drugs: Comparison of key clinical trials. Epilepsia 1999;40:590–600.
4. McAuley JW, Biederman T, Smith J, et al. Newer therapies in the drug treatment of epilepsy. Ann Pharmacother 2002;36:119–129.
5. Pack AM, Morrell MJ. Adverse effects of antiepileptic drugs on bone structure: Epidemiology, mechanisms and therapeutic implications. CNS Drugs 2001;15: 633–642.
6. French JA, Kanner AM, Bautista J, et al. Efficacy and tolerability of the new antiepileptic drugs II. Treatment of refractory epilepsy. Neurology 2004;62:1261–1273.

60 GENERALIZED TONIC–CLONIC SEIZURES

▶ Mrs. Johnson's Son (Level I)

Monica A. Summers, PharmD
Sharon M. Tramonte, PharmD

▶ After completing this case study, students should be able to:

- Define epilepsy.
- Differentiate seizure types based on clinical presentation and description.
- Recommend drugs of choice and alternative therapies for different types of seizures.
- Identify appropriate dosing, the most common adverse effects, and monitoring parameters for anticonvulsants.
- Develop an appropriate pharmaceutical care plan for a patient with epilepsy.

PATIENT PRESENTATION

Chief Complaint

"My son is still having a lot of seizures."

HPI

Dale Johnson is a 34 yo man brought into the epilepsy clinic for routine follow-up by his mother. He currently has two to three seizures per week. Mrs. Johnson describes her son's seizures as involving his whole body. "His arms and legs stick out and shake. Sometimes he loses control of his bladder or yells out. Then he is out of it for 10 to 15 minutes after he stops shaking."

Anticonvulsants tried in the past include primidone, phenytoin, carbamazepine, valproic acid, felbamate, gabapentin, and lamotrigine. The patient has never been seizure-free. For the last 2 years he has averaged 10 to 12 seizures per month. Monotherapy with primidone, phenytoin, carbamazepine, and valproic acid was ineffective in controlling his seizures. A combination of phenytoin and valproic acid was unsuccessful due to inability to achieve therapeutic concentrations of valproic acid. Addition of carbamazepine to valproic acid reduced the number of seizures to three to five seizures per month but valproic acid had to be discontinued because of thrombocytopenia. Addition of gabapentin and later lamotrigine did not appear to improve seizure control. It appears that carbamazepine has been the most effective anticonvulsant for this patient. However, monotherapy did not completely control his seizures. Past carbamazepine levels have been as high as 16 mcg/mL with 8 to 12 seizures/month. A summary of his medication regimen and the number of seizures per month for the last year are included in the following table:

Months Ago	Number of Seizures	Lamotrigine Oral Dose	Carbamazepine Oral Dose	Carbamazepine Plasma Conc.
11	7	200 mg BID	300 mg TID	7.4 mcg/mL
10	11	200 mg BID	300 mg TID	
9	3	200 mg BID	400 mg TID	8.6 mcg/mL
8	12	250 mg BID	400 mg TID	
7	10	250 mg BID	400 mg TID	
6	11	250 mg BID	400 mg TID	
5	10	300 mg BID	400 mg TID	
4	5	300 mg BID	400 mg TID	
3	14	300 mg BID	400 mg TID	8.5 mcg/mL
2	9	300 mg BID	400 mg TID	
1	19	350 mg BID	400 mg TID	
Current	11	350 mg BID	400 mg TID	

PMH

Birth followed a relatively normal pregnancy with no prenatal care. Delayed developmental milestones were noticed by 3 months. Dale was diagnosed with mental retardation and cerebral palsy. Seizures developed some time during infancy, but the exact time they started is unclear. PMH is also significant for scoliosis, poor feeding resulting in weight loss and subsequent PEG tube placement (5 years ago), hypothyroidism (4 years ago), and a benign colon polyp (1 year ago).

FH

Negative for seizures. Both parents are alive and in good health; mother has osteoarthritis treated with PRN NSAIDs. He has no siblings.

SH

Never attended school. Requires close supervision by family or aides hired by the family. No tobacco or EtOH use.

Meds

Levothyroxine 0.05 mg GT once daily
Multivitamins with minerals 15 mL GT once daily
Lactulose 45 mL GT BID
Carbamazepine 400 mg GT TID
Lamotrigine 350 mg GT BID
Lorazepam 2 mg IM PRN for 3 seizures in 24 hours or seizures lasting more than 5 minutes (not to exceed 3 doses/day)

All

NKDA

Adverse Drug Effect History

Primidone (excessive sedation)
Felbamate (elevated LFTs)
Valproic acid (thrombocytopenia)
Carbamazepine (hyponatremia)

PE

Gen

Exam reveals a thin 34 yo man in NAD

VS

BP 125/79, P 70, RR 12, T 37°C; Ht 5′1″, Wt 40.8 kg

HEENT

Head circumference 53 cm; atraumatic; PERRL

Neck/LN

No thyromegaly, lymphadenopathy, or carotid bruits

Chest/Lungs

Chest deformed secondary to scoliosis; left thoracic scar with depression deformity; lungs CTA

CV

RRR, no m/r/g

Abd

Soft, non-tender; no HSM; (+) BS, PEG in situ

MS/Ext

Muscles hypotonic, pulses present bilaterally

Neuro

CN II–XII intact, reflexes 1+ and symmetric throughout

Labs

Na 130 mEq/L	Hgb 13.5 g/dL	AST 21 IU/L
K 4.7 mEq/L	Hct 41%	ALT 19 IU/L
Cl 97 mEq/L	RBC 4.5 × 10^6/mm^3	T. bili 0.8 mg/dL
CO_2 25 mEq/L	WBC 5.1 × 10^3/mm^3	Alk Phos 71 IU/L
BUN 10 mg/dL	Diff WNL	GGT 136 IU/L
SCr 0.4 mg/dL	MCV 97 μm^3	TSH 0.9 mIU/L
Glu 100 mg/dL	RDW 11.6%	

EEG

Generalized background slowing and paroxysmal bihemispheric sharp-wave activity. Photic stimulation failed to produce any other changes.

Assessment

34 yo mentally retarded man with difficult-to-control seizures. His seizures have never been adequately controlled despite numerous trials of multiple anticonvulsant regimens.

Questions

Problem Identification

1. a. *What are this patient's drug therapy problems?*
   b. *What additional information is needed to fully assess the patient's problems related to epilepsy or his drug therapy?*

Desired Outcome

2. *What are the goals of pharmacotherapy in this case?*

Therapeutic Alternatives

3. a. *What nonpharmacologic interventions may be helpful for this patient?*
   b. *Given the patient's lack of success with previous antiepileptic drugs, what other pharmacotherapeutic options are available to treat his epilepsy?*

Optimal Plan

4. *What is the best pharmacotherapeutic plan for this patient?*

Outcome Evaluation

5. *Which clinical and laboratory parameters are needed to evaluate the therapy to ensure the best possible outcome?*

Patient Education

6. *What information should the patient and/or caregiver have to ensure successful therapy and to minimize adverse effects?*

Clinical Course

One month after your recommendation was taken, the patient returns to the clinic with symptoms of an upper respiratory tract infection. The physician asks for your advice on whether clarithromycin would interact with his antiepileptic drug therapy.

Follow-Up Questions

1. *What information should be given to the physician in this situation?*

Self-Study Assignments

1. Smoking can affect serum concentrations of drugs. Perform a literature search to determine why this occurs and what effect it might have on anticonvulsants.
2. Perform a literature search to identify articles that have concluded that seizure medications can be withdrawn after a certain seizure-free interval.
3. Write a concise paper outlining the current recommendations for assisting a person who is having a seizure.
4. Assume that a patient taking valproic acid has poorly controlled seizures and a decision is made to add lamotrigine. What precautions, if any, should be taken? How should you initiate lamotrigine therapy?
5. Is there a potential role for the vagus nerve stimulator (VNS) device in this patient? What information should be given to patients and caregivers who are considering this option?

Clinical Pearl

A normal EEG does not guarantee that the patient will remain seizure free; many patients with epilepsy have perfectly normal EEGs between seizures.

References

1. Commission on Classification and Terminology of the International League Against Epilepsy. Proposal for revised classification of epilepsies and epileptic syndromes. Epilepsia 1989;30:389–399.
2. Garnett WR. Antiepileptic drug treatment: Outcomes and adherence. Pharmacotherapy. 2000;20(8 Pt 2):191S–199S.
3. Biton V, Montouris GD, Ritter F, et. al. A randomized, placebo-controlled study of topiramate in primary generalized tonic-clonic seizures. Topiramate YTC Study Group. Neurology 1999;52:1330–1337.
4. Pellock JM. Important changes in the treatment of epilepsy. Pharmacotherapy 2001;21(4):517–518.
5. Topamax (topiramate) tablets [product information]. Raritan, NJ: Ortho-McNeil Pharmaceuticals, Inc; 2003.
6. Pellock JM, Morton LD. Treatment of epilepsy in the multiply handicapped. Ment Retard Dev Disabil Res Rev. 2000;6(4):309–323.

---

61 STATUS EPILEPTICUS

Not Just Another Seizure (Level I)

Monica A. Summers, PharmD
Sharon M. Tramonte, PharmD

After completing this case study, students should be able to:

- Define status epilepticus and its precipitating causes.
- Identify measures that should be taken in the ED for a patient in status epilepticus.
- Recommend appropriate drug treatment for status epilepticus.
- Recommend an appropriate pharmaceutical care plan for a patient with status epilepticus.

PATIENT PRESENTATION

Chief Complaint

As given by a friend of the patient: "About a half hour ago we were playing tennis and she cried out, fell to the ground, and started having a seizure and wet herself. I couldn't wake her up so her husband and I brought her here. She started this seizure about 10 minutes ago while we were on the way here, and it hasn't stopped."

HPI

Michelle Stillman is a 29 yo woman brought to the ED by her husband and best friend. She is non-responsive, currently exhibits tonic–clonic activity (bilateral arm and leg shaking/jerking), and has foaming saliva at her mouth. Her husband reports that he thinks she stopped taking her medication a few days ago because she hasn't had seizures in years, the side effects bother her, and she thinks she doesn't need medicine anymore.

PMH

Medical records revealed that the patient developed generalized tonic–clonic seizures in childhood. Phenobarbital was initiated and controlled the seizures for many years. Withdrawal of phenobarbital was attempted 15 years ago after several years of being seizure free. The drug was restarted when seizures occurred during the attempted taper. Phenobarbital was then replaced with carbamazepine because of sedation and lethargy. Phenytoin was added 8 years ago because of frequent and prolonged breakthrough seizures. The carbamazepine was tapered and discontinued six years ago. According to her husband, she has remained seizure-free on phenytoin monotherapy.

Six months ago, Michelle was diagnosed with moderate depression following her mother's death. Her husband and friend agree that her medication has helped her and that she is recovering well.

FH

Negative for epilepsy; the patient has five siblings, all alive and well. Both parents are deceased. No other information on family history was obtained.

SH

Married with no children; no tobacco use; "occasional glass of red wine with dinner"

Meds

Phenytoin 200 mg po BID
Escitalopram 10 mg po once daily

All

NKDA
Adverse Drug Effect History
- Phenobarbital (sedation, lethargy)
- Carbamazepine (sedation, lethargy)
- Phenytoin (mild gingival hyperplasia, mild hirsutism, acne)

PE

Gen

WDWN woman who is unarousable; clothes are wet from urinary incontinence

VS

BP 150/90, P 150, RR 25, T 37.5°C; Ht 5′3″, Wt 63.5 kg

Skin

Warm, dry and pale; nail beds are pale

HEENT

Mucous membranes are dry, mild gingival hyperplasia, mild hirsutism

Neck/LN

Supple; no thyromegaly or lymphadenopathy

Chest/Lungs

Symmetric, lungs CTA

CV

RRR, no m/r/g

Abd

Soft, no HSM, (+) BS

MS/Ext

Muscle mass normal, full ROM

Neuro

Unarousable; reflexes 3+ bilaterally

Labs

Na 136 mEq/L	Hgb 12.8 g/dL	Drug Screen: pending
K 4.5 mEq/L	Hct 38%	Phenytoin: pending
Cl 97 mEq/L	Plt 320 × 10^3/mm^3	
CO_2 28 mEq/L	WBC 9.0 × 10^3/mm^3	
BUN 16 mg/dL	Diff WNL	
SCr 1.0 mg/dL		
Glu 60 mg/dL		

EEG

Baseline from medical record (six years ago): Diffuse background slowing; no focal changes or epileptiform activity present

Assessment

29 yo woman with a history of tonic–clonic seizures now in status epilepticus

---

Questions

Problem Identification

1. a. *What are this patient's drug therapy problems?*
   b. *What steps should be taken when the patient is first seen in the ED?*

Desired Outcome

2. *What are the goals of pharmacotherapy in this case?*

Therapeutic Alternatives

3. *What pharmacotherapeutic options are available to treat status epilepticus?*

Optimal Plan

4. a. *What is the best pharmacotherapeutic plan for this patient to treat status epilepticus?*
   b. *What is the best outpatient pharmacotherapeutic plan for this patient (following hospital discharge)?*

Outcome Evaluation

5. *Which clinical and laboratory parameters are needed to evaluate the therapy to ensure the best possible outcome?*

Patient Education

6. *What information should the patient receive to ensure successful therapy and to minimize adverse effects?*

▶ Self-Study Assignments

1. There are several drug interactions with phenytoin and other antiepileptic drugs. Describe the effects that these drugs have on one another. What, if anything, should be done to compensate for these drug interactions?
2. There are sports in which patients with epilepsy should not participate. What are some of these sports, and why should these individuals not participate in them?
3. Prepare a short paper summarizing the hematologic adverse effects of all of the antiepileptic drugs.
4. Women with epilepsy who take antiepileptic drugs may consider self-discontinuing their medication when they become or want to become pregnant. Describe the potential risks to the mother and baby from antiepileptic drugs and from uncontrolled seizures. What can be done to minimize these risks?

▶ Clinical Pearl

In non-convulsive status epilepticus, it is often impossible to determine whether seizures have stopped without obtaining an EEG.

References

1. Lowenstein DH, Alldredge BK. Status epilepticus. N Engl J Med 1998;338:970–976.
2. Weise KL, Bleck TP. Status epilepticus in children and adults. Crit Care Clin 1997;13:629–646.
3. Bone RC, ed. Treatment of convulsive status epilepticus. Recommendations of the Epilepsy Foundation of America's Working Group on Status Epilepticus. JAMA 1993;270:854–859.
4. Treiman DM, Meyers PD, Walton NY, et al. A comparison of four treatments for generalized convulsive status epilepticus. Veterans Affairs Status Epilepticus Cooperative Study Group. N Engl J Med 1998;339:792–798.
5. Sinha S, Naritoku DK. Intravenous valproate is well tolerated in unstable patients with status epilepticus. Neurology 2000;55:722–724.
6. Kumar A, Bleck TP. Intravenous midazolam for the treatment of refractory status epilepticus. Crit Care Med 1992;20:483–488.
7. Dansky LV, Rosenblatt DS, Andermann E. Mechanisms of teratogenesis: Folic acid and antiepileptic therapy. Neurology 1992;42(4 Suppl 5):32–42.
8. Morrell M. Reproductive and metabolic disorders in women with epilepsy. Epilepsia 2003;44(Suppl 4):11–20.

62 ACUTE MANAGEMENT OF THE BRAIN INJURY PATIENT

▶ Bowled Over (Level III)

Denise H. Rhoney, PharmD

▶ After completing this case study, students should be able to:

- Discuss the goals of cerebral resuscitation.
- Identify parameters beneficial in assessing the severity of the brain injury.
- Discuss the therapeutic management of increased intracranial pressure.
- Recommend appropriate therapy to prevent medical complications after brain injury.

PATIENT PRESENTATION

Chief Complaint

Not available—the patient was brought in by EMS as a trauma code.

HPI

Jonathan Bowle is a 25 yo, 80-kg man who was involved in an MVA in which his car veered off the road and into a tree about 45 minutes PTA. He was not wearing a seat belt at the time of the collision. Witnesses report that he was initially lucid at the scene but has become progressively less responsive since then.

PMH

Unknown

FH

Unknown

SH

Unknown, but possible alcohol abuse

ROS

Unobtainable

Meds

Unknown

All

Unknown

PE

Gen

Well-developed male who is unresponsive with extensor posturing; heavy smell of alcohol. Mood and affect are not assessable.

VS

BP 85/55, P 140, RR 40, T 38.4°C; Wt 80 kg, Ht 6′2″

Skin

Several abrasions noted

HEENT

Inspection of conjunctivae and lids reveal bilateral periorbital ecchymoses. The left pupil is 6 mm and nonreactive and the right pupil is 3 mm and nonreactive. EOMs are not reactive and not moving. External inspection of ears and nose reveals no acute abnormalities. There is some dried blood in both nares and mouth. Internal inspection of the ears reveals evidence of hemotympanum. Battle's sign and raccoon eyes are present. The head has a 4-cm scalp laceration over the left frontal region of the skull with some swelling. Neck is in a cervical collar, therefore movement was not attempted. There is no bony step-off noted and no gross masses in the neck.

Lungs

Increased respiratory effort with retractions and rhonchi noted diffusely

Heart

Auscultation reveals a tachycardic rhythm with no abnormal sounds

Abd

Soft with no masses or tenderness but decreased bowel sounds. There is no gross HSM

Ext

No non-traumatic edema is noted

Neuro

There is no response other than extensor posturing to pain

Labs

Na 145 mEq/L	Hgb 13.4 g/dL	Ca 8.7 mg/dL	ABG
K 3.8 mEq/L	Hct 40.7%	Mg 1.2 mg/dL	pH 7.5
Cl 109 mEq/L	Plt 101 × 10^3/mm^3	Phos 1.4 mEq/L	HCO_3 18 mEq/L
CO_2 21 mEq/L	WBC 16.0 × 10^3/mm^3	Alb 2.4 g/dL	pCO_2 28 mm Hg
BUN 15 mg/dL	Diff N/A	Ethanol 312 mg/dL	pO_2 71 mm Hg
SCr 1.2 mg/dL			O_2 sat 80% on RA
Glu 235 mg/dL			

Portable Chest X-Ray

No evidence of pneumothorax, hemothorax, or rib fractures; the ET tube is above the carina

Head CT

Small, left frontal-parietal acute subdural hematoma with subarachnoid blood and a non-depressed linear skull fracture

Assessment

1. S/P MVA
2. Intracranial bleed
3. Coma
4. Respiratory distress

▶ Clinical Course

Upon arrival in the ED, IV access was initiated, and the patient was intubated orally using a rapid sequence intubation technique (10 mg IV vecuronium followed by 100 mg IV lidocaine, 2 mg IV midazolam, and 100 mg IV succinylcholine). The patient was taken to the operating room immediately for evacuation of the hematoma and ventriculostomy placement for monitoring of ICP. The patient will then be transferred to the neurotrauma unit for monitoring.

▶ Questions

Problem Identification

1. a. *Which information (signs, symptoms, laboratory values) indicates the severity of this patient's brain injury?*
   b. *What is the Glasgow coma score for this patient?*
   c. *Does this patient have any factors that may complicate assessment of the neurologic examination?*
   d. *What poor prognostic indicators does this patient exhibit?*

Desired Outcome

2. a. *What are the goals of therapy for this patient?*
   b. *What are the goals of fluid resuscitation and hemodynamic monitoring for this patient?*

Therapeutic Alternatives

3. a. *What therapeutic alternatives are available for fluid resuscitation, and which would be the most appropriate for this patient?*
   b. *What nondrug therapies may be useful in preventing or treating increased ICP?*
   c. *What pharmacotherapeutic alternatives are available for the treatment of increased ICP?*

Optimal Plan

4. a. *Develop an optimal pharmacotherapeutic plan to treat the patient's increased ICP.*
   b. *Outline a pharmacotherapeutic plan for prevention of medical complications that may occur in this patient.*

Outcome Evaluation

5. *Which monitoring parameters should be instituted to ensure efficacy and prevent toxicity for the therapy recommended for treating increased ICP?*

Patient Education

6. *What medication information should this patient receive if he is discharged on phenytoin?*

▶ Self-Study Assignments

1. Review the different types of neurologic monitoring devices that are available and how drug therapy might influence these monitoring parameters.
2. Review cerebral autoregulation in the normal brain and injured brain and discuss the potential use of hypertensive cerebral perfusion pressure as a treatment modality for increased ICP.

▶ Clinical Pearl

There are only three standards of care for severe brain injury patients: (a) use of corticosteroids is not recommended for improving outcome or reducing ICP; (b) in the absence of increased ICP, chronic prolonged hyperventilation ($Paco_2 < 25$ mm Hg) should be avoided; and (c) prophylactic use of antiepileptic drugs is not recommended for preventing late posttraumatic seizures (> 7 days).

References

1. The Brain Trauma Foundation. Early indicators of prognosis in severe traumatic brain injury. J Neurotrauma 2000;1(6–7 Pt 2):557–627.
2. Muizelaar JP, Marmarou A, Ward JD, et al. Adverse effects of prolonged hyperventilation in patients with severe head injury: A randomized clinical trial. J Neurosurg 1991;75:731–739.
3. The Brain Trauma Foundation. Guidelines for the management of severe head injury. J Neurotrauma 2000;17(6–7 Pt 1):453–556.
4. Kelly DF, Goodale DB, Williams J, et al. Propofol in the treatment of moderate and severe head injury: A randomized, prospective double-blinded pilot trial. J Neurosurg 1999;90:1042–1052.
5. Hsiang JK, Chesnut RM, Crisp CB, et al. Early, routine paralysis for intracranial pressure control in severe head injury: Is it necessary? Crit Care Med 1994;22:1471–1476.
6. Doyle JA, Davis DP, Hoyt DB. The use of hypertonic saline in the treatment of traumatic brain injury. J Trauma 2001;50:367–383.
7. Rovlias A, Kotsou S. The influence of hyperglycemia on neurological outcome in patients with severe head injury. Neurosurgery 2000;46:335–342.
8. Temkin NR, Dikmen SS, Wilensky AJ, et al. A randomized, double-blind study of phenytoin for the prevention of post-traumatic seizures. N Engl J Med 1990;323:497–502.
9. Reusser P, Gyr K, Scheidegger D, et al. Prospective endoscopic study of stress erosions and ulcers in critically ill neurosurgical patients: Current incidence and effect of acid-reducing prophylaxis. Crit Care Med 1990;18:270–274.
10. Black PM. Baker MF, Snook CP. Experience with external pneumatic calf compression in neurology and neurosurgery. Neurosurgery 1986;18:440–444.
11. Mascia L, Andrews PJ, McKeating EG, et al. Cerebral blood flow and metabolism in severe brain injury: The role of pressure autoregulation during cerebral perfusion pressure management. Intensive Care Med 2000;26:202–205.
12. Juul N, Morris GF, Marshall SB, et al. Intracranial hypertension and cerebral perfusion pressure: influence on neurological deterioration and outcome in severe head injury. The Executive Committee of the International Selfotel Trial. J Neurosurg 2000;92:1–6.

63 PARKINSON'S DISEASE

▶ On Shaky Ground (Level II)

Mary Louise Wagner, MS, PharmD
Margery H. Mark, MD

▶ After completing this case study, students should be able to:

- Recognize motor and non-motor symptoms of Parkinson's disease (PD).
- Develop an optimal pharmacotherapeutic plan for a patient with PD.
- Recommend alterations in therapy for a patient experiencing adverse drug effects.
- Educate patients with PD about the disease and its drug therapy.

PATIENT PRESENTATION

Chief Complaint

"I have trouble writing and I have no motivation."

HPI

Paul Muller is a 60-year-old right-handed man who presents to the neurology clinic because of a tremor in his right hand for the last 6 months. He also complains of stiffness on the right side. For the last year, he feels more apathetic and sad at times. He also complains of poor appetite and occasional constipation. He has trouble falling asleep and wakes up early due to excessive worrying. He reports difficulty reading because his vision seems blurry. His wife says that he kicks her during the night and that the bedding is all tangled in the morning. They both awake tired in the morning.

PMH

BPH × 4 years
Restless legs syndrome × 2 years

FH

Mother died at age 74 of complications associated with Alzheimer's disease; father died of colon cancer; two daughters and wife are alive and in good health

SH

(–) Alcohol, (–) tobacco, married for 38 years.

ROS

The patient has no complaints other than those noted in the HPI. He denies any other symptoms of autonomic dysfunction such as problems with swallowing, urination, sweating spells, drooling, or dizziness. He also denies any other psychological problems such as panic attacks, vivid dreams, hallucinations, paranoia, or memory problems.

Meds

Terazosin 1 mg po daily
Ferrous sulfate 325 mg po TID
Vitamin C 500 mg TID
Oxycodone 5 mg when RLS symptoms are bothersome (2–3 times per month)

Allergies

Shellfish (shortness of breath and rash)

PE

Gen

The patient is a Caucasian man who appears his stated age

VS

BP 118/76 sitting, 114/70 standing; P 70; RR 13; T 36.8°C; Wt 66 kg, Ht 5′8″

Skin

Small amount of dry yellow scales on forehead

HEENT

Decreased volume of speech, decreased facial expression, decreased eye blinking; PERRLA; EOMI

Neck/LN

Supple, no masses, normal thyroid, no bruits

Lungs/Thorax

Clear, Normal breath sounds, CTA

CV

RRR, no murmurs, no bruits

Abd

Soft, non-tender, no palpable masses

Genit/Rect

Enlarged prostate, but no nodules palpated; no rectal polyps

MS/Ext

Resting tremor only in right hand and foot. Mild rigidity in right arm. Decreased fine motor coordination on the right. Normal peripheral pulses and postural stability. No CCE.

Neuro

General neurologic exam intact, Folstein MMSE 30/30
Unified Parkinson's Disease Rating Scale (UPDRS):

Part 1: Mentation, Behavior, and Mood score 2/16 (Mild problems with depression and apathy but no problems with memory or behavior).

Part 2: ADL score 3/52 (Mild trouble with speech, handwriting, and tremor. No problems with salivation, swallowing, dressing, cutting food, hygiene, turning in bed, falling, freezing, walking, or sensory effects).

Part 3: Motor Exam 10/108 (Mild problems with speech, facial expression, right-sided rest tremor, rigidity in right limbs, rapid alternating movements in his right hand, and bradykinesia. No problems with leg agility, arising from a chair, posture, gait, or postural stability).

Handwriting sample: Somewhat slow and progressively smaller in size indicating signs of micrographia.

Labs

Na 136 mEq/L	Hgb 13.5 g/dL	AST 20 IU/L
K 4.3 mEq/L	Hct 30.0%	ALT 24 IU/L
Cl 101 mEq/L	RBC 4.42 × 10^6	Alk phos 80 IU/L
CO_2 23 mEq/L	WBC 5.0 × 10^3/mm^3	GGT 18 IU/L
BUN 8 mg/dL	Plt 395 × 10^3/mm^3	Ferritin 50 ng/mL
SCr 1.0 mg/dL		TSH 2.0 mIU/L
Glu 95 mg/dl		T4 total 7.5 mcg/dL

Assessment

Based on the HPI and UPDRS, the patient's symptoms are consistent with early, mild Parkinson's disease. His other medical conditions are stable.

▶ Questions

Problem Identification

1. a. *Create a list of the patient's drug-related problems.*
   b. *What signs and symptoms of PD are present in this patient?*
   c. *According to the Hoehn–Yahr Scale, what stage is his disease?*

Desired Outcome

2. *What are the goals of therapy for PD?*

Therapeutic Alternatives

3. a. *What nonpharmacologic alternatives may be beneficial for the treatment of PD in this patient?*
   b. *Based on the patient's signs and symptoms, what pharmacotherapeutic alternatives are viable options for him at this time?*

Optimal Plan

4. *What drug, dosage form, dose, schedule, and duration of therapy are best for this patient?*

Outcome Evaluation

5. *Which monitoring parameters should be used to evaluate the patient's response to medications and to detect adverse effects?*

Patient Education

6. *How would you educate this patient to ensure successful therapy, enhance compliance, and minimize adverse effects?*

▶ Clinical Course

Seven years later, the patient returns to the neurology clinic for a routine follow-up visit. He feels that he has good and bad days, but overall his PD medications don't last as long as they used to. All his medications are the same as the initial visit except now he is also taking pramipexole 1 mg po TID (for 7 years) and carbidopa/levodopa 25/100 TID (for 3 years). He takes both medications with meals (7:00 a.m., noon, and 6:00 p.m.).

His symptoms are now bilateral. He reports that he is fine until his noon dose; around 4:00 p.m., he has a 2-hour off period. His 6:00 PM dinner dose has a delayed onset. He is afraid to drive because he heard that pramipexole causes sleep attacks. His UPDRS scores while "on" are: Mood 3, ADL 12, and Motor 33. Generally, his depression has remained the same with increased episodes during prolonged off periods. He now reports mild intellectual impairment, as he is more forgetful (MMSE 27/30). He is less able to handle activities of daily living as handwriting is more difficult and his tremor is more bothersome. He also now reports that he is slower and clumsier in almost all activities but especially when driving, handling utensils, dressing, shaving, turning in bed, and getting out of a chair. He now has some difficulty walking and reports some mild body aches. He still has good postural stability without falls. He also reports no difficulties with autonomic symptoms. His neurologist decides to change each Sinemet® dose to two Stalevo® tablets (each tablet contains carbidopa 37.5 mg, levodopa 150 mg, and entacapone 200 mg) TID.

Four days later, the patient's wife calls the neurologist complaining that her husband has nausea and vomiting. He has jerky movements of his face, shoulders, and hips that last for about 2 hours after each dose. He also has been unable to sleep due to severe nightmares awakening him during the night. She admits that her husband is experiencing less wearing-off periods and is able to move around with greater ease. She does report an improvement in his mood, so much so, that "he dances around the house with his imaginary friend."

▶ Follow-Up Questions:

1. *What side effects of therapy does the patient now manifest?*
2. *What adjustments in drug therapy do you recommend at this time?*
3. *What new patient education should be provided to the patient?*

▶ Self-Study Assignments

1. Evaluate the use of apomorphine in the treatment of PD.
2. Evaluate the use of liquid Sinemet in the treatment of PD.
3. Investigate the use of over-the-counter medications in the treatment of PD.

▶ Clinical Pearl

As Parkinson's disease progresses, the timing of medications needs to coincide with symptoms. Evaluate the onset and duration of each dose and make dose modifications accordingly. Patient symptoms may worsen when they are forced to receive their medications at predetermined dosing times such as those used in hospitals and nursing homes. Thus, let the patient's symptoms guide the dosing times.

References

1. Olanow CW, Watts RL, Koller WC. An algorithm (decision tree) for the management of Parkinson's disease (2001): treatment guidelines. Neurology 2001; 56(11 Suppl 5):S1–S88.
2. Berchou RC. Maximizing the benefit of pharmacotherapy in Parkinson's disease. Pharmacotherapy 2000:20(1 pt 2):33S–42S.
3. Olanow CW. The role of dopamine agonists in the treatment of early Parkinson's disease. Neurology 2002;58(4 Suppl 1):S33–S41.
4. Clarke CE, Guttman M. Dopamine agonist monotherapy in Parkinson's disease. Lancet 2002;360:1767–1769.
5. Van Camp G, Flamez A, Cosyns B, et al. Heart valvular disease in patients with Parkinson's disease treated with high-dose pergolide. Neurology 2003;61: 859–861.
6. Dewey RB, Baseman DG, OSuilleabhain PE, et al. Chronic treatment with pergolide for Parkinson's disease is associated with significant cardiac valve regurgitation. Neurology 2004;62(Suppl 5):A331–A332.
7. Paus S, Brecht HM, Koster J, et al. Sleep attacks, daytime sleepiness, and dopamine agonists in Parkinson's disease. Mov Disord 2003;18:659–667.
8. Arnulf I, Konofal E, Merino-Andreu M, et al. Parkinson's disease and sleepiness: an integral part of PD. Neurology 2002;58:1019–1024.
9. Nieves AV, Lang AE. Treatment of excessive daytime sleepiness in patients with Parkinson's disease with modafinil. Clin Neuropharmacol 2002;25:111–114.
10. Driver-Dunckley E, Samanta J, Stacy M. Pathological gambling associated with dopamine agonist therapy in Parkinson's disease. Neurology 2003;61:422–423.
11. Schapira A, Obeso J, Olanow CW. The place of COMT inhibitors in the armamentarium of drugs for the treatment of Parkinson's disease. Neurology 2000:55(11 Suppl 4):S65–S71.
12. Metman LV, Del Dotto P, LePoole K, et al. Amantadine for levodopa-induced dyskinesias: a 1-year follow-up study. Arch Neurol 1999;56:1383–1386.
13. Miller JW, Selhub J, Nadeau MR, et al. Effect of L-dopa on plasma homocysteine in PD patients: relationship to B-vitamin status. Neurology 2003;60:1125–1129.
14. Rogers JD, Sanchez-Saffon A, Frol AB, et al. Elevated plasma homocysteine levels in patients treated with levodopa: association with vascular disease. Arch Neurol 2003;60:59–64.
15. Goetz CG, Blasucci L, Stebbins GT. Switching dopamine agonists in advanced Parkinson's disease: is rapid titration preferable to slow? Neurology 1999;52: 1227–1229.
16. Lang AE. Clinical rating scales and videotape analysis. In: Koller WC, Paulson G, eds. Therapy of Parkinson's Disease, 2nd ed. New York, Marcel Dekker, 1995: 21–46.
17. Fernandez HH, Trieschmann ME, Friedman JH. Treatment of psychosis in Parkinson's disease: safety considerations. Drug Saf 2003;26:643–659.

64 PAIN MANAGEMENT

▶ Oh, My Aching Back! (Level II)

Christine K. O'Neil, PharmD, BCPS

▶ After completing this case study, students should be able to:

- Define the goals for pain management in a patient with chronic non-malignant pain.

- Define a pharmacotherapeutic pain management plan.
- Understand the use of NSAIDs, other non-opioids, and opioid analgesics in the treatment of chronic non-malignant pain.
- Establish monitoring parameters for safety and efficacy when managing analgesic therapy.

PATIENT PRESENTATION

Chief Complaint
"I have a constant pain in my lower back with occasional tingling in my left leg. Can I take more Percodan?"

HPI
Mary Miller is a 78 yo woman who has had a history of lower back pain since an automobile accident 10 years ago. Details regarding the accident are limited, but the patient reported that she had an operation (laminectomy) to relieve the pain shortly after the accident. Records were unclear as to whether she had a herniated or ruptured disc. She has tried numerous pain therapies including local anesthetic injections and a TENS unit without relief.

PMH
Type 2 diabetes mellitus × 8 years
HTN × 15 years
Lymphedema of legs and arms
Sciatica on the left side × 20 years
Insomnia
Depression
History of "heart attack" per patient report (no records available)

SH
Lives at home with her husband. She is very sedentary, remaining in bed or a chair for most of the day. She does not smoke and denies alcohol use.

FH
Non-contributory

Meds
Lanoxin 0.125 mg po once daily
Atenolol 25 mg po every other day
Aspirin 325 mg po once daily
Maxzide 25/50 po once daily
OsCal 500 mg po BID
Humulin 70/30 30 units Q AM and 40 units Q PM (previously on glyburide)
Zoloft 75 mg po at bedtime
Percodan 2 tablets Q 6 H
Halcion 0.25 mg po at bedtime

All
Meperidine → bronchospasm, hives; PCN → allergy as a child; flurbiprofen → GI intolerance

ROS
Positive for moderate to severe lower back pain with tingling in the left leg. No other complaints.

PE

Gen
Patient is a 78 yo woman with no signs of discomfort

VS
BP 104/72, P 72, RR 15, T 37.4°C, Wt 68 kg, Ht 5′0″

HEENT
PERRLA, EOMI, TMs intact

Neck
Supple, no JVD, no bruits

Resp
CTA & P; no crackles or wheezes

Thorax
Localized kyphosis with an exaggerated lordosis of the lumbar spine. Tenderness to palpation of the low lumbar region. Flexion of the lumbosacral spine was 60 degrees with 0 degrees of lumbar extension. Lateral bend to the right and left and trunk rotation was limited.

CV
NSR without m/r/g

Breasts
Negative

Abd
Soft, NT, liver and spleen not palpable, (+) BS

Genit/Rect
Heme (–) stool, other exam deferred

Ext
Lymphedema of the arms and thighs. Wide-based gait. Hips with full range of motion. Toe and heel walk were difficult to perform.

Neuro
A & O × 3; knee jerk was 2+ bilaterally; ankle jerk diminished on the left side; straight leg raising test in the seated and supine position were normal. Sensation was intact.

Labs

Na 144 mEq/L	CBC & diff: WNL	AST 30 IU/L
K 3.9 mEq/L	HbA_{1c} 9.1%	ALT 15 IU/L
Cl 103 mEq/L	Ca 9.8 mg/dL	Alk phos 182 IU/L
CO_2 31 mEq/L	T. bili 0.2 mg/dL	
BUN 16 mg/dL	T. prot 8.1 g/dL	
SCr 1.6 mg/dL	Alb 3.8 g/dL	
Glu 53 mg/dL (fasting)		

MRI of spine

Slight degenerative disc disease; no evidence of spinal stenosis or herniated disc

DEXA Scan

Lumbar spine T score: −3.73
Left hip T score: −3.57

Assessment

1. Chronic moderate to severe lower back pain related to a past automobile accident with increasing requests for pain control
2. Poorly-controlled diabetes
3. Osteoporosis, currently untreated; will start alendronate
4. Lymphedema of the arms and thighs
5. Hx HTN, insomnia, depression, and questionable MI

Questions

Problem Identification

1. a. *Create a list of the patient's drug therapy problems.*
   b. *Which information indicates the presence or severity of chronic non-malignant pain?*
   c. *Could any of the patient's problems have been caused by drug therapy?*
   d. *What additional information is needed to satisfactorily assess this patient's pain?*

Desired Outcome

2. *What are the goals of pharmacotherapy in this case?*

Therapeutic Alternatives

3. a. *What nondrug therapies might be useful for this patient?*
   b. *Compare the pharmacotherapeutic alternatives available for treatment of this patient's pain.*

Optimal Plan

4. a. *What drug, dosage, form, schedule, and duration of therapy are best for treating this patient's pain?*
   b. *What alternatives would be appropriate if the initial therapy fails or cannot be used?*

Outcome Evaluation

5. *Which clinical and laboratory parameters are necessary to evaluate the therapy for achievement of the desired therapeutic outcome and to detect or prevent adverse effects?*

Patient Education

6. *What information should be provided to the patient to enhance compliance, ensure successful therapy, and minimize adverse effects?*

Clinical Course

The physician accepted your initial plan of care. At her 2-week follow-up appointment the patient complained of minimal pain relief and worsening of her edema. She describes her pain as a 7 on scale of 1 to 10. She was also very resistant to reducing the dose of Percodan. She stated that she was sleeping better since starting the antidepressant. She complained of headache since starting the alendronate and expressed concerns about continuing this treatment.

Follow-Up Questions

1. *How would you alter your treatment plan for this patient?*

Additional Case Questions

1. *What drug therapy suggestions could be made to optimize this patient's antihypertensive regimen?*
2. *If this patient were to require a surgical procedure, what would be your general recommendations for postoperative pain management?*
3. *What changes or additions to her diabetes regimen would you suggest?*

Self-Study Assignments

1. Prepare a list of opioids and their corresponding equianalgesic dosing.
2. Prepare a set of guidelines for the management of chronic malignant/cancer pain.

Clinical Pearl

Antidepressants, particularly tricyclic antidepressants, are effective first-line therapy for neuropathic pain.

References

1. Agency for Health Care Policy and Research. Management of cancer pain: Adults. Am J Hosp Pharm 1994;51:1643–1656.
2. Portenoy RK. Opioid therapy for chronic nonmalignant pain: A review of critical issues. J Pain Symptom Manage 1996;11(4):203–217.
3. McCarberg BH, Barkin RL. Long-acting opioids for chronic pain: Pharmacotherapeutic opportunities to enhance compliance, quality of life, and analgesia. Am J Ther 2001;8:181–186.
4. Rowbotham MC, Twilling L, Davies PS, et al. Oral opioid therapy for chronic peripheral and central neuropathic pain. N Engl J Med 2003;348;1223–1232.
5. Ripamonti C, Groff L, Brunelli C, et al. Switching from morphine to oral methadone in treating cancer pain: What is the equianalgesic dose ratio? J Clin Oncol 1998;16:3216–3221.
6. Ahmad M. Goucke CR. Management strategies for the treatment of neuropathic pain in the elderly. Drugs Aging 2002;19:929–945.
7. Ansari A. The efficacy of newer antidepressants in the treatment of chronic pain: A review of current literature. Harv Rev Psychiatry 2000;7(5):257–277.
8. Gammaitoni AR, Alvarez NA, Galer BS. Safety and tolerability of the lidocaine patch 5%, a targeted peripheral analgesic: A review of the literature. J Clin Pharmacol 2003:43:111–117.

65 HEADACHE DISORDERS

► The Migraineur (Level II)

Tejal Patel, PharmD
Susan R. Winkler, PharmD, BCPS

► After completing this case study, students should be able to:

- Develop pharmacotherapeutic goals for the treatment and prevention of migraine headaches.
- Make recommendations regarding pharmacotherapeutic regimens for an individual patient based on information concerning the patient's headache type and severity, medical history, previous drug therapy, concomitant problems, and pertinent laboratory data.
- Provide education to patients on the use of abortive and prophylactic agents for migraine headaches.
- Describe the appropriate use of a headache diary and how it may be used to refine headache treatment.

PATIENT PRESENTATION

Chief Complaint

"This new medication is not working for my headaches."

HPI

Caroline Parker is a 36 yo woman who presents to the Neurology Clinic for follow-up of migraine headaches. She states that she used to get about two migraines every month; however, she recently got divorced and started a new job. Since then, the frequency of her migraines has increased to about four to five per month. She states her migraines usually occur in the morning, and there is no identifiable relationship with her menses. Her typical headache evolves quickly (within 1 hour) and involves severe throbbing pain, which is unilateral and temporal in distribution and preceded by an aura, which consists of nausea and pastel lights flashing throughout her visual field. It frequently involves photophobia as well. Vomiting may occur with an extreme headache. If untreated, the migraine attacks last from 7 to 72 hours. She typically has to retreat to a dark room and avoid any noise, or the severity of the migraine increases. She rates her migraines as 7 to 8 on a headache scale of 1 to 10, with 10 being the worst. At her previous visit to the Neurology Clinic two months ago, she was prescribed sumatriptan 50 mg po to be taken at the onset of headache. However, sumatriptan has not been effective for five of the seven migraines she has had in the last two months. During two of the attacks, she experienced partial pain relief, with the pain returning later in the day. She mentions that she was prescribed sumatriptan when the Cafergot she was taking stopped working. She states she has taken her medications exactly as advised. She prefers to use medications that can be taken orally.

PMH

Migraine with aura since age 33; previous medical work-up, including an EEG and a head MRI, demonstrated no PVD, CVA, brain tumor, infection, cerebral aneurysm, or epileptic component. Drug therapies have included the following.

Abortive therapies

1. Simple analgesics, NSAIDs, and Cafergot (good efficacy until two months ago)
2. Narcotics (good efficacy, but puts her "out of commission for days")
3. Midrin (no efficacy)
4. Sumatriptan (minimal efficacy)

Prophylactic therapies

1. Amitriptyline 50 mg at bedtime (increased daytime drowsiness with no reduction in migraine frequency or severity; discontinued several months ago)
2. Propranolol 20 mg BID (increased episodes of dizziness and light-headedness; patient self-discontinued medication)

Other medical problems include chronic mild depression for 8 months.

FH

Positive for migraines (both parents); hypertension and type 2 diabetes (mother).

SH

Secretary. Recently divorced; mother of two boys, ages 6 and 9. Denies tobacco or alcohol use. Occasional caffeine intake.

ROS

Complains of increased frequency of headaches starting about 6 months ago and limited efficacy with sumatriptan; no nausea, vomiting, diarrhea, or flashing lights at present.

Meds

Sumatriptan 50 mg tablets, 1 tablet po at onset of migraine, repeat dose of 50 mg po in 2 hours if partial response or if headache returns. Maximum dose 200 mg (4 tablets per 24 hours).
Metoclopramide 10 mg po at onset of migraine
Sertraline 50 mg po at bedtime

All

NKDA

PE

Gen

WDWN woman in mild distress

VS

BP 132/86, HR 76, RR 18, T 37.2°C; Ht 5′0″, Wt 70 kg

Skin

Normal skin turgor; no diaphoresis

HEENT

PERRLA; EOMI; no funduscopic exam performed

Neck

Supple; no masses, thyroid enlargement, adenopathy, bruits, or JVD

Chest

Good breath sounds bilaterally; clear to A & P

CV

RRR, S_1, S_2 normal, no m/r/g

Abd

Soft, NT/ND, no hepatosplenomegaly, (+) BS

Genit/Rect

Deferred

MS/Ext

UE/LE strength 5/5 with normal tone; radial and femoral pulses 3 bilaterally; no edema; no evidence of thrombophlebitis; full ROM

Neuro

A & O × 3; no dysarthria or aphasia; memory intact; no nystagmus; no fasciculations, tremor, or ataxia; (–) Romberg; CN II–XII intact; sensory intact; DTRs 2+ throughout; Babinski (–) bilaterally

Labs

Na 138 mEq/L	Hgb 13 g/dL	AST 23 IU/L
K 4.5 mEq/L	Hct 40%	ALT 25 IU/L
Cl 101 mEq/L	Plt 302 × 10^3/mm^3	Alk Phos 35 IU/L
CO_2 23 mEq/L	WBC 8 × 10^3/mm^3	Urine pregnancy test (–)
BUN 8 mg/dL	Differential WNL	
SCr 0.6 mg/dL		
Glu 95 mg/dL		

Assessment

1. Increase in frequency of migraines related to an increase in stress
2. Minimal efficacy of sumatriptan 50 mg po as an abortive treatment
3. Previous prophylactic treatments have been unsuccessful

▶ Questions

Problem Identification

1. a. *Create a list of the patient's drug therapy problems at this clinic visit.*
   b. *What clinical information is consistent with a diagnosis of migraines in this patient?*
   c. *Could any of the patient's problems have been caused or exacerbated by her drug therapy?*

Desired Outcomes

2. *What are the goals of therapy for this patient?*

Therapeutic Alternatives

3. a. *What pharmacotherapeutic alternatives are available for treatment of the patient's nausea, and how will they impact potential abortive therapies?*
   b. *What pharmacotherapeutic alternatives are available for the abortive treatment of this patient's migraine attacks?*
   c. *What pharmacotherapeutic alternatives are available for prophylaxis of this patient's migraine attacks?*

Optimal Plan

4. a. *Considering this patient's past successes and failures in treating her migraine attacks, design an optimal pharmacotherapeutic plan for aborting her migraine headaches.*
   b. *Design an optimal pharmacotherapeutic plan for prophylaxis of her migraine headaches.*

Outcome Evaluation

5. *Which clinical and/or laboratory parameters should be assessed regularly to evaluate the therapy for achievement of the desired therapeutic outcome and to detect or prevent adverse effects?*

Patient Education

6. *What information should be provided to the patient regarding her new abortive and prophylactic therapies?*

▶ Follow-Up Questions

1. *Describe how a headache diary could help the treatment of this patient's migraine headaches (see Figure 65–1).*

▶ Self-Study Assignments

1. Review the literature regarding intravenous agents (e.g., dihydroergotamine, valproate sodium) that are used for aborting migraines.
2. Familiarize yourself with different strategies (stratified and step-care) used in the treatment of migraine.
3. Prepare a report highlighting antiepileptic drugs used for the prophylaxis of migraines.

▶ Clinical Pearl

Migraines are three times more prevalent in women and are associated with estrogen levels. Sixty percent of women migraineurs report menstrually associated migraines, and 7% to 14% have migraines exclusively with menses.

References

1. Mannix LK. Relieving migraine pain: sorting through the options. Cleve Clin J Med 2003;70:8–28.
2. Eadie MJ. Clinically significant drug interactions with agents specific for migraine attacks. CNS Drugs 2001;15:105–118.
3. Tepper SJ. Drug interactions and the triptans. CNS News 2001;3:43–46.

Name: ________________ **Month:** __________ **Year:** __________

Date of Headache														
Headache Intensity														
Excruciating pain	10	10	10	10	10	10	10	10	10	10	10	10	10	10
	9	9	9	9	9	9	9	9	9	9	9	9	9	9
Severe pain	8	8	8	8	8	8	8	8	8	8	8	8	8	8
	7	7	7	7	7	7	7	7	7	7	7	7	7	7
Severe pain	6	6	6	6	6	6	6	6	6	6	6	6	6	6
	5	5	5	5	5	5	5	5	5	5	5	5	5	5
Moderate pain	4	4	4	4	4	4	4	4	4	4	4	4	4	4
	3	3	3	3	3	3	3	3	3	3	3	3	3	3
Mild pain	2	2	2	2	2	2	2	2	2	2	2	2	2	2
Aura only	1	1	1	1	1	1	1	1	1	1	1	1	1	1
Headache Duration (hours)														
Level of Disability														
Hospitalized														
Treatment by healthcare professional														
Bedrest required														
Decrease in activity by 50%														
Decrease in activity by 25%														
Normal activity														
Other (comment below)														
Associated Symptoms														
Nausea														
Vomiting														
Visual disturbances														
Menstrual period														
Neurological														
Other (comment below)														
Medications Taken														
1.														
2.														
3.														
4.														
5.														
Treatment Results														
Complete relief														
75% relief														
50% relief														
25% relief														
No relief														
Other (comment below)														
General Comments														

Note: A normal diary includes space to record a full month of headache activity. This form has been truncated for space purposes.

Figure 65–1. A headache diary.

4. Snow V, Weiss K, Wall EM, et al. Pharmacologic management of acute attacks of migraine and prevention of migraine headache. Ann Intern Med 2002;137:840–849.
5. Goadsby PJ, Lipton RB, Ferrari MD. Migraine – Current understanding and treatment. N Engl J Med 2002;346:257–270.
6. Ferrari MD, Roon KI, Lipton RB, et al. Oral triptans (serotonin 5–HT 1B/1D agonists) in acute migraine treatment: A meta-analysis of 53 trials. Lancet 2001;358:1668–1675.
7. Edwards KR, Glantz MJ, Norton A, et al. Prophylactic treatment of episodic migraine with topiramate: A double-blind, placebo-controlled trial in 30 patients. Cephalalgia 2000;20:316. Abstract.
8. Storey JR, Calder CS, Hart DE, et al. Topiramate in migraine prevention: A double-blind, placebo-controlled study. Headache 2001;41:968–975.
9. Mathew NT, Schmitt J, Jacobs D, et al. Topiramate in migraine prevention (MIGR-001): Effect on migraine frequency. Neurology 2003;60(Suppl 1):A336. Abstract.
10. Brandes JL, Jacobs D, Neto W, et al. Topiramate in the prevention of migraine headache: A randomized, double-blinded, placebo-controlled, parallel study (MIGR-002). Neurology 2003;60(Suppl 1):A238. Abstract.
11. Silberstein SD. Practice parameter: Evidence-based guidelines for migraine headache (an evidence-based review): Report of the Quality Standards Subcommittee of the American Academy of Neurology. Neurology 2000;55:754–762.

SECTION 7

Psychiatric Disorders

66 ATTENTION-DEFICIT HYPERACTIVITY DISORDER

▶ Bouncing Off the Walls (Level I)

William H. Benefield, Jr., PharmD, BCPP, FASCP

▶ After completing this case study, students should be able to:

- Identify the target symptoms of attention-deficit hyperactivity disorder (ADHD).
- Describe the advantages and limitations of the therapeutics options available for the treatment of ADHD
- Recommend appropriate therapeutic plans for patients with ADHD.
- Perform patient assessment to determine the effectiveness of ADHD pharmacotherapy and identify major side effects.

PATIENT PRESENTATION

Chief Complaint

"He never listens to me and just won't sit still!"

HPI

Timothy Johnson is a 5-year-old boy who presents to psychiatry clinic with his mother. She states that over the last several months Timothy has been having more hyperactive, impulsive behavior and he always seems to be "on the go." Teachers complain that he does not listen to them, does not follow instructions like the other kids, gets bored during activities, does not wait his turn, and has difficulty engaging in games for longer periods of time. During the interview you find out that Timothy's behavior has been so severe that Ms. Johnson has not been able to find a day care center that will accept him. This is a major concern because she works outside the home and has not been able to return to work as a paralegal. Timothy is moving constantly, will not sit still, is easily distracted by noise, and interrupts you and his mother repeatedly.

PMH

No previous psychiatric history; medical history is insignificant except for complex partial seizures that are well controlled. Mother had a normal pregnancy and delivery. Vaccinations are up to date.

FH

Both his father and paternal uncle have a history of hyperactivity during childhood and were diagnosed with ADHD. His mother has migraine headaches. Both mother and aunt suffered from febrile seizures as infants.

SH

Lives with sister and both parents in an upper middle-class suburb

ROS

Occasional GI upset

Meds

Carbamazepine "chewtabs" 100 mg po Q AM and 200 mg po at bedtime
Hydroxyzine 25 mg po PRN for "allergies"

All

Cats and dust mites cause sneezing and rhinorrhea. Sulfa drugs resulted in a rash.

Limited PE

Gen

He is a healthy-appearing, well-nourished boy

VS

BP 110/60, P 62; Wt 16.8 kg (within the 50th and 75th percentile, Ht 3′7″ (within the 25th and 50th percentile)

Labs

Na 130 mEq/L	Hgb 14.2 g/dL	AST 33 IU/L	Cl 106 mEq/L	WBC 12.0 × 103/mm^3	Alk Phos 5.3 mg/dL
K 3.8 mEq/L	Hct 44.7%	ALT 24 IU/L	CO_2 23 mEq/L	Neutros 64%	T. bili 0.8 mg/dL
			BUN 18 mg/dL	Lymphs 25%	Carbamazepine 7.8 mcg/mL
			SCr 1.0 mg/dL	Monos 8%	
			Glu 103 mg/dL	Eos 2%	
				Baso 1%	
				Platelets 256 × 10^3/mm^3	

Assessment

ADHD

▶ Questions

Problem Identification

1. a. *Create a list of the patient's drug therapy problems.*
   b. *Which information (signs, symptoms, laboratory values) indicates the presence or severity of ADHD?*

Desired Outcome

2. *What are the goals of nondrug and drug therapy in this case?*

Therapeutic Alternatives

3. a. *What nondrug therapies might be useful for this patient?*
   b. *What feasible pharmacotherapeutic approaches are available for treatment of ADHD in this patient?*

Optimal Plan

4. a. *What drug, dosage form, dose, schedule, and duration of therapy are best for this patient?*
   b. *What alternatives would be appropriate if the initial therapy fails or cannot be used?*

Outcome Evaluation

5. *Which clinical and laboratory parameters are necessary to evaluate the therapy for achievement of the desired therapeutic outcome and to detect or prevent adverse effects?*

Patient Education

6. *What information should be provided to the patient's mother to enhance compliance, ensure successful therapy, and minimize adverse effects?*

▶ Clinical Course

Timothy returns to the clinic 2 weeks later and is taking methylphenidate 5 mg po Q AM. Mom reports that he is improved during the morning hours but his behavior starts to worsen after lunch. Timothy has had no problems with his appetite and is sleeping well at night. No tics are present or reported. He has been seizure-free.

▶ Follow-Up Question

1. *Given this new information, what interventions, if any, would you recommend at this time?*

▶ Self-Study Assignments

1. Perform a literature search and write a brief paper related to the concerns about growth suppression in children taking stimulants for ADHD.
2. Perform a literature search and compose a paper on the effects of stimulants on seizure threshold.
3. What is the role of pemoline in the treatment of ADHD?
4. Are serotonin-selective reuptake inhibitors (SSRIs) effective for ADHD symptoms?
5. Which herbal therapies have been studied in ADHD, and what have the results shown? Are any dietary therapies effective for treating ADHD?
6. What drug may is most likely responsible for his hyponatremia?

References

1. Spencer T, Biederman J, Wilens T, et al. Pharmacotherapy of attention-deficit hyperactivity disorder across the life cycle. J Am Acad Child Adolesc Psychiatry 1996;35:409–432.
2. Clinical Practice Guideline: Diagnosis and evaluation of the child with attention-deficit/hyperactivity disorder. American Academy of Pediatrics. Pediatrics 2000;105:1158–1170.
3. Pliszka SR, Greenhill LL, Crismon ML et al. The Texas Children's Medication Algorithm Project: Report of the Texas Consensus Conference Panel on Medication Treatment of Childhood Attention-Deficit/Hyperactivity Disorder. Part II. Tactics. Attention-Deficit/Hyperactivity Disorder. J Am Acad Child Adolesc Psychiatry 2000;39:920–927.
4. Kratochvil CJ, Heiligenstein JH, Dittmann R, et al. Atomoxetine and methylphenidate treatment in children with ADHD: A prospective, randomized, open-label trial. J Am Acad Child Adolesc Psychiatry 2002;41:776–784.
5. Popper CW. Antidepressants in the treatment of attention-deficit/hyperactivity disorder. J Clin Psychiatry 1997;58(Suppl 14):14–29.

67 EATING DISORDERS: ANOREXIA NERVOSA

▶ Sweet Sixteen (Level I)

Libby S. Schindler, PharmD, BCPP

▶ After completing this case study, students should be able to:

- Identify specific factors that differentiate anorexia nervosa from bulimia nervosa.
- Describe physiologic symptoms that may be associated with anorexia nervosa.
- Describe secondary medical complications that may occur as a consequence of the starvation activities associated with anorexia nervosa.
- Develop a treatment plan that addresses selection of psychotherapy and pharmacotherapy, defining patient goals, and monitoring for achievement of the desired outcome.

PATIENT PRESENTATION

Chief Complaint

"I am tired of being fat and tired all the time."

HPI

Jennifer Carter is a 16 yo young woman who is in 11th grade at Epperson High School. This is her first visit to the Eating Disorder Clinic (EDC). She was referred to the EDC by her family physician, who had seen her for amenorrhea that has lasted for several months. When she was younger she was of normal height and weight and ate freely from all food groups. Her parents both work full time and she is frequently responsible for preparing meals for her siblings. At the age of 12 she was 5′5″ tall, weighed between 56.7 and 58 kg, and entered menarche. At that time, she did not feel that she was overweight but recalls her father teasing her about her "baby fat." At her mother's urging, she tried out for and made the cheerleading squad at her Junior High School. At the age of 14 she weighed 61.7 kg (her highest weight) and began to run cross-country and track on the High School JV team. Two years ago she attended a "healthy eating" seminar after school, sponsored by the High School. She began to prepare family meals using low-fat diets she found on the Internet. By spring break, about 4 months later, her weight had dropped to 54.9 kg.

That summer, she began to restrict her food intake (eating only half-portions of any food) and felt that she needed to lose several more pounds before HS cheerleading try-outs, but would not define the exact number. Because of her family's hectic schedules, meals were rarely eaten together and she was able to skip meals. The family has a membership at a local gym enabling her to exercise significantly everyday. She would spend an hour lifting weights, then spend another hour and one-half on one of the cardio machines. This was in addition to the daily runs she does for track.

She admits to taking a diet supplement, Metabolife, in the past. She felt like it gave her more energy and helped her not feel hungry. She stopped taking it when it became "Ephedra Free," stating that it didn't work like it did before. The last time she took any was about a year ago. She denies using any laxatives or ipecac. She denies any forced vomiting. Both parents state that they have noticed that she has seemed anxious, irritable and withdrawn, rarely going out with friends from school. They state that this behavior is not like her. They describe her as meticulous with schoolwork and housework; that she always does what is expected of her (e.g., looking out for her brothers). Jennifer denies having any suicidal ideation.

PMH

Negative for surgeries or hospitalizations
Negative for serious injuries or bone fractures
Chickenpox at the age of 6

FH

Oldest child of three siblings, the only daughter. Her father is a lawyer, her mother works in public relations for a local record label. Mother was treated for depression with fluoxetine for 1 year 3 years ago. Maternal grandmother has been diagnosed with depression; her paternal grandfather is an alcoholic.

SH

An "A/B" student, would like to be a lawyer like dad, "that would make him proud of me." Active in student activities, including track and cheerleading; and was a class officer on the student council last year. Denies use of tobacco, alcohol, or illicit substances.

ROS

She complains of dizziness and difficulty concentrating. She states that sometimes her bones ache when she exercises. No history of seizures. She reports a decrease in appetite and energy and has felt fatigued over the last 2 to 3 weeks. She has no c/o epigastric or abdominal pain. She usually has a bowel movement every other day, but admits that she has not had one in a week. She has intolerance to cold. Her last menses was 7 months ago. She denies any sexual activity.

Meds

No prescribed medications
Daily OTC multivitamin

All

NKDA

PE

Gen

The patient is a cooperative, pleasant, young female. She is dressed in a loose sweater and jeans and behaves like she is cold. Appears to be low weight. Easily engaged in conversation. She is not guarded in responses, and makes occasional eye contact with interviewer. Answers all questions in a low quiet voice. No odd or inappropriate motor behavior.

VS

BP 104/78, P 55, RR 16, T 36.6°C; Ht 5′6″, Wt 47 kg (lowest to date)

Skin
Dry, some scaling; negative for rashes; skin tone normal in color; acne on forehead; no hirsutism.

HEENT
PERRLA; EOMI; TMs intact; teeth show no signs of erosion; throat without erythema or soreness. Hair is thin and dry

Neck/LN
Neck supple without lymphadenopathy or thyromegaly

Breasts
Normal without masses

CV
Heart RRR, no m/r/g

Abd
Soft, NT, hypoactive bowel sounds, no organomegaly

Genit/Rect
Refused exam

MS/Ext
No CCE; range of motion intact; good peripheral pulses bilaterally

Neuro
A & O × 3; CN II–XII intact; DTRs 2+ throughout; Babinski (–)

Labs

Na 144 mEq/L	Hgb 13.0 g/dL	AST 17 IU/L
K 4.8 mEq/L	Hct 39%	ALT 23 IU/L
Cl 104 mEq/L	Plt 200 × 10^3/mm^3	Alk phos 51 IU/L
CO_2 24 mEq/L	WBC 5.0 × 10^3/mm^3	GGT 20 IU/L
BUN 7 mg/dL	Ca 10.5 mg/dL	TSH 1.834 mIU/L
SCr 0.9 mg/dL	Mg 1.4 mg/dL	HCG neg
Glu 83 mg/dL	Phos 2.6 mg/dL	

Assessment
Anorexia nervosa, Malnutrition, Depression Symptoms

► Questions

Problem Identification

1. a. *Create a list of this patient's drug therapy problems.*
   b. *What information from the history and physical exam is consistent with a diagnosis of anorexia nervosa?*
   c. *What signs and symptoms of malnutrition often seen in anorexia nervosa are not exhibited by this patient?*
   d. *Classify this patient's subtype of anorexia nervosa. How severe is the disorder at this point?*
   e. *What physical signs or other evidence would warrant inpatient treatment for anorexia nervosa?*

Desired Outcome

2. a. *What are the goals of treatment for this patient?*
   b. *What secondary complications do you want to avoid in this patient?*

Therapeutic Alternatives

3. a. *What nonpharmacologic interventions must be considered for this patient?*
   b. *What pharmacologic interventions may be considered for this patient?*

Optimal Plan

4. a. *Design an optimal therapeutic regimen for this patient.*

Outcome Evaluation

5. *How should the therapy you recommended be monitored for efficacy and side effects?*

Patient Education

6. *What information should be provided to the patient about her nondrug and drug therapies?*

► Follow-Up Question

1. *What is the likelihood of relapse or resistance to therapy?*

► Self-Study Assignments

1. Regulation of hunger and feeding involve the interregulation of several neurotransmitters (norepinephrine, serotonin, dopamine) and neuropeptides (CCK and pancreatic polypeptides). Review how these interrelate with each other and the proposed mechanism of action. How would this aid in the future development of medications to target these systems?
2. Compare and contrast the symptoms and signs of anorexia nervosa to bulimia nervosa. Does pharmacotherapy improve outcomes any better in bulimia nervosa?

► Clinical Pearl

The primary treatment modalities for anorexia nervosa are weight restoration, behavior modification, and psychotherapy. Pharmacotherapy remains adjunctive and has had limited success in treatment of anorexia nervosa.

References

1. American Psychiatric Association Working Group on Eating Disorders. Practice guidelines for the treatment of patients with eating disorders (Revision). Am J Psychiatry 2000;157(1 Suppl):1–39.

2. Mehler PS. Diagnosis and care of patients with anorexia nervosa in primary care settings. Ann Intern Med 2001;134:1048–1059.
3. Rock CL, Curran-Celentano J. Nutritional management of eating disorders. Psychiatr Clin North Am 1996;19:701–713.
4. Rosenblum J, Forman S. Evidence-based treatment of eating disorders. Curr Opin Pediatr 2002;14:379–383.
5. Vaswani M, Kalra H. Selective serotonin reuptake inhibitors in anorexia nervosa. Expert Opin Investig Drugs 2004;13:349–357.
6. Kaye W, Gendall K, Strober M. Serotonin neuronal function and selective serotonin reuptake inhibitor treatment in anorexia and bulimia nervosa. Biol Psychiatry 1998;44:825–838.
7. Jimerson DC, Wolfe BE, Brotman AW, et al. Medications in the treatment of eating disorders. Psychiatr Clin North Am 1996;19:739–754.
8. Kruger S, Kennedy SH. Psychopharmacotherapy of anorexia nervosa, bulimia nervosa and binge-eating disorder. J Psychiatry Neurosci 2000;25:497–508.
9. Pederson KJ, Roerig JL, Mitchell JE. Towards the pharmacotherapy of eating disorders. Expert Opin Pharmacother 2003;4(10):1659–1678.
10. Steinhausen H. The outcome of anorexia nervosa in the 20th century. Am J Psychiatry 2002;159:1284–1293.

68 ALZHEIMER'S DISEASE

▶ Agitated, Not Stirred (Level I)

Cynthia P. Koh-Knox, PharmD
Robert W. Bennett, MS

▶ After completing this case study, students should be able to:

- Recognize cognitive deficits and noncognitive/behavioral symptoms of Alzheimer's disease (AD).
- Recommend pharmacotherapy to manage the cognitive and behavioral symptoms of AD.
- Provide education and counseling to patients and caregivers about AD, the possible benefits and adverse effects of pharmacotherapy for the disorder, and the importance of adherence to therapy.
- List at least 3 theories of AD etiologies and agents under investigation based on those theories.

PATIENT PRESENTATION

Chief Complaint

"Mom thinks she's doing fine, but she seems to pace around the house a lot lately. She often checks the doors and windows several times to see if they are closed or locked."

HPI

Norma Dale is a 71 yo woman who presents to the geriatric care clinic for a routine visit accompanied by her daughter, Ann. Norma was diagnosed with Alzheimer's disease 4 years ago when her children reported short-term memory loss and noticeable cognitive symptoms, which included forgetting times and dates easily, misplacing and losing items, repeating questions and current events, inability to answer questions, and increasing difficulty with managing finances.

At that time, Mrs. Dale and 4 of her children met with the geriatric care team and discussed the diagnosis of probable Alzheimer's disease. It was explained that Mrs. Dale was in the early, moderate stage and it was to be expected that she would have waxing and waning of symptoms that would result in good and bad days. Tacrine was initiated for cognitive symptoms, and sertraline was started for depression.

At the 1-year follow-up visit, the patient reported that she had missed taking some of her medication because she was confused about how to take it. During her initial therapy with tacrine, she developed GERD, lost 8 pounds in 5 months, and had elevated liver enzymes. However, her children reported that she had been participating more actively in family and social functions. Her depression was less frequent and she felt happy most of the time. However, tacrine and sertraline were discontinued and Aricept 5 mg po at bedtime was started.

At last year's clinic visit, Norma was restarted on sertraline for mild depression and maintained on Aricept. She also started using Depends™ undergarments as extra protection for urinary incontinence. Norma lives with her daughter, Ann, who reports that this living arrangement is tolerable. However, her mother seems to be been pacing around the house more frequently and often checks the doors and windows to see if they are locked. Ann asks about newer Alzheimer's disease agents and therapy to treat her mother's behavior.

PMH

Osteoarthritis in both knees × 6 years
Alzheimer's disease diagnosed 4 years ago
Hx GERD—noncontributory since discontinuation of tacrine 3 years ago

FH

Noncontributory, both parents deceased. Five children, 4 who live nearby

SH

Lives with daughter; has been widowed for 5 years (husband died of cancer)

Meds

Aricept 10 mg po at bedtime
Sertraline 50 mg po once daily
Vitamin E 400 IU once daily
Pepcid AC 20 mg po at bedtime PRN
Ensure® drinks PRN
Tylenol PRN
Maalox PRN

All

NKA

ROS

Reports occasional bladder incontinence and knee pain; no c/o heartburn, chest pain, or shortness of breath

PE

Gen
WD woman who appears her stated age

VS
BP 122/80 sitting, 126/76 standing; P 76; RR 18; T 37°C; Wt 120 lb., Ht 5′6″

Skin
Normal texture and color

HEENT
WNL, TMs intact

Neck/LN
Neck supple without thyromegaly or lymphadenopathy

Lungs/Thorax
Clear, normal breath sounds

Breasts
No masses or tenderness

CV
RRR, no murmurs or bruits

Abd
Soft, NTND

Genit/Rect
Normal external female genitalia

MS/Ext
No CCE, normal ROM

Neuro
Motor, sensory, CNs, cerebellar, and gait normal. Folstein MMSE score 17/30, compared to a score of 19/30 at the initial diagnosis. Disoriented to season, month, date, and day of week. Disoriented to country. Good registration but impaired attention and very poor short-term memory. Unable to remember any of 3 items after 3 minutes. Able to follow commands. Stood up from chair four times during MMSE.

Labs

Na 139 mEq/L	Hgb 13.5 g/dL	T. bili 0.9 mg/dL	Ca 9.7 mg/dL
K 3.7 mEq/L	Hct 39.0%	D. bili 0.3 mg/dL	Phos 4.5 mg/dL
Cl 108 mEq/L	AST 25 IU/L	T. prot 7.5 g/dL	TSH 3.6 mIU/L
CO_2 25.5 mEq/L	ALT 24 IU/L	Alb 4.5 g/dL	T_4 5.9 ng/dL
BUN 16 mg/dL	Alk phos 81 IU/L	Chol 212 mg/dL	UA 6.8 mg/dL
SCr 1.1 mg/dL	GGT 22 IU/L	Trig 155 mg/dL	
Glu 102 mg/dL	LDH 85 IU/L		

CT Scan (4 years ago)
Mild to moderate generalized cerebral atrophy

Assessment

1. Alzheimer's disease, stage 4 to 5 on the Global Deterioration Scale (moderate AD—early dementia)
2. Increasing agitation reported as pacing and checking doors and windows; slightly agitated during MMSE interview
3. Mild symptoms of depression
4. Occasional urinary incontinence
5. Occasional knee pain

Questions

Problem Identification

1. a. *Create a list of the patient's drug therapy problems.*
   b. *What information (signs, symptoms, laboratory values) indicates the presence or severity of the cognitive and noncognitive problems of this patient with Alzheimer's disease?*

Desired Outcome

2. *What are the goals of pharmacotherapy in this case?*

Therapeutic Alternatives

3. a. *What nondrug therapies might be useful for this patient?*
   b. *What feasible pharmacotherapeutic alternatives are available for the treatment of the cognitive deficits of Alzheimer's disease?*
   c. *What pharmacologic treatments may be useful to treat the noncognitive symptoms and behaviors of this patient?*
   d. *What economic and psychosocial considerations are applicable to this patient?*

Optimal Plan

4. a. *What drug, dosage form, dose, schedule, and duration of therapy are best for the cognitive and noncognitive symptoms of this patient?*
   b. *What alternatives would be appropriate if the initial therapy fails or cannot be used?*

Outcome Evaluation

5. *What clinical and laboratory parameters are necessary to evaluate the therapy for achievement of the desired therapeutic outcome and to detect or prevent adverse effects?*

Patient Education

6. *What information should be provided to the patient to enhance compliance, ensure successful therapy, and minimize adverse effects?*

▶ Self-Study Assignments

1. Describe neurofibrillary tangles and neuritic plaques and their roles in AD development.
2. List at least 3 theories of the etiology of AD. What therapies are under investigation to support these theories?
3. What are the stages of cognitive decline as defined by the global deterioration scale? At what stage is AD identified?
4. Differentiate cognitive deficits from noncognitive/psychiatric symptoms and behaviors.

▶ Clinical Pearl

When counseling caregivers on Alzheimer's disease, encourage them to plan activities and daily tasks to help the person with Alzheimer's organize his/her day and focus on enjoyment, not achievement.

References

1. Gauthier S. Advances in the pharmacotherapy of Alzheimer's disease. CMAJ 2002; 166(5): 616–623.
2. Doody RD, Stevens JC, Beck C, et al. Practice parameter: Management of dementia (an evidence-based review). Report of the quality standards subcommittee of the American Academy of Neurology. Neurology 2001;56:1154–1166.
3. Adams LL, Gatchel RJ, Gentry C. Complementary and alternative medicine: Applications and implications for cognitive functioning in elderly populations. Altern Ther Health Med 2001;7(2):52–61.
4. Trinh NH, Hoblyn J, Mohanty S, et al. Efficacy of cholinesterase inhibitors in the treatment of neuropsychiatric symptoms and functional impairment in Alzheimer disease: A meta-analysis. JAMA 2003;289:210–216.
5. Reisberg B, Doody R, Stoffler A, et al. Memantine in moderate-to-severe Alzheimer's disease. N Engl J Med 2003;348:1333–1341.
6. Hartmann S, Mobius HJ. Tolerability of memantine in combination with cholinesterase inhibitors in dementia therapy. Int Clin Psychopharmacol 2003;18:881–885.
7. Doraiswamy PM. Non-cholinergic strategies for treating and preventing Alzheimer's disease. CNS Drugs 2002;16:811–824.
8. Aisen PS, Schafer KA, Grundman M, et al. Effects of rofecoxib or naproxen vs placebo on Alzheimer disease progression: A randomized controlled trial. JAMA 2003;289:2819–2826.
9. Engelhart MJ, Geerlings MI, Ruitenberg A, et al. Dietary intake of antioxidants and risk of Alzheimer disease. JAMA 2002;287: 3223–3229.

69 ALCOHOL WITHDRAWAL

▶ No More Drinking and Driving (Level I)

Rob Maher, PharmD, BCPS

▶ After completing this case study, students should be able to:

- Identify the signs and symptoms of alcohol dependence.
- Recognize the common signs and symptoms of alcohol withdrawal.
- Recognize the common laboratory abnormalities seen in an alcohol-dependent patient.
- Develop a treatment plan for alcohol withdrawal.

PATIENT PRESENTATION

Chief Complaint

"I have been sweating, shaking, vomiting, and running a fever for 2 days."

HPI

Aaron Jackson is a 69 yo man who presents to the ED stating that he drinks too much and needs alcohol rehabilitation. He states that he was released yesterday after spending 2 days in jail for driving while intoxicated. The patient states that he has been drinking one 750-mL bottle of vodka per day for 7 to 8 years. He had become increasingly depressed over the time prior to his arrest because his wife had left him. He states that he was on a drinking binge for 7 days prior to being arrested. The patient has not had any alcohol since the arrest.

PMH

Alcohol dependence
Hx depression (unknown history and duration)
Posttraumatic stress disorder (PTSD) S/P Korean War veteran
HTN ×10 years
BPH × 5 years

FH

Patient has three brothers and a sister, their medical histories unknown. Parents are deceased; patient is unable to give medical histories.

SH

Currently unemployed and has had sporadic employment (frequently fired because of call-offs) over the last 9 years. The patient has attended the PTSD group therapy on a monthly basis for several years. Divorced two times; current wife moved out 2 weeks ago; drinks 750 mL vodka/day for 7 to 8 years; (+) tobacco 1.5 ppd for 20 years; denies any illicit drug use.

ROS

Normal except for sweating, tremors in both hands, and fever. Patient states that he is feeling nervous and anxious.

Meds

Flomax 0.4 mg po at bedtime
Norvasc 10 mg po once daily
Cozaar 50 mg po once daily
Colace 100 mg po BID
Ibuprofen 600 mg po Q 6 H PRN headaches
Gaviscon 1–2 tablets po QID PRN GI upset

All

Penicillin

PE

Gen

Patient is a WDWN African-American man lying comfortably on a gurney; there is an odor of alcohol, sweat, and urine in the room. Patient's clothes are soiled with urine. Upon interview, the patient's mental status fluctuated from confusion to coherence. Patient also stated that he heard "female voices" talk to him last night, even though he now lives alone.

VS

BP 166/80, P 84 supine; 140/82, P 110 standing; RR 20; T 102°F

Skin

Moist secondary to diaphoresis

HEENT

Normal; unable to visualize fundi

Neck/LN

No lymphadenopathy, JVD, or carotid bruits

Lungs

Clear bilaterally, no crackles

CV

Normal S_1 and S_2; no m/r/g; occasional premature beats

Abd

Soft, obese; NT; (+) bowel sounds; (+) hepatomegaly; (–) splenomegaly

Genit/Rect

(+) Enlarged prostate, (–) occult blood in stool

MS/Ext

Tremor in both hands (R > L), pulses 1+ dorsalis pedis, none in posterior tibial

Neuro

A & O × 3, (+) tremors in both hands, CN II–XII intact; DTRs are exaggerated, gait unsteady when walking in the room.

Labs

Na 135 mEq/L	AST 254 IU/L	Ca 9.8 mg/dL
K 2.6 mEq/L	ALT 113 IU/L	Mg 1.2 mg/dL
Cl 87 mEq/L	Alk phos 41 IU/L	Phos 2.5 mg/dL
CO_2 23 mEq/L	GGT 265 IU/L	UA 10.8 mg/dL
BUN 28 mg/dL	LDH 321 IU/L	Alb 3.1 g/dL
SCr 1.0 mg/dL	T. bili 1.1 mg/dL	PT 12.2 sec
Glu 136 mg/dL	D. bili 0.4 mg/dL	INR 1.03

Post-Exam Note

The patient became very agitated and started having auditory hallucinations; he had to be physically restrained in the ED after his physical exam.

Toxicology Screen

(–) illicit drugs, (–) alcohol

Assessment

The patient appears to be going through alcohol withdrawal with delirium tremens.

▶ Questions

Problem Identification

1. a. *Create a list of the patient's drug therapy problems.*
   b. *What information (signs, symptoms, laboratory values) indicates that the patient is going through alcohol withdrawal?*
   c. *What signs and symptoms are consistent with delirium tremens?*
   d. *What signs, symptoms, and history are consistent with alcohol dependence in this patient?*
   e. *What laboratory abnormalities may be expected in a patient with a history of alcohol abuse?*

Desired Outcome

2. *What are the short-term and long-term goals of pharmacotherapy in this case?*

Therapeutic Alternatives

3. *What pharmacotherapeutic alternatives are available for the treatment of alcohol withdrawal and to prevent further alcohol withdrawal complications?*

Optimal Plan

4. *Design an optimal pharmacotherapeutic plan to rapidly control withdrawal symptoms in this patient and to prevent further withdrawal complications. Explain the rationale for your selections.*

Outcome Evaluation

5. *Which clinical and laboratory parameters are necessary to evaluate your chosen therapy for the achievement of desired outcome and to detect or prevent adverse effects?*

Patient Education

6. *What information should be provided to the patient to enhance compliance, ensure successful therapy, and to minimize adverse effects?*

▶ Clinical Course

After 1 week of detoxification and taper, Mr. Jackson's tremor has disappeared, vital signs are within normal limits, and his auditory hallucinations have disappeared. He is calm and able to think clearly. He still craves alcohol but has entered Alcoholics Anonymous and has agreed to increase his visits at the PTSD discussion group, as well as to enroll in individual psychiatric therapy for his depression. The patient vows to try to maintain sobriety in the future.

▶ Self-Study Assignments

1. Design an outpatient pharmacotherapeutic plan for this patient after discharge.
2. Describe the Alcoholics Anonymous 12-step approach to staying sober.
3. Discuss the pharmacologic options that are currently marketed in the United States (FDA-approved drugs) for the treatment of alcohol dependence.

▶ Clinical Pearl

In a patient with chronic alcoholism, parenteral thiamine of 100 mg should be administered before or concurrently with dextrose-containing intravenous fluids to prevent Wernicke's encephalopathy, a neurologic disorder common in alcoholics caused by thiamine deficiency.

References

1. Kosten TR, O'Connor PG. Management of drug and alcohol withdrawal. N Engl J Med 2003;348:1786–1795.
2. Fiellin DA, Reid MC, O'Connor PG. Outpatient management of patients with alcohol problems. Ann Intern Med 2000;133:815–827.
3. Swift FM. Drug therapy for alcohol dependence. N Engl J Med 1999;340:1482–1490.
4. Mayo-Smith MF. Pharmacological management of alcohol withdrawal: A meta-analysis and evidence-based practice guideline. The American Society of Addiction Medicine Working Group on Pharmacological Management of Alcohol Withdrawal. JAMA 1997;278:144–151.
5. Saitz R, O'Malley SS. Pharmacotherapies for alcohol abuse: Withdrawal and treatment. Med Clin North Am 1997:81;881–907.
6. McCowan C, Marik P. Refractory delirium tremens treated with propofol: A case series. Crit Care Med 2000;28:1781–1784.
7. Sullivan JT, Sykora K, Schneiderman J, et al. Assessment of alcohol withdrawal: The revised clinical institute withdrawal assessment for alcohol scale (CIWA-Ar). Br J Addict 1989;84:1353–1357.

Acknowledgement: This case is based on the case written for the Fifth Edition by Jill Slimick-Ponzetto, PharmD, BCPS.

70 NICOTINE DEPENDENCE

▶ The Cunning, Wicked Weed (Level II)

Julie C. Kissack, PharmD, BCPP

▶ After completing this case study, students should be able to:

- Identify the pharmacist's role in promoting smoking cessation and nicotine abstinence by using the 5A plan.
- Provide patient-specific recommendations for initiating lifestyle modifications and pharmacologic treatments to encourage smoking cessation.
- Recommend alternative treatments for nicotine dependence if the initial plan fails.
- Provide patient education on the use of pharmacotherapeutic agents used to treat nicotine dependence.

PATIENT PRESENTATION

Chief Complaint

"I can't breathe and my back really hurts."

HPI

I.M. Diene is a 55 yo man who presents to the community pharmacy with complaints of breathing difficulties that have become increasingly worse during the past week. He lost his inhaler last month and now requests a refill for his inhaler.

PMH

S/P MI 3 months prior to this visit
Emphysema diagnosed at age 52
Hyperlipidemia diagnosed at age 48
Chronic back pain diagnosed at age 40

FH

Mother died at age 38 of a heart attack. Father is alive and suffers from diabetes and arthritis. Patient is the second child of six siblings. All close family members are cigarette smokers.

SH

Lived alone for past 5 years since his wife's death. Wife was a nonsmoker who died from lung cancer. Three weeks ago his 13 yo granddaughter moved into his home. He is a retired textile mill worker; smokes 3 ppd (has smoked for the past 40 years); drinks 6 cups of coffee each day and 1 to 2 glasses of wine each night; does not exercise on a regular basis. Three adult children and seven grandchildren live in the local area. The 13 yo granddaughter started smoking daily this year.

ROS

Negative except for the problems described above.

Meds

Zocor 10 mg po once daily
Atrovent inhaler 2 inhalations QID
MS Contin 100 mg po BID
Amitriptyline 50 mg po at bedtime
Enteric-coated aspirin 325mg po once daily
Propranolol 10 mg po TID

All

NKDA

PE

Gen
Well-groomed, thin man who looks his stated age, with a flushed face and in obvious respiratory distress. Sitting during the interview with chest forward and hands resting on his knees

VS
BP 118/75, P 122 obtained at the pharmacy

Skin
Pale

HEENT
Wears dentures

Lungs
Breathing through pursed lips
No other PE information is available.

Labs
None available

Assessment
Patient's quality of life is greatly compromised by untreated emphysema exacerbated by cigarette smoking, exposure to second hand smoke (SHS), and inadequately-treated back pain.

▶ Questions

Problem Identification

1. a. *Create a list of this patient's drug therapy problems.*
   b. *What information in the patient's history can be identified as disease or symptomatology directly related to the patient's smoking history (see Figure 70–1)?*
   c. *List the 5A intervention plan for smokers. Describe your intervention plan for this patient.*
   d. *Describe aspects of the case that reveal the severity of nicotine dependence.*
   e. *List questions used to evaluate a patient's nicotine dependence.*

Desired Outcome

2. *What are the goals of smoking cessation pharmacotherapy?*

Therapeutic Alternatives

3. a. *Describe nondrug therapies that may help this patient quit smoking.*
   b. *What pharmacotherapeutic alternatives are available for the treatment of the nicotine dependence?*
   c. *What economic, psychosocial, racial, and ethical issues need to be considered in this patient's treatment?*

Optimal Plan

4. *What drug, dosage form, dose, schedule, and duration of therapy are best for this patient?*

Outcome Evaluation

5. *What clinical and laboratory parameters are necessary to evaluate the therapy for achievement of the desired therapeutic outcome and to detect or prevent adverse effects?*

Patient Education

6. *What information should be provided to the patient to enhance compliance, ensure successful therapy, and minimize adverse effects?*

A Cigarette and Select Smoke Components

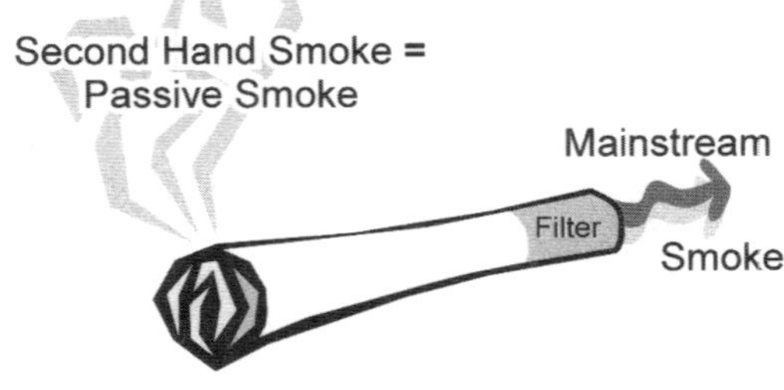

Cigarette Smoke

Gaseous Component	*Particulate Component*
Carbon monoxide	Nicotine
Hydrogen cyanide	Tobacco alkaloids
Toluene	Tar
Methanol	Polynuclear Aromatic Hydrocarbons (PAH)
Acetone	

Figure 70–1. A cigarette and select smoke components.

▶ Clinical Course

The patient complains of a rash at the patch site 3 days after starting the nicotine transdermal patch you recommended. He informs you that he can't stand the itching and would rather quit using the patch than continue if it is going to mean this much misery. In addition, he can't sleep at night and has noticed a large increase in his appetite and fears gaining a lot of weight.

▶ Follow-Up Questions

1. *What is the risk of smoking relapse now?*
2. *Has the treatment goal changed at this point?*
3. *Evaluate the patient's complaints and recommend alternative treatments.*
4. *Design an alternative pharmacotherapeutic plan to address the patient's nicotine addiction.*
5. *Describe clinical monitoring parameters for the patient.*

▶ Clinical Course

The patient stopped smoking while wearing the nicotine transdermal patch for 8 weeks. Five months later, he returns to your pharmacy to have prescriptions filled. He has been hospitalized twice in the past 6 weeks to treat respiratory infections and he is feeling very down about his ill health. He has begun smoking. He wants to know why it is so hard for him to quit smoking and if there are any new medications available that will help him "stay off the wicked weed." He states that he had a strong craving to smoke even when he wore the nicotine patch.

▶ Follow-Up Questions

1. *To determine what pharmacotherapy may be beneficial at this point, evaluate the positive and negative factors of this case that may affect the ultimate goal of smoking abstinence.*
2. *Describe the patient's complaints and recommend options to deal with the problems.*
3. *Design an alternative pharmacotherapeutic plan to address his nicotine dependence.*
4. *What information should be provided to the patient to enhance compliance, ensure successful therapy, and minimize adverse effects?*

▶ Self-Study Assignments

1. Perform a literature search to determine whether an alcoholic patient in recovery will need a different smoking cessation intervention plan than a person who is not an alcoholic. (Hint: You may wish to use the terminology "nicotine use and dependence" in the literature search). Write a two-page paper outlining the differences that might be required.
2. Visit the smokefree.gov website and determine whether or not your state has a nicotine quit line. What is the name of the program? Describe other resources that are available on this website. Devise a plan to use this website to help a family member or friend achieve a lifestyle free of cigarette smoking.
3. Identify the manufacturers of two nicotine lozenges that are available over-the-counter: Commit and Ariva. Write a one-page paper describing the different market focus for each company that produces a nicotine lozenge.
4. What was the original name of the company known as Altria? Identify nicotine and non-nicotine products produced by this company. Write a one-page personal opinion paper about the Altria name change and how it might impact your personal buying habits.

▶ Clinical Pearl

Nicotine dependence is a chronic, relapsing disease. Smoking cessation is achieved through a dynamic process; thus, an intervention with a smoker must be personalized and relevant to the smoker's current status.

References

1. Silagy C, Lancaster T, Stead L, et al. Nicotine replacement therapy for smoking cessation (Cochrane Review). In: *The Cochrane Library,* Issue 1, 2003. Oxford: Update Software.
2. The Tobacco Use and Dependence Clinical Practice Guideline Panel, Staff, and Consortium Representatives. A clinical practice guideline for treating tobacco use and dependence. A US Public Health Service Report. JAMA 2000;283:3244–3254.
3. Wongwiwatthananukit S, Jack HM, Popovich NG. Smoking cessation: Part 1. An overview. J Am Pharm Assoc 1998;38:58–70.
4. Rustin TA. Assessing nicotine dependence. Am Fam Physician 2000;62;579–584, 591–592.

71 SCHIZOPHRENIA

▶ A Thousand Worms Inside My Body (Level I)

William H. Benefield, Jr., PharmD, BCPP, FASCP
Lawrence J. Cohen, PharmD, BCPP, FASHP, FCCP

▶ After completing this case study, students should be able to:

- Identify the target symptoms of schizophrenia.
- Manage an acutely psychotic patient with appropriate pharmacotherapy.
- Manage adverse effects of the antipsychotics.
- Discuss the role of atypical antipsychotics in the treatment of schizophrenia.

PATIENT PRESENTATION

Chief Complaint

"I want to see my lawyer."

HPI

This is the first admission for Anita Gonzalez, a 32 yo woman who was brought to the state hospital by the police. The patient apparently has been delusional and believes people sneak into her room at night when she is asleep and place a thousand worms inside her body. She also believes that she is being raped by passing men on the street. She is quite preoccupied about having massive wealth. She claims to have bought some gold and left it at the grocery store. She believes that her ideas have been given to a Cuban communist who has had plastic surgery to look like her and is using her ID to take possession of all of her property. She states that she is having difficulty getting her property back.

Apparently, the precipitating event causing her hospitalization was that she created a disturbance at a local fast-food restaurant, claiming that she owned it. Because of the disturbance, police were called and she subsequently was sent here on an order of protective custody. According to the patient, she bought a hamburger and sat down to eat it, and for some reason somebody called the police and charged her with illegal trespassing. She claims that 6 years ago she was raped by a relative of a sister and broke her hip in the process. She states that her feet were cut off because she would not do what her impostors wanted her to do, and her feet were subsequently sent back to her from Central America and were reattached.

Her speech is quite rambling, and she speaks of having been part of an experiment in Monterey, Mexico, in which 38 eggs were taken from her body, and children were produced from them and then killed by the government. She claims that she has worms in her that are the type that kill dogs and horses, and says that they have been put there by the government. She also claims that at one time she had transmitters in her backbone and that it took 3 years to have them taken out by the government. She claims to have had surgery in the past, and the surgeon didn't know what he was doing and took out her gallbladder and put it in the intestines where it exploded. The patient also states that on one occasion a physician was removing the snakes from her abdominal cavity, and the snakes killed the doctor and a nurse. She also claims that she worked as a surgeon herself before 1963.

Past Psychiatric History

The patient denies any prior hospitalization for mental problems, and denies any street drugs or significant substance use. There is some history of her having frequent visits to the local hospital. She denies any drug or alcohol use. She smokes two packs of cigarettes per day.

PMH

- The patient's past records indicate that she did have gallbladder surgery (cholecystectomy) 2 months ago
- There is no record of her ever being raped or having a broken hip
- No further medical history is known

Family Psychiatric History

The patient claims that her alleged family is not really her family and that she is not sure who is her family

Meds

None noted

All

Penicillin → rash

Legal/Social Status

Divorced, heterosexual; lives in an apartment alone; employment history unknown.

Mental Status Exam

The patient is a white female of Hispanic ethnicity, modestly dressed with some disarray. She is morbidly obese. Her hair is black and unwashed. She is alert, oriented, and in no acute distress. Her speech is clear, constant, pressured, with many grandiose delusions and illogical thoughts. She is quite rambling, going from one subject to the other without interruption. Her affect is mood congruent, her mood is euphoric, and there is a marked degree of grandiosity. Her thought processes are quite illogical with marked delusional thinking. There is no evidence of auditory hallucinations, and she denies visual hallucinations. She denies any suicidal or homicidal ideation, but she is quite verbal and pressured in her thought content, verbalizing a great deal about the things that have been taken away from her illegally by people impersonating her. She has marked delusional symptoms with paranoid ideation prominent. Her memory (immediate, recent, and remote) is fair. Her cognition and concentration are adequate. Her intellectual functioning is within the average range. Insight and judgment are markedly impaired.

ROS

Reports occasional GI upset; complains that worms are inside her stomach. Otherwise negative.

PE

VS

BP 140/85, P 80, RR 17, T 37.1°C; Wt 97 kg; Ht 5′3″

HEENT

PERRLA; EOMI; fundi benign; throat and ears clear; TMs intact

Skin

Scratches on both hands

Neck

Supple, no nodes; normal thyroid

CV

RRR, normal S_1 and S_2

Lungs

CTA & P

Abd

(+) BS, non-tender

Ext

Full ROM, pulses 2+ bilaterally

Neuro

A & O × 3; reflexes symmetric; toes downgoing; normal gait; normal strength; sensation intact; CN II–XII intact

Labs

Na 140 mEq/L	Hgb 14.6 g/dL	WBC $11.0 \times 103/mm^3$	AST 34 IU/L	Ca 9.6 mg/dL
K 3.9 mEq/L	Hct 45.7%	Neutros 66%	ALT 22 IU/L	Phos 5.1 mg/dL
Cl 104 mEq/L	RBC $4.7 \times 10^6/mm^3$	Lymphs 24%	Alk phos 89 IU/L	TSH 4.5 mIU/L
CO_2 22 mEq/L	MCV 90.2 μm^3	Monos 8%	GGT 38 IU/L	RPR negative
BUN 19 mg/dL	MCH 31 pg	Eos 1%	T. bili 0.9 mg/dL	Urine pregnancy (–)
SCr 1.1 mg/dL	MCHC 34.5 g/dL	Basos 1%	Alb 3.6 g/dL	
Glu 100 mg/dL		Plt $232 \times 10^3/mm^3$	T. chol 208 mg/dL	

UA

Color, yellow; appearance, slightly cloudy; glucose (–); bili (–); ketones, trace; SG 1.025; blood (–); pH 6.0; protein (–); nitrites (–); leukocyte esterase (–)

Assessment

Axis I: Schizophrenia, paranoid type, acute exacerbation
Axis II: None
Axis III: Patient allergic to penicillin by history, S/P gallbladder surgery 2 months ago, obesity
Axis IV: Unemployment
Axis V: Global Assessment of Functioning (GAF) Scale = 32

▶ Questions

Problem Identification

1. a. *Create a list of the patient's drug therapy problems.*
   b. *Which information (signs, symptoms, laboratory values) indicates the presence or severity of an acute exacerbation of schizophrenia, paranoid type?*

Desired Outcome

2. *What are the goals of pharmacotherapy in this case?*

Therapeutic Alternatives

3. a. *What nondrug therapies might be useful for this patient?*
   b. *What pharmacotherapeutic options are available for the treatment of this patient?*

Optimal Plan

4. a. *What drug, dosage form, dose, schedule, and duration of therapy are best for this patient?*
   b. *What alternatives would be appropriate if the initial therapy fails or cannot be used?*

Outcome Evaluation

5. *What clinical and laboratory parameters are necessary to evaluate the therapy for achievement of the desired therapeutic outcome and to detect or prevent adverse effects?*

Patient Education

6. *What information should be provided to the patient to enhance compliance, ensure successful therapy, and minimize adverse effects?*

▶ Self-Study Assignments

1. Perform a literature search regarding weight gain with each of the atypical antipsychotics currently marketed. Which ones are more likely to cause weight gain? Which ones are less likely to cause weight gain?
2. Perform a literature search regarding QTc changes with both typical and atypical antipsychotics. Which antipsychotics are more likely to alter the QT interval?
3. Review the pharmacoeconomic literature for the atypical antipsychotics. For your geographic area, compare costs for the average daily doses of haloperidol, aripiprazole, clozapine, olanzapine (oral, rapid-dissolving formulation and IM), risperidone (oral, rapid-dissolving formulation and long-acting injection), quetiapine, and ziprasidone (oral and IM).

▶ Clinical Pearl

A benzodiazepine (lorazepam) can be scheduled routinely during the initiation of an antipsychotic to minimize aggression and allow time for the antipsychotic to take effect. The addition of lorazepam may also allow lower initial dosages to be used initially and during the maintenance phase of treatment.

References

1. Marder SR. Facilitating compliance with antipsychotic medication. J Clin Psychiatry 1998; 59(Suppl 3):21–25.
2. Freedman R. Schizophrenia. N Engl J Med 2003;349:1738–1749.
3. Expert consensus panel for optimizing pharmacologic treatment of psychotic disorders. Expert consensus guideline series. Optimizing pharmacologic treatment of psychotic disorders. J Clin Psychiatry 2003;64 (Suppl 12):2–97.
4. Revicki DA. Methods of pharmacoeconomic evaluation of psychopharmacologic therapies for patients with schizophrenia. J Psychiatry Neurosci 1997;22:256–266.
5. Glazer WM. Olanzapine and the new generation of antipsychotic agents: Patterns of use. J Clin Psychiatry 1997; 8(Suppl 10):18–21.
6. Kinon BJ, Basson BR, Gilmore JA, et al. Long-term olanzapine treatment: Weight change and weight-related health factors in schizophrenia. J Clin Psychiatry 2001;62:92–100.
7. Conley RR, Kelly DL, Richardson CM, et al. The efficacy of high-dose olanzapine versus clozapine in treatment-resistant schizophrenia: A double-blind crossover study. J Clin Psychopharmacol 2003;23: 668–671.
8. Nelson MW, Reynolds R, Kelly DL, et al. Safety and tolerability of high dose quetiapine in treatment refractory schizophrenia: Preliminary results from an open-label trial. Schizophrenia Res 2003;60(Suppl):363. Abstract.
9. Sharma T, Mockler D. The cognitive efficacy of atypical antipsychotics in schizophrenia. J Clin Psychopharmacol 1998;18(Suppl 1):12S–19S.
10. Taylor DM, McAskill R. Atypical antipsychotics and weight gain—A systematic review. Acta Psychiatr Scand 2000;101:416–432.

72 MAJOR DEPRESSION

▶ A Life Worth Living (Level I)

Brian L. Crabtree, PharmD, BCPP
Victor G. Dostrow, MD

▶ After completing this case study, students should be able to:

- Identify the signs and symptoms of depression.
- Develop a pharmacotherapy plan for a patient with depression.
- Compare side-effect profiles of various antidepressant drugs.
- Discuss pharmacoeconomic considerations in antidepressant therapy.

PATIENT PRESENTATION

Chief Complaint

"I don't think I can go on like this. I can't sleep. I can't eat. I can't think straight. Sometimes I wonder if life is worth living."

HPI

Ella Mae Hodges is a 38 yo woman who presents to her family physician with the above complaint. She separated from her husband 3 months previously. She has felt down, sad, and worried for more than a year, but her symptoms have become worse over the last couple of months.

Ella Mae left her husband, Robert, after 5 years of marriage. This was her second marriage. Violent arguments between them, during which her husband beat her, had occurred for the last 4 years of their marriage. They had daily arguments during which Robert hit her hard enough to leave bruises on her face and arms. During their final argument, about Ella Mae buying a gift for a favorite niece, Robert threatened to take the gift away from the niece and destroy it if she didn't agree to return it to the store for a refund. Ella Mae has obtained a court order of protection that prevents Robert from having any contact with her. She has moved in with her parents.

In the 3 months since she left her husband, Ella Mae has become increasingly depressed. Her appetite has been poor, she has little interest in food, and she has lost 14 pounds. She cries frequently and wakes up around 3:00 AM, unable to get back to sleep. She lies awake at night when she goes to bed, crying and tossing and turning for hours before falling asleep. She experiences nightmares about the previous deaths of her sisters. In these nightmares, the sisters summon her to join them. She is unable to concentrate as well as before. She has tried to read the Bible to comfort herself, but she finds herself just reading the same lines over and over. Most recently, she has had thoughts that she wishes she could just go to sleep and not wake up.

PMH

Childhood illnesses—she has had all of the usual childhood illnesses.

Adult illnesses—no current nonpsychiatric adult illnesses; no previous psychiatric treatment, but reports a life-long history of occasional periods of intense sadness lasting several weeks. During these times, she would lose interest in her usual activities, sometimes missing school or work as a result.

Trauma—fractured arm due to bicycle accident at age 9, otherwise unremarkable.

Surgeries—hx childbirth by CS; tonsillectomy at age 6.

Travel—no significant travel history.

Diet—no dietary restrictions; recently has had a poor appetite and eats only sporadically, skipping many meals.

Exercise—no regular exercise program.

Immunizations—no personal records of childhood vaccinations; had tetanus booster 9 years ago.

FH

Mother has history of anxiety and depression, takes antidepressant medication; Ella Mae doesn't know its name. Father is in good health except for well-controlled HTN. Two sisters, both deceased. One committed suicide by stepping in front of a train.

SH

High school graduate with 2 years education at a community college; now unemployed but worked as a secretary before getting married. Married for 5 years, now separated for 3 months. Lives with her parents. Health insurance is through husband's employer (he services photocopiers for an office supply business). Attended church occasionally (Baptist) in the past, but not in the last year or so.

Drinks alcohol (wine and beer) once or twice a month; denies drinking to intoxication. Smokes about 1 ppd with about 14 pack-year history. Drinks 3 to 4 cups of caffeinated coffee per day; usually drinks iced tea with evening meal; drinks colas as leisure beverage. Used marijuana a few times after high school, denies any use in more than 10 years; denies use of other illicit substances.

ROS

General Appearance—Pt c/o feeling tired much of the time.

HEENT—wears contact lenses; no tinnitus, ear pain, or discharge; no c/o nasal congestion; hx of dental repair for caries.

Chest —no hx of asthma or other lung disease.

CV—reports occasional feelings of "racing heartbeat." No hx of heart disease.

GI—reports infrequent constipation, takes MOM PRN. Has lost 6.4 kg in last 3 months.

GU—has regular menses associated with some cramping.

Neuromuscular—has frequent bifrontal non-pulsatile headaches for last several weeks; often feels stiff and tense in neck and shoulders; no c/o dizziness.

Skin—no complaints.

Meds

Ortho-Novum 1/35–28, 1 po daily; hasn't taken for 2 months

Took Tranxene (unknown dosage) for about 2 weeks while in college, Rx by family MD

St. John's wort 300 mg po TID for the last month or so (purchased at health food store; someone told her it would "lift my spirits")

OTC ibuprofen 400 mg (2 × 200-mg tablets) PRN for headache pain or menstrual cramps, not daily

Uses OTC antihistamines and decongestants for colds or allergies; none in recent months

MOM 2 tbsp PRN for occasional constipation

All

NKDA

PE

Performed by nurse practitioner.

Gen

Thin WF, slightly unkempt, and no makeup

VS

BP 112/68, P 92, RR 22, T 36.9°C; Wt 50.3 kg, Ht 5′6″

Skin

Normal skin, hair, and nails

Neck/LN

Supple without thyromegaly or lymphadenopathy

HEENT

PERRLA; EOM intact, no nystagmus. Fundus—disks sharp, no retinopathy; no nasal discharge or nasal polyps; TMs gray and shiny bilaterally; minor accumulation of cerumen

Chest/Lungs

Frequent sighing during examination, but no tachypnea or SOB; chest CTA

Heart

RRR without murmur

Breasts

No masses or tenderness

Abdomen

Soft, non-tender; (+) BS; no organomegaly

Genit/Rect

Deferred

Ext

Unremarkable

Neuro

CN: no evidence of facial paresis or anesthesia. Casual gait normal. Finger-to-nose normal. Motor—normal symmetric grip strength. DTRs 2+ and equal. Sensory—intact bilaterally.

Mental Status

The patient is pale and thin, dressed in worn-out jeans and dark blue sweater. Her hair looks unwashed, and she appears older than her stated age. She speaks slowly, describing her depressed mood and lack of energy. She says that she has no pleasure in her life. She has no social contacts other than with her parents. She feels worthless and blames herself for her marital discord. She is often anxious and worries about the future. Speech and thought are logical, coherent, and goal-oriented. No active suicidal ideas, but admits to wishing she could "just pass away." No homicidal ideas. She denies hallucinations. Paranoid delusions, flight of ideas, ideas of reference, and looseness of associations are absent.

Labs (collected 11:45 AM)

Na 139 mEq/L	Hgb 14.0 g/dL	AST 34 IU/L
K 4.2 mEq/L	Hct 46.2%	ALT 42 IU/L
Cl 102 mEq/L	MCV 92 μm^3	GGT 38 IU/L
CO_2 24 mEq/L	MCH 29 pg	T. bili 0.8 mg/dL
BUN 12 mg/dL	Plt 234 × $10^3/mm^3$	T. prot 7.0 g/dL
SCr 0.9 mg/dL	WBC 7.3 × $10^3/mm^3$	Alb 4.4 g/dL
Glu 98 mg/dL	Segs 49%	CK 57 IU/L
Ca 9.5 mg/dL	Bands 1%	T_4 8.6 mcg/dL
Mg 1.7 mEq/L	Lymphs 42%	T_3 uptake 29%
Uric acid 4.0 mg/dL	Monos 2%	TSH 2.8 mIU/L
	Eos 6%	

UA

Glucose (–); ketones (–); pH 5.8; SG 1.016; bilirubin (–); WBC 1/hpf, protein (–), amorphous—rare, epithelial cells 1/hpf; color yellow; blood (–), RBC 0/hpf; mucus—rare; bacteria—rare; casts 0/lpf; appearance clear

Assessment

Major depressive disorder, recurrent, with melancholic features

Plan

Refer for support group, psychotherapy; begin antidepressant medication

▶ Questions

Problem Identification

1. a. *Create a list of this patient's drug therapy problems.*
   b. *What signs, symptoms, and laboratory values indicate depression in this patient?*
   c. *What factors in the family history support a diagnosis of depression?*
   d. *Why is this patient's depression considered to be recurrent even though this is her first psychiatric treatment?*
   e. *Is there anything in the patient's medication history that could cause or worsen depression?*

Desired Outcome

2. *What are the goals of pharmacotherapy in this case?*

Therapeutic Alternatives

3. a. *What nonpharmacologic treatments are important in this case? Should nonpharmacologic treatments be tried before beginning medication?*
   b. *What pharmacotherapeutic options are available for the treatment of depression?*

Optimal Plan

4. a. *What drug regimen (drug, dosage, schedule, and duration) is best for this patient?*

b. *How should the patient be advised about the herbal therapy, St. John's wort?*

c. *What alternatives would be appropriate if the patient fails to respond to initial therapy?*

Outcome Evaluation

5. *What clinical and laboratory parameters are necessary to evaluate the therapy for efficacy and adverse effects?*

Patient Education

6. *What information should be provided to the patient to enhance compliance, ensure successful therapy, and minimize adverse effects?*

▶ Follow-Up Question

1. *For questions related to the use of St. John's wort for the treatment of depression, please see Section 19 of this Casebook.*

▶ Self-Study Assignments

1. Because the SSRI antidepressants are commonly used and have the same reuptake pharmacology, contrast the agents in this class, considering relative side effects, dosing, and drug interactions.
2. Discuss pharmacoeconomic considerations in antidepressant therapy, including choice of agents for inclusion in the formulary of a hospital or health maintenance organization.
3. Review the medical literature and evaluate the scientific evidence for the efficacy of St. John's wort in the treatment of depression.

▶ Clinical Pearl

Although the newer antidepressants are more expensive than older antidepressants such as the tricyclic antidepressants, cost of therapy may be the same or less because of fewer adverse effects, fewer follow-up office visits, improved compliance, and less need for other concurrent medications.

References

1. Perry PJ. Pharmacotherapy for major depression with melancholic features: Relative efficacy of tricyclic versus selective serotonin reuptake inhibitor antidepressants. J Affect Disord 1996;39:1–6.
2. Peretti S, Judge R, Hindmarch I. Safety and tolerability considerations: Tricyclic antidepressants vs. selective serotonin reuptake inhibitors. Acta Psychiatr Scand Suppl 2000;403:17–25.
3. Hemeryck A, Belpaire FM. Selective serotonin reuptake inhibitors and cytochrome P-450 mediated drug interactions: An update. Curr Drug Metab 2002;3:13–37.
4. Homsi J, Nelson KA, Sarhill N, et al. A phase II study of methylphenidate for depression in advanced cancer. Am J Hosp Palliat Care. 2001;18:403–407.
5. Ferguson JM. SSRI antidepressant medications: Adverse effects and tolerability. Primary Care Companion J Clin Psychiatry 2001;3:22–27.
6. Schmidt ME, Fava M, Robinson JM, et al. The efficacy and safety of a new enteric-coated formulation of fluoxetine given once weekly during the continuation treatment of major depressive disorder. J Clin Psychiatry 2000;61:851–857.
7. Barbui C, Percudani M, Hotopf M. Economic evaluation of antidepressive agents: A systematic critique of experimental and observational studies. J Clin Psychopharmacol 2003; 3:145–154.
8. Geddes JR, Carney SM, Davies C, et al. Relapse prevention with antidepressant drug treatment in depressive disorders: A systematic review. Lancet 2003;361:653–661.
9. Lecrubier Y, Clerc G, Didi R, et al. Efficacy of St. John's wort extract WS5570 in major depression: A double-blind, placebo-controlled trial. Am J Psychiatry 2002;159:1361–1366.
10. Shelton RC, Keller MB, Gelenberg A, et al. Effectiveness of St. John's wort in major depression: A randomized controlled trial. JAMA 2001;285:1978–1986.
11. Glisson JK, Rogers HE, Abourashed EA, et al. Clinic at the health food store? Employee recommendations and product analysis. Pharmacotherapy 2003;23:64–72.
12. Markowitz JS, Donovan JL, DeVane CL. Effect of St John's wort on drug metabolism by induction of cytochrome P450 3A4 enzyme. Obstet Gynecol Surv 2004;59:358–359.
13. Kornbluh R, Papakostas GI, Petersen T, et al. A survey of prescribing preferences in the treatment of refractory depression: Recent trends. Psychopharmacol Bull 2001;35:150–156.
14. McIntyre RS, Muller A, Mancini DA, et al. What to do if an initial antidepressant fails? Can Fam Physician. 2003;49:449–457.

73 BIPOLAR DISORDER

▶ Don't Hate Me Because I'm Beautiful (Level II)

Lawrence J. Cohen, PharmD, BCPP, FASHP, FCCP
William H. Benefield, Jr., PharmD, BCPP, FASCP

▶ After completing this case study, students should be able to:

- Outline a mental status examination and identify target symptoms of bipolar disorder when given patient interview information.
- Recommend appropriate pharmacotherapy for patients with acute mania.
- Generate parameters for monitoring anticonvulsant therapy for bipolar disorder.
- Identify the pharmacotherapeutic options for treating the subtypes of bipolar disorder.

PATIENT PRESENTATION

Chief Complaint

"There are hundreds of vampires in this city, and I have the documents to prove it."

HPI

Michael Harrison is a 25 yo man who was brought to the hospital by police. This is his third psychiatric admission. According to neighbors who called the police, the patient has been acting increasingly strangely. The lights in the house are left on all night, and spiritual music is played at all hours. Last evening, he dug a trench around his front yard with an electric lawn edger and filled it with garlic cloves. This evening, he painted crosses on the front of the house and threw furniture into his yard and the street. When approached by neighbors, he apparently began screaming and preaching at them. When the police arrived, they found the patient standing naked on the dining room table in his front yard preaching. When the police approached he began throwing garlic tablets at them and screaming, "Become naked in the eyes of the Lord and you will be saved." He became increasingly hostile during the arrest shouting, "Don't hate me because I'm beautiful." He then tried to bite one of the officers.

PMH

- Manic episodes first occurred while he was in college, leading to psychiatric admissions at ages 21 and 23 for acute mania. Patient was treated with haloperidol 5 mg po once daily and lithium 600 mg po Q AM and 900 mg po at bedtime, with adequate response and discharged on both occasions after about a month.
- Medical problems include migraine headaches.

Patient Interview

Patient is disheveled with pungent body odor. He is pacing the room, waving his hands in the air and preaching in an elated, loud, sing-songy voice. He is dressed flamboyantly in a brightly colored bathrobe and appears to be wearing a garlic necklace. He is carrying a Bible. When asked how he felt, he stated, "Playful, with intense clarity, sharp, spiffy, and clean." He then became angry, insisting that he be discharged before sunrise or he would "face the light of the right and mighty and burn in 'demonocratic' hell." He then asked for a priest to exorcise the homosexual demons from his body. He believes that vampires live in the city. He stated he has the documents to prove it, and that the vampires are pursuing him to keep him from exposing their existence to Christians everywhere. He spoke in long run-on sentences with many political, religious, and sexual references. He was very difficult to interrupt. For example, at one point he stated, "Can't you see, or are you an idiot?! I am being persecuted by the right, 100 points of light, Republicans, redeeming the public, for the republic, under which I stand because I have no one to lean on, one gay man, bitten by the democrat, the demoncrat, doomed and miserable for loving the company I keep, and that's why misery loves company, and if you don't get that you're an idiot."

When asked about his sleep, he angrily replied, "Would you sleep at a time like this? If I sleep, America will fall, and it will all be on my shoulders. The towers in New York City have already fallen because I didn't get there in time." The patient stated that he has not been eating and has not taken his lithium in several days because, "Lithium is of the ground, the underworld. The Lord will sustain me."

Through his verbose conversation, it becomes apparent that a man he picked up in a gay bar last week bit him on the neck. He also seems to believe that he has been given a mission from God as penance for visiting this bar. Several times during the interview, he began crying and wailing loudly begging to be saved, and shouting, "I'm sorry." He said something about the trials of Job and that he would be the next to die. He sang "Swing Low Sweet Chariot" in a very loud voice. When told that he might need to stay at the hospital so we could help him with his problems, he screamed, "You can't help me! Only the Lord can help me! They have drunk from the fruit of the vine. I am that fruit."

Abnormal Involuntary Movement Scale (AIMS)

Excessive eye-blinking and mild grimacing; unclear whether abnormal (patient states this is the "demon blood" trying to take over his body). He is bothered by it in that to him it represents "his sinful nature."

FH

Father has a history of depression, paternal grandmother was placed in an "asylum" for hysteria secondary to childbirth. Mother and brother have type 2 diabetes.

SH

Recently fired from his job as a nurse at a local hospital. Patient is a single homosexual. Religious upbringing as a Southern Baptist. Smokes 1 ppd for 5 years. Patient states that he drinks "only occasionally," but he was noted to be intoxicated with a BAC 0.14% on a previous admission.

Meds

Ergotamine and ibuprofen PRN for migraines

All

NKA

ROS

Migraine headaches about twice a month, no aura, (+) nausea and photophobia. Occasional GI upset with no clear relationship to meals or time of day; frequent loose stools.

PE

VS

BP 118/73, P 83, RR 16, T 37.1°C; Wt 94 kg, Ht 5′2″

HEENT

PERRLA, EOMI, fundi benign, throat and ears clear, TMs intact; rapid eye-blinking and facial grimacing (may indicate early tardive dyskinesia)

Skin

Psoriasis evident on both elbows

Neck

Supple, bite mark, no nodes

Cor

RRR; S_1, S_2 normal; no m/r/g

Lungs

CTA & P

Abd

(+) BS, non-tender

Ext

Full ROM, pulses 2+ bilaterally

Neuro

A & O × 3, reflexes symmetric, toes downgoing, normal gait, normal strength, sensation intact, CN II–XII intact

Labs

Na 141 mEq/L	Hgb 14.6 g/dL	WBC $12.0 \times 10^3/mm^3$	AST 32 IU/L	Ca 9.7 mg/dL
K 3.8 mEq/L	Hct 45.7%	Neutros 67%	ALT 21 IU/L	Phos 5.3 mg/dL
Cl 103 mEq/L	RBC $4.73 \times 10^6/mm^3$	Lymphs 23%	Alk Phos 87 IU/L	TSH 4.1 μIU/mL
CO_2 24 mEq/L	MCV 90.2 μm^3	Monos 7%	GGT 46 IU/L	RPR: Neg
BUN 19 mg/dL	MCH 31 pg	Eos 2%	T. bili 0.9 mg/dL	Lithium 0.1 mEq/L
SCr 1.1 mg/dL	MCHC 34.4 g/dL	Basos 1%	Alb 3.7 g/dL	
Glu 89 mg/dL	Plt $256 \times 10^3/mm^3$		T. chol 218 mg/dL	

UA

Color yellow; appearance slightly cloudy; glucose (–), bili (–), ketones trace; SG 1.025, blood (–), pH 6.0, protein (–), nitrites (–), leukocyte esterase (–)

Assessment

Axis I: Bipolar disorder, current episode mixed
Axis II: Deferred
Axis III: Migraine headache by history

► Questions

Problem Identification

1. a. *From the case information and patient interview, write a mental status examination for this patient.*
   b. *Create a list of this patient's drug therapy problems.*
   c. *What information (target symptoms, laboratory values) indicates the presence and severity of bipolar disorder, mixed episode?*

Desired Outcome

2. *What are the goals of pharmacotherapy in this patient?*

Therapeutic Alternatives

3. a. *What nondrug therapies might be useful for this patient?*
   b. *What feasible pharmacotherapeutic alternatives are available for treatment of bipolar disorder?*

Optimal Plan

4. a. *What drug, dosage form, dose, schedule, and duration of therapy are best for this patient?*
   b. *What alternatives would be appropriate if the initial therapy fails or cannot be used?*

Outcome Evaluation

5. *Which clinical and laboratory parameters are necessary to evaluate response to therapy and to detect or prevent adverse effects?*

Patient Education

6. *What information should be provided to the patient to enhance compliance, ensure successful therapy, and minimize adverse effects?*

► Self-Study Assignments

1. Perform a literature search and explore the role of the newer anticonvulsants (lamotrigine, gabapentin, oxcarbazepine, and topiramate) in the treatment of bipolar disorder.
2. Perform a literature search on once-daily dosing of antimanic agents. How would you go about changing a patient's dosing regimen to increase compliance? Based on the literature, which patients are most suitable for conversion to once- or twice-daily dosing with lithium, carbamazepine, or valproate? Can regular-release products be used, or must the patient be converted to extended-release products?
3. Design an algorithm for the treatment of bipolar disorder. Include treatment strategies for acute mania, rapid cycling, depression, and mixed states.

► Clinical Pearl

When a patient admitted with acute mania is taking an antidepressant, the antidepressant should be tapered and withdrawn. In some patients, antidepressants may activate mania or increase the rate of cycling, and potentially prolong response to antimanic medication.

References

1. Swann AC, Bowden CL, Morris D, et al. Depression during mania: Treatment response to lithium or divalproex. Arch Gen Psychiatry 1997;54:37–42.
2. Freeman TW, Clothier JL, Pazzaglia P, et al. A double-blind comparison of valproate and lithium in the treatment of acute mania. Am J Psychiatry 1992;149:108–111.
3. Goldberg JF, Garno JL, Leon AC, et al. Rapid titration of mood stabilizers predicts remission from mixed or pure mania in bipolar patients. J Clin Psychiatry 1998;59:151–158.
4. Tohen M, Jacobs TG, Grundy SL, et al. Efficacy of olanzapine in acute bipolar mania: A double-blind, placebo-controlled study. The Olanzapine HGGW Study Group. Arch Gen Psychiatry 2000;57:841–849.
5. Tohen M, Sanger TM, McElroy SL, et al. Olanzapine versus placebo in the treatment of acute mania. Olanzapine HGEH Study Group Trial. Am J Psychiatry 1999;156:702–709.
6. Sachs G, Mullen JA, Devine NA. Quetiapine vs placebo as adjunct to mood stabilizer for the treatment of acute mania. Bipolar Disord 2002;4(S1);Abstract 61:133.
7. Bowden CL, Calabrese JR, Sachs G, et al. A placebo-controlled 18-month trial of lamotrigine and lithium maintenance treatment in recently manic or hypomanic patients with bipolar I disorder. Arch Gen Psychiatry. 2003;60:392–400.
8. Goldsmith DR, Wagstaff AJ, Ibbotson T, et al. Spotlight on lamotrigine in bipolar disorder. CNS Drugs. 2004;18:63–67.
9. Algorithm for patient management of acute manic states: Lithium, valproate, or carbamazepine? J Clin Psychopharmacol 1992;12:57S–63S.
10. Hartong EG, Moleman P, Hoogduin CA, et al. Prophylactic efficacy of lithium versus carbamazepine in treatment-naive bipolar patients. J Clin Psychiatry 2003;64:144–151.
11. McElroy SL, Keck PE, Tugrul KC, et al. Valproate as a loading treatment in acute mania. Neuropsychobiology 1993;27:146–149.
12. Sachs GS, Printz DJ, Kahn DA, et al. The Expert Consensus Guideline Series: Medication Treatment of Bipolar Disorder 2000. Postgrad Med 2000 Apr; Spec No:1–104.

13. Ghaemi SN. New treatments for bipolar disorder: The role of atypical neuroleptic agents. J Clin Psychiatry 2000;61(Suppl 14):33–42.
14. Calabrese JR, Vieta E, Sheldon MD. Latest maintenance data on lamotrigine in bipolar disorder. Eur Neuropsychopharmacol 2003;13(Suppl 2):S57–S66.

74 GENERALIZED ANXIETY DISORDER

▶ Worried Sick (Level I)

Sarah T. Melton, PharmD, BCPP
Cynthia K. Kirkwood, PharmD, BCPP

▶ After completing this case study, the student should be able to:

- Identify target symptoms associated with generalized anxiety disorder (GAD).
- Establish treatment goals of pharmacotherapy for GAD.
- Recommend appropriate pharmacotherapy and duration of treatment for the acute, continuation, and maintenance phases of GAD.
- Educate patients and consult with providers about the pharmacotherapy used in the treatment of GAD.
- Develop a monitoring plan for a patient treated for GAD based on the treatment regimen.

PATIENT PRESENTATION

Chief Complaint
"I worry so much I feel sick."

HPI
Caroline Long is a 31 yo woman who presents to her family physician with complaints of irritability, feelings of "being on edge," and inability to fall asleep at night. She states that she always feels tense and exhausted with constant muscle tension and body aches. She has been employed as an elementary school teacher for 3 years. Over the past school year she has had difficulty concentrating when preparing lessons and her mind often "goes blank" in the classroom. She has frequent abdominal pain and diarrhea. She constantly worries about the children in her class, her teaching ability, finances, and her relationship with her husband. She is afraid she will receive a poor evaluation and be asked to leave the school. She states that she cannot control her worry and her anxiety has increased in intensity over the past 6 months. She denies having obsessive-compulsive thoughts or behaviors, or symptoms of panic disorder. She recently discontinued hydroxyzine 12.5 mg BID and 25 mg at bedtime PRN for anxiety secondary to excessive sedation and dry mouth. She tried kava kava from an herbal store a few months ago. It was not effective and she discontinued it after 2 weeks because of severe abdominal pain.

PMH
Records from the nurse practitioner indicate frequent visits over the past year for headaches, abdominal pain, and diarrhea.
After a recent visit to the ED, she was prescribed hydroxyzine to be taken at night for sleep and during the day as needed for anxiety.
No past psychiatric history.

FH
Father, 62 yo, on "nerve medication" for several years. Mother, 59 yo, with history of major depression, now doing well. Patient has one brother who has no known psychiatric or medical problems.

SH
Married for 5 years, no children, master's degree in elementary education, no tobacco use, little exercise because of time constraints, drinks 4–5 cups of coffee per day. She drinks 1 alcoholic drink every evening to help her "calm down and sleep."

Meds
Pseudoephedrine 30 mg po QID PRN nasal congestion
Loperamide 2 mg po Q 6 H PRN diarrhea

All
Penicillin (hives), iodine

ROS
Positive only for paresthesias and mild diaphoresis; negative for dizziness, palpitations, SOB, chest pain.

PE

Gen
Nervous, thin woman sitting on exam table, cooperative, oriented × 3.

VS
BP 100/65, P 90, RR 18, T 36.5°C; Wt 50 kg, Ht 5′5″

Skin
Clammy, no rashes, lesions, or track marks

HEENT
EOMI, PEERLA; fundi benign, ear and nose clear, dentition intact, tonsils 1+

Neck/LN
Supple, no lymphadenopathy; thyroid symmetrical and of normal size

Lungs/Chest
Symmetrical chest wall movement, BS equal bilaterally, no rub; clear to A&P

Breasts
No masses or tenderness

CV
RRR, normal S_1 and S_2, no M/R/G

Abd
Symmetric, NT/ND, normal BS, no organomegaly or masses

MS/Ext

Small frame; normal bones, joints, & muscles

Neuro

CN II–XII intact, motor and sensory grossly normal, coordination intact

MSE

Appearance and Behavior: Well-groomed, good eye contact, wringing hands and bouncing legs
Speech: Well-spoken, coherent with normal rate and rhythm
Mood: Anxious, worried about what is wrong with her and if she can get better
Affect: Full
Thought processes: Linear, logical, and goal-directed
Thought content: Negative for suicidal or homicidal ideations, obsessions/compulsions, delusions, or hallucinations
Memory: 3/3 at 0 minutes, 2/3 at five minutes; spelled "steak" backwards
Abstractions: Good
Judgment: Good by testing
Insight: Fair
Score on Hamilton Anxiety Scale = 28 points (see Appendix A)

Labs

Na 142 mEq/L	Hgb 14.0 g/dL
K 4.3 mEq/L	Hct 38%
Cl 105 mEq/L	TSH 3 mIU/L
CO_2 28 mEq/L	AST 23 IU/L
BUN 15 mg/dL	ALT 20 IU/L
SCr 0.9 mg/dL	Alk Phos 23 IU/L
Glu 80 mg/dL	

EKG

NSR, rate 88 bpm
Urine toxicology screen: Negative

Assessment

Generalized anxiety disorder

Questions

Problem Identification

1. a. *Create a list of the patient's drug therapy problems.*
   b. *Is there anything in the patient's medication history that could cause or worsen anxiety?*
   c. *What information (signs, symptoms, laboratory values) indicates the presence or severity of GAD?*

Desired Outcome

2. *What are the goals of pharmacotherapy in this case?*

Therapeutic Alternatives

3. a. *What nonpharmacologic therapies might be useful for this patient?*
   b. *What pharmacotherapeutic alternatives are available for the treatment of GAD?*

Optimal Plan

4. a. *What drug, dosage form, dose, schedule, and duration of therapy are best for this patient?*
   b. *What pharmacotherapeutic alternatives would be appropriate if the optimal plan fails?*

Outcome Evaluation

5. *Which clinical and laboratory parameters are necessary to evaluate the therapy for achievement of the desired therapeutic outcome and to detect or prevent adverse effects?*

Patient Education

6. *What information should be provided to the patient to enhance compliance, ensure successful therapy, and minimize adverse effects?*

▶ Follow-Up Question

1. For questions related to the use of kava kava for the treatment of anxiety, please see Section 20 of the Casebook.

▶ Self-Study Assignments

1. Perform a literature search to obtain recent information about GAD in the elderly. Write a two-page paper detailing how the elderly present with GAD and the most appropriate pharmacotherapy for treating this special population.
2. Perform a literature search to obtain recent information about the use of SSRIs for the treatment of GAD. Write a brief critical overview of the controlled trials that support the use of SSRIs in the treatment of GAD.
3. Benzodiazepines were once prescribed on long-term basis for the treatment of GAD. Write a critical review detailing the historical basis and reasoning for the current recommendation to use benzodiazepines only in the acute treatment of GAD.

Clinical Pearl

With effective pharmacotherapy available for the acute and long-term therapy of GAD, the treatment goal for anxiety is remission. Many patients exhibit treatment response but still have anxiety symptoms and social and functional impairment. Remission is a more rigorous treatment goal that requires a HAM-A score of less than or equal to 7 or reduction of at least 70% in baseline levels of symptoms.

References

1. Hamilton M. Hamilton Anxiety Scale. In Guy W, ed. ECDEU Assessment Manual for Psychopharmacology. Rockville, MD: US Department of Health, Education, and Welfare, 1976:193–198.

2. Ballenger JC, Davidson JRT, Lecrubier Y, et al. Consensus statement on generalized anxiety disorder from the International Consensus Group on Depression and Anxiety. J Clin Psychiatry 2001;62(Suppl 11):53–58.
3. Kapczinski F, Lima MS, Souza N, et. al. Antidepressants for generalized anxiety disorder (Cochrane Review). Cochrane Database Syst Rev 2003;2:CD003592.
4. Davidson JR, DuPont RL, Hedges D, et al. Efficacy, safety, and tolerability of venlafaxine extended release and buspirone in outpatients with generalized anxiety disorder. J Clin Psychiatry 1999;60:528–535.
5. Stocchi F, Nordera G, Jokinen RH, et al. Efficacy and tolerability of paroxetine for the long-term treatment of generalized anxiety disorder. J Clin Psychiatry 2003;64:250–258.
6. Llorca PM, Spadone C, Sol O, et al. Efficacy and safety of hydroxyzine in the treatment of generalized anxiety disorder: A 3-month double-blind study. J Clin Psychiatry 2002;63:1020–1027.
7. Pollack MH. Optimizing pharmacotherapy of generalized anxiety disorder to achieve remission. J Clin Psychiatry 2001;62(Suppl 19):20–25.

APPENDIX A. THE RESULTS OF THE HAMILTON ANXIETY (HAM-A) SCALE (ECDEU VERSION)[1] FOR THIS PATIENT.

Mark and score as follows: 0=Not present; 1 = Mild; 2 = Moderate; 3 = Severe; 4 = Very severe

ANXIOUS MOOD

4 Worries, anticipation of the worst, fearful anticipation, irritability

TENSION

3 Feelings of tension, fatigability, startle response, moved to tears easily, trembling, feelings of restlessness, inability to relax

FEARS

2 Of dark, of strangers, of being left alone, of animals, of traffic, of crowds

INSOMNIA

3 Difficulty in falling asleep, broken sleep, unsatisfying sleep and fatigue on waking, dreams, nightmares, night terrors

INTELLECTUAL

3 Difficulty in concentration, poor memory

DEPRESSED MOOD

0 Loss of interest, lack of pleasure in hobbies, depression, early waking, diurnal swing

SOMATIC (Muscular)

2 Pains and aches, twitchings, stiffness, myoclonic jerks, grinding of teeth, unsteady voice, increased muscular tone

SOMATIC (Sensory)

1 Tinnitus, blurring of vision, hot and cold flushes, feelings of weakness, pricking sensation

CARDIOVASCULAR SYMPTOMS

1 Tachycardia, palpitations, pain in chest, throbbing of vessels, fainting feelings, sighing, dyspnea

RESPIRATORY SYMPTOMS

1 Pressure or constriction in chest, choking feelings, sighing, dyspnea

GASTROINTESTINAL SYMPTOMS

3 Difficulty in swallowing, wind, abdominal pain, burning sensations, abdominal fullness, nausea, vomiting, borborygmi, looseness of bowels, loss of weight, constipation

GENITOURINARY SYMPTOMS

1 Frequency of micturition, urgency of micturition, amenorrhea, menorrhagia, development of frigidity, premature ejaculation, loss of libido, impotence

AUTONOMIC SYMPTOMS

1 Dry mouth, flushing, pallor, tendency to sweat, giddiness, tension, headache, raising of hair

BEHAVIOR AT INTERVIEW

3 Fidgeting, restlessness or pacing, tremor of hands, furrowed brow, strained face, sighing or rapid respiration, facial pallor, swallowing, etc.

Total Score : 28

75 OBSESSIVE-COMPULSIVE DISORDER

▶ Five is the Magic Number (Level I)

Sarah T. Melton, PharmD, BCPP
Cynthia K. Kirkwood, PharmD, BCPP

▶ After completing this case study, the student should be able to:

- Identify target symptoms associated with obsessive-compulsive disorder (OCD).
- Discuss treatment goals of pharmacotherapy for OCD.
- Recommend nonpharmacologic therapies for OCD.
- Recommend appropriate pharmacotherapy and duration of treatment for management of OCD.
- Educate patients and consult with providers about the pharmacotherapy used for OCD.
- Develop a monitoring plan for a patient treated for OCD based on the treatment regimen.

PATIENT PRESENTATION

Chief Complaint
"I am afraid that I'm going to hurt my baby."

HPI
Kayla Mitchell is a 27 yo woman presenting to her family physician for a 6-week postpartum check-up with complaints of anxiety and feelings of unease for the past two weeks. She reports that she is having intrusive thoughts of harming her baby. Because these thoughts are becoming more frequent, she feels she is a bad mother and may actually harm her baby. She has started checking all appliances in the house multiple times during the day to make sure they are turned off because she fears starting a fire that will harm her baby. At first, she incessantly checked on the baby but now is beginning to avoid the baby because of her fears. She states that she knows that these thoughts are irrational. She is concerned because the checking behavior consumes 2 to 3 hours each day. She has stopped going out with the baby because she has to check and recheck the car seat safety belts so often that she usually does not make it to her destination. She also reports rubbing her arm in multiples of 5 to feel some relief from the overwhelming anxiety that develops throughout the day from the intrusive thoughts. She states that she has tried to hide this behavior from her husband, but it has become so time-consuming and distressful that she asked him to accompany her on this visit to the physician.

PMH
G_1P_1 now at 6 weeks postpartum, normal spontaneous vaginal delivery with 1° perineal tear
Small external hemorrhoids s/p delivery
H/O chronic sinusitis

PPH
No hospitalizations or outpatient psychiatric treatment, but she recalls from childhood doing strange counting rituals while lying in bed or watching TV. She has always felt a need to "control things."

FH
Father, 68 yo with history of major depression. Mother, 65 yo with multiple sclerosis. Older brother is a "perfectionist" and has to have everything "just right."

SH
Married for 3 years, bachelor's degree in business, presently on maternity leave from the bank where she works; undecided about returning to work, no tobacco or alcohol use. Breast-fed infant for 4 weeks, now bottle-feeding. She had excessive worrying that the baby was starving because he was not getting enough breast milk. Has prescription drug coverage through her husband's insurance program at work.

Meds
Docusate sodium 100 mg po BID

All
Sulfa (hives), adhesive bandages

ROS
No fatigue, change in appetite, sleep pattern, difficulty concentrating, crying spells. No palpitations, dyspnea

PE

Gen
Anxious, WDWN woman sitting on exam table rubbing her arm up and down in multiples of 5, cooperative, oriented × 3

VS
BP 120/75, P 80, RR 19, T 36.5°C; Wt 60 kg, Ht 5′5″

Skin
Left arm red and slightly inflamed from elbow to wrist; no rashes, lesions, track marks. Normal hair growth and distribution.

HEENT
EOMI, PEERLA; fundi benign, ear and nose clear, dentition intact, tonsils 1+

Neck/LN
Supple, no lymphadenopathy; thyroid symmetrical and of normal size

Lungs/Chest
Symmetrical chest wall movement, BS equal bilaterally, no rub; clear to A&P

Breasts
Slight tenderness s/p weaning from breastfeeding

CV
RRR, normal S_1 and S_2, no M/R/G

Abd
Symmetric, NT/ND, normal BS, no organomegaly or masses

Gyn

Normal hair distribution and external genitalia, normal urethra, well-healed perineum. Parous cervix with no lesions or discharge. Uterus normal; no adnexal masses or tenderness

MS/Ext

Small frame, normal bones, joints, muscles

Neuro

CN II–XII intact, motor and sensory grossly normal, coordination intact, no tremor

MSE

Appearance and Behavior: Well-groomed, poor eye contact, rubbing arm up and down in a slow methodical manner

Speech: Well-spoken, coherent with normal rate and rhythm

Mood: Anxious, worried that she is a bad mother and will harm her baby

Affect: Anxious, frightened

Thought processes: Linear, logical, and goal-directed

Thought content: Negative for suicidal or homicidal ideations. Positive for obsessions about harming her child, compulsions including checking and rubbing arm in multiples of 5, denies delusions and hallucinations

Memory: 3/3 at 0 minutes, 3/3 at five minutes (ball, purple, chair); spelled "horse" backwards

Abstractions: Fair

Judgment: Good by testing

Insight: Good

Score on Yale-Brown Obsessive Compulsive Scale = 28 points

Labs

Na 140 mEq/L	Hgb 15.0 g/dL
K 3.7 mEq/L	Hct 40%
Cl 107 mEq/L	TSH 2.8 mIU/L
CO_2 28 mEq/L	AST 28 IU/L
BUN 14 mg/dL	ALT 25 IU/L
SCr 0.8 mg/dL	Alk Phos 42 IU/L
Glu 75 mg/dL	

EKG

NSR, rate 80 bpm

Urine toxicology screen

Negative

Assessment

Obsessive-Compulsive Disorder

Questions

Problem Identification

1. a. *Create a list of the patient's drug therapy problems.*
   b. *Is there anything in the patient's history that could be considered a risk factor for the development of OCD?*
   c. *What information (signs, symptoms, laboratory values) indicates the presence or severity of OCD?*

Desired Outcome

2. *What are the goals of pharmacotherapy for OCD in this case?*

Therapeutic Alternatives

3. a. *What nonpharmacologic therapies might be useful for this patient?*
   b. *What pharmacotherapeutic alternatives are available for the treatment of OCD?*

Optimal Plan

4. a. *What drug, dosage form, dose, schedule, and duration of therapy are best for this patient?*
   b. *What pharmacotherapeutic alternatives would be appropriate if the optimal plan fails?*
   c. *When is a patient with OCD considered to be "treatment refractory?" What other pharmacologic alternatives are available if this patient is determined to be refractory to standard pharmacotherapy?*

Outcome Evaluation

5. *Which clinical and laboratory parameters are necessary to evaluate the therapy for achievement of the desired therapeutic outcomes and to detect or prevent adverse effects?*

Patient Education

6. *What information should be provided to the patient to enhance compliance, ensure successful therapy, and minimize adverse effects?*

Follow-Up Questions

1. *When is a decrease in the Y-BOCS score considered clinically significant?*
2. *If this patient had presented to the physician desiring to continue breastfeeding, what would your recommendations be regarding pharmacotherapy?*

Self-Study Assignments

1. Prepare a short paper evaluating the risks and benefits of using SSRIs in the pharmacotherapy of OCD in a female who is pregnant or breastfeeding.

2. Perform a literature search and write a short paper describing Pediatric Autoimmune Neuropsychiatric Disorders Associated with Streptococcus (PANDAS) and current recommendations for therapy.
3. Discuss the pharmacotherapeutic agents used to augment antidepressant therapy in the treatment of OCD in patients who have a partial response to antidepressant monotherapy.
4. Using the Internet, find and report on several OCD or mental health foundations that provide valuable information and support for patients and families affected by OCD.

▶ Clinical Pearl

Higher dosages of antidepressant medication than those typically used for depression are often required to obtain antiobsessional effects. A response to pharmacotherapy may not occur until a therapeutic dose has been maintained for at least 10 to 12 weeks.

References

1. Arnold LM. A case series of women with postpartum-onset obsessive-compulsive disorder. Primary Care Companion J Clin Psychiatry 1999;1:103–108.
2. Levine RE, Oandasan AP, Primeau LA, et al. Anxiety disorders during pregnancy and postpartum. Am J Perinatol 2003;20:239–248.
3. Jenike MA. Obsessive-compulsive disorder. N Engl J Med 2004;350:259–265.
4. Goodman WK, Price LH, Rasmussen SA, et al. The Yale-Brown Obsessive Compulsive Scale. I. Development, use, and reliability. Arch Gen Psychiatry 1989;46:1006–1011.
5. March JS, Frances A, Kahn DA, et al, eds. The Expert Consensus Guideline Series: Treatment of Obsessive-Compulsive Disorder. J Clin Psychiatry 1997;58 (Suppl 4):4–72. www.psychguides.com/gl-treatment_of_obsessive-compulsive_disorder.html (accessed June 20, 2004).
6. Denys D, van der Wee N, van Megen HJ, et al. A double blind comparison of venlafaxine and paroxetine in obsessive-compulsive disorder. J Clin Psychopharmacol 2003;23:568–575.
7. Kaplan A, Hollander E. A review of pharmacologic treatments for obsessive-compulsive disorder. Psychiatr Serv 2003;54:1111–1118.
8. Hollander E, Allen A, Steiner M, et al. Acute and long-term treatment of prevention of relapse of obsessive-compulsive disorder with paroxetine. J Clin Psychiatry 2003;64:1113–1121.

76 INSOMNIA

▶ In Search of Rest (Level II)

Mollie Ashe Scott, PharmD, BCPS, CPP
Amy M. Lugo, PharmD, CDM, CPP

▶ After completing this case study, students should be able to:

- Identify the psychosocial, disease-related, and drug-induced causes of insomnia.
- Educate a patient regarding nonpharmacologic treatments for insomnia.
- Design a therapeutic plan for treatment of insomnia.

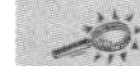 PATIENT PRESENTATION

Chief Complaint

"I haven't slept for years."

HPI

Jane Parker is a 72 yo woman who is referred by her primary care physician to a Pharmacotherapy Clinic for a medication review. She is noticeably tired. Her daughter accompanies her. The patient states that she has not slept well since the death of her husband three years ago, despite taking flurazepam 15 mg po at bedtime since that time. She is currently taking flurazepam for sleep 3 to 4 times weekly. She is concerned that she might be taking too many medications and she feels that she is a burden to her daughters.

PMH

Insomnia
Osteoarthritis (right hip, right knee, and hands)
Dyslipidemia treated with diet and exercise
DM type 2 for 12 years
Peripheral neuropathy
HTN for 10 years
H/O tobacco abuse
COPD
Recent fall with arm fracture

FH

Mother died of CVA at age 65, had breast cancer; father lived until his late 80s

SH

Married for 52 years, recently widowed 3 years ago, lives alone. Mother of two and grandmother of three. One daughter lives next door and the other lives in the same town. She has a good support system with her family. She reports having financial stressors since her only income currently is Social Security and a small pension from her husband's job. Patient was a stay-at-home mother, has Medicare, and pays out-of-pocket for her medications. She has a 30 pack-year smoking history but quit 10 years ago and denies any alcohol use.

ROS

Patient reports difficulty going to sleep and staying asleep for several years. She admits that flurazepam worked initially and then quit working, however, she states she "still needs it to sleep." She complains of constipation since starting her pain pills for her broken arm, which was fractured last month after falling in her home when she got up in the middle of the night to go to the bathroom. Her verbal pain scale for her fractured arm is 3/10. Additionally, she reports a 10-lb. weight loss over the past few months since she doesn't feel like eating. She denies a "blue mood" or any thoughts of suicide; however, her daughter feels like she may be depressed. She states she uses incontinence pads and reports urinary frequency, urgency, and often doesn't make it in time to the bathroom. She has stopped going to church and to lunch with her friends for fear of being incontinent.

She has right knee pain and stiffness, particularly upon awakening and after sitting. Her hand and wrist pain have caused her to stop quilting, which she truly enjoys. Her verbal pain scale regarding her OA in her hip, knee and hands is 5/10. She frequently has SOB and coughing with exertion throughout the day, but denies nighttime SOB.

Meds

Flurazepam 15 mg po at bedtime PRN sleep
Acetaminophen 500 mg po QID PRN
Glucosamine 500 mg po TID
Amitriptyline 50 mg po at bedtime
HCTZ 25mg po Q AM
Metformin 1000 mg po BID
Combivent MDI 2 puffs QID PRN
Vicodin 1–2 Q 4–6 hours PRN pain

PE (from the last visit with her PCP)

Gen
Elderly WDWN woman who walks with a cane and looks her stated age

VS
BP 140/92, P 76, RR 12, T 37°C; Wt 48 kg; Ht 5′5″

Skin
Normal skin color and turgor, no lesions noted

HEENT
Normocephalic, PERRLA, EOMI

Neck/LN
Supple with normal size thyroid, (–) adenopathy

Lungs
CTA bilaterally

CV
Normal S_1, S_2; no m/r/g

Abd
NTND, no HSM

GU/Rect
Deferred

Ext
No C/C/E; normal muscle bulk and tone; muscle strength 5/5 and equal in all extremities; 1+ popliteal and dorsalis pedis pulses; decreased lower extremity sensation to monofilament bilaterally; rotation of the right hip produced pain in her groin indicative of hip OA. Right knee demonstrates bony changes indicative of knee OA; (–) for effusions of the knee; DIP joints demonstrate bony changes associated with OA including Heberden's nodes.

Neuro
Oriented to person, place, and time; CN II–XII intact; Mini Mental Status Examination results: 27/30

Labs

Na 140 mEq/L	Hgb 14 g/dL	AST 34 IU/L	*Lipid Panel*
K 4.2 mEq/L	Hct 43%	ALT 32 IU/L	TC 212 mg/dL
Cl 105 mEq/L	RBC 4.7 × 10^6/mm^3	LDH 112 IU/L	LDL 137 mg/dL
CO_2 28 mEq/L	Plt 262 × 10^3/mm^3	GGT 47 IU/L	HDL 45 mg/dL
BUN 11 mg/dL	WBC 6.2 × 10^3/mm^3	T. Bili 0.3 mg/dL	TG 180 mg/dL
SCr 1.4 mg/dL	TSH 0.25 mIU/L	T. prot 7.1 g/dL	HbA_{1C} 9.2%
Glu 192 mg/dL	Free T_4 4.1 ng/dL	Alb 4.0 g/dL	

Assessment

1. Insomnia
2. Untreated urge incontinence
3. OA
4. Dyslipidemia
5. Recent falls
6. Possible depression
7. HTN
8. DM type 2
9. Peripheral neuropathy
10. Obesity
11. COPD
12. Renal insufficiency
13. Constipation
14. At risk for osteoporosis

▶ Questions

Problem Identification

1. a. *Create a drug-related problem list for the patient.*
   b. *Which information (signs, symptoms, laboratory values) indicates the presence or severity of insomnia?*
   c. *Could any of the patient's problems have been caused by drug therapy?*
   d. *What additional information is needed to satisfactorily assess this patient?*

Desired Outcome

2. *What are the goals of pharmacotherapy in this case?*

Therapeutic Alternatives

3. a. *What nonpharmacologic therapies might be useful for this patient?*
   b. *What feasible pharmacotherapeutic alternatives are available for treatment of insomnia?*

Optimal Plan

4. a. *What drug, dosage form, dose, schedule, and duration of therapy are best for this patient?*

b. What alternatives would be appropriate if the initial therapy fails or cannot be used?

Outcome Evaluation

5. Which clinical and laboratory parameters are necessary to evaluate the therapy for achievement of the desired therapeutic outcome and to detect or prevent adverse effects?

Patient Education

6. What information should be provided to the patient to enhance compliance, ensure successful therapy, and minimize adverse effects?

▶ Follow-Up Questions

1. What other medication adjustments should be made at this time?

▶ Self-Study Assignments

1. Describe how aging affects normal sleep architecture.
2. Develop a pharmacotherapy plan for the treatment of her urge incontinence.
3. Develop a nonpharmacologic plan to help her prevent falls in her home.
4. List medications that increase the risk for falls in the elderly.

▶ Clinical Pearl

Insomnia is often caused by an acute stressor or underlying medical or psychiatric condition. Hypnotics should be prescribed on a short-term basis as part of a comprehensive treatment plan that addresses any underlying causes of poor sleep.

References

1. National Heart, Lung, and Blood Institute Working Group on Insomnia. Insomnia: assessment and management in primary care. Am Fam Physician 1999;59:3029–3038.
2. Holbrook AM, Crowther R, Lotter A, et al. Meta-analysis of benzodiazepine use in the treatment of insomnia. CMAJ 2000;162:225–233.
3. Fick DM, Cooper JW, Wade WE, et al. Updating the Beers Criteria for potentially inappropriate medication use in older adults: Results of a US consensus panel of experts. Arch Intern Med 2003;163:2716–2724.
4. Dooley M, Plosker GL. Zaleplon: A review of its use in the treatment of insomnia. Drugs 2000;60:413–445.
5. Montplaisir J, Hawa R, Moller C, et al. Zopiclone and zaleplon vs benzodiazepines in the treatment of insomnia: Canadian consensus statement. Hum Psychopharmacol 2003;18:29–38.
6. Terzano MG, Rossi M, Palomba V, et al. New drugs for insomnia: Comparative tolerability of zopiclone, zolpidem and zaleplon. Drug Saf 2003;26: 261–282.
7. Krystal AD, Walsh JK, Laska E, et al. Sustained efficacy of eszopiclone over 6 months of nightly treatment: Results of a randomized, double-blind, placebo-controlled study in adults with chronic insomnia. Sleep 2003;26:793–799.
8. Wortelboer U, Cohrs S, Rodenbeck A, et al. Tolerability of hypnosedatives in older patients. Drugs Aging 2002;19:529–539.
9. Olde Rikkert MG, Rigaud AS. Melatonin in elderly patients with insomnia. A systematic review. Z Gerontol Geriatr 2001;34:491–497.
10. Donath F, Quispe S, Diefenbach K, et al. Critical evaluation of the effect of valerian extract on sleep structure and sleep quality. Pharmacopsychiatry 2000;33:47–53.
11. Schweizer E, Rickels K, Case WG, et al. Long-term therapeutic use of benzodiazepines. II. Effects of gradual taper. Arch Gen Psychiatry 1990;47:908–915.

SECTION 8

Endocrinologic Disorders

77 TYPE 1 DIABETES MELLITUS AND KETOACIDOSIS

► Emergency Room Honeymoon (Level II)

Amy S. Nicholas, PharmD, CDE
Holly S. Divine, PharmD, CGP, CDE

► After completing this case study, students should be able to:

- Recognize signs and symptoms of diabetic ketoacidosis (DKA).
- Establish laboratory parameters for the diagnosis and monitoring of DKA.
- Identify anticipated electrolyte abnormalities associated with DKA and their treatment.
- Recommend appropriate initial IV insulin doses and insulin infusion concentrations for treating DKA.
- Identify therapeutic decision points in DKA treatment and provide parameters for altering therapy at those points.
- Determine when patients may be converted from IV to subcutaneous insulin therapy and calculate the dose of insulin that should be administered.
- Provide patient education for sick day management of patients with diabetes mellitus.
- Provide patient education about lifestyle modifications to help control type 1 diabetes.

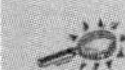

PATIENT PRESENTATION

Chief Complaint

"It burns when I urinate and my lower abdomen hurts."

HPI

Sherry Sutherland is a 26 yo woman with a history of type 1 DM of 16 years duration. She recently graduated from pharmacy school. Sherry and her husband just returned from their honeymoon in Hawaii two days ago, and she states that she has been under a "lot of stress" in the last two months preparing for the wedding and studying for the boards. She began having suprapubic pain and felt like she had a fever about 5 days ago but dismissed it, not wanting to "ruin" their trip by complaining. Last night before supper (5:00 PM), she took her usual dose of insulin lispro. She began feeling nauseated with some stomach pains several hours after supper, and she began vomiting at 10:00 PM. Her blood glucose at that time was 370 mg/dL. She took her usual bedtime insulin glargine and supplemented this with additional insulin lispro to compensate for the hyperglycemia. She tried sipping water and clear diet soda but was unable to keep any fluids down. She vomited six more times that evening before falling asleep for several hours. Her husband (who is also a pharmacist) had trouble waking her the next morning. She tried eating and drinking but was unable to keep anything down again and vomited another three times. Her husband was concerned after he helped her back to bed because he noticed a pink tinge in the toilet after she last urinated. He contacted her physician by phone after he noted heavy breathing (and timed it to be 30 breaths/minute). Her physician instructed them to seek transportation to the hospital ED. She did not test her urine for ketones but did take her insulin lispro for the hyperglycemia (glucose 500 mg/dL) at breakfast time, even though she was unable to eat.

Sherry had a visit with her ophthalmologist 9 months ago and was told there was nothing abnormal after receiving a dilated eye examination. Her last screen for microalbuminuria 3 months ago was positive, although she has not had additional screenings to confirm those results. She has no paresthesias of the feet or hands and has never had a foot ulcer. She denies any chest pain, history of hypertension, and intermittent claudication. Her last lipid panel was obtained 3 months ago and was suboptimal. She has had a history of hypoglycemic coma but no episodes in the past 3 years. Her glucose control has been suboptimal with an A1C performed 3 months ago of 9.5%. She infrequently sees a dietitian and admits that she has had difficulty with carbohydrate counting due to the demands of pharmacy school, a busy schedule while planning the wedding and studying for the boards.

PMH

Type 1 DM diagnosed 16 years ago; hospitalized 3 times for DKA in the past 10 years

PSH

Appendectomy 1997

FH

Father age 50 has HTN and hyperlipidemia; mother deceased at 47 from colon CA; one brother age 36 with type 1 DM, HTN and hyperlipidemia; one other healthy sibling.

SH

Recently married. Does not smoke, or abuse drugs. Occasional wine 1 to 3 glasses/week with dinner.

Meds

Insulin glargine 24 units subQ at bedtime
Insulin lispro 6 units subQ before meals
Yasmin one tablet po daily

All

NKDA

ROS

HEENT—Awakened with blurry vision and dizziness on postural change but denies vertigo, head trauma, ear pain, tinnitus, dysphagia, odynophagia.

CV—No complaints of chest pain, orthopnea, peripheral edema, or heart murmur.

Resp—No complaints of cough, wheezing, dyspnea.

GI—Vomiting as noted above; complains of lower abdominal pain; denies constipation, diarrhea, or food intolerance.

GU—Had polyuria (large volumes every 2 hours) last night; urinated × 1 since awakening. Complains of dysuria and hematuria (noted × 1 per husband).

OB-GYN—G_0P_0. Denies current pregnancy and has ongoing menses. Menses flows for 5 days and is regular every 28 days. Sexually active and denies any vaginal discharge, pain, or itching.

Neuro—Has never had a seizure or weakness in an arm or leg. No complaints of headache, paresthesias, dysesthesias, or anesthesias.

Derm—No history of chronic rashes, sweating abnormalities, or recent skin lesions. Has had mild lipohypertrophy at old thigh injection sites but tries to avoid these areas.

Endo—Denies a history of goiter and has no heat or cold intolerance. She has gained 15 pounds in the last 4 years.

PE

Gen

Mildly overweight white woman with a female body habitus looking her stated age, with deep respirations, alcohol or ketones on her breath and not confused, but questionably appropriate

VS

BP 114/79 supine, 105/69 sitting; P 128; RR 30; T 38.0°C; Ht 5′5″; Wt 75 kg

Skin

Lipohypertrophy is present on both lateral thighs

HEENT

NCAT, PERRLA, EOM intact. Mucous membranes are dry; pharynx is erythematous without tonsillar exudates. Ears are unremarkable

Neck

Thyroid is palpable but not enlarged. No masses

LN

Cervical, axillary, and femoral lymph nodes are not palpable

CV

PMI is normal and non-displaced. S_1 and S_2 are normal without S_3, S_4, murmur, or rub. RRR. Carotid, femoral, and dorsalis pedis pulses are 2+ throughout. There are no carotid, abdominal or femoral bruits.

Chest

Lungs are CTA & P. There is full chest excursion

Abd

Soft, without organomegaly or masses; guarding noted upon palpation of suprapubic area. Bowel sounds are decreased

Rect

Anus is normal. No masses or hemorrhoids are noted. Stool is heme (–)

Ext

There is no pretibial edema. Feet are without ulcers; calluses noted on heals bilaterally

Neuro

DTRs bilaterally 2+ for the biceps, brachioradialis, quadriceps, and Achilles. Plantars are downgoing bilaterally. Vibratory perception at the 1st MTP bilaterally is slightly depressed. Muscle strength is 5/5.

Labs

			Fasting Lipid Panel
Na 126 mEq/L	Hgb 16 g/dL	WBC $5.9 \times 10^3/mm^3$	T. Chol 230 mg/dL
K 6.0 mEq/L	Hct 44%	Neutros 50%	LDL 133 mg/dL
Cl 98 mEq/L	RBC $5.3 \times 10^6/mm^3$	Bands 17%	HDL 38 mg/dL
CO_2 6.0 mEq/L	Plt $270 \times 10^3/mm^3$	Lymphs 28%	Trig 250 mg/dL
Anion gap 26 mEq/L	MCV 90 μm^3	Monos 5%	Serum pregnancy: negative
BUN 23 mg/dL	MCHC 35 g/dL		
SCr 1.3 mg/dL			
Glu 735 mg/dL			

ABG

On room air: pH 7.2; pCO_2 7.6; pO_2 139; HCO_3 2.0, O_2 sat 97%

UA

SG 1.020, pH 6, glu 3+, protein 2+, ketones 3+, blood 3+, nitrite +; leukocyte esterase +; 80 WBC/hpf; 89 RBC/hpf

Chest X-Ray

Normal

ECG

Sinus tachycardia

Assessment

1. Diabetic ketoacidosis precipitated by UTI
2. Type 1 DM complicated by hypercholesterolemia and microalbuminuria
3. Overweight

▶ Questions

Problem Identification

1. a. *What signs, symptoms, and laboratory findings indicate the presence and severity of DKA in this patient?*
   b. *What are the diagnostic criteria for DKA?*
   c. *What problems beyond hyperglycemia are encountered in DKA that may require intervention?*

Desired Outcome

2. *What are the goals of therapy for this patient?*

Therapeutic Alternatives

3. *What therapies are available to correct the metabolic derangements of DKA?*

Optimal Plan

4. *Outline your specific plan for providing the IV fluids and medications that should be administered to this patient.*

Outcome Evaluation

5. a. *What monitoring is necessary for the therapeutic plan that you developed for the patient?*
   b. *What changes in the therapeutic regimen should be considered when the blood glucose drops below 250 mg/dL or the potassium drops into the range of 3.3 to 5.0 mEq/L? Provide the rationale for your answer.*
   c. *When is the DKA considered to be resolved, and when can IV insulin therapy be converted to subcutaneous therapy?*
   d. *Outline a plan for converting the patient from IV to subcutaneous insulin after resolution of the DKA.*

Patient Education

6. *How should patients be informed about self-management on a "sick day" (i.e., when they are anorectic, nauseated, or vomiting)?*

▶ Follow-Up Questions

1. *Are there any other medications that should be added to her regimen based on her presenting laboratory values and/or HPI? What, if any, lifestyle recommendations would you make?*
2. *Describe the nonpharmacologic approaches that should be taken to prevent further complications associate with diabetes, including the prevention of future episodes of UTI.*

▶ Self-Study Assignments

1. Describe the medical complications associated with DKA and DKA treatment.
2. Persons with type 1 diabetes are at risk for developing cardiovascular disease and end-stage renal disease. Describe therapeutic approaches to prevent these two complications.
3. DKA and hyperosmolar hyperglycemic nonketotic coma are metabolic disorders commonly encountered in patients with diabetes. Compare these two disorders with respect to precipitating factors, signs/symptoms, pathophysiology, and treatment strategies.

▶ Clinical Pearl

Obtaining a hemogram is crucial in patients presenting with DKA because up to 25% of patients have emesis that may be "coffee-ground" in appearance and guaiac-positive.

References

1. DeFronzo RA, Matsuda M, Barrett EJ. Diabetic ketoacidosis: A combined metabolic-nephrologic approach to therapy. Diabetes Rev 1994;2:209–238.
2. Morris LR, Murphy MB, Kitabchi AE. Bicarbonate therapy in severe diabetic ketoacidosis. Ann Intern Med 1986;105:836–840.
3. Kitabchi AE, Umpierrez GE, Murphy MB, et al. Management of hyperglycemic crises in patients with diabetes. Diabetes Care 2001;24:131–153.
4. Ennis ED, Stahl EJB, Kreisberg RA. The hyperosmolar hyperglycemic syndrome. Diabetes Rev 1994;2:115–126.
5. Kitabchi AE, Umpierrez GE, Murphy MB, et al. American Diabetes Association. Hyperglycemic crises in diabetes. ADA Clinical Practice Recommendations. Diabetes Care 2004;27(Suppl 1):S94–S102.

Acknowledgement: This case is based in part on the case written for the Fifth Edition by Scott Jacober, DO, CDE, and Linda A. Jaber, PharmD.

78 TYPE 2 DIABETES MELLITUS: NEW ONSET

▶ An American Epidemic (Level III)

Scott R. Drab, PharmD, CDE, BC-ADM

▶ Learning Objectives

▶ After completing this case study, the student should be able to:

- Recognize the signs, symptoms and risk factors associated with type 2 diabetes mellitus (DM).
- Identify the comorbidities in type 2 DM associated with insulin resistance (metabolic syndrome, Syndrome X).
- Compare the pharmacotherapeutic options in the management of type 2 DM including mechanism of action, contraindications, and side effects.
- Describe the role of self-monitoring of blood glucose (SMBG) and identify factors to enhance patient adherence.
- Develop a patient-specific pharmacotherapeutic plan for the treatment and monitoring of type 2 DM.

PATIENT PRESENTATION

Chief Complaint
"Lately I feel extremely tired and now my vision is blurred."

HPI
William Jenkins is a 67 yo man who presents to the family medicine clinic complaining of periodic blurred vision for the past 3 weeks. He further complains of severe fatigue and lack of energy, which limits his daily activities. He states that he started taking a multiple vitamin 1 week ago but has not noticed any improvement in his energy level.

PMH
HTN × 7 years
Hyperlipidemia × 5 years

FH
Diabetes present in both father and paternal grandfather. Father died suddenly of a massive stroke at age 62; mother died of breast cancer at age 49; 2 younger siblings are alive and apparently well.

SH
Married × 43 years with 2 children. Works full-time as a parking lot attendant. No alcohol or tobacco use. Rarely exercises and admits to trying fad diets for weight loss with little success.

Meds
Propranolol LA 80 mg po once daily
MVI po once daily

All
NKDA

ROS
Occasional polydipsia, polyphagia, fatigue, weakness, blurred vision. Denies chest pain, dyspnea, tachycardia, dizziness or lightheadedness upon standing, tingling or numbness in extremities, leg cramps, peripheral edema, changes in bowel movements, GI bloating or pain, nausea or vomiting, urinary incontinence, or presence of skin lesions.

PE

Gen
The patient is an obese African-American man who seems restless and in mild distress

VS
BP 149/96 without orthostasis; P 80; RR 18; T 37.2°C; Wt 111.5 kg; Ht 65″; BMI 41 kg/m^2

Skin
Dry with poor skin turgor; no ulcers or rash

HEENT
PERRLA; EOMI; TMs intact; no hemorrhages or exudates on funduscopic examination; mucous membranes normal; nose and throat clear w/o exudates or lesions

Neck/LN
Supple; without lymphadenopathy, thyromegaly, or JVD

CV
RRR; normal S_1 and S_2; no S_3, S_4, rubs, murmurs, or bruits

Lungs
CTA

Abd
Soft, NT, central obesity; normal BS; no organomegaly, or distention

GU/Rect
Normal external male genitalia

Ext
Normal ROM and sensation; peripheral pulses 2+ throughout; no lesions, ulcers, or edema

Neuro
A&O × 3, CN II–XII intact; DTRs 2+ throughout; feet with normal vibratory and pinprick sensation (5.07/10 g monofilament)

Labs

Na 141 mEq/L	Ca 9.9 mg/dL
K 4.0 mEq/L	Phos 3.2 mg/dL
Cl 96 mEq/L	AST 21 IU/L
CO_2 22 mEq/L	ALT 15 IU/L
BUN 24 mg/dL	Alk phos 45 IU/L
SCr 1.6 mg/dL	T. bili 0.9 mg/dL
Random Glu 260 mg/dL	T. chol 285 mg/dL

UA

(–) ketones, (–) protein, (–) microalbuminuria

Assessment

1. Elevated random glucose; presumed newly-diagnosed type 2 diabetes mellitus. Will obtain a fasting blood glucose level to confirm the diagnosis and also check A1c.
2. Elevated total cholesterol. Will obtain fasting lipid profile to evaluate LDL, HDL, and triglycerides.
3. Hypertension
4. Obesity

▶ Clinical Course:

The patient returned to clinic 3 days later for lab work, which revealed: FBG 177 mg/dL; A1c 9.1%; FLP: T. chol 280 mg/dL, HDL 27 mg/dL, LDL 176 mg/dL, Trig 302 mg/dL.

▶ Questions

Problem Identification

1. a. *What risk factors for type 2 DM are present in this patient?*
   b. *What information (signs, symptoms, laboratory values) supports the diagnosis of type 2 DM?*
   c. *What information presented indicates the presence of insulin resistance?*
   d. *Create a list of this patient's drug therapy problems.*

Desired Outcome

2. a. *What are the desired goals for the treatment of this patient's diabetes?*
   b. *Considering his other medical problems, what other treatment goals should be established?*

Therapeutic Alternatives

3. a. *What nonpharmacologic therapies might be useful in the management of this patient?*
   b. *What feasible pharmacotherapeutic alternatives are available for the treatment of this patient's DM? Identify the factors that will influence your choice of initial therapy.*

Optimal Plan

4. a. *Outline a complete pharmacotherapeutic plan to manage this patient's current problems including drug, dosage form, dose, schedule, and rationale for your selections.*
   b. *What changes in therapy would you recommend if your initial plan fails to achieve adequate glycemic control?*

Outcome Evaluation

5. a. *What clinical and laboratory parameters will you monitor to evaluate glycemic efficacy and to detect or prevent adverse effects?*
   b. *The patient's physician suggested that he obtain a blood glucose meter for self-testing. What are the healthcare provider's responsibilities with respect to patients and self-monitoring of blood glucose (SMBG)?*
   c. *Identify at least four potential situations in which the information provided by SMBG would be useful to patients and healthcare providers.*
   d. *What factors should be considered in the selection of an appropriate blood glucose meter? (See example in Figure 78–1.)*

Patient Education

6. a. *What information should be provided to the patient about diabetes and its treatment to enhance compliance, ensure successful therapy, minimize adverse effects, and prevent future complications?*
   b. *How would you educate the patient regarding how and when to check his blood glucose?*

▶ Follow-Up Questions

1. *Which over-the-counter products could be recommended for patients to use in treating hypoglycemic episodes?*
2. *List several potential sources of error in SMBG.*
3. *When starting patients on insulin, the use of combination oral antihyperglycemic agents and insulin offers several advantages over switching entirely to insulin:*
   a. *What are the advantages of adding insulin to existing therapies with oral agents?*
   b. *List an appropriate method of starting insulin therapy to adequately control fasting hyperglycemia in patients on combination oral agents.*

▶ Self-Study Assignments

1. Describe how you would evaluate and monitor this patient's quality of life.
2. Characterize the relationship between insulin resistance and the risk for atherosclerotic vascular disease.
3. Prepare a list of medications that have been associated with increasing blood glucose. Provide literature evidence on the strength of the association with each medication.
4. Review the literature and conduct a comparative review of the efficacy of inhaled insulin therapy relative to the insulin products commercially available for subcutaneous injection.

▶ Clinical Pearl

More than 18 million Americans have diabetes, and approximately 1.3 million new cases are diagnosed each year. From 1990–2003, the CDC reported

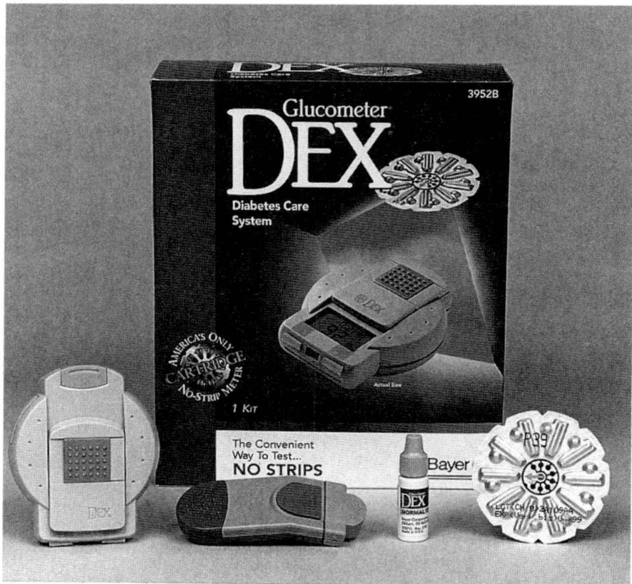

Figure 78–1. The Glucometer DEX System for self-monitoring of blood glucose by patients with diabetes mellitus. *(Photo courtesy of Bayer Corporation, Diagnostics Division. Glucometer and DEX are registered trademarks of Bayer Corporation, Diagnostics Division).*

that the number of Americans with diabetes rose 94 percent providing further evidence that diabetes is a major public health threat of epidemic proportions. Excess caloric intake, low physical activity, and increasing levels of obesity are the main contributors to the increased incidence.

References

1. American Diabetes Association. Screening for diabetes. Diabetes Care 2003; 26(Suppl 1):S21–S24.
2. American Diabetes Association. Report of the expert committee on the diagnosis and classification of diabetes mellitus. Diabetes Care 2003;26(Suppl 1):S5–S20.
3. Frohlich M, Imhof A, Berg G, et al. Association between C-reactive protein and features of the metabolic syndrome: A population-based study. Diabetes Care. 2000;23:1835–1839.
4. Bloomgarden ZT. Insulin Resistance: Current concepts. Clin Ther. 1998; 20: 216–231.
5. Elliott WJ, Stein PP, Black HR. Drug treatment of hypertension in patients with diabetes. Diabetes Rev 1995;3:447–497.
6. American Diabetes Association. Standards of medical care for patients with diabetes mellitus. Diabetes Care 2003;26(Suppl 1):S33–S50.
7. American Diabetes Association. Evidence-based nutrition principles and recommendations for the treatment and prevention of diabetes and related complications. Diabetes Care 2003;26(Suppl 1):S51–S61.
8. American Diabetes Association. The pharmacological treatment of hyperglycemia in NIDDM. Diabetes Care. 1996;19(Suppl 1):S54–S61.
9. Campbell RK, White JR, Biguanides. In: Medications for the treatment of diabetes. Alexandria, VA: American Diabetes Association; 2000:100–112.
10. American Diabetes Association. Hypertension management in adults with diabetes. Diabetes Care 2004;27(Suppl 1):S65–S67.
11. National Cholesterol Education Program (NCEP) Expert Panel: Executive Summary of the third report of the NCEP expert panel on detection, evaluation, and treatment of high blood cholesterol in adults (Adult Treatment Panel III). JAMA 2001;285;2486–2497.
12. Garg A. Dyslipoproteinemia and diabetes. Endocrinol Metab Clin North Am 1998;27:613–625.
13. American Diabetes Association. Influenza and pneumococcal immunization in diabetes. Diabetes Care. 2004;27(Suppl 1):S111–S113.
14. American Diabetes Association. Aspirin therapy in diabetes. Diabetes Care 2004;27(Suppl 1):S72–S73.

Acknowledgement: This case is based in part on the case written for the Fifth Edition by Scott R. Drab, PharmD, CDE, BC-ADM, and Linda A. Jaber, PharmD.

79 TYPE 2 DIABETES MELLITUS: EXISTING DISEASE

▶ Establishing Optimal Control (Level II)

Kelly P. Jones, PharmD
Jean-Venable (Kelly) R. Goode, PharmD, BCPS

▶ After completing this case study, students should be able to:

- Identify the goals of therapy for the treatment of type 2 diabetes mellitus (DM).
- Discuss the risk factors and comorbidities associated with type 2 DM.
- Compare options for drug therapy management of type 2 DM including mechanisms of action, combination therapies, comorbidities, and patient-friendly treatment plans.
- Develop an individualized drug therapy management plan including dosage regimens, therapeutic endpoints, and monitoring parameters.

- Provide patient education regarding medications, adherence to the treatment plan, monitoring the disease state, blood glucose control, and seeking advice from health care providers when necessary.

PATIENT PRESENTATION

Chief Complaint:

"I would like to get my blood pressure and blood sugar checked."

HPI

Lauren Johnson is a 46 yo woman who comes to the pharmacy for a regularly-scheduled wellness day (a wellness day is an open clinic day for pharmacy-based screening services). She would like for the pharmacist to check her blood sugar and blood pressure. She was diagnosed with type 2 diabetes mellitus two years ago. She has been controlling her disease with diet and exercise. She has lost 100 pounds over the past two years and states that she feels a lot better. Ms. Johnson's log book indicates that she has been monitoring her blood glucose levels twice a day (before breakfast and dinner) with a range of 150 to 200 mg/dL. Her fasting levels average 170 mg/dL. She has been able to lose weight by going to the gym 3 times a week and minimizing her carbohydrate intake.

PMH

Type 2 DM × 2 years
HTN × 10 years
Breast CA 1996
Depression × 7 years
Osteoarthritis in both knees
Carpal tunnel syndrome (bilateral)

SH

Married for 30 years, keeps children in her home during the day; denies any use of tobacco and quit drinking alcohol about 10 years ago

FH

Maternal grandmother and fraternal grandfather had DM; father has HTN; mother died at 63 from MI; daughter has asthma

ROS

Denies nocturia, polyuria, polydipsia, nausea, constipation, diarrhea, signs or symptoms of hypoglycemia, paresthesias, and dyspnea

Meds

Effexor 25 mg ½ tab po BID
Prinivil 10 mg po once daily
Glucosamine/chondroitin 500 mg po TID
Chromium 10 mcg po TID
EC ASA 81 mg po once daily
B-100 Complex, 1 capsule po BID
Aleve 220 mg, 2 tablets po Q 12 H PRN

All

Codeine – hives, headache
Penicillin – hives

PE

Gen

WDWN severely obese, white woman in NAD

VS

BP 142/88, P 84, RR 18, T 38.6°C; Wt 111 kg, Ht 5′5″

HEENT

PERRLA, EOMI, R&L fundus exam without retinopathy

CV

RRR, no m/r/g

Lungs

Clear to A & P

Abd

NT/ND

Genit/Rect

Deferred

MS/Ext

Carotids, femorals, popliteals, and right dorsalis pedis pulses 2+ throughout; left dorsalis pedis 1+; feet show thick calluses on MTPs

Neuro

DTRs 2+ throughout, feet with normal sensation (5.07 monofilament) and vibration

Labs

		Fasting Lipid Profile
Na 139 mEq/L	Ca 9.4 mg/dL	T. chol 163 mg/dL
K 3.6 mEq/L	Phos 3.3 mg/dL	LDL 96 mg/dL
Cl 103 mEq/L	AST 15 IU/L	HDL 32 mg/dL
CO_2 31 mEq/L	ALT 18 IU/L	Trig 173 mg/dL
BUN 15 mg/dL	Alk Phos 62 IU/L	TC/HDL ratio 5.1
SCr 0.8 mg/dL	T. bili 0.4 mg/dL	
Gluc (random) 249 mg/dL	A1c 8.5%	

UA

2+ Protein, (+) microalbuminuria

Assessment

The patient reports adherence to diet, exercise, and drug therapy as prescribed. Her glycemic control has improved somewhat (A1c previously was 10.1%) with lifestyle modifications and weight reduction. BP has remained consistent for the past year. She has lost 45 kg in the last 2 years. Her glycemic control and blood pressure have not improved adequately despite her nutritional and drug therapy.

Questions

Problem Identification

1. a. *What are this patient's drug therapy problems?*
   b. *What findings indicate poorly-controlled diabetes in this patient?*

Desired Outcome

2. a. *What are the goals of treatment for type 2 diabetes in this patient?*
   b. *What individual patient characteristics should be considered in determining the treatment goals?*

Therapeutic Alternatives

3. a. *What nonpharmacologic interventions should be recommended for this patient's drug therapy problems?*
   b. *What pharmacologic interventions could be considered for this patient's drug therapy problems?*

Optimal Plan

4. *What pharmacotherapeutic regimen would you recommend for each of the patient's drug therapy problems?*

Outcome Evaluation

5. *What parameters should be monitored to evaluate the efficacy and possible adverse effects associated with the optimal regimens you selected?*
6. *What information should be given to the patient regarding diabetes mellitus, hypertension, and hyperlipidemia, and her treatment plan to increase adherence, minimize adverse effects, and improve outcomes? Include information on use of a glucagon emergency kit (see Figure 79–1).*

Follow-Up Question

1. *What alternative therapies might be appropriate if the initial plan for diabetes treatment fails?*

Self-Study Assignments

1. Discuss the phenomenon known as the metabolic syndrome (syndrome X) and the role that insulin resistance is postulated to play in its sequelae.
2. Explore and discuss the importance of monitoring postprandial blood glucose levels and its impact on overall glucose control, A1c levels, and progression of diabetes complications.
3. Research the various blood glucose monitors available including features that meet the needs of individual patients and improve adherence to testing regimens.

Clinical Pearl

Initial therapy for a patient with diabetes should be selected based on several factors including medical nutrition therapy, exercise, A1c, weight, and comorbid conditions.

References

1. American Diabetes Association. Standards of medical care in diabetes. Diabetes Care 2004;27(Suppl 1);S15–S35.
2. Grundy SM, Cleeman JI, Merz CN, et al. Implications of recent clinical trials for the National Cholesterol Education Program Adult Treatment Panel III Guidelines. Circulation 2004;110:227–39.
3. Expert Panel on Detection, Evaluation, and Treatment of High Blood Cholesterol in Adults. Executive Summary of the third report of the National Cholesterol Education Program (NCEP) Expert Panel on detection, evaluation, and

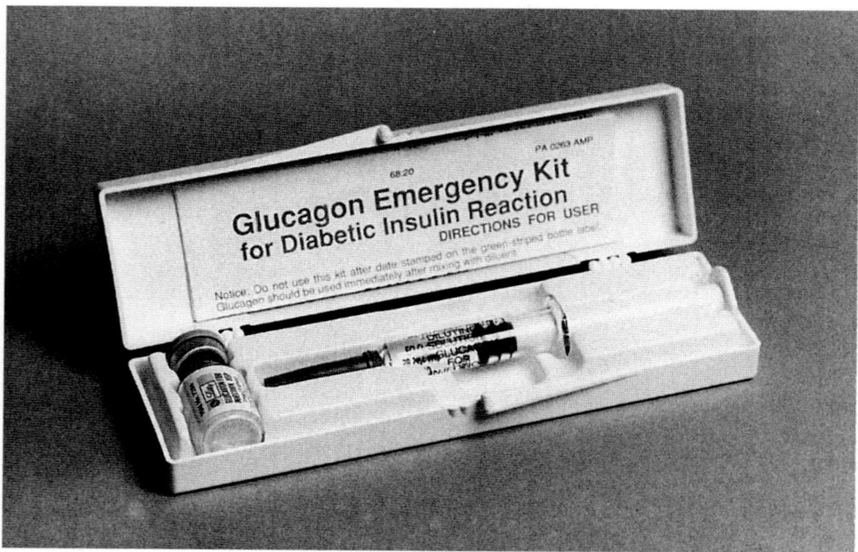

Figure 79–1. The Glucagon Emergency Kit for the treatment of hypoglycemia.

treatment of high blood cholesterol in adults (Adult Treatment Panel III). JAMA 2001;285:2486–2497.

4. Joint National Committee on Prevention, Detection, Evaluation, and Treatment of High Blood Pressure. The seventh report of the Joint National Committee on Prevention, Detection, Evaluation, and Treatment of High Blood Pressure. Arch Intern Med 2003;42:1206–1252.
5. Melander A. Oral antidiabetic drugs: An overview. Diabet Med 1996;13(9 Suppl 6):S143–S147.
6. Saltiel AR, Olefsky JM. Thiazolidinediones in the treatment of insulin resistance and type II diabetes. Diabetes 1996;45:1661–1669.
7. Horton ES, Clinkingbeard C, Gatlin M, et al. Nateglinide alone and in combination with metformin improves glycemic control by reducing mealtime glucose levels in type 2 diabetes. Diabetes Care 2000;23:1660–1665.
8. DeFronzo RA. Pharmacologic therapy for type 2 diabetes mellitus. Ann Intern Med 1999;131:281–303.
9. EUCLID Study Group. Randomized placebo-controlled trial of lisinopril in normotensive patients with insulin-dependent diabetes and normoalbuminuria. Lancet 1997;349:1787–1792.
10. Pepine CJ, Handberg EM, Cooper-DeHoff RM. A calcium antagonist vs a non-calcium antagonist hypertension treatment strategy for patients with coronary artery disease: The International Verapamil-Trandolapril Study (INVEST): A randomized control trial. JAMA 2003;290:2805–2816.
11. Estacio RO, Jeffers BW, Hiatt WR, et al. The effect of nisoldipine as compared with enalapril on cardiovascular outcomes in patients with non-insulin-dependent diabetes and hypertension. N Engl J Med 1998;338:645–652.
12. Tatti P, Pahor M, Byington RP, et al. Outcome results of the Fosinopril Versus Amlodipine Cardiovascular Events Randomized Trial (FACET) in patients with hypertension and NIDDM. Diabetes Care 1998;21:597–603.

80 HYPERTHYROIDISM: GRAVES' DISEASE

▶ Gland Central (Level II)

Kristine S. Schonder, PharmD

▶ After completing this case study, students should be able to:

- Describe the signs, symptoms, and laboratory parameters associated with hyperthyroidism and relate them to the pathophysiology of the disease.
- Select and justify appropriate patient-specific initial and follow-up pharmacotherapy for patients with hyperthyroidism.
- Develop a plan for monitoring the pharmacotherapy for hyperthyroidism.
- Provide appropriate education information to patients receiving drug therapy for hyperthyroidism.

PATIENT PRESENTATION

Chief Complaint

"My heart feels like it is racing and beating out of my chest."

HPI

Elaine Marywood is a 58 yo woman who presents with her daughter to the walk-in clinic with complaints of palpitations that started a few months ago. She stated that they would come and go until the past couple of weeks when they began occurring more frequently, almost daily. She denies CP, but occasionally notes shortness of breath when she walks for a distance. She reports a 9-kg weight loss over the past 2 months, despite a good appetite. She has also had difficulty swallowing solid food for the past few months and has been unable to sleep for the past 3 days. She has noticed that her neck feels swollen and sometimes "pulsates." Her daughter reports that the patient is "more nervous and hyper than usual."

PMH

Entered menopause 10 years ago

FH

She has a half-sister with Graves' disease. Her father had arthritis and multiple MIs; her mother had breast cancer; her grandmother had leukemia.

SH

She lives with her husband and smokes ½ ppd × 35 years (she may have smoked more in the past). She does not drink alcohol.

ROS

She notes that her hair has become more fine and thinner in distribution recently. She has no visual changes, CP, or dyspnea. She has occasional N/V/D.

Meds

None (She used to take a combination estrogen/progesterone hormonal supplement for 5 years, but stopped it 1 year ago.)

All

PCN (rash)

PE

Gen

The patient is a thin, tan-appearing WF in NAD.

VS

BP 150/90, P 120–160 irreg, RR 18, T 37.1°C; Wt 53.5 kg, Ht 5′2″

Skin

Hyperpigmented on upper back and lower extremities; warm and moist. Hair is fine and sparse on crown of head

HEENT

PERRL, EOMI, (+) lid lag, mild proptosis (no ophthalmoplegia), mild lid retraction

Neck/LN

Supple, (+) smooth, symmetrically enlarged thyroid, (+) thyroid bruit, (+) JVD to jaw, prominent pulsations in neck vessels

Lungs

CTA bilaterally, no wheezes or rales

CV

Irregularly irregular rhythm, tachycardic without murmurs; (+) carotid bruits bilaterally

Abd

Soft, NT/ND; (+) BS; no HSM or masses. Aortic pulsations palpable

Rect

Guaiac (–) stool

Ext

2+ DP pulses bilaterally, no calf tenderness. No cyanosis. Fingernails and toenails are flaking. Thumbnails have prominent ridges

Neuro

A & O × 3; fine tremor with outstretched hands; hyperreflexia at knees; no proximal muscle weakness

Labs

Na 140 mEq/L	Hgb 14.5 g/dL	RDW 16.4%	AST 16 IU/L	Total T_4 18.1 mcg/dL
K 3.8 mEq/L	Hct 42.1%	WBC 5.5 × 10^3/mm^3	ALT 26 IU/L	TSH < 0.018 mIU/L
Cl 106 mEq/L	RBC 3.48 × 10^6/mm^3	Polys 54%	T. bili 0.8 mg/dL	T_3 resin uptake 42%
CO_2 28 mEq/L	Plt 249 × 10^3/mm^3	Lymphs 39%	Amylase 54 IU/L	Total T_3 428 ng/dL
BUN 9 mg/dL	MCV 91.4 μm^3	Monos 4%	Ca 8.5 mg/dL	Free thyroxine index 31.9
SCr 0.7 mg/dL	MCH 31.1 pg	Eos 2%	Mg 1.8 mEq/L	
Glu 113g/dL	MCHC 31.1 g/dL	Basos 1%	Phos 3.7 mg/dL	

ECG

Atrial fibrillation; sinus tachycardia (rate of 118)

Assessment

58 yo woman with goiter, probable hyperthyroidism, and new onset atrial fibrillation. Most likely cause is Graves' disease.

Questions

Problem Identification

1. a. *Create a list of the patient's drug therapy problems.*
   b. *What signs, symptoms, and laboratory values indicate the presence or severity of hyperthyroidism?*

Desired Outcome

2. *What are the goals of pharmacotherapy in this case?*

Therapeutic Alternatives

3. a. *What nondrug therapies and counseling might be useful for this patient?*
   b. *What feasible pharmacotherapeutic alternatives are available for the treatment of hyperthyroidism in this patient?*

Optimal Plan

4. *What drug, dosage form, dose, schedule, and duration of therapy are best for this patient?*

Outcome Evaluation

5. *What clinical and laboratory parameters are necessary to evaluate the response to therapy and to detect or prevent adverse effects?*

Patient Education

6. *What information should be provided to the patient to enhance compliance, ensure successful therapy, and minimize adverse effects?*

Clinical Course

The patient is started on the treatment you recommended and returns for a 1-month follow-up visit. The following information is obtained:

VS: BP 135/80, P 98 irreg, RR 18, T 37.0°C.

Labs

Hgb 14.0 g/dL	WBC 4.6 × 10^3/mm^3	AST 18 IU/L	Total T_4 16.2 mcg/dL
Hct 40.5%	Polys 61%	ALT 24 IU/L	TSH <0.018 mIU/L
MCV 92 μm^3	Lymphs 31%	Alk Phos 326 IU/L	*Thyroid Antibodies*
MCH 30.1 pg	Monos 5%	T. bili 1.0 mg/dL	Thyroglobulin 176 IU/mL
MCHC 32.1 g/dL	Eos 2%	PT 14.4 sec	T_{perox} 158 IU/mL
RDW 16.7%	Basos 1%	INR 1.3	

Follow-Up Questions

1. *What interventions, if any, would you suggest at this point?*
2. *If the patient subsequently becomes hypothyroid but clinical signs indicate that the patient still has Graves' disease, what plan should be implemented?*

Self-Study Assignments

1. Develop a monitoring protocol for the pharmacotherapy of hyperthyroidism.
2. Design a systematic approach for a patient education technique for the drug therapy of hyperthyroidism.

Clinical Pearl

Hyperthyroidism in pregnant women must be treated to avoid fetal complications or death. Surgery and radioactive iodine are contraindicated in pregnancy. PTU is preferred because it does not cross the placental barrier as efficiently as methimazole. The lowest dose possible should be used to avoid fetal hypothyroidism and goiter. Free T_4 levels should be used to monitor therapy and should be maintained within the upper limit or slightly above normal to mimic the slightly elevated free T_4 levels seen in euthyroid pregnancies. TSH and free T_3 levels can be misleading when used to monitor therapy.

References

1. Ginsberg J. Diagnosis and management of Graves' Disease. CMAJ 2003;168: 575–585.
2. Leech NJ, Dayan CM. Controversies in the management of Graves' Disease. Clin Endocrinol (Oxf) 1998;49:273–280.

81 HYPOTHYROIDISM

▶ It's Always Sweater Weather (Level II)

Michael A. Oszko, PharmD, BCPS, FASHP

▶ After completing this case study, the student should be able to:

- Recognize the signs and symptoms of hypothyroidism.
- Identify the goals of therapy for hypothyroidism.
- Develop an appropriate treatment plan for thyroid replacement based on individual patient characteristics.
- Select an appropriate agent for thyroid replacement therapy.
- Thoroughly educate a patient taking thyroid replacement therapy.

PATIENT PRESENTATION

Chief Complaint

"I still feel very tired, even after my gynecologist said my iron levels are normal."

HPI

Abigail Simpson is a 55 yo woman who presents to her PCP complaining of feeling tired for the last 6 months. During the past year, she has had significant dysfunctional uterine bleeding and complained of worsening fatigue. Six months ago, she was found to have a hemoglobin of 8.5 g/dL and an MCV of 61 μm^3. She was diagnosed with iron-deficiency anemia and was placed on ferrous sulfate. Two months ago, she underwent a total abdominal hysterectomy. At that time, her hemoglobin was 11.6 g/dL and her MCV was 75 μm^3. Despite the improvement in anemia, she still continues to complain of significant fatigue, as well as what she describes as "persistent depression." In addition, she has noticed that her skin seems more dry and itchy in the scalp, breast, abdomen, and buttock area. She also states that she has difficulty keeping warm and frequently wears a sweater, even in warm weather.

PMH

Iron-deficiency anemia × 6 months
Depression × 2 years
Post-menopausal × 6 years

FH

Positive for CVD, CAD; father died of CVA at age 55, mother is alive with HTN and had an MI at 60; she has one brother with type 2 DM and a sister with HTN.

SH

Married, lives with her husband of 30 years; has 4 children who are now healthy adults. Works as a secretary in a middle school × 20 years. Social drinker; (–) tobacco or illicit drug use.

ROS

Occasional headaches relieved with non-aspirin pain reliever; (–) tinnitus, vertigo, or infections; frequent body aches which she attributes to lack of exercise; (–) change in urinary frequency, but she has noticed an increase in the number of episodes of constipation in the past year; reports cold extremities; (–) history of seizures, syncope, or LOC.

Meds

MOM 30 mL daily PRN constipation
Paroxetine 20 mg daily
$FeSO_4$ 300 mg po BID
Acetaminophen 325–650 mg PRN headache, body aches

All

NKDA

PE

Gen

Well-appearing, middle-aged, moderately obese, Caucasian woman in NAD

VS

BP 130/82, P 64, RR 18, T 36.4°C; Wt 80 kg, Ht 5′2″

Skin

Dry appearing skin and scalp; (–) rashes or lesions

HEENT

NCAT; PERRLA, trace periorbital edema; (–) sinus tenderness; TMs appear normal. Upper dentures in place.

Neck/LN

(–) thyroid nodules or goiter; (–) lymphadenopathy

Lungs/Thorax

CTA

Breasts

(–) lumps/masses; last mammogram (2 years ago) was normal

CV

RRR, normal S_1, S_2; (–) S_3 or S_4

Abd

NT/ND

Neuro

A & O × 3; CN II–XII intact; DTRs 2+

Labs

Na 145 mEq/L	Hgb 12.6 g/dL	Serum Fe 50 mcg/dL
K 4.0 mEq/L	Hct 42%	TIBC 250 mcg/dL
Cl 101 mEq/L	RBC 4.2×10^6/mm^3	T. sat 35%
CO_2 26 mEq/L	WBC 6.0×10^3/mm^3	TSH 14.2 mIU/L
BUN 10 mg/dL	MCV 80 μm^3	Free T_4 0.52 ng/dL
SCr 0.8 mg/dL	MCH 29 pg	T. chol 225 mg/dL
Glu 96 mg/dL	MCHC 33 g/dL	

Assessment

Middle-aged woman with signs, symptoms, and laboratory tests that are suggestive of hypothyroidism.

▶ Questions

Problem Identification

1. a. *Identify this patient's drug therapy problems.*
   b. *What information (signs, symptoms, laboratory values) indicates the presence of hypothyroidism?*
   c. *Could any of the patient's complaints have been caused by drug therapy?*

Desired Outcome

2. *What are the goals of pharmacotherapy in this patient?*

Therapeutic Alternatives

3. a. *What nondrug therapies might be useful for this patient?*
   b. *What feasible pharmacotherapeutic alternatives are available for treatment of hypothyroidism?*

Optimal Plan

4. *What drug, dosage form, dose, schedule, and duration of therapy are best for this patient?*

Outcome Evaluation

5. *What clinical and laboratory parameters are necessary to evaluate thyroid replacement therapy to achieve euthyroidism and prevent adverse effects?*

Patient Education

6. *What information should be provided to the patient to enhance compliance, ensure successful therapy, and minimize adverse effects?*

▶ Follow-Up Questions

1. *How should this patient's elevated cholesterol be handled at this point?*
2. *Assume that the patient returns for a routine exam in 6 months and her cholesterol is still elevated. How should this be assessed?*
3. *Evaluate this patient's continued need for ferrous sulfate therapy. Can it be discontinued? If not, what potential problems (if any) might be expected once thyroid replacement therapy is started?*
4. *Evaluate this patient's depression. Is it primary or secondary? What modifications in this patient's drug regimen would you consider at this point?*

▶ Self-Study Assignments

1. Which levothyroxine products have been deemed to be bioequivalent by the Food and Drug Administration? Is there a consensus regarding the substitution of levothyroxine products?
2. What are the potential cardiovascular effects of thyroid replacement therapy in patients with coronary heart disease? How should these effects be managed or minimized?

▶ Clinical Pearl

In general, the TSH is the only thyroid function test that needs to be monitored on a long-term basis. Routine monitoring of the total T_4 is no longer recommended due to its lack of sensitivity and specificity. The Free T_4 (in addition to the TSH) may be helpful when (1) initially evaluating a patient's thyroid status, (2) the patient's thyroid status is unstable, (3) the patient is suspected to be noncompliant with the medication regimen.

References

1. Dong BJ, Hauck WW, Gambertoglio JG, et al. Bioequivalence of generic and brand-name levothyroxine products in the treatment of hypothyroidism. JAMA 1997;277:1205–1213.
2. Bunevicius R, Kazanavicius G, Zalinkevicius R, et al. Effects of thyroxine as compared with thyroxine plus triiodothyronine in patients with hypothyroidism. N Engl J Med 1999;340:424–429.
3. Walsh JP, Shiels L, Lim EM, et al. Combined thyroxine/liothyronine treatment does not improve well-being, quality of life, or cognitive function compared to thyroxine alone: A randomized controlled trial in patients with primary hypothyroidism. J Clin Endocrinol Metab 2003;88:4543–4550.
4. Sawka AM, Gerstein HC, Marriott MJ, et al. Does a combination regimen of thyroxine (T_4) and 3,5,3'-triiodothyronine improve depressive symptoms better than T_4 alone in patients with hypothyroidism? Results of a double-blind, randomized, controlled trial. J Clin Endocrinol Metab 2003;88:4551–4555.

5. Clyde PW, Harari AE, Getka EJ, et al. Combined levothyroxine plus liothyronine compared with levothyroxine alone in primary hypothyroidism: A randomized controlled trial. JAMA 2003;290:2952–2958.
6. AACE Thyroid Task Force. American Association of Clinical Endocrinologists medical guidelines for clinical practice for the evaluation and treatment of hyperthyroidism and hypothyroidism. Endocr Pract 2002;8(6):457–469.
7. Expert Panel on Detection, Evaluation, and Treatment of High Blood Cholesterol in Adults. Executive Summary of the Third Report of the National Cholesterol Education Program (NCEP) Expert Panel on Detection, Evaluation, and Treatment of High Blood Cholesterol in Adults (Adult Treatment Panel III). JAMA 2001;285:2486–2497.
8. Campbell NR, Hasinoff BB, Stalts H, et al. Ferrous sulfate reduces thyroxine efficacy in patients with hypothyroidism. Ann Intern Med 1992;117:1010–1013.

82 CUSHING'S SYNDROME

▶ When One Gland Affects Another (Level II)

Christopher M. Terpening, PharmD
John G. Gums, PharmD

▶ After completing this case study, students should be able to:

- Recognize and differentiate the signs, symptoms, and laboratory changes associated with the various forms of Cushing's syndrome.
- Recognize the biochemical, anatomic, and emotional changes that can occur with Cushing's syndrome.
- Recommend appropriate treatment regimens for patients with Cushing's syndrome.
- Suggest appropriate adjunctive pharmacotherapy to other health care providers for patients with Cushing's disease.
- Provide patient education on proper dosing, administration, and adverse effects of treatment for Cushing's disease.

PATIENT PRESENTATION

Chief Complaint
"I have been tired and weak lately."

HPI
Susan Taylor is a 31 yo woman who presents to her family physician complaining of fatigue and weakness. She also reports weight gain (50 lb. over 2 years) and depression with insomnia.

PMH
Patient has been healthy with no other major medical illnesses. She had two healthy children by uncomplicated vaginal deliveries.

FH
Mother is alive at age 54 with type 2 DM; father is living at age 56 with HTN. She has two sisters, one is healthy, and the other has depression.

SH
Patient does not smoke, and drinks occasionally. She is a photographer. Children are ages 6 and 3.

ROS
(+) For fatigue, weakness, occasional back pain, and weight gain; also reports episodes of sadness, depressed mood, and insomnia; skin bruises easily; occasional headache, blurred vision, and heartburn; no CP, wheezing, or SOB. Normal menstruation with regular periods.

Meds
Triphasil-21 as directed
Unisom PRN sleep
Advil PRN headache

All
Sulfa → rash

PE

Gen
WDWN obese, Cushingoid-appearing white woman in NAD

VS
BP 160/100, HR 85, RR 14, T 37.0°C; Wt 82.1 kg, Ht 5′3″

Skin
Thin skin with some bruising and scratches; purple striae visible on abdomen

HEENT
Rounded face; moderate facial hair; PERRLA; EOMI; funduscopic exam shows normal retinal background, optic cup-to-disk ratios 0.4; visual fields appear to be grossly intact; OP moist and pink

Neck/LN
Supple; (–) JVD, bruits, adenopathy, or thyromegaly

Chest
CTA bilaterally

Breasts
No lumps or masses

CV
RRR, no m/r/g

Abd
Obese, soft, NT, (–) masses or organomegaly

Genit/Rect
Guaiac (–); normal external genitalia; no masses

MS/Ext
Appears to have decreased strength bilaterally; DTR 1–2+ and symmetric throughout all four extremities; no CCE

Neuro

Oriented × 3; flat affect; CN II–XII intact

Labs

Na 138 mEq/L	Hgb 13.4 g/dL	AST 9 IU/L	TSH 2.33 mIU/L
K 3.3 mEq/L	Hct 38.5%	ALT 7 IU/L	HbA1c7.1%
Cl 105 mEq/L	RBC 4.0 × 10^6/mm^3	Alk Phos 180 IU/L	*Fasting Lipid Profile*
CO_2 25 mEq/L	Plt 264 × 10^3/mm^3	T. bili 0.5 mg/dL	T. chol 261 mg/dL
BUN 12 mg/dL	WBC 5.8 × 10^3/mm^3	Alb 4.5 g/dL	HDL 62 mg/dL
SCr 0.9 mg/dL		UA 5.6 mg/dL	LDL 120 mg/dL
Glu 160 mg/dL			Trig 396 mg/dL

Assessment

Patient appears to have Cushing's syndrome and should be evaluated by an endocrinologist.

▶ Clinical Course

The patient was seen by an endocrinologist for further evaluation. Baseline 24-hour UFC was 156 and 162 mcg on separate days. A midnight salivary cortisol level was 0.54 mcg/dL. An overnight 1-mg DST showed a plasma cortisol of 9.2 mcg/dL. Plasma ACTH levels on 2 consecutive days at 1:00 PM were 103 and 110 pg/mL. A 2-day high-dose DST resulted in a UFC of 13 mcg. A CRH stimulation test revealed a baseline plasma cortisol of 10.4 mcg/dL and ACTH of 108 pg/mL, with an increase to a plasma cortisol of 13.5 mcg/dL and ACTH of 187 pg/mL following CRH administration. An MRI revealed an enlarged pituitary gland; the same finding was seen on a focused repeat MRI. There was no focal inhomogeneity that would suggest an isolated adenoma (i.e., the tumor cannot be localized).

The risks and benefits of all the treatments were explained to Ms. Taylor. She preferred to undergo radiation treatments rather than exploratory-type surgery. She indicated that she would like to have more children and would prefer to try other treatments prior to surgery.

▶ Questions

Problem Identification

1. a. *Create a list of this patient's drug therapy problems.*
   b. *What information (signs, symptoms, laboratory values) indicates the presence or severity of Cushing's syndrome?*

Desired Outcome

2. *What are the goals of pharmacotherapy in this case?*

Therapeutic Alternatives

3. a. *What nondrug therapies might be useful for this patient?*
   b. *What feasible pharmacotherapeutic alternatives are available for the treatment of Cushing's disease?*

Optimal Plan

4. a. *What drug, dosage form, dose, schedule, and duration of therapy are best for treating this patient's Cushing's disease?*
   b. *In addition to treatment for Cushing's disease, what other changes in this patient's drug therapy may be beneficial?*

Outcome Evaluation

5. *What clinical and laboratory parameters are necessary to evaluate the therapy for achievement of the desired therapeutic outcome and to detect or prevent adverse events?*

Patient Education

6. *What information should be provided to the patient to enhance compliance, ensure successful therapy, and minimize adverse events?*

▶ Follow-Up Questions

1. *How do the dexamethasone dosage and procedures for collecting urinary/plasma steroid levels differ in the 2-day versus the overnight dexamethasone suppression test for the diagnosis of Cushing's syndrome?*
2. *What advantages does measuring late-night salivary cortisol have over measuring late-night serum cortisol levels?*

▶ Self-Study Assignments

1. Many of the tests used in the differential diagnosis of Cushing's syndrome require drug therapy (e.g., DST, CRH). Create a table to assist health care providers in performing these tests correctly (include possible adverse events, timing, critical values, and evaluation of the results).
2. Compare the retail costs in your area for each of the pharmacotherapeutic alternatives for the treatment of Cushing's syndrome. Write a brief summary of your findings, and describe whether this information would cause you to change your recommendation for the initial drug therapy for this patient.
3. Describe methods that may be used to minimize drug-induced Cushing's syndrome.

▶ Clinical Pearl

Most patients with Cushing's disease are treated with transphenoidal surgery because of its high cure rate (80% to 90%). Pharmacotherapy is usually used as adjunctive therapy rather than primary therapy.

References

1. Boscaro M, Barzon L, Fallo F, et al. Cushing's syndrome. Lancet 2001;357:783–791.
2. Sonino N, Boscaro M. Medical therapy for Cushing's disease. Endocrinol Metab Clin North Am 1999;28:211–222.
3. Raff H, Findling JW. A physiologic approach to diagnosis of the Cushing syndrome. Ann Intern Med 2003;138:980–991.

83 ADDISON'S DISEASE

▶ What, Me on Steroids? (Level II)

Cynthia P. Koh-Knox, PharmD
Bruce C. Carlstedt, PhD

▶ After completing this case study, students should be able to:

- Recognize the clinical presentation, symptoms, and laboratory changes associated with Addison's disease.
- Optimize pharmacologic and nonpharmacologic therapy for patients with Addison's disease.
- Provide education to patients and family members about Addison's disease and the proper administration, side effects, and adverse effects of corticosteroids and mineralocorticoids, and the importance of adherence to therapy.
- Provide education about common side effects associated with high and low cortisol levels.
- Compare corticosteroids with respect to relative glucocorticoid and mineralocorticoid potencies.

PATIENT PRESENTATION

Chief Complaint

"I haven't been able to watch my children play soccer and softball because I'm just too tired. I've tried to drink more coffee but it doesn't help."

HPI

Carla Stanley is a 43 yo woman who presents to the clinic for her annual visit. She reports feeling fatigued with bouts of nausea and anorexia for several days. She has not felt well enough to take her children to their games or even to watch them.

PMH

Hypothyroidism × 15 years

FH

Father had DM for 50 years; mother has HTN and osteoporosis; has three sisters with hypothyroidism and one sister with hyperthyroidism.

SH

Married to a professor; works as an occupational therapist; has three teenaged children; drinks wine with dinner occasionally and socially; nonsmoker.

Meds

Levothyroxine 0.088 mg po once daily
Citracal daily

All

NKDA

ROS

Reports several days of profound fatigue, nausea, anorexia, and 5-pound weight loss. She has significant tanning of her skin despite her denial of recent participation in her children's outdoor activities. Denies fever, night sweats, visual disturbances, or changes in menstrual cycle.

PE

Gen

Tired-looking, tanned woman in NAD

VS

BP 100/78, P 88, RR 22; T 96.8°F; Ht 5′6″, Wt 60 kg

Skin

Normal texture; slightly dry, no cracks, pigmented skin creases on palms of hand; generalized tan appearance even in unexposed areas. Darkened scar on right forearm.

HEENT

WNL except dry mucous membranes; TMs intact

Neck

Supple without thyromegaly or adenopathy

Lungs

Clear, normal breath sounds

Breasts

No masses

CV

RRR, no m/r/g

Abd

NT; no HSM

GU

Normal external female genitalia

MS/Ext

No CCE; normal ROM

Neuro

A & O × 3

Labs (fasting, drawn at 9:00 AM):

Na 127 mEq/L	TSH 4.8 mIU/L
K 5.0 mEq/L	Free T_4 1.3 ng/dL
Cl 99 mEq/L	Cortisol 1.4 mcg/dL
CO_2 27 mEq/L	ACTH 2096 pg/mL
BUN 15 mg/dL	
SCr 1.0 mg/dL	
Glu 102 mg/dL	

Reference range: cortisol AM: 8–25 mcg/dL, PM 4–20 mcg/dL.

UA
Clear, yellow, SG 1.015, pH 7.0

Other
No CT scan or ECG performed.

Assessment

1. Primary adrenal insufficiency, most likely due to an autoimmune disease
2. History of hypothyroidism, currently treated with levothyroxine

▶ Questions

Problem Identification

1. a. *Create a list of the patient's drug therapy problems.*
   b. *What information (signs, symptoms, laboratory values) indicates the presence or severity of Addison's disease?*

Desired Outcome

2. *What are the goals of pharmacotherapy in this case?*

Therapeutic Alternatives

3. a. *What nondrug therapies might be useful for this patient?*
   b. *What feasible pharmacotherapeutic alternatives are available for the treatment of Addison's disease?*
   c. *What psychosocial considerations are applicable to this patient?*

Optimal Plan

4. *What drug, dosage form, dose, schedule, and duration of therapy are best for this patient?*

Outcome Evaluation

5. *What clinical and laboratory parameters are necessary to evaluate the therapy for achievement of the desired therapeutic outcome and to detect or prevent adverse effects?*

Patient Education

6. *What information should be provided to the patient to enhance compliance, ensure successful therapy, and minimize adverse effects?*

▶ Self-Study Assignments

1. What are the signs and symptoms of an acute adrenal crisis, and what is the treatment?
2. Differentiate the glucocorticoids with respect to duration of activity, glucocorticoid potency, and mineralocorticoid potency.
3. What are the biologic functions of cortisol and aldosterone?
4. Explain why the skin becomes pigmented in adrenal insufficiency.

▶ Clinical Pearl

Osteoporosis is common among patients with Addison's disease due to long-term use of steroids and low levels of dehydroepiandrosterone (DHEA). Recommend osteoporosis prevention, including calcium and vitamin D supplementation, appropriate weight-bearing exercise, and proper diet.

References

1. Living with Addison's Disease: an owner's manual for individuals with the disease. www.adshg.org.uk/info/manual/ADSHGGUIDELINES.pdf (Accessed July 1, 2004).
2. Lovas K, Husebye ES, Holsten F, et al. Sleep disturbances in patients with Addison's disease. Eur J Endocrinol 2003;148:449–456.
3. Arlt W, Allolio B. Adrenal insufficiency. Lancet 2003;361:1881–1893.
4. Flemming TG, Kristensen LO. Quality of self-care in patients on replacement therapy with hydrocortisone. J Intern Med 1999:246:497–501.
5. Jódar E, Valdepeñas MP, Martinez G, et al. Long-term follow-up of bone mineral density in Addison's disease. Clin Endocrinol (Oxf) 2003;58:617–620.
6. Gebre-Medhin G, Husebye ES, Mallmin H, et al. Oral dehydroepiandrosterone (DHEA) replacement therapy in women with Addison's disease. Clin Endocrinol (Oxf) 2000;52:775–780.

84 HYPERPROLACTINEMIA

▶ Preconceived Ideas (Level I)

Amy Heck Sheehan, PharmD
Karim Anton Calis, PharmD, MPH, BCPS, BCNSP, FASHP, FCCP

▶ After completing this case study, students should be able to:

- Recognize the signs and symptoms of hyperprolactinemia.
- Recommend appropriate treatment options for hyperprolactinemia.
- Outline a plan to monitor the response to the pharmacologic treatment of hyperprolactinemia.

PATIENT PRESENTATION

Chief Complaint

"I haven't had my period for almost a year."

HPI

Laura Barnett is a 31 yo woman with a history of oligomenorrhea (menstrual cycle every 2 to 6 months) since menarche at age 14. She presents to her gynecologist after 11 months of amenorrhea and a small amount of milky discharge from her left breast, which she first noticed 1 to 2 months ago. The patient and her husband would like to start a family, but she is concerned that she may be unable to have children. The patient states that she and her husband have not used birth control for more than 1 year, and she has had several negative home pregnancy tests.

PMH

GERD
Migraine headaches (one to two episodes per month)

FH

Father died at age 58 from an AMI; mother (age 62) has type 2 DM and HTN. Patient has two brothers (ages 33 and 35) who are alive and well.

SH

The patient is employed as a fifth-grade elementary school teacher. She does not smoke and has less than one drink of alcohol per month. She has been married for 18 months and lives with her husband.

ROS

Galactorrhea of the left breast and amenorrhea for 11 months as described above. No visual defects. No active GERD or migraine symptoms.

Meds

Omeprazole 20 mg po once daily
Sumatriptan 6 mg SubQ PRN migraine
Acetaminophen 500 mg po PRN
Ginseng tea occasionally at bedtime to relieve stress

All

PCN (hives)

PE

Gen

The patient is a WDWN white woman in NAD

VS

BP 118/68, P 70, RR 12, T 37.1°C, Ht 5′7″, Wt 65 kg

Skin

Normal, intact, warm and dry

HEENT

PERRLA, EOMI, normal funduscopic exam, normal visual fields

Neck/LN

Normal thyroid, no lymphadenopathy

CV

RRR, S_1 and S_2 normal, no m/r/g

Lungs/Chest

Clear to A & P

Breasts

Galactorrhea of left breast, no masses

Abd

Soft, non-tender, no organomegaly, (+) bowel sounds

GU

LMP 11 months ago, normal pelvic exam and Pap smear

MS/Ext

Normal range of motion, no edema, pulses 2+ throughout

Neuro

A & O × 3, bilateral reflexes intact, normal gait, CN II–XII intact

Labs

Na 139 mEq/L	AST 21 IU/L	TSH 2.2 mIU/L
K 4.1 mEq/L	ALT 36 IU/L	T_3 110 ng/dL
Cl 102 mEq/L	Alk Phos 110 IU/L	Total T_4 7.6 mcg/dL
CO_2 26 mEq/L	T. bili 0.4 mg/dL	Free T_4 1.2 ng/dL
BUN 12 mg/dL		Serum β-HCG negative
SCr 0.7 mg/dL		
Glu 86 mg/dL		

Serum prolactin on 3 separate days: 151, 163, and 147 mcg/L

Other

MRI of the pituitary gland revealed a 6-mm pituitary adenoma.

Assessment

Hyperprolactinemia due to a microprolactinoma.

▶ Questions

Problem Identification

1. a. *Create a list of this patient's drug therapy problems.*
   b. *What signs, symptoms, and laboratory values indicate the presence of hyperprolactinemia?*
   c. *Could this patient's hyperprolactinemia be drug-induced?*

Desired Outcome

2. *What are the goals of treatment for a woman with hyperprolactinemia?*

Therapeutic Alternatives

3. a. *What nondrug therapies can be considered for the treatment of hyperprolactinemia?*
   b. *What pharmacotherapeutic options are available for the treatment of hyperprolactinemia in this woman?*

Optimal Plan

4. *What medication regimen would you recommend for this patient?*

Outcome Evaluation

5. a. *What clinical and laboratory parameters are necessary to monitor the patient's response to therapy?*
   b. *If the initial therapy you recommend is effective, how soon can the patient hope to become pregnant?*

Patient Education

6. *What information should be provided to the patient to enhance compliance, ensure successful therapy, and minimize adverse effects?*

▶ Clinical Course

The patient was started on the regimen that you recommended, and she returned to the clinic 4 weeks later complaining of significant nausea and abdominal pain that was temporally associated with medication administration. Serum prolactin concentrations measured 10 minutes apart were 141 mcg/L, 147 mcg/L, and 145 mcg/L. Galactorrhea and amenorrhea were unchanged.

▶ Follow-Up Questions

1. *Identify the possible reasons for the patient's poor initial response to therapy.*
2. *Given the new patient information, what alternative therapies should be considered?*
3. *How long will this patient require drug treatment for the prolactinoma?*

▶ Clinical Pearl

Although dopamine agonists are the mainstay of therapy for hyperprolactinemia, approximately 5% to 10% of patients do not respond to these agents because of poor compliance, suboptimal dosing, or the presence of a treatment-resistant prolactinoma.

▶ Self-Study Assignments

1. If this patient eventually becomes pregnant, should dopamine agonist therapy be continued?
2. Is this patient a candidate for hormone replacement therapy?
3. How would the management of hyperprolactinemia be different if the patient were diagnosed with a macroprolactinoma instead of a microprolactinoma?

References

1. Webster J. A comparative review of the tolerability profiles of dopamine agonists in the treatment of hyperprolactinaemia and inhibition of lactation. Drug Saf 1996;14:228–238.
2. Verhelst J, Abs R, Maiter D, et al. Cabergoline in the treatment of hyperprolactinemia: A study of 455 patients. J Clin Endocrinol Metab 1999;84:2518–2522.
3. Molitch ME. Disorders of prolactin secretion. Endocrinol Metab Clin North Am 2001;30:585–609.
4. DiSarno A, Landi ML, Cappabianca P, et al. Resistance to cabergoline as compared with bromocriptine in hyperprolactinemia: Prevalence, clinical definition, and therapeutic strategy. J Clin Endocrinol Metab 2001;86:5256–5261.
5. Colao A, DiSarno A, Landi ML, et al. Macroprolactinoma shrinkage during cabergoline treatment is greater in naïve patients than in patients pretreated with other dopamine agonists: A prospective study in 110 patients. J Clin Endocrinol Metab 2000;85:2247–2252.
6. Molitch ME. Medical management of prolactin-secreting pituitary adenomas. Pituitary 2002;5:55–65.
7. Mah PM, Webster J. Hyperprolactinemia: Etiology, diagnosis and management. Semin Reprod Med 2002;20:365–373.

SECTION 9

Gynecologic Disorders

85 CONTRACEPTION

▶ I Need the Pill (Level II)

Julia M. Koehler, PharmD

▶ After completing this case study, students should be able to:

- Discuss the advantages and disadvantages of the various forms of contraception.
- Compare and contrast the marketed oral contraceptive (OC) combinations and be able to select the best product for an individual patient.
- Develop strategies for managing the possible side effects of OCs and prepare appropriate alternative treatment plans.
- Provide specific patient education on the administration, expected side effects, and potential drug interactions with OCs.

PATIENT PRESENTATION

Chief Complaint

"I need the pill."

HPI

Sarah Jackson is an 18 yo high school senior who presents to the Family Practice Center for contraceptive counseling. She has been dating her 19 yo boyfriend for a year, and they have been having unprotected sex for a few months with occasional condom use. The patient began menses at age 13, with irregular cycles of 25 to 36 days in length. Her last menses was 2 weeks ago.

PMH

Seizure disorder beginning at age 4 following a minor MVA in which she sustained a head injury. She is currently controlled on seizure medications and has been seizure-free for 4½ years.

FH

Mother has type 1 diabetes, HTN, and migraine headaches. Grandmother died from complications of breast cancer, which was diagnosed at age 60. Paternal family history is positive for hyperlipidemia and cardiovascular disorders; father (age 42) has familial hypercholesterolemia, and grandfather died at age 52 of MI.

SH

Lives at home with mother, father, and two younger brothers. She is typically a "B" to "C" student. Sexually active for about 5 months. She denies smoking, alcohol, or drug abuse. At age 14 she became a vegetarian. Participates on high school track team as a long-distance runner and also runs cross-country.

ROS

Menstrual periods are the most irregular during cross-country season when she runs 30 to 50 miles per week. No complaints of headache. No symptoms of diabetes (no polyuria or urinary frequency) or cardiovascular disorders (BP has always been normal to low, no palpitations).

Meds

Tegretol XR 200 mg po BID

All

NKDA

PE

Gen
WDWN female, thin and pale in appearance, muscular legs

VS
BP 126/68, P 58, RR 14, T 37°C; Ht 5′4″, Wt 49 kg

HEENT
NC/AT; PERRLA; EOMI; TMs intact; oral mucosa clear

Breasts
Equal in size without nodularity or masses, non-tender

CV
NSR without murmurs, rubs or gallops

Lungs
CTA, no wheezing

Abd
Soft, NT, no masses or organomegaly

GU
Normal vaginal exam w/o tenderness or masses

Ext
Normal ROM; muscle strength 5/5 throughout; pulses 2+

Neuro
A & O × 3; CN II–XII intact; DTRs 2+; Babinski (–)

Labs
Negative Pap smear and UPT; carbamazepine level 8 mcg/mL

Assessment
Sexually active teenager requesting birth control

▶ Questions

Problem Identification

1. a. *Create a list of this person's potential drug therapy problems.*
   b. *What medical problems are absolute contraindications to hormonal contraceptive use, and do any of these conditions apply to this patient?*
   c. *What medical problems are relative contraindications to hormonal contraceptive use, and do any of these apply to this patient?*
   d. *What other information should be obtained before creating a pharmacotherapeutic plan?*

Desired Outcome

2. *What are the goals of pharmacotherapy in this case?*

Therapeutic Alternatives

3. a. *What nondrug methods of contraception might be useful for this patient, considering the advantages and disadvantages of each?*
   b. *What pharmacotherapeutic alternatives are available for prevention of pregnancy in this patient, and what are the advantages or disadvantages of each? (See Table 85–1 and Figure 85–1)*

Optimal Plan

4. *What method, dose, schedule, and duration of therapy are best for this patient?*

Outcome Evaluation

5. *What clinical and laboratory parameters are necessary to evaluate the therapy for efficacy and adverse effects?*

Patient Education

6. *What information should be provided to the patient to enhance compliance, ensure successful therapy, and minimize adverse effects?*

▶ Clinical Course

Sarah returns to the clinic in 3 months complaining of never having a period since beginning the pill.

TABLE 85–1. Comparative First-Year Contraceptive Failure Rates With Typical Use Versus Perfect Use[a]

Method	Percent of Women Experiencing an Accidental Pregnancy Within the First Year of Use		Percent of Women Continuing Use at 1 Year
	Typical Use	***Perfect Use***	
Chance	85	85	—
Spermicides	26	6	40
Cervical cap	20–40	9–26	42–56
Diaphragm	20	6	56
Female condom	21	5	56
Male condom	14	3	61
Combined OCs	3	0.1	72
Progestin-only OCs	3	0.5	72
IUD	0.1–2.0	0.1–1.5	81
Depo-Provera	0.3	0.3	70
Female sterilization	0.5	0.5	100

[a]Trussel J, Kowal D. The essentials of contraception: Efficacy, safety, and personal considerations. In: Hatcher RA, Trussell J, Stewart F, et al., eds. Contraceptive Technology, 17th ed. New York, Ardent Media, 1998:216.

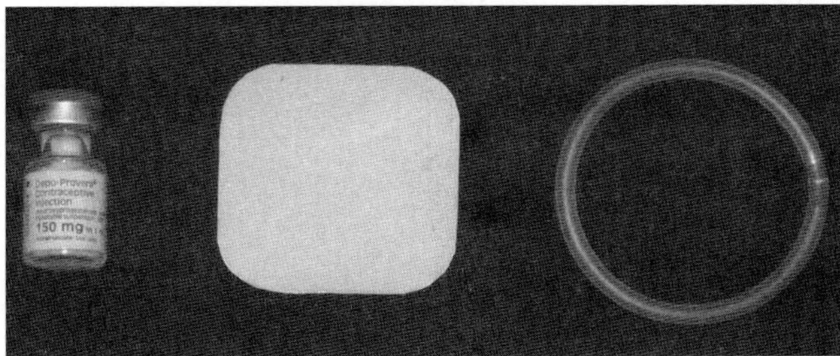

Figure 85–1. Three non-oral contraceptive products: Medroxyprogesterone acetate injectable suspension (Depo-Provera) for IM injection *(left)*, norelgestromin/ethinyl estradiol (Ortho Evra) transdermal system for topical application *(middle)*, and etonogestrel/ethinyl estradiol (NuvaRing) ring for intravaginal use *(right)*.

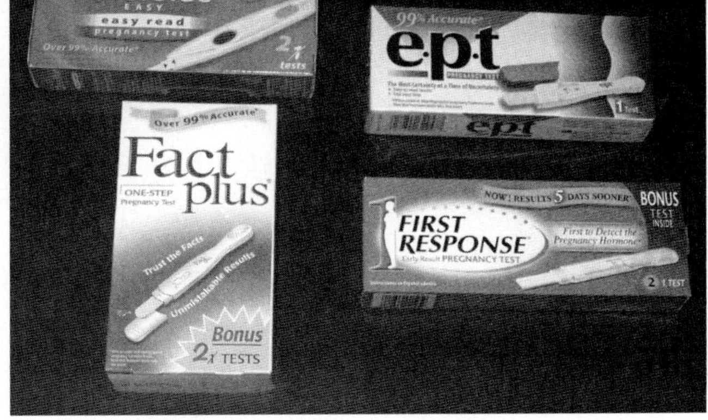

Figure 85–2. Several examples of home pregnancy test kits.

▶ Follow-Up Questions

1. *What are the most likely causes of amenorrhea in this patient?*
2. *How could this problem be evaluated?*
3. *If her pregnancy and other diagnostic tests are negative, what are the pharmacotherapeutic alternatives for treating the amenorrhea?*
4. *If she had developed breakthrough bleeding when she initiated her OC, what could be some of the possible causes?*
5. *If breakthrough bleeding is not caused by a concomitant medical condition, how can it be managed?*

▶ Self-Study Assignments

1. In a case such as the one described, review what might be done to adjust the patient's seizure medication to avoid drug interactions.
2. Compare the costs of each method of birth control and prepare a report that contains your conclusions as to which method provides the best efficacy at the most reasonable cost.
3. Visit a pharmacy and review the various home pregnancy tests; determine how you would educate a patient to use each one, and evaluate them for ease of use (see Figure 85–2 for examples).

▶ Clinical Pearl

Caution patients taking oral contraceptives about the potential for drug interactions. Drugs that reduce absorption, induce metabolism, or alter gut bacterial flora can reduce oral contraceptive efficacy.

References

1. Hatcher RA, Guillebaud J. The pill: Combined oral contraceptives. In: Hatcher RA, Trussell J, Stewart F, et al, eds. Contraceptive Technology, 17th ed. New York, Ardent Media, 1998:405–465.
2. Lewis MA, Spitzer WO, Heinemann LA, et al. Third generation oral contraceptives and risk of myocardial infarction: An international case-control study. Transitional Research Group on Oral Contraceptives and the Health of Young Women. BMJ 1996;312:88–90.
3. American Diabetes Association. Report of the expert committee on the diagnosis and classification of diabetes mellitus. Diabetes Care 2002;25(Suppl 1):S5–S20.
4. Joint National Committee on Prevention, Detection, Evaluation, and Treatment of High Blood Pressure. The seventh report of the Joint National Committee on Prevention, Detection, Evaluation, and Treatment of High Blood Pressure. JAMA 2003;289:2560–2572.
5. Audet M, Moreau M, Koltun WD, et al. Evaluation of contraceptive efficacy and cycle control of a transdermal contraceptive patch vs an oral contraceptive: A randomized controlled trial. JAMA 2001;285:2347–2354.
6. Bjarnadottir RI, Tuppurainen M, Killick SR. Comparison of cycle control with a combined contraceptive vaginal ring and oral levonorgestrel/ethinyl estradiol. Am J Obstet Gynecol 2002;186:389–395.
7. Executive Summary of the Third Report of the National Cholesterol Education Program (NCEP) Expert Panel on Detection, Evaluation, and Treatment of High Blood Cholesterol in Adults (Adult Treatment Panel III). JAMA 2001;285:2486–2497.

86 PREMENSTRUAL DYSPHORIC DISORDER

▶ Dual Identity (Level II)

Martha P. Fankhauser, MS, BCPP, FASHP
Donna M. Jermain, PharmD, BCPP

▶ After completing this case study, students should be able to:

- Recognize and differentiate the symptoms of premenstrual dysphoric disorder (PMDD) from other psychiatric disorders.
- Develop a pharmacotherapeutic plan for treatment of PMDD.
- Recommend alternative treatment options for patients with PMDD.

- Discuss the signs and symptoms of the perimenopause phase and its impact on PMDD and treatment approaches.
- Educate patients on the expected benefits and possible adverse effects of the drugs used to treat PMDD.

PATIENT PRESENTATION

Chief Complaint

"My family is frightened by me."

HPI

Sharon Beck is a 42 yo woman who was referred to the Women's Mental Health clinic by her primary care provider. She states that she is frightened because for some months she has felt suicidal just prior to her menses. Upon further questioning, she states that approximately 12 days prior to menses she becomes extremely irritable with everyone around her. She feels as if she is out of control. She describes feeling tired, uncoordinated, anxious, and depressed. She also has irresistible chocolate cravings and experiences weight gain, bloating, backaches, cramps, breast tenderness, and headaches. Other concerns include inability to concentrate, confusion, and mood swings. During the past year she has noticed a decrease in libido and more sleep awakenings secondary to hot flashes.

She relates the story of how severe her irritability can become. She states that her son came home with his report card and received poor marks in language arts. Her son has never been strong in this subject so this is nothing out of the ordinary. However, during this time of her menstrual cycle she began screaming at him, calling him an "idiot" and tell him that he is grounded for a week. She feels significant remorse soon after as she has said hurtful things to her son and she feels like she can not control herself. Within 1 to 2 days of starting her menses, her mood improves, and her symptoms resolve. "I am normally a happy person," she says. She describes her PMS symptoms as getting worse with age and much worse after the birth of her third child. She brought to clinic the daily calendars she has completed to document her symptoms (see Table 86–1).

TABLE 86–1. A Portion of the Daily Calendar Used by the Patient to Document Her PMDD Symptoms.[a]

Symptom	Before Treatment	After Treatment
Fatigue, lack of energy	4	1
Poor coordination	3	1
Feeling out of control, overwhelmed	3	1
Crying	4	1
Headache	3	0
Anxiety	3	0
Aches	4	0
Irritability, persistent anger	3	1
Mood swings	3	1
Bloating, weight gain	4	0
Food cravings, increased appetite	4	0
Nervous tension	3	1
Cramps	3	0
Depression, feeling sad or blue	3	1
Breast tenderness	2	0
Insomnia or hypersomnia	3	1
Confusion, difficulty concentrating	3	1
How much distress or concern have your symptoms caused you today?	3	1

[a] Data shown are the last day before the onset of menses. Scale: 0, not present; 1, mild; 2, moderate; 3, severe; 4, very severe.

PMH

Gestational diabetes

FH

Her sister has been diagnosed with postpartum depression. Her mother has HTN and diabetes.

SH

She has been married for 21 years. She has 3 children: a 17 yo daughter, a 13 yo daughter, and a 9 yo son. She denies tobacco use but admits to drinking alcohol socially. She works as an accountant.

ROS

She states she has had a headache for the past 2 days and that she feels somewhat nauseated.

Meds

Ibuprofen 800 mg PRN for headaches

All

She develops rash with penicillin

PE

Gen

She is a healthy appearing, mildly overweight female in NAD

VS

BP 114/60, P 83, RR 18, T 99.0°F; Ht 5′6,″ Wt 77.3 kg

Skin

Warm and dry

HEENT

PERRLA, throat pink, no nasal discharge

Neck/LN

Supple; no palpable nodes, thyroid not enlarged

Lungs

CTA

Breasts
Mild fibrocystic changes

CV
RRR; S_1, S_2 normal; no S_3 or S_4 heard; no murmurs or rubs

Abd
Mildly obese, NT/ND

Genit/Rect
She declined examination, as she just had a pelvic exam 1 week ago

MS/Ext
Normal ROM, pedal pulses strong

Neuro
WNL; CN II–XII intact, DTRs 2+ throughout

Labs

		Fasting Lipid Profile	
Hgb 13.2 g/dL	WBC $5.2 \times 10^3/mm^3$	T. Chol 240 mg/dL	TSH 1.7 mIU/L
Hct 38.1%	Neutros 73%	LDL 175 mg/dL	Estradiol (serum) 48 pg/mL
RBC $4.4 \times 10^6/mm^3$	Lymphs 18%	HDL 41 mg/dL	FSH 45 mIU/mL
MCV 97.7 μm^3	Monos 9%	Trig 151 mg/dL	Testosterone (free) 2.7 pg/mL
MCH 33.0 pg	Eos 0%	Glu 92 mg/dL	
MCHC 33.7 g/dL	Basos 0%	A1c 4.9%	
RDW 12.8%			
Plt $155 \times 10^3/mm^3$			

Assessment

1. PMDD
2. Premenopausal
3. Mild obesity
4. Elevated fasting lipid panel
5. History of headaches

▶ Questions

Problem Identification

1. a. *What are the patient's drug therapy and medical problems?*
   b. *What pattern of symptoms does this patient have that are consistent with PMDD requiring treatment?*
   c. *Which symptoms does this patient have that are amenable to drug therapy?*

Desired Outcome

2. *What are the goals of treatment for PMDD in this case?*

Therapeutic Alternatives

3. *What nonpharmacologic and pharmacotherapeutic choices are available for persons with PMDD?*

Optimal Plan

4. *Outline a pharmacotherapeutic plan to treat this patient's PMDD.*

Outcome Evaluation

5. *What clinical parameters are necessary to evaluate the therapy for achievement of the desired therapeutic outcome and to detect or prevent adverse effects?*

Patient Education

6. *What information should be provided to the patient to enhance compliance, ensure successful therapy, and minimize adverse effects?*

▶ Clinical Course

The patient was asked to return to clinic 1 month after being started on the treatment you recommended. During the initial 2 to 3 days of treatment, she had some nausea but considered it to be mild. She noted that her irritability, depressive feelings, and feelings of losing control were markedly decreased. She states that her husband and children noted the improvement because she responded to them as she would have during her "non-PMS" days. She even notes that her cramps and breast tenderness did not seem as severe. Her daily calendars also reflect the improvement (see Table 86–1).

▶ Follow-Up Questions

1. *What is your assessment of the patient's response to the intervention?*
2. *How long would you recommend that she continue therapy?*

▶ Self-Study Assignments

1. Review the textbook chapter on hyperlipidemia and outline your recommendations for lowering her total and LDL cholesterol and triglyceride levels.
2. Based upon the individual's PMDD and perimenopausal symptoms, develop a monitoring tool that would allow the patient and you to record and track the changes in her individual symptoms. This monitoring tool should also include space for her to document adverse effects.

▶ Clinical Pearl

The diagnosis and recommendation for luteal phase dosing of PMDD should be based on prospective daily calendars to assure that there is no comorbidity such as a depressive disorder.

References

1. American Psychiatric Association: Diagnostic and Statistical Manual of Mental Disorders, 4th ed, Text Revision. Washington, DC: American Psychiatric Press, 2000:771–774.

2. Bastian LA, Smith CM, Nanda KI. Is this woman perimenopausal? JAMA 2003;289:895–902.
3. Haywood A, Slade P, King H. Assessing the assessment measures for menstrual cycle symptoms: A guide for researchers and clinicians. J Psychosom Res 2002; 52:223–237.
4. Freeman EW, Sammel MD, Liu L, et al. Psychometric properties of a menopausal symptom list. Menopause. 2003;10:258–265.
5. Pearlstein T. Selective serotonin reuptake inhibitors for premenstrual dysphoric disorder: The emerging gold standard? Drugs 2002;62:1869–1885.
6. Archer JS. Relationship between estrogen, serotonin, and depression. Menopause 1999;6:71–78.
7. Mitwally MF, Kahn LS, Halbreich U. Pharmacotherapy of premenstrual syndromes and premenstrual dysphoric disorder: Current practices. Expert Opin Pharmacother 2002;3:1577–1590.
8. Pearlstein T, Steiner M. Non-antidepressant treatment of premenstrual syndrome. J Clin Psychiatry 2000;61(Suppl 12):22–27.
9. Bäckstrom T, Andreen L, Birzniece V, et al. The role of hormones and hormonal treatments in premenstrual syndrome. CNS Drugs 2003;17:325–342.
10. Luisi AF, Pawasauskas JE. Treatment of premenstrual dysphoric disorder with selective serotonin reuptake inhibitors. Pharmacotherapy 2003;23(9):1131–1140.

87 MANAGING MENOPAUSAL SYMPTOMS

▶ The Change (Level II)

Melissa A. Somma, PharmD, CDE
Jonathan D. Ference, PharmD

▶ After completing this case study, students should be able to:

- Identify the signs and symptoms of menopause.
- List the risks and benefits associated with hormone replacement therapy (HRT) and identify appropriate candidates for HRT.
- Describe the differences among HRT products.
- List nondrug and pharmacologic alternatives to HRT for menopausal symptoms.
- Design a comprehensive pharmacotherapeutic plan for a patient on HRT including treatment options and monitoring.
- Educate patients on the treatment options, benefits, risks, and monitoring of HRT.

PATIENT PRESENTATION

Chief Complaint

"I have been having hot flashes for the past few months and they are becoming very bothersome."

HPI

Susan Franklin is a 50 yo woman who reports experiencing hot flashes for the past 3 months, sometimes associated with nausea. She states that her mother was prescribed a pill for this, but she is afraid to take the same thing because she has heard on the news and from friends that the medication may not be safe. She wants to avoid getting her periods back if possible. Successfully treated for depression in the past, she is currently controlled on paroxetine therapy. She currently exercises three times a week and tries to follow a low-cholesterol diet.

PMH

Depression
GERD
Hypercholesterolemia × 1 year; controlled by diet

FH

Mother died of stroke at age 67; father deceased of lung cancer at age 62. Patient has one brother, 52, and one sister, 46, who are alive and well, but both with HTN.

SH

Married, mother of two healthy daughters, ages 21 and 25. She completed nursing school at a local hospital and is an RN in a neighboring physician's office. She walks on her treadmill three times a week and is trying to follow a dietitian-designed low-cholesterol diet. She does not smoke and occasionally drinks alcohol.

Meds

Ranitidine 150 mg po at bedtime
Paroxetine 20 mg po once daily

All

NKDA

ROS

Noncontributory except for hot flashes and nausea noted above. LMP 9 months ago.

PE

Gen
WDWN female in NAD

VS
BP 122/86, P 78, RR 15, T 36.4°C; Wt 76.2 kg, Ht 5′6″

Skin
Warm, dry, no lesions

HEENT
WNL

Neck/LN
Supple, no bruits, no adenopathy

Breasts
Supple; no masses

CV
RRR, normal S_1 and S_2; no m/r/g

Abd
Soft, NT/ND, (+) BS; no masses

Genit/Rect
Pelvic exam normal except (+) mucosal atrophy; stool guaiac (–)

Ext
(–) CCE; pulses intact

Neuro
Normal sensory and motor levels

Labs

Na 136 mEq/L	Hgb 12.7 g/dL	Ca 9.3 mg/dL	*Fasting Lipid Profile*
K 3.9 mEq/L	Hct 39.3%	AST 32 IU/L	T. chol 227 mg/dL
Cl 104 mEq/L	WBC 6.5×10^3/mm^3	ALT 30 IU/L	LDL 140 mg/dL
CO_2 25 mEq/L	Plt 208×10^3/mm^3	TSH 2.46 mIU/L	HDL 46 mg/dL
BUN 10 mg/dL		FSH 87.8 mIU/mL	Trig 205 mg/dL
SCr 0.7 mg/dL		UPT (–)	
Random Glu 112 mg/dL			

Other
Pap smear and mammogram: Normal

Assessment
50 yo symptomatic postmenopausal woman considering HRT vs. other treatment options.

Questions

Problem Identification

1. a. *Create a list of the patient's drug therapy problems.*
   b. *What information (signs, symptoms, laboratory values) indicates the presence or severity of this patient's problems as she begins menopause?*

Desired Outcome

2. *What are the goals of therapy for this patient's menopausal symptoms?*

Therapeutic Alternatives

3. a. *What nondrug therapies might be useful for this patient?*
   b. *What are the benefits and risks of hormone replacement therapy (HRT) for this patient?*
   c. *What pharmacotherapeutic hormonal alternatives are available for treatment of menopause (see Figure 87–1)?*
   d. *What non-hormonal therapies may be used to manage menopausal symptoms?*

Optimal Plan

4. *What drug, dosage form, dose, schedule, and duration are best for this patient?*

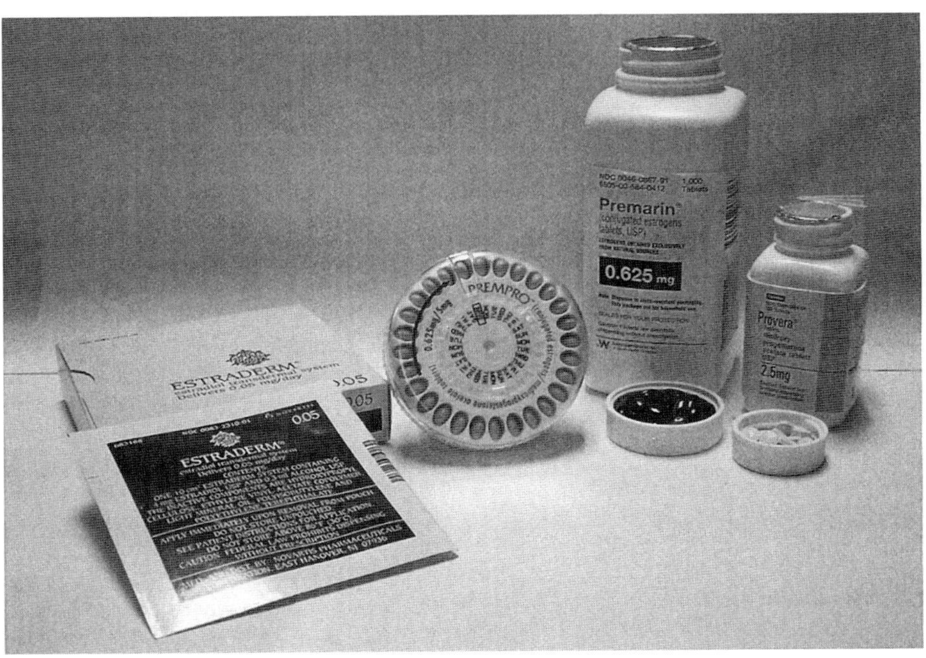

Figure 87–1. Estraderm, Prempro, Premarin, and Provera products for hormone replacement therapy.

Outcome Evaluation

5. *What clinical and laboratory parameters are necessary to evaluate the therapy for achievement of the desired therapeutic outcome and to detect or prevent adverse effects?*

Patient Education

6. *What information should be provided to the patient to enhance compliance, ensure successful therapy and minimize adverse effects?*

▶ Clinical Course

The patient returns to her physician after taking HRT for 1 year. She reports that her hot flashes and nausea have subsided and she would like to know how long she should continue taking the HRT regimen.

▶ Follow-Up Questions

1. *What is the optimal length of time for a patient to continue on HRT?*

▶ Self-Study Assignments

1. Research the dietary supplements that have been used for menopausal symptoms and compare the scientific evidence of their efficacy to traditional medications.
2. Review the results of the Women's Health Initiative (WHI) study and provide a summary of the findings regarding estrogen replacement therapy and cardiovascular risk.

▶ Clinical Pearl

Transdermal estrogens increase triglycerides to a lesser extent than oral estrogen replacement products.

References

1. Manson JE, Martin KA. Postmenopausal hormone-replacement therapy. N Engl J Med 2001;345:34–40.
2. Hulley S, Grady D, Bush T, et al. Randomized trial of estrogen plus progestin for secondary prevention of coronary heart disease in postmenopausal women. Heart and Estrogen/progestin Replacement Study (HERS) Research Group. JAMA 1998;280:605–613.
3. Writing group for the PEPI Trial. Effects of estrogen or estrogen/progestin regimens on heart disease risk factors in postmenopausal women. The Postmenopausal Estrogen/Progestin Interventions (PEPI) Trial. JAMA 1995;273:199–208.
4. Mosca L, Grundy SM, Judelson D, et al. Guide to preventive cardiology for women. AHA/ACC Scientific Statement Consensus panel statement. Circulation 1999;99:2480–2484.
5. Rossouw JE, Anderson GL, Prentice RL, et al. Writing Group for the Women's Health Initiative Investigators. Risks and benefits of estrogen plus progestin in healthy postmenopausal women: Principal results from the Women's Health Initiative randomized controlled trial. JAMA 2002;288:321–33.
6. Loprinzi CL, Kugler JW, Sloan JA, et al. Venlafaxine in management of hot flashes in survivors of breast cancer: A randomized controlled trial. Lancet 2000;356:2059–2063.
7. Goldberg RM, Loprinzi CL, O'Fallon JR, et al. Transdermal clonidine for ameliorating tamoxifen-induced hot flashes. J Clin Oncol 1994;12:155–158.
8. Pandya KL, Raubertas RF, Flynn PJ, et al. Oral clonidine in postmenopausal patients with breast cancer experiencing tamoxifen-induced hot flashes: A University of Rochester Cancer Center Community Clinical Oncology Program study. Ann Intern Med 2000;132:788–793.

SECTION 10

Urologic Disorders

88 ERECTILE DYSFUNCTION

▶ A Sensitive Issue (Level III)

Cara L. Liday, PharmD

▶ After completing this case study, students should be able to:

- Identify the different etiologies of erectile dysfunction (ED).
- Recognize risk factors for the development of ED.
- Provide brief descriptions of the advantages and disadvantages of the common methods available for the treatment of ED.
- Recommend appropriate therapy and alternative treatments for ED.
- Educate patients on treatment options, proper administration of selected treatments, and possible side effects.

PATIENT PRESENTATION

Chief Complaint

"I've been having some problems with my sex life."

HPI

Roy Johnson is a 39 yo man who presents to his PCP with the above complaint. Upon questioning, he states that for the last 10 months he has only been able to achieve partial erections that are insufficient for intercourse. He notices occasional nocturnal penile tumescence, but these are also only partial erections.

PMH

Type 2 DM × 6 years
HTN × 27 years
COPD × 4 years
GERD × 2 years
Carpal tunnel release surgery in both wrists 2 years ago
No history of STDs

FH

Strong for polyps of the colon. Brother had colitis. Father recently died at age 64 of COPD and cardiac arrest.

SH

Patient is single and lives alone. Has a girlfriend and desires a monogamous sexual relationship. Has a 25 pack-year smoking history but quit smoking 2 years ago. Drinks alcohol only around holidays.

ROS

Denies significant life stressors, nausea, vomiting, sweating, blurry vision, dizziness, nocturia, urgency, or symptoms of prostatitis. Complains of slight SOB, cold and hypersensitive feet, difficulty achieving and maintaining erections, and seasonal allergies (not active at present).

Meds

Lotensin 20 mg po once daily
Coreg 12.5 mg po BID
HCTZ 12.5 mg po once daily
Metformin 850 mg po TID
Glyburide 1.25 mg po Q AM
Prilosec 20 mg po once daily
Albuterol MDI PRN

All
NKDA

PE

Gen
Alert, cooperative, anxious, obese man in NAD

VS
BP 146/88, P 64, RR 20, T 37.2°C; Wt 128 kg, Ht 5′10″

Skin
Warm, dry; no lesions

HEENT
NC/AT; EOMI; PERRLA; funduscopic exam shows no arteriolar narrowing, hemorrhages, or exudates; TMs WNL bilaterally

Neck/LN
Supple without lymphadenopathy, masses, or goiter

Lungs/Chest
Clear to A & P bilaterally

CV
RRR; normal S_1 and S_2; no m/r/g

Abd
Soft, obese; NT/ND; normal bowel sounds; no masses or organomegaly

Genit/Rect
Normal scrotum, testes descended; NT w/o masses. Penis without discharge or curvature

MS/Ext
Muscle strength 5/5 throughout; full ROM in all extremities; pulses 2+ throughout; ingrown toenail on left great toe

Neuro
CN II–XII intact; DTRs 2+ and equal bilaterally. No sensory/motor deficits; reduced sensation in extremities bilaterally

Labs

			Fasting Lipid Profile
Na 137 mEq/L	Hgb 15.0 g/dL	Ca 9.4 mg/dL	T. chol 216 mg/dL
K 4.0 mEq/L	Hct 48%	Mg 1.6 mEq/L	HDL 30 mg/dL
Cl 100 mEq/L	WBC $7.6 \times 10^3/mm^3$	Phos 4.0 mg/dL	LDL 138 mg/dL
CO_2 27 mEq/L		A1c 11.8%	TG 189 mg/dL
BUN 9 mg/dL		Testosterone 700 ng/dL	
SCr 0.6 mg/dL			
Glu (nonfasting) 223 mg/dL			

UA
SG 1.015, pH 5.0, leukocyte esterase (–), nitrite (–), protein 100 mg/dL, ketones (–), urobilinogen normal, bilirubin (–), blood 10 RBC/μL.

Assessment
1. Erectile dysfunction
2. Poor long-term control of type 2 DM
3. Poor control of hypertension
4. Dyslipidemia

▶ Questions

Problem Identification

1. a. *Create a list of the patient's drug therapy problems.*
   b. *What risk factors for ED are present in this patient?*
   c. *What are the etiologies of ED, and what is this patient's most likely etiology?*
   d. *Could any of the patient's problems have been caused by drug therapy?*

Desired Outcome

2. *What are the goals of therapy in this case?*

Therapeutic Alternatives

3. a. *What nonpharmacologic alternatives are available for the treatment of ED?*
   b. *What pharmacologic alternatives are available for the treatment of ED?*

Optimal Plan

4. *What therapy is most appropriate and effective for initial treatment of this patient? If drug therapy is indicated, list the drug, dosage form, dose, schedule, and duration of therapy.*

Outcome Evaluation

5. *What clinical parameters are necessary to evaluate the therapy for achievement of the desired therapeutic outcome and to detect or prevent adverse effects?*

Patient Education

6. *What information should be provided to the patient to enhance compliance, ensure successful therapy, and minimize adverse effects?*

▶ Self-Study Assignments

1. Investigate the treatments for priapism and write a two-page report that includes your conclusion about the most effective treatment.

2. Review the components of the initial assessment of a patient with ED, and describe how each type of dysfunction (psychogenic, organic, or mixed) is diagnosed.
3. Perform a literature search to identify new oral therapies and alternative routes of medication delivery for ED. Compare the potential advantages and disadvantages of each treatment.

▶ Clinical Pearl

Some degree of erectile dysfunction is experienced by about 50% of American men, but many do not receive effective treatment because they are hesitant to discuss the issue with their physicians. The advent of oral therapies has revolutionized the treatment of erectile dysfunction and has opened the door for communication between provider and patient.

References

1. Wagner G, Saenz de Tejada I. Update on male erectile dysfunction. BMJ 1998; 316:678–682.
2. Guay AT, Spark RF, Bansal S. AACE Male Sexual Dysfunction Task Force. American Association of Clinical Endocrinologists medical guidelines for clinical practice for the evaluation and treatment of male sexual dysfunction: A couple's problem – 2003 update. Endocr Pract 2003;9:77–95.
3. Carvajal A, Martin Arias LH. Gynecomastia and sexual disorders after the administration of omeprazole. Am J Gastroenterol 1995;90:1028–1029. Letter.
4. Ralph D, McNicholas T. For the Erectile Dysfunction Alliance. UK management guidelines for erectile dysfunction. BMJ 2000;321:499–503.
5. Gresser U, Gleiter CH. Erectile dysfunction: Comparison of efficacy and side effects of the PDE-5 inhibitors sildenafil, vardenafil and tadalafil – Review of the literature. Eur J Med Res 2002;7:435–446.
6. Cohen JS. Is the sildenafil product information adequate to facilitate informed therapeutic decisions? Ann Pharmacother 2001;35:337–342.
7. Padma-Nathan H, Hellstrom WJ, Kaiser FE, et al. Treatment of men with erectile dysfunction with transurethral alprostadil. Medicated Urethral System for Erection (MUSE) Study Group. N Engl J Med 1997;336:1–7.
8. Soderdahl DW, Thrasher JB, Hansberry KL. Intracavernosal drug-induced erection therapy versus external vacuum devices in the treatment of erectile dysfunction. Br J Urol 1997;79:952–957.

89 BENIGN PROSTATIC HYPERPLASIA

▶ For Whom the Bathroom Tolls... (Level II)

Kevin W. Cleveland, PharmD
Catherine A. Heyneman, PharmD, MS, CGP, FASCP
Richard S. Rhodes, PharmD

▶ After completing this case study, students should be able to:

- Recognize the clinical manifestations of BPH.
- Differentiate between obstructive and irritative symptoms.
- Recommend appropriate pharmacotherapeutic treatment for BPH.
- Recognize when surgical therapies should be considered.
- Understand how some drugs can exacerbate BPH symptoms.

PATIENT PRESENTATION

Chief Complaint

"I can't sleep at night. I'm up 4 or 5 times feeling that I have to urinate, and then when I get to the bathroom all I can do is dribble. Sometimes I don't even make it to the bathroom in time. I've been really depressed lately."

HPI

Hugh Rowlett is a 79 yo man with a long-standing history of UTIs. He has been hospitalized twice in the past 3 years for urosepsis. He is currently being evaluated because of a guaiac-positive stool detected last week and complaints of the recent-onset of urinary hesitancy, nocturia, and dribbling.

PMH

Severe OA with L total hip replacement 9 years ago and R total hip replacement 3 years ago
Laminectomy 10 years ago
BPH with urge incontinence
Chronic UTIs
Type 2 DM (well controlled with tolbutamide)
Hypertension
UGI bleed 2 months ago
Obesity
Hx Headaches
CHD
Lipoma of the lower back
Chronic major depression diagnosed 15 years ago

FH

White male educated through the sixth grade. Father died of massive MI at age 72; mother died of natural causes at age 94.

SH

Worked for 35 years as a railroad diesel refrigeration mechanic; retired 17 years ago. Married twice. Second wife deceased 5 years ago (stroke); one daughter, two granddaughters. Admitted to a long-term care facility 3 years ago; was living with one granddaughter who could no longer care for him because of his fading memory and walking/hearing limitations. He has a strained relationship with that granddaughter; he recently changed his power of attorney to his other granddaughter. Used smokeless tobacco × 55 years; heavy EtOH in the past, none now. He is socially active; is chairman of the resident council at the nursing home.

ROS

In conversation, he seems alert, friendly, and courteous but complains that his depression is getting significantly worse. He has no c/o dyspepsia, dysphagia, abdominal pain, hematemesis, or visible blood in the stool.

Meds

Cimetidine 400 mg po BID for PUD
Tolbutamide 500 mg po TID for DM
Amitriptyline 50 mg po at bedtime for HA prophylaxis
Ibuprofen 800 mg po BID for OA
Trazodone 50 mg 4½ tabs po at bedtime for depression
Lisinopril 40 mg po daily for HTN and prevention of diabetic nephropathy

All

NKDA

PE

Gen
Elderly white man in NAD; well-kept appearance; A & O × 3; poor historian

VS
BP 142/90, P 72, RR 24, T 37°C; Wt 115.2 kg, Ht 6′0″

Skin
Vertical scars on neck and lower back from laminectomies

HEENT
PERRLA, EOMI, TMs WNL, nose and throat clear w/o exudate or lesions

Neck/LN
Supple w/o LAD or masses; thyroid in midline

Lungs/Thorax
CTA, distant sounds

CV
RRR w/o murmurs

Abd
Soft, NT/ND w/o masses or scars; (+) BS

Genit/Rect
Testes ↓↓, penis circumcised w/o DC

MS/Ext
Neurovascular intact, distal pulses 1–2+

Neuro
DTRs 2+; CN II–XII grossly intact

UA

Color straw; appearance clear; SG 1.010; pH 6.5; glucose (–), bilirubin (–), ketones (–), blood (–), urobilinogen 0.2 mg/dL, nitrite (–), leukocyte esterases (–), epithelial cells—occasional per hpf; WBC—occasional per hpf; RBC—none seen; bacteria—trace; amorphous—none seen; crystals—1+ calcium oxalate; mucous—none seen. Culture not indicated.

GU Consult

Patient treated for UTI 2 weeks ago with Cipro 250 mg Q 12 H for 3 days. Urine clear, negative for glucose. Bladder exam with ultrasound revealed postvoid residual estimate of 20 mL. Prostate approximately 25 g, moderately enlarged, benign.

Assessment

BPH with urge incontinence
Normocytic anemia possibly secondary to UGI bleed
Chronic major depression

Labs

Na 136 mEq/L	Hgb 12.6 g/dL	WBC 5.6 × 10^3/mm^3	AST 12 IU/L	Ca 8.5 mg/dL
K 4.1 mEq/L	Hct 37.9%	Neutros 75%	ALT 16 IU/L	Phos 3.5 mg/dL
Cl 103 mEq/L	MCV 92.5 μm^3	Lymph 16%	Alk Phos 55 IU/L	Uric Acid 3.5 mg/dL
CO_2 41 mEq/L	MCH 30.8 pg	Monos 5%	LDH 121 U/L	T_4 7.3 mcg/dL
BUN 9 mg/dL	MCHC 33.3 g/dL	Eos 3%	T. bili 0.6 mg/dL	TSH 1.04 mIU/L
SCr 0.7 mg/dL	Plt 191 × 10^3/mm^3	Basos 1%	T. prot 6.1 g/dL	A1c 7.5%
Glu 120 mg/dL			T. chol 146 mg/dL	

▶ Questions

Problem Identification

1. *a. Create a list of the patient's drug therapy problems.*
   b. Describe the natural history and epidemiologic characteristics of BPH.
   c. Which of this patient's complaints are consistent with obstructive symptoms of BPH? Which are consistent with irritative symptoms?
   d. What steps are recommended in the initial evaluation of all patients presenting with BPH? (See Figure 89–1)
   e. What other medical conditions should be ruled out before treating this patient for BPH?
   f. Could any of this patient's problems have been exacerbated by drug therapy?
   g. Are any of this patient's problems amenable to pharmacotherapy?

Desired Outcome

2. *What are the goals of pharmacotherapy in this case?*

Therapeutic Alternatives

3. *What are the treatment alternatives for BPH?*

Optimal Plan

4. *What drug, dosage form, dose, schedule, and duration of therapy are best for this patient?*

Outcome Evaluation

5. *Which clinical and laboratory parameters are necessary to evaluate the therapy for achievement of the desired therapeutic outcome and to detect or prevent adverse effects?*

Patient Name: ______	DOB: ______	ID: ______	Date of assessment: ______			
Initial Assessment ( ) Monitor during: ______	Therapy ( ) after: ______	Therapy/surgery ( ) ______				

AUA BPH Symptom Score

	Not at all	Less than 1 time in 5	Less than half the time	About half the time	More than half the time	Almost always	
1. Over the past month, how often have you had a sensation of not emptying your bladder completely after you finished urinating?	0	1	2	3	4	5	
2. Over the past month, how often have you had to urinate again less than two hours after you finished urinating?	0	1	2	3	4	5	
3. Over the past month, how often have you found you stopped and started again several times when you urinated?	0	1	2	3	4	5	
4. Over the past month, how often have you found it difficult to postpone urination?	0	1	2	3	4	5	
5. Over the past month, how often have you had a weak urinary stream?	0	1	2	3	4	5	
6. Over the past month, how often have you had to push or strain to begin urination?	0	1	2	3	4	5	
	None	1 time	2 times	3 times	4 times	5 or more times	
7. Over the past month, how many times did you most typically get up to urinate from the time you went to bed at night until the time you got up in the morning?	0	1	2	3	4	5	
				Total Symptom Score			

Figure 89–1. The American Urologic Association (AUA) Symptom Index for Benign Prostatic Hyperplasia (BPH). *(Reprinted with permission from* ***BPH, Main Report:*** *Claus G. Roehrborn, MD; John D. McConnell, MD; Michael J. Barry, MD; Elie A. Benaim, MD; Michael L. Blute, MD; Reginald Bruskewitz, MD; H. Logan Holtgrewe, MD, FACS; Steven A. Kaplan, MD; John L. Lange, MD; Franklin C. Lowe, MD, MPH; Richard G. Roberts, MD, JD; and Barry Stein, MD. AUA Guideline on the Management of Benign Prostatic Hyperplasia. American Urological Association Education and Research, Inc., © 2003. http://auanet.org/guidelines/bph.cfm. Viewed October 4, 2004.)*

Patient Education

6. *What information should be provided to the patient to enhance compliance, ensure successful therapy, and minimize adverse effects?*

▶ Follow-Up Question

1. *For questions related to the use of saw palmetto for the treatment of BPH, please see Section 20 of this Casebook.*

▶ Clinical Course

Mr. Rowlett's BPH symptoms improved within days after discontinuation of two of his medications. He required no further drug therapy for BPH. However, 6 months later, his symptoms returned and he opted for laser prostatectomy. This procedure was successful in alleviating his symptoms but left him impotent. The resolution of urge incontinence was such a relief to him that he considered his situation greatly improved.

▶ Self-Study Assignments

1. Compare the efficacy of saw palmetto (Serenoa repens) to finasteride and α_1-antagonists for the treatment of BPH.
2. Perform a literature search for evidence that supports the use of finasteride and α_1-antagonists as combination therapy for BPH.
3. Compare treatment options for hypertension in patients with BPH. Discuss the risks and liabilities of using a diuretic compared to an α_1-antagonist for BP control.

▶ Clinical Pearl

Physiologic measurements such as postvoid residuals, uroflowmetry, and pressure-flow studies often do not correlate well with the patient's perception of symptom severity.

References

1. AUA Practice Guidelines Committee. AUA guideline on management of benign prostatic hyperplasia (2003). Chapter 1: Diagnosis and treatment recommendations. J Urol 2003;170(2 Pt 1):530–547.
2. Narayan P, Evans CP, Moon T. Long-term safety and efficacy of tamsulosin for the treatment of lower urinary tract symptoms associated with benign prostatic hyperplasia. J Urol 2003;170 (2 Pt 1):498–502.
3. McConnell JD, Bruskewitz R, Walsh P, et al. The effect of finasteride on the risk of acute urinary retention and the need for surgical treatment among men with benign prostatic hyperplasia. N Engl J Med 1998;338:557–563.
4. Lowe FC, McConnell JD, Hudson PB, et al. Finasteride Study Group. Long-term

6-year experience with finasteride in patients with benign prostatic hyperplasia. Urology 2003;61:791–796.
5. Roehrborn CG, Boyle P, Nickel JC, et al. Efficacy and safety of a dual inhibitor of 5-alpha-reductase types 1 and 2 (dutasteride) in men with benign prostatic hyperplasia. Urology 2002;60:434–441.
6. McConnell JD, Roehrborn CG, Bautista OM, et al. Medical Therapy of Prostatic Symptoms (MTOPS) Research Group. The long-term effect of doxazosin, finasteride, and combination therapy on the clinical progression of benign prostatic hyperplasia. N Engl J Med 2003;349:2387–2398.
7. Dvorkin L, Song KY. Herbs for benign prostatic hyperplasia. Ann Pharmacother 2002;36:1443–1452.

90 NEUROGENIC BLADDER AND URINARY INCONTINENCE

▶ Bladder Matters (Level III)

Mary Lee, PharmD, BCPS, FCCP

▶ After completing this case study, students should be able to:

- Distinguish among four types of urinary incontinence: urge, stress, overflow, and functional incontinence.
- Define overactive bladder syndrome.
- Determine when anticholinergic and muscle relaxant drugs should be recommended for the management of urge incontinence based on their mechanism of action and adverse effects.
- Differentiate the adverse reactions associated with anticholinergic and muscle relaxant drugs used for urge incontinence.
- Recognize concomitant drug therapy that may exacerbate urge incontinence.
- Recommend appropriate nondrug therapy for the management of urge incontinence.
- Explain why anticholinergic and muscle relaxant drugs should be used cautiously in elderly patients with bladder outlet obstruction.

PATIENT PRESENTATION

Chief Complaint

"I can't seem to get to the bathroom on time because I can't control my urinary stream."

HPI

John Brown is a 74 yo man with urinary urgency and frequency for 6 weeks after a CVA. He reports soiling his underwear at least four times during the day and several times during the night, and has resorted to wearing adult diapers. The patient has curtailed much of his volunteer work and social activities because of this problem.

PMH

HTN for many years, treated with medications for 20 years
CVA 6 weeks ago, appears to have no residual neurologic deficits except for urinary incontinence

FH

Non-contributory

SH

Non-smoker, social drinker, married

Meds

Hydrochlorothiazide 25 mg po once daily with supper
Terazosin 10 mg po once daily
Aspirin 325 mg po Q AM

All

NKDA

ROS

Complains that he can't control his urinary stream and leaks urine repeatedly throughout the day. He reports good control of his BP and has no complaints of weakness, fatigue, dizziness, or headaches.

PE

Gen

WDWN man who looks healthy but smells of urine

VS

BP 150/90, P 90, RR 16, T 37°C; Wt 80 kg, Ht 5′6″

Skin

No rashes, wounds, or open sores

HEENT

PERRLA, EOMI; no A-V nicking or hemorrhages

Neck/LN

No palpable thyroid masses; no lymphadenopathy

CV

Regular S_1, S_2; (+) S_4; (–) S_3, murmurs, or rubs

Pulm

Clear to A & P

Abd

Soft, NT/ND, (+) bowel sounds

Rect

External hemorrhoids; heme (–) stool; prostate mildly enlarged; external genitalia normal

Ext

Normal; equal motor strength in both arms and legs

Neuro

A & O × 3, CN II–XII grossly intact; DTRs 3/5 bilaterally; negative Babinski

Labs

Na 137 mEq/L
K 3.7 mEq/L
Cl 102 mEq/L
CO_2 28 mEq/L
BUN 30 mg/dL
SCr 1.4 mg/dL
Glu 139 mg/dL

Hgb 13 g/dL
Hct 40%
Plt 400 × $10^3/mm^3$
WBC 5.6 × $10^3/mm^3$

UA

No bacteria; no WBC

Cystoscopy

No urethral or bladder abnormalities noted; prostate does not appear to cause bladder outlet obstruction. Urinary flow rate is 16 mL/s, which is normal.

Cystometrogram (CMG)

Bladder capacity 130 mL with maximal detrusor pressure of 75 cm Hg at time of bladder emptying. During the CMG, uninhibited detrusor muscle contractions documented at lower detrusor muscle pressures of 40–60 cm Hg. Bladder sensation is intact.

Assessment

Urge incontinence secondary to CVA and possibly exacerbated by drug therapy.

▶ Questions

Problem Identification

1. a. *Create a list of the patient's drug therapy problems.*
   b. *What information (signs, symptoms, medical history, laboratory values, other test results) indicates the presence or severity of urge incontinence?*
   c. *Differentiate urge incontinence from stress incontinence, overflow incontinence, and functional incontinence.*
   d. *Define overactive bladder syndrome.*
   e. *In addition to the medications the patient is currently taking, what other drugs could exacerbate urge incontinence?*

Desired Outcome

2. *What are the goals of pharmacotherapy in this case?*

Therapeutic Alternatives

3. a. *What nondrug therapies might be useful for this patient?*
   b. *What feasible pharmacotherapeutic alternatives are available for treatment of urge incontinence?*
   c. *Propantheline bromide is a quaternary ammonium anticholinergic agent, whereas hyoscyamine and tolterodine are tertiary amines. What are the potential advantages of propantheline because of this chemical difference?*

Optimal Plan

4. *What drug, dosage form, dose, schedule, and duration of therapy are best for this patient?*

Outcome Evaluation

5. *What clinical and laboratory parameters are necessary to evaluate the therapy for achievement of the desired therapeutic outcome and to detect or prevent adverse effects?*

Patient Education

6. *What information should be provided to the patient to enhance compliance, ensure successful therapy, and minimize adverse effects?*

▶ Clinical Course

The patient was started on propantheline bromide 15 mg Q 6 H but experienced severe constipation and excessive sedation. Adverse effects did not abate despite continuation of therapy for 1 week. For this reason, therapy was changed to a drug with a different mechanism of action. The patient had complete relief of symptoms of urinary leakage with this regimen and continued to take it for 1½ years. During the last 6 months of treatment, the patient noted that he was developing a slower urinary stream. He seemed to have greater difficulty emptying his bladder completely and always felt that his bladder was still full despite having just voided. He has required antibiotic treatment regularly for relapsing urinary tract infections.

He sought medical attention and was referred to a urologist. Rectal examination revealed a significantly enlarged 30-g smooth prostate (normal, 15–20 g). A PSA was 10 ng/dL; BUN and serum creatinine were unchanged from the last visit. Repeat cystoscopy showed a large obstructing prostate at the bladder neck and a hypertrophied, noncontractile detrusor muscle. Peak urinary flow rate was 3 mL/s. Postvoid residual bladder volume is 1,200 mL.

▶ Follow-Up Questions

1. *Why has the patient developed new and different voiding symptoms?*
2. *How should this patient's voiding problem now be managed?*
3. *Assume that the patient refuses surgery and wants drug treatment only to relieve his symptoms. The patient states that he was on terazosin before and he was told this caused his initial urinary leakage a few years ago, so he refuses to be restarted on this. How should you respond to the patient's concern?*
4. *Based on the patient's current medical condition and his refusal to restart terazosin, what other similar therapeutic alternatives are available? Design an effective alternative regimen for this patient.*

▶ Self-Study Assignments

1. Conduct a literature search to identify current studies that compare the efficacy and safety of the investigational drug terodiline for treatment of urge incontinence.
2. Tricyclic antidepressants have been used to treat stress incontinence. Explain the rationale for the use of this class of drugs for this disorder.
3. Other drugs that have been used for urge incontinence include terbutaline and indomethacin. Conduct a literature search and interpret what you read. Explain how these drugs can relieve the symptoms of urge incontinence.

▶ Clinical Pearl

Proper classification of the type of urinary incontinence is key to selecting appropriate drug therapy. Urge incontinence responds to anticholinergics or muscle relaxants. Overflow urinary incontinence may respond to α-adrenergic antagonists or to cholinergic stimulants, based on the pathologic cause of the disorder in a particular patient. Stress incontinence responds to α-adrenergic stimulants.

References

1. Sullivan J, Abrams P. Pharmacological management of incontinence. Eur Urol 1999;36(Suppl 1):89–95.
2. Hampel C, Wienhold D, Benken N, et al. Definition of overactive bladder and epidemiology of urinary incontinence. Urology 1997;50 (Supple 6A): 4–14.
3. Ouslander JG, Schnelle JF, Uman G, et al. Does oxybutynin add to the effectiveness of prompted voiding for urinary incontinence among nursing home residents? A placebo-controlled trial. J Am Geriatr Soc 1995;43:610–617.
4. Hills CJ, Winter SA, Balfour JA. Tolterodine. Drugs 1998;55(6):813–820.
5. Abrams P. Evidence for the efficacy and safety of tolterodine in the treatment of overactive bladder. Expert Opin Pharmacother 2001;2:1685–1701.
6. Dmochowski RR, Davila GW, Zinner NR, et al. For the Transdermal Oxybutynin Study Group. Efficacy and safety of transdermal oxybutynin in patients with urge and mixed urinary incontinence. J Urol 2002;168:580–586.
7. Van Kerrebroeck P, Kreder K, Jonas U, et al. the Tolterodine Study Group. Tolterodine once-daily: Superior efficacy and tolerability in the treatment of overactive bladder. Urology 2001;57:414–421.
8. AUA Practice Guidelines Committee. AUA guideline on the management of benign prostatic hyperplasia (2003). Chapter 1: Diagnosis and treatment recommendations. J Urol 2003;170(2 Pt 1):530–547.
9. Lee M. Tamsulosin for the treatment of benign prostatic hypertrophy. Ann Pharmacother 2000;34:188–199.

Acknowledgment

The author would like to acknowledge the assistance and kind help of Dr. Roohollah Sharifi, Professor of Urology, University of Illinois at Chicago College of Medicine.

SECTION 11

Immunologic Disorders

91 SYSTEMIC LUPUS ERYTHEMATOSUS

► More Than Just Skin Deep (Level II)

Ralph E. Small, PharmD, FCCP, FASHP, FAPhA
Nicole M. Paolini, PharmD

► After completing this case study, students should be able to:

- Describe the clinical and laboratory features of lupus nephritis.
- Recommend appropriate therapy for lupus nephritis.
- Define the monitoring parameters for disease activity, drug efficacy, and drug toxicity.

PATIENT PRESENTATION

Chief Complaint

"I've had a red rash on my arms for the past 3 days."

HPI

Linda Fields is a 46 yo woman admitted from Rheumatology Clinic with increased serum creatinine. She was diagnosed with SLE 2 years ago after she presented with arthralgias and rash. At the beginning of this year, she was found to have proteinuria with RBCs and RBC casts in her urine. Her BUN and creatinine were 20 and 0.9 mg/dL, respectively. Renal biopsy revealed segmental proliferative glomerulonephritis and membranous glomerulonephritis compatible with lupus nephritis. She was treated with prednisone without significant improvement in her proteinuria. At this visit, she complains of a 3-day history of erythematous rash on her arms. She denies taking OTC drugs or NSAIDs.

PMH

HTN × 7 years
Acute sinusitis 1 year ago
Ovarian cyst removal 20 years ago

FH

Father died of MI; mother alive in her seventies.

SH

Employed as a teacher; married 20 years; no tobacco use; occasional EtOH use.

Meds

Enalapril 10 mg po BID
Prednisone 10 mg po once daily

All

PCN (rash)

ROS

No fever, chills, or sweats; no arthralgias or myalgias.

PE

Gen

Slightly obese woman in NAD

VS

BP140/80, P 70, RR 20, T 38.2°C; Wt 64 kg

Skin
Erythematous rash on upper extremities

HEENT
PERRLA; EOMI; disks flat, no hemorrhages or exudates; oropharynx without lesions

Neck/LN
Supple without adenopathy

CV
RRR, grade IV systolic murmur

Abdomen
Soft, non-tender

Ext
Peripheral pulses intact; joint examination reveals no active synovitis or arthritis; no CCE

Neuro
A & O × 3; sensory and motor levels normal; CN II–XII intact; DTRs 2+; Babinski negative

Labs

Na 140 mEq/L	Hgb 10.5 g/dL	C4 14 mg /dL
K 4.9 mEq/L	Hct 32%	C3 66 mg/dL
Cl 107 mEq/L	WBC 6.3×10^3/mm^3	Anti-ds DNA antibody 584 mg/dL
CO_2 24 mEq/L	Plt 280×10^3/mm^3	
BUN 52 mg/dL	ESR 53 mm/h	
SCr 2.0 mg/dL		
Uric acid 8.3 mg/dL		

UA
Many RBCs, RBC casts, 3+ proteinuria

Renal biopsy
Much more proliferative changes than on previous biopsy and increased interstitial fibrosis

Assessment
Acute worsening of lupus nephritis; exacerbation of SLE.

▶ Questions

Problem Identification

1. a. *Create a list of the patient's drug therapy problems.*
   b. *What information indicates worsening lupus nephritis?*

Desired Outcome

2. *What are the goals of pharmacotherapy for lupus nephritis in this patient?*

Therapeutic Alternatives

3. a. *What nonpharmacologic therapies might be useful in this patient?*
   b. *What pharmacotherapeutic alternatives are used to manage patients with lupus nephritis?*

Optimal Plan

4. *Outline a specific pharmacotherapeutic plan for treating lupus nephritis in this patient.*

Outcome Evaluation

5. *How should this patient be monitored for efficacy and adverse effects?*

Patient Education

6. *What information should be provided to the patient regarding her drug therapy?*

▶ Clinical Course

The patient experienced a remission in her renal disease following the drug therapy you recommended, but her proteinuria failed to improve, suggesting that her mesangial renal histology was irreversible. She also tapered her prednisone but experienced a lupus flare with complications from vasculitis and reemergence of her lupus nephritis. Her prednisone dosage was increased and treatment of her lupus nephritis was reinstituted.

▶ Follow-Up Questions

1. *What other medications can be used to control this patient's non-renal disease manifestation (i.e., erythematous rash)?*
2. *What is your recommendation for the patient's other current medications?*

▶ Self-Study Assignments

1. Recent animal experiments have suggested a number of strategies for treating lupus nephritis. Perform a literature search on experimental treatments for lupus nephritis.
2. Glucocorticoid-induced osteoporosis is a serious complication associated with long-term prednisone therapy. Perform a literature search and suggest strategies for ameliorating the long-term effects of prednisone.
3. The investigational drug prasterone (Aslera) showed some positive results in increasing response rates, improving bone mineral density, and decreasing triglyceride levels when compared to placebo in patients with mild to moderate SLE. Perform a literature search and determine its FDA approval status as well as its potential benefits and risks.
4. Recent case reports have linked immunizations to the onset of systemic lupus erythematosus (SLE). Perform a literature search and determine whether the temporal relationship between time of immunization and onset of symptoms is valid and worthy of further investigation.

5. Traditional NSAIDs serve as a useful treatment modality in mild SLE. Perform a literature search to assess the usefulness of COX-2 selective inhibitors.

▶ Clinical Pearl

Because UV light exacerbates SLE, drugs that induce photosensitivity should be avoided.

References

1. Austin HA III, Klippel JH, Balow JE, et al. Therapy of lupus nephritis. Controlled trial of prednisone and cytotoxic drugs. N Engl J Med 1986;314:614–619.
2. Bijl M, Horst G, Bootsma H, et al. Mycophenolate mofetil prevents a clinical relapse in patients with systemic lupus erythematosus at risk. Ann Rheum Dis 2003;62:534–539.
3. Chan TM, Li FK, Tang CSO, et al. Efficacy of mycophenolate mofetil in patients with diffuse proliferative lupus nephritis. N Engl J Med 2000;343:1156–1162.
4. Dooley MA, Cosio FG, Nachman PH, et al. Mycophenolate mofetil therapy in lupus nephritis: clinical observations. J Am Soc Nephrol 1999,10:833–839.
5. Briggs WA, Choi MJ, Scheel PJ Jr.: Successful mycophenolate mofetil treatment of glomerular disease. Am J Kidney Dis 1998, 31:213–217.
6. Gescuk BD, Davis JC. Novel therapeutic agents for systemic lupus erythematosus. Curr Opin Rheumatol 2002;14:515–521.
7. Llorente L, Richaud-Patin Y, Garcia-Padilla C, et al. Clinical and biological effects of anti-interleukin-10 monoclonal antibody administration in systemic lupus erythematosus. Arthritis Rheum 2000;43:1790–1800.
8. van Vollenhoven RF, Park JL, Genovese MC, et al. A double-blind, placebo-controlled, clinical trial of dehydroepiandrosterone in severe systemic lupus erythematosus. Lupus 1999;8:181–187.
9. van Vollenhoven RF, Morabito LM, Engleman EG, et al. Treatment of systemic lupus erythematosus with dehydroepiandrosterone: 50 patients treated up to 12 months. J Rheumatol 1998;25:285–289.
10. Ostensen M, Villiger PM. Nonsteroidal anti-inflammatory drugs in systemic lupus erythematosus. Lupus 2001;10:135–139.
11. Ginzler EM, Aranow C, Buyon J et al. A multicenter study of mycophenolate mofetil (MMF) vs. intravenous cyclophosphamide (IVC) as induction therapy for severe lupus nephritis (LN): Preliminary results. Arthritis Rheum 2003;48(9):S647. Abstract.
12. Kanekura T, Yoshii N, Terasaki K, et al. Efficacy of topical tacrolimus for treating the malar rash of systemic lupus erythematosus. Br J Dermatol 2003;148: 353–356.
13. Yoshimasu T, Ohtani T, Sakamoto T, et al. Topical FK506 (tacrolimus) therapy for facial erythematous lesions of cutaneous lupus erythematosus and dermatomyositis. Eur J Dermatol 2002;12:50–52.

92 SOLID ORGAN TRANSPLANTATION

▶ A New Kidney for Mary (Level III)

Kristine S. Schonder, PharmD

▶ After completing this case study, students should be able to:

- Develop a patient-specific therapeutic plan for complications associated with solid organ transplantation.
- Educate a transplant recipient on the importance of medication adherence and implement mechanisms to enhance adherence.
- Describe possible adverse effects to immunosuppressive medications and develop a plan to resolve these effects.
- Assess a transplant medication regimen for potential drug interactions and develop a plan to resolve any identified interactions.

PATIENT PRESENTATION

Chief Complaint
"I have had diarrhea for the past 3 days."

HPI
Mary Johnson is a 42 yo female who presents to the renal transplant clinic for evaluation of diarrhea.

PMH
2 months s/p cadaveric kidney transplant
ESRD secondary to SLE glomerulonephritis

FH
Mother is 60 yo with HTN; father died 2 years ago from MI. Mrs. Johnson is married with 3 children, Michael, James and Catherine, who are alive and well.

SH
She drinks an occasional glass of wine on holidays, but has not since her transplant. She does not smoke cigarettes or use tobacco products. She has no history of IVDA.

ROS
She has been having significant diarrhea 3 to 4 times a day and occasional N/V and nocturia.

Meds
Tacrolimus 5 mg po BID (last dose taken last night at 8:00 PM)
Prednisone 15 mg po once daily
Mycophenolate mofetil 750 mg po BID
Sulfamethoxazole 400 mg/trimethoprim 80 mg po once daily
Acyclovir 200 mg po BID
ASA 81 mg po daily
Docusate sodium 100 mg po BID
Sodium bicarbonate 1300 mg po TID
Ferrous sulfate 300 mg po TID

All
NKDA

PE

Gen
WDWN Caucasian female in NAD

VS

BP 170/95; BP readings have been elevated (> 140/90) on the last 4 clinic visits; P 80 reg; RR 18; T 37.9°C; Ht 5′ 5″, Wt 70 kg

Skin

Warm and dry

HEENT

PERRLA; EOMI

Chest

CTA & P

CV

Normal S_1 and S_2; no m/r/g

Abd

Soft, NT with palpable, non-tender graft; incisional wound is healing; liver size normal

Ext

1+ pitting edema in LE; 2+ DP pulses bilaterally. No cyanosis.

Neuro

A & O × 3; CN II–XII intact; DTRs 2+ throughout

Labs

At 8:00 AM today (fasting):

Na 135 mEq/L	Hgb 11.5 g/dL	Ca 8.2 mg/dL	*Fasting Lipid Panel*
K 4.1 mEq/L	Hct 35.1%	Phos 1.8 mg/dL	T. chol 296 mg/dL
Cl 104 mEq/L	RBC 3.35 × 10^6/mm^3	Mg 1.1 mEq/L	LDL-C 187 mg/dL
CO_2 28 mEq/L	WBC 6.1 × 10^3/mm^3	FK 10.3 ng/mL[a]	HDL-C 47 mg/dL
BUN 20 mg/dL	Plt 160 × 10^3/mm^3		Trig 310 mg/dL
SCr 1.0 mg/dL			CMV antigenemia test: Positive (59/200,000 leukocytes)
FBS 254 mg/dL			

[a] Tacrolimus whole blood concentration (therapeutic range, 5–20 ng/mL)

Assessment

CMV infection

▶ Questions

Problem Identification

1. a. *Create a list of the patient's drug therapy problems.*
   b. *Which signs, symptoms, and laboratory values indicate the presence of CMV infection?*
   c. *What are the potential causes of hypertension in this patient?*

Desired Outcome

2. *What are the goals of pharmacotherapy in this case?*

Therapeutic Alternatives

3. a. *What nonpharmacologic therapies and education might be useful for this patient?*
   b. *What feasible pharmacotherapeutic alternatives are available for the treatment of CMV infection?*
   c. *What feasible pharmacotherapeutic alternatives are available for the treatment of hypertension in this patient?*
   d. *What feasible pharmacotherapeutic alternatives are available for the treatment of dyslipidemia in this patient?*

Optimal Plan

4. *Design a pharmacotherapeutic regimen to treat this patient's CMV infection, hypertension, dyslipidemia, and other medical problems.*

Outcome Evaluation

5. *What clinical and laboratory parameters are necessary to evaluate the response to therapy and to detect or prevent adverse effects?*

Patient Education

6. *What information should be provided to the patient to enhance adherence, ensure successful therapy, and minimize adverse effects?*

▶ Clinical Course

The patient is started on the treatment you recommended and returns for a 1-month follow-up visit. She now complains that she has a headache almost daily. Her hands are shaking uncontrollably and she has trouble sleeping.

Meds

Tacrolimus 5 mg po BID (last dose taken last night at 8:00 PM)
Prednisone 12.5 mg po once daily
Mycophenolate mofetil 750 mg po BID
Sulfamethoxazole 400 mg/trimethoprim 80 mg po once daily
Ganciclovir 350 mg IV BID
ASA 81 mg po daily
Sodium bicarbonate 650 mg po TID
Ferrous sulfate 300 mg po TID
Glyburide 5 mg po once daily
Nifedipine ER 30 mg po once daily
Clarithromycin 500 mg po BID for sinus infection (she is on day 6 of a 10-day course prescribed by her PCP.)

PE

Unremarkable, except for tremors in upper extremities

VS

BP 158/90; P 84 reg; RR 20; T 36°C; Wt 69 kg

Labs

At 8:00 AM today:

Na 139 mEq/L	Hgb 12.3 g/dL	Ca 8.9 mg/dL	AST 17 IU/L
K 4.8 mEq/L	Hct 35.9 %	Phos 3.2 mg/dL	ALT 6 IU/L
Cl 103 mEq/L	RBC 3.45 × 10^6/mm^3	Mg 1.3 mEq/L	T. bili 0.4 mg/dL
CO_2 31 mEq/L	WBC 4.0 × 10^3/mm^3	FK 29.0 ng/mL	Alb 3.2 g/dL
BUN 29 mg/dL	Plt 203 × 10^3/mm^3		CMV Antigenemia Test: Negative (The test was also negative one week ago)
SCr 1.4 mg/dL			
FBS 78 mg/dL			

► Follow-Up Questions

1. *What is the most likely cause for the patient's tremors?*
2. *What new information should be provided to the patient about her medications regarding drug interactions and adverse effects?*
3. *What changes (if any) should be made to the patient's CMV treatment?*
4. *Develop a pharmacotherapeutic plan to manage the patient's tremors.*

► Self-Study Assignments

1. Develop a pharmacotherapeutic plan for the different strategies to prevent and manage CMV infection in solid organ transplant recipients.
2. Design a systematic approach for patient education for a new solid organ transplant recipient focusing on immunosuppressive therapies, adverse effects and drug interactions, and strategies to manage patient compliance with a complicated regimen.

► Clinical Pearl

It is estimated that 75% to 90% of people are CMV-seropositive. Solid organ transplant recipients are at risk of active CMV infection due to immunosuppressive therapy. The greatest risk of CMV infection occurs in CMV-seronegative recipients who receive an allograft from a CMV-seropositive donor. Recipients who are CMV-seropositive are also at risk for reactivation of CMV.

References

1. Sia IG, Patel R. New strategies for prevention and therapy of cytomegalovirus infection and disease in solid-organ transplant recipients. Clin Microbiol Rev 2000;13:83–121.
2. Tylicki L, Habicht A, Watschinger B, et al. Treatment of hypertension in renal transplant recipients. Curr Opin Urol 2003;13:91–98.
3. K/DOQI clinical practice guidelines for managing dyslipidemias in chronic kidney disease. http://www.kidney.org/professionals/kdoqi/guidelines_lipids/index.htm. Accessed July 4, 2004.
4. Andany MA, Kasiske BL. Dyslipidemia and its management after renal transplantation. J Nephrol 2001;14(Suppl 4):S81–S88.
5. Kletzmayr J, Kreuzwieser E, Klauser R. New developments in the management of cytomegalovirus infection and disease after renal transplantation. Curr Opin Urol 2001;11:153–158.
6. Zhang R, Leslie B, Boudreaux JP, et al. Hypertension after kidney transplantation: Impact, pathogenesis and therapy. Am J Med Sci 2003;325:202–208.

SECTION 12

Bone and Joint Disorders

93 OSTEOPOROSIS

▶ These Brittle Bones (Level II)

Julia M. Koehler, PharmD

▶ After completing this case study, students should be able to:

- Identify the risk factors for the development of osteoporosis.
- Recommend appropriate nonpharmacologic measures for the prevention and treatment of osteoporosis.
- Recommend the correct amount and form of calcium supplementation required for the prevention and treatment of osteoporosis.
- Design an appropriate pharmacologic regimen for the treatment of osteoporosis in postmenopausal women.
- Provide appropriate patient education regarding osteoporosis and its therapy.

PATIENT PRESENTATION

Chief Complaint

"That calcium supplement you recommended makes me nauseated."

HPI

Emma West is a 74 yo woman with a history of HTN, hyperlipidemia, COPD, hypothyroidism, and osteoporosis. She presents to the family medicine clinic for a follow-up visit for HTN and osteoporosis. She has been experiencing episodes of nausea without vomiting since she began taking Os-Cal 500 after her last clinic visit.

PMH

HTN first diagnosed at age 50
S/P MI 12 years ago
Hyperlipidemia × 13 years; patient modified diet and took cholestyramine for several years
Hypothyroidism × 27 years, treated with levothyroxine
Osteoporosis diagnosed by DXA scan 2 years ago
COPD diagnosed several years ago; stable on multiple inhalers
Appendectomy at age 15
Breast cancer with mastectomy of left breast and radiation therapy at age 40
Menopause at age 48
Right carotid endarterectomy 2 years ago

FH

Paternal history(+) for CAD; father died at age 60 of "heart trouble." Maternal history (+) for stroke and vascular disorders; mother became menopausal before age 45.

SH

Widowed; G_2P_3; 2½ ppd smoker, quit after MI; non-drinker.

ROS

Mild headaches and chronic back pain, treated with acetaminophen; vaginal dryness; hot flushes and night sweats occasionally; has noticed that her height has decreased by 2″ since she was 35 years old; cold intolerant; denies shortness of breath or chest pain.

Meds

Ramipril 10 mg po BID × 2 years
Atrovent MDI 2 puffs QID × 2 years
Advair 250/50 1 puff BID × 3 months
Albuterol MDI 2 puffs Q 6 H PRN

Synthroid 100 mcg po once daily × 20 years
Atenolol 50 mg po daily x 10 years
Aspirin 325 mg po daily x 12 years
Lipitor 10 mg po daily x 3 months
Os-Cal 500 po TID × 3 months

All

NKDA

PE

Gen

WDWN white woman in NAD

VS

BP 168/86, P 64, RR 17, T 37°C; Ht 5′3″, Wt 64.4 kg

Skin

Fair complexion, color good, no lesions

HEENT

Normocephalic; smooth, red tongue; mucous membranes moist; PERRLA; EOMI; eyes and throat clear; funduscopic exam reveals mild arteriolar narrowing, with AV ratio 1:3; no hemorrhages, exudates, or papilledema

Neck/LN

Supple, without obvious nodes; no JVD

Chest

Decreased breath sounds bilaterally; air movement decreased; no rales or rhonchi

Breasts

Mastectomy scar left breast; right breast normal

CV

RRR; no murmurs; normal S_1 and S_2, no S_3 or S_4

Abd

Soft, NT/ND, (+) BS

Genit/Rect

Deferred

MS/Ext

Prominent saphenous vein visible in left leg, with multiple varicosities bilaterally; tendon xanthoma noted in left Achilles; good pulses bilaterally

Neuro

CN II–XII intact; DTRs 2+; sensory and motor levels intact; toes downgoing

Labs

Na 141 mEq/L	TSH 3.492 mIU/L	
K 4.1 mEq/L	*Fasting lipid profile*	*Lipids 3 months ago*
Cl 104 mEq/L	T. chol 224 mg/dL	T. chol 253 mg/dL
CO_2 25 mEq/L	Trig 260 mg/dL	Trig 320 mg/dL
BUN 17 mg/dL	HDL 43 mg/dL	HDL 30 mg/dL
SCr 1.1 mg/dL	LDL 165 mg/dL	LDL 180 mg/dL
Glu 98 mg/dL		

Other

DXA scan of lumbar spine (4 mo. ago): L2–4 = 0.780 g/cm² (T score: –3.5 SD); right femoral neck = 0.615 g/cm² (T score: –3.04 SD)

Assessment

1. Nausea caused by Os-Cal 500
2. Severe osteoporosis requiring further intervention
3. Hypertension not adequately controlled
4. Familial combined hyperlipidemia responding to therapy
5. COPD stable on present regimen
6. Hypothyroidism well controlled on present regimen

▶ Questions

Problem Identification

1. a. *Create a list of the patient's drug therapy problems.*
   b. *What information (signs, symptoms, laboratory values) indicates the presence or severity of the patient's osteoporosis? What are the patient's risk factors for developing osteoporosis?*
   c. *What additional information would be useful in determining the extent of the patient's osteoporosis and the need for aggressive therapy?*

Desired Outcome

2. *What are the goals of pharmacotherapy for osteoporosis in this case?*

Therapeutic Alternatives

3. a. *What nondrug therapies might be useful for this patient's osteoporosis?*
   b. *What feasible pharmacotherapeutic alternatives are available for treatment of the osteoporosis?*

Optimal Plan

4. a. *What drug, dosage form, dose, schedule, and duration of therapy are best for treating this patient's osteoporosis?*
   b. *What alternatives would be appropriate if the initial therapy fails or cannot be used?*

Outcome Evaluation

5. *Which clinical and laboratory parameters are necessary to evaluate the therapy for achievement of the desired therapeutic outcome and to detect or prevent adverse effects?*

Patient Education

6. *What information should be provided to the patient to enhance compliance, ensure successful therapy, and minimize adverse effects?*

▶ Self-Study Assignments

1. Investigate the new drugs and drug classes under development for the treatment of osteoporosis.
2. Complete a pharmacoeconomic analysis of the various drugs used to treat osteoporosis. Which therapy is the most cost effective?
3. Develop an exercise plan to prevent osteoporosis.

▶ Clinical Pearl

In elderly patients, use calcium gluconate, citrate, or lactate instead of calcium carbonate, as these salt forms do not require an acidic gastric pH for dissolution.

References

1. The Women's Health Initiative Steering Committee. Effects of conjugated equine estrogen in postmenopausal women with hysterectomy: The Women's Health Initiative randomized controlled trial. JAMA 2004;291:1701–1712.
2. Feskanich D, Willett WC, Stampfer MJ, et al. A prospective study of thiazide use and fractures in women. Osteoporos Int 1997;7:79–84.
3. Goldstein MF, Fallon JJ Jr, Harning R. Chronic glucocorticoid therapy-induced osteoporosis in patients with obstructive lung disease. Chest 1999;116:1733–1749.
4. NIH Consensus Development Panel on Osteoporosis Prevention, Diagnosis, and Therapy. Osteoporosis prevention, diagnosis, and therapy. JAMA 2001;285:785–795.
5. Rossouw JE, Anderson GL, Prentice RL. Writing Group for the Women's Health Initiative Investigators. Risks and benefits of estrogen plus progestin in healthy postmenopausal women: Principal results from the Women's Health Initiative randomized controlled trial. JAMA 2002;288:321–333.
6. Grady D, Herrington D, Bittner V, et al. Cardiovascular disease outcomes during 6.8 years of hormone therapy: Heart and Estrogen/progestin Replacement Study follow-up (HERS II). JAMA 2002;288:49–57.
7. Greenspan SL, Resnick NM, Parker RA. Combination therapy with hormone replacement and alendronate for prevention of bone loss in elderly women: A randomized controlled trial. JAMA 2003;289:2525–2533.
8. Reginster J, Minne HW, Sorensen OH, et al. Randomized trial of the effects of risedronate on vertebral fractures in women with established postmenopausal osteoporosis. Vertebral Efficacy with Risedronate Therapy (VERT) Study Group. Osteoporos Int 2000;11:83–91.
9. Ettinger B, Black DM, Mitlak BH, et al. Reduction of vertebral fracture risk in postmenopausal women with osteoporosis treated with raloxifene: Results from a 3-year randomized clinical trial. Multiple Outcomes of Raloxifene Evaluation (MORE) Investigators. JAMA 1999;282:637–645.
10. Barrett-Connor E, Grady D, Sashegyi A, et al. MORE Investigators. Raloxifene and cardiovascular events in osteoporotic postmenopausal women: Four-year results from the MORE (Multiple Outcomes of Raloxifene Evaluation) randomized trial. JAMA 2002;287:847–857.
11. Neer RM, Arnaud CD, Zanchetta JR, et al. Effect of parathyroid hormone (1–34) on fractures and bone mineral density in postmenopausal women with osteoporosis. N Engl J Med 2001;344:1434–1441.

94 RHEUMATOID ARTHRITIS

▶ Joint Project (Level II)

Amy L. Whitaker, PharmD
Ralph E. Small, PharmD, FCCP, FASHP, FAPhA

▶ After completing this case study, students should be able to:

- Identify the signs and symptoms of rheumatoid arthritis (RA).
- Recommend appropriate drug therapy for the management of RA.
- Recognize alternative therapies for the treatment of pain and inflammation in patients with RA.
- Recommend appropriate nonpharmacologic options for managing patients with RA.
- Educate patients about the drug therapy used to treat RA.

PATIENT PRESENTATION

Chief Complaint

"I have pain in all of my joints, a swollen left knee, and stiffness every morning."

HPI

Janet Hobbs is a 58 yo woman who presents to her rheumatologist with generalized arthralgias, a swollen left knee, and morning stiffness. These symptoms have been occurring with increasing severity for the past several weeks. She presented with similar symptoms 3 months ago, at which time her methotrexate dosage was increased.

PMH

RA × 6 years
S/P hysterectomy 4 years ago
HTN × 10 years

FH

Father died from complications after a traumatic fall at age 65. Mother died of hip fracture and pneumonia at age 78. No siblings.

SH

Housewife; married for 32 years; has two grown children with no known medical problems. Denies alcohol or tobacco use. Volunteers in the community extensively, but has been doing less in the past 2 months.

ROS

Swelling in left knee; decreased ROM in hands; morning stiffness every day for about 1½ hours; fatigue experienced daily during afternoon hours; denies HA, chest pain, SOB, bleeding episodes, or syncopal attacks; denies nausea, vomiting, diarrhea, loss of appetite or weight loss; reports minor visual changes corrected with stronger prescription glasses.

Meds

HCTZ 25 mg po Q AM
Norvasc 10 mg po once daily
Celebrex 200mg BID
Prednisone 5 mg, ½ tab po Q AM
Methotrexate 2.5 mg, 6 tabs po once a week
Folic acid 1 mg po once daily

Patient receives medications at a local community pharmacy. Medication profile indicates that she refills her medications on time the first of each month.

All

Penicillin (rash 25 years ago)

PE

Gen

Pleasant middle-aged white woman in moderate distress because of pain and swelling in left knee

VS

BP 138/80, P 82, RR 14, T 37.1°C; Ht 5′6″, Wt 65.3 kg

Skin

No rashes; normal turgor; no breakdown or ulcers

HEENT

Atraumatic; moon facies; PERRLA; EOMI; A-V nicking visible bilaterally; pale conjunctiva bilaterally; TMs intact; xerostomia

Neck/LN

Supple, no JVD or thyromegaly; no bruits; palpable lymph nodes

Chest

CTA

CV

RRR; normal S_1, S_2; no m/r/g

Abd

Soft, NT/ND; (+) BS

Breasts

Normal; no lumps

GU/Rect

Deferred

MS/Ext

Hands: mild RA changes; swelling of the 3rd, 4th, and 5th PIP joints bilaterally; pain in the 3rd and 4th MCP joints on left; Boutonniere deformity of the 3rd and 4th digits bilaterally; ulnar deviation bilaterally; decreased grip strength, L > R (patient is left-handed)
Wrists: good ROM
Elbows: good ROM; slight permanent contracture on right; fixed nodule at pressure point
Shoulders: decreased ROM (especially abduction) bilaterally
Hips: decreased ROM on right; atrophy of quadriceps, L > R
Knees: pain bilaterally; decreased ROM on left; effusion/edema on left
Feet: no edema; full plantar flexion and dorsiflexion; 3+ pedal pulses

Neuro

CN II–XII grossly intact; muscle strength 5/5 UE, 4/5 LE, DTRs 2/4 biceps & triceps, 1/4 patella

Labs

Na 135 mEq/L	Hgb 10.0 g/dL	AST 15 IU/L	CK < 20 IU/L	*Fasting Lipid Profile*
K 4.1 mEq/L	Hct 31%	ALT 12 IU/L	ANA negative	T. Chol 219 mg/dL
Cl 101 mEq/L	WBC 13. × $10^3/mm^3$	Alk phos 56 IU/L	Wes ESR 47 mm/hr	LDL 106 mg/dL
CO_2 22 mEq/L	Plt 356 × $10^3/mm^3$	T. bili 0.8 mg/dL	RF (+) 1:1280	HDL 50 mg/dL
BUN 12 mg/dL	Ca 9.1 mg/dL	Alb 4.2 g/dL	Anti-CCP (+)	TG 150 mg/dL
SCr 0.8 mg/dL	Urate 5.1 mg/dL	HbsAg (–)	aPTT 31 sec	
Glu 103 mg/dL	TSH 0.74 mIU/L	Anti-HCV (–)	INR 1.0	

UA

Normal

Chest X-Ray

No fluid, masses, or infection; no cardiomegaly

Hand X-Ray

Erosion of MCP and PIP joints bilaterally; measurable joint space narrowing from previous x-ray 6 months ago

Synovial Fluid

From left knee; white cells 23.0 × $10^3/mm^3$, turbid in appearance

Assessment

58 yo woman in moderate distress with acute flare of RA (functional class II). RA not adequately controlled with current therapy. Patient is adherent with current medication regimen. HTN is controlled on present therapy.

Questions

Problem Identification

1. a. *List the patient's drug therapy problems.*
   b. *What information (signs, symptoms, laboratory values) indicates the presence and severity of rheumatoid arthritis?*
   c. *What additional information is needed to assess the patient?*

Desired Outcome

2. *What are the goals of pharmacotherapy in this case?*

Therapeutic Alternatives

3. a. *What nonpharmacologic modalities may be beneficial for this patient?*
   b. *What pharmacologic alternatives are available for the treatment of RA?*
   c. *What economic and psychosocial considerations are applicable to this patient?*

Optimal Plan

4. *What drug, dosage form, dose, schedule, and duration of therapy are best for this patient?*

Outcome Evaluation

5. *What clinical and laboratory parameters are necessary to evaluate the patient's drug therapy?*

Patient Education

6. *What information should be provided to the patient to enhance adherence, ensure successful therapy, and minimize adverse effects?*

▶ Self-Study Assignments

1. Perform a literature search and assess the current efficacy and toxicity information about COX-2 selective inhibitors.
2. Create a list of the clinically significant drug interactions for NSAIDs and DMARDs, including methotrexate.
3. Compare the biologic agents used to treat rheumatoid arthritis with respect to class of agent, route of administration, efficacy, and incidence of side effects.

▶ Clinical Pearl

Treat with high-dose corticosteroids to obtain short-term benefit and relieve the flare of rheumatoid arthritis. Concurrently, or shortly thereafter, begin an NSAID and a DMARD to obtain long-term benefit and prevent disease flares and progression.

References

1. American College of Rheumatology Subcommittee on Rheumatoid Arthritis Guidelines. Guidelines for the management of rheumatoid arthritis: 2002 Update. Arthritis Rheum 2002;46:328–346.
2. Moreland LW, Schiff MH, Baumgartner SW, et al. Etanercept therapy in rheumatoid arthritis. A randomized controlled trial. Ann Intern Med 1999;130:478–486.
3. Weinblatt ME, Kremer JM, Bankhurst AD, et al. A trial of etanercept, a recombinant tumor necrosis factor receptor:Fc fusion protein in patients with rheumatoid arthritis receiving methotrexate. N Engl J Med 1999;340:253–259.
4. Maini R, St. Clair EW, Breedveld F, et al. Infliximab (chimeric anti-tumor necrosis factor-alpha monoclonal antibody) versus placebo in rheumatoid arthritis patients receiving concomitant methotrexate: A randomized phase III trial. ATTRACT Study Group. Lancet 1999;354:1932–1939.
5. Weinblatt ME, Keystone EC, Furst DE, et al. Adalimumab, a fully human anti-tumor necrosis factor alpha monoclonal antibody, for the treatment of rheumatoid arthritis in patients taking concomitant methotrexate: the ARMADA trial. Arthritis Rheum 2003;48:35–45.
6. Cohen S, Hurd E, Cush J, et al. Treatment of rheumatoid arthritis with anakinra, a recombinant human interleukin-1 receptor antagonist, in combination with methotrexate: Results of a twenty-four-week, multicenter, randomized, double-blind, placebo-controlled trial. Arthritis Rheum 2002;46:614–624.
7. O'Dell JR, Haire C, Erikson N, et al. Efficacy of triple DMARD therapy in patients with RA with suboptimal response to methotrexate. J Rheumatol 1996;23(Suppl 44):72–74.
8. Keystone EC. Tumor necrosis factor-alpha blockade in the treatment of rheumatoid arthritis. Rheum Dis Clin North Am 2001;27(2):427–443.

95 OSTEOARTHRITIS

▶ Murder by Joints (Level II)

Michael A. Oszko, PharmD, BCPS, FASHP

▶ After completing this case study, students should be able to:

- Recognize the most common signs and symptoms of osteoarthritis.
- Design an appropriate pharmacotherapeutic regimen for treating osteoarthritis, taking into account a patient's other medical problems and drug therapy.
- Incorporate potential adjunctive therapies (pharmacologic, nonpharmacologic, and alternative) into the regimen of a patient with osteoarthritis.
- Assess and evaluate the efficacy of an analgesic regimen for a patient with osteoarthritis, and formulate an alternative plan if the regimen is inadequate or causes unacceptable toxicity.

PATIENT PRESENTATION

Chief Complaint

"My joints are killing me, and nobody want to help."

HPI

Diane Webster is a 49 yo woman who presents to the Family Medicine Clinic for the first time complaining of increasing pain in her lower back, hips, and right knee. She has a long history of OA and had most recently been seen by a local rheumatologist, who tried a variety of NSAIDs without apparent success. She began insisting that the rheumatologist provide her with increasing quantities of opioid analgesics, which he subsequently refused to do. She is now seeking medical care from the Family Medicine Clinic.

Last fall, she broke her right ankle and a bone in her foot. Her foot was in a cast for 4 weeks, and she was on crutches for 2 months. During this time, she noted that her arthritic symptoms were becoming increasingly more bothersome. In addition, she states that although her arthritis usually improves with warmer weather, it didn't improve at all this past summer. She is a rather poor historian.

PMH

OA × 18 years
Morbid obesity × 21 years
Type 2 DM, insulin-requiring × 9 years
Hypercholesterolemia × 5 years
HTN × 10 years
DVT 3 years ago
"Anxiety disorder"—unspecified, × many years

PSH

Appendectomy 27 years ago
TAH-BSO 14 years ago
Right lateral maleolus and first metatarsal fracture repair 9 months ago

FH

Mother alive with DM; father died at age 69 secondary to pancreatic cancer; no siblings.

SH

Unemployed; disabled, on Medicaid; no other health insurance; occasional alcohol, no tobacco or illicit drug use.

ROS

Positive for pain in left shoulder; low back pain with "shooting pains" radiating to the buttocks and groin area; "deep, boring" pain originating in the right pretibial area and extending distally to the right ankle and toes. Negative for headache, neck stiffness, joint swelling, or erythema; no SOB or palpitations; denies urinary frequency or burning, constipation, diarrhea, or tarry stools. Fingerstick blood glucose concentrations are usually in the mid-200s (although she admits to rarely checking them); occasional polyuria, but no blurred vision.

Meds

- Lisinopril 10 mg po Q AM
- Novolin N, 25 units subQ Q AM and 15 units subQ Q PM
- Evista 60 mg po Q AM
- Warfarin 5 mg po once daily
- OxyContin 20 mg po TID
- Lortab 10/650, 1–2 tabs po PRN pain
- Ambien 10 mg po at bedtime PRN sleep
- Xanax 0.5 mg po TID PRN anxiety
- Claritin 10 mg po PRN

All

Demerol—"makes me goofy"
Sulfa—hives
Various pain meds (unspecified)—nausea, "passes out"

PE

Gen

Well developed, obese, Caucasian woman slightly anxious, but otherwise in NAD

VS

BP 134/88, P 84, RR 16, T 37.1°C; Ht 5′3″, Wt 201 lb. No orthostatic changes

Skin

Warm, dry; LE—shiny, somewhat discolored areas on the pre-tibial area bilaterally, consistent with venous stasis dermatitis; feet—Stage I skin changes on the plantar aspect of the right first metatarsal.

HEENT

NC/AT; PERRLA; funduscopic exam reveals sharp disks; mild A-V nicking, but no hemorrhages or exudates; no scleral icterus; TMs intact; mucous membranes moist; poor dentition with gingival erythema; no lateral deviation of tongue; no pharyngeal edema or erythema.

Neck

Supple; unable to assess thyromegaly or lymphadenopathy secondary to body habitus; no carotid bruits.

Lungs

CTA

Breasts

Difficult to examine due to size; symmetrical; no apparent masses

CV

Distant heart sounds, Normal S_1 and S_2; PMI at 5th ICS/MCL; RRR; no m/r/g; no JVD or HJR

Abdomen

Obese, soft, non-tender; no guarding; (+) BS; unable to assess liver size upon palpation

GU/Rect

Normal female genitalia; some mild vaginal atrophy; normal sphincter tone; guaiac (–) stool in rectal vault

MS/Ext

Back pain radiating to right buttock with straight leg raising at 60°; right hip pain with flexion > 90° and with internal and external rotation > 45°; both hips tender to palpation; right knee (+) crepitus; right ankle with full ROM, no swelling or edema

Neuro

Oriented × 3; flat affect; appears at times to alternate between apathy and anger/frustration; CN II–XII intact; DTRs equal bilaterally except for slightly diminished Achilles reflexes bilaterally; no focal deficits; gait impaired secondary to hip pain. Slightly decreased sensation to pinprick and vibration on the distal half of right foot. Babinski's downgoing.

Labs

Na 135 mEq/L	Hgb 13.7 g/dL	RDW 14.4%	Ca 11.2 mg/dL
K 4.8 mEq/L	Hct 39.7%	AST 38 IU/L	Phos 4.5 mg/dL
Cl 98 mEq/L	WBC 4.5 × 10^3/mm^3	Alk Phos 106 IU/L	Uric acid 7.2 mg/dL
CO_2 26 mEq/L	Plt 286 × 10^3/mm^3	T. prot 7.4 g/dL	ESR 18 mm/hour
BUN 9 mg/dL	MCV 85.3 μm^3	Alb 4.4 g/dL	CRP 0.2 mg/dL
SCr 0.9 mg/dL	MCH 29.4 pg	T. chol 254 mg/dL	INR 1.8
Glu 248 mg/dL	MCHC 34.5 g/dL	HbA1c 14.4%	

UA

SG 1.011; pH 6.5; WBC (–), RBC (–), leukocyte esterase (–), nitrite (–). Microscopic examination reveals 2 to 5 epithelial cells/hpf and occasional bacteria.

X-rays

Lumbar spine: advanced degenerative changes at L3–4 and at L4–5.
Right hip: moderate degenerative changes with some spurring of the femoral head and slight decrease in joint space.
Right knee: moderate degenerative changes. No effusion.
Right foot: completely healed lateral maleolus and first metatarsal bone.

Assessment

1. Pain secondary to moderate to severe OA of the lumbar spine, hips, and right knee
2. Morbid obesity (175% of IBW, BMI = 35.7 kg/m^2)
3. DM
4. Hypercholesterolemia
5. HTN
6. Unspecified depressive or anxiety disorder
7. R/O possible narcotic abuse

Questions

Problem Identification

1. a. *Create a list of the patient's drug therapy problems.*
   b. *What information (symptoms, signs, laboratory values) indicates the presence or severity of the primary problem (osteoarthritis)?*
   c. *What additional information is needed to satisfactorily assess this patient's major medical problems?*

Desired Outcome

2. *What are the goals of pharmacotherapy for each of this patient's drug-related problems?*

Therapeutic Alternatives

3. a. *What nondrug therapies might be useful for this patient?*
   b. *What feasible pharmacotherapeutic alternatives are available for treatment of this patient's osteoarthritis?*

Optimal Plan

4. a. *What drug, dosage form, schedule, and duration of therapy are best for treating this patient's osteoarthritis?*
   b. *What alternatives would be appropriate if the initial therapy fails or cannot be used?*

Outcome Evaluation

5. *What clinical and laboratory parameters are necessary to evaluate the therapy for achievement of the desired therapeutic outcome and to detect or prevent adverse effects?*

Patient Education

6. *What information should be provided to the patient to enhance compliance, ensure successful therapy, and minimize adverse effects?*

Additional Case Questions

1. *Evaluate this patient's continued need for warfarin therapy, taking into account benefit vs. risk, potential drug interactions, and any other important considerations.*
2. *Evaluate this patient's therapy for diabetes mellitus. What additional information do you need to determine the adequacy of therapy? What modifications to the diabetes treatment should be considered?*
3. *Is this patient a candidate for pharmacotherapy to treat her morbid obesity? If so, what treatment(s) would you recommend?*
4. *For additional questions related to the use of glucosamine for the treatment of osteoarthritis, please see Section 20 of this Casebook.*

Self-Study Assignments

1. Patients whose arthritis is poorly or inadequately controlled often turn to alternative, homeopathic, or herbal remedies for relief. Develop a list of nontraditional therapies that have been used for treating arthritis.
2. Identify an Internet website that provides useful information to patients about osteoarthritis. Identify one site that you think provides misleading or potentially dangerous information to patients.

Clinical Pearl

Pain relief is the top priority when treating osteoarthritis. Use a systematic approach to assessing and treating pain in order to achieve total (or near-total) pain relief, avoid wasting resources, and prevent drug misuse/addiction. Remember, "Pain is what the patient tells you it is."

References

1. Simon LS, Lipman AG, Jacox AK, et al. Pain in osteoarthritis, rheumatoid arthritis and juvenile chronic arthritis. 2nd ed. Glenview (IL): American Pain Society (APS); 2002;1–179. (Clinical practice guideline; no. 2). Available on the Internet at www.guideline.gov. (Accessed July 5, 2004).
2. Recommendations for the medical management of osteoarthritis of the hip and knee: 2000 update. American College of Rheumatology Subcommittee on Osteoarthritis Guidelines. Arthritis Rheum 2000;43:1905–1915.
3. Arroll B, Goodyear-Smith F. Corticosteroid injections for osteoarthritis of the knee: Meta-analysis. BMJ 2004;328:869. Available on the Internet at http://bmj.bmjjournals.com. (Accessed July 5, 2004).
4. Lo GH, LaValley M, McAlindon T, et al. Intra-articular hyaluronic acid in the treatment of knee osteoarthritis: A meta-analysis. JAMA 2003;290:3115–3121.
5. Richy F, Bruyere O, Ethgen O, et al. Structural and symptomatic efficacy of glucosamine and chondroitin in knee osteoarthritis: A comprehensive meta-analysis. Arch Intern Med 2003;163:1514–1422.
6. Towheed TE, Anastassiades TP. Glucosamine and chondroitin for treating symptoms of osteoarthritis: Evidence is widely touted but incomplete. JAMA 2000;283:1483–1484. Editorial.

96 GOUT AND HYPERURICEMIA

▶ The Party's Over (Level II)

Ralph E. Small, PharmD, FCCP, FASHP, FAPhA

▶ After completing this case study, students should be able to:

- Identify the risk factors for hyperuricemia.
- Recommend appropriate treatment for an acute attack of gouty arthritis.
- Recognize the importance of determining the presence of an overproducer versus underexcretor of uric acid.
- Recommend appropriate therapy for the treatment of chronic gouty arthritis.

PATIENT PRESENTATION

Chief Complaint

"My toe hurts so bad, I can't put my shoe on!"

HPI

Harvey Jones is a 53 yo man seen in the clinic by his physician for severe pain in his left great toe. The pain began the day after his 35th high school class reunion 2 nights ago. The morning after the reunion he noticed that his toe was sore and the pain got increasingly worse throughout the day. Last night the pain kept him awake most of the night. He states that he is unable to bear any weight on that foot and came into the clinic without a shoe on. He has no history of injury to that foot.

PMH

HTN × 5 years
Hyperlipidemia × 5 years
Seasonal allergic rhinitis (since adolescence)

FH

Father deceased from MI at age 70; mother alive and healthy.

SH

Married with adult children. He is self-employed as a construction worker. He is a non-smoker (5 years) and occasionally uses alcohol (4 to 5 drinks per week).

ROS

No HA, dizziness, SOB, rhinorrhea, sneezing, itching, or generalized swelling or tenderness of the joints.

Meds

HCTZ 25 mg po once daily
ASA 325 mg po once daily
Atorvastatin 20 mg po once daily
Loratadine 10 mg po once daily PRN

All

NKDA

PE

Gen

Healthy white man in acute distress

VS

BP 134/84, HR 90, RR 22, T 37.9°C, Wt. 102.1 kg, Ht. 6′0″

Neck/LN

Normal with no swelling, thyromegaly, or JVD

HEENT

PERRLA; no A-V nicking, hemorrhages, or exudates

Lungs

CTA

CV

RRR, no m/r/g

Abd

Non-tender; obese; no HSM

MS/Ext

Left first MTP swollen, hot, tender, erythematous (see Figure 96–1)

Neuro

A & O × 3; CN II–XII intact; DTRs 2+, Babinski (–)

Labs

Na 142 mEq/L	Hgb 15.5 g/dL	Uric acid 11.7 mg/dL
K 3.8 mEq/L	Hct 45%	Westergren ESR 18 mm/h
Cl 100 mEq/L	WBC 12.0 × 10^3/mm^3	*Fasting Lipid Profile*
CO_2 23 mEq/L	60% PMNs	T. chol 174 mg/dL
BUN 10 mg/dL	3% Bands	HDL 42 mg/dL
SCr 1.0 mg/dL	35% Lymphs	LDL 138 mg/dL
Glu 95 mg/dL	2% Eos	Trig 126 mg/dL

UA

Negative

X-Ray

Left great toe: some soft tissue swelling; normal joint space

Other

Left great toe synovial fluid aspirate: PMNs and monosodium urate crystals (see Figure 96–2).

Assessment

1. Primary presentation of gout
2. HTN controlled on medical therapy
3. Hyperlipidemia controlled on medical therapy
4. Allergic rhinitis controlled on medical therapy

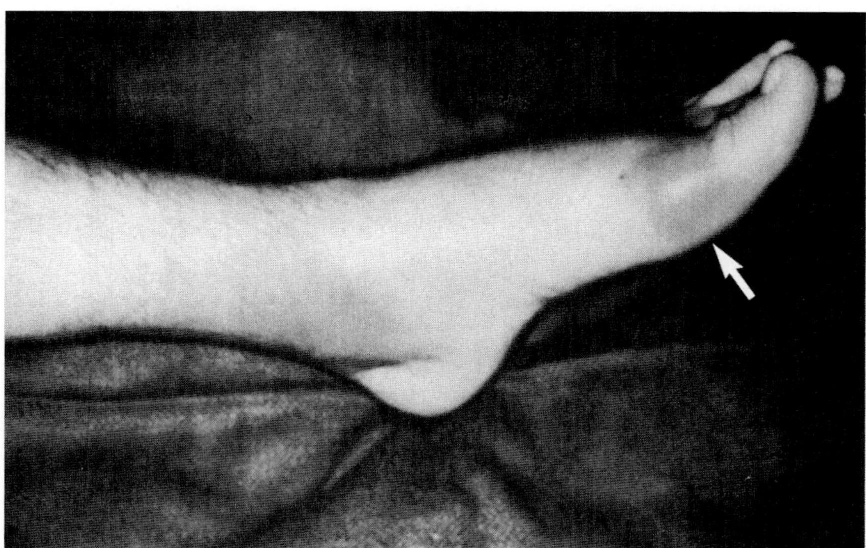

Figure 96–1. Swollen, erythematous, and painful left great toe caused by an acute attack of gout. *(Reprinted from the Clinical Slide Collection on the Rheumatic Diseases, copyright 1991. Used by permission of the American College of Rheumatology.)*

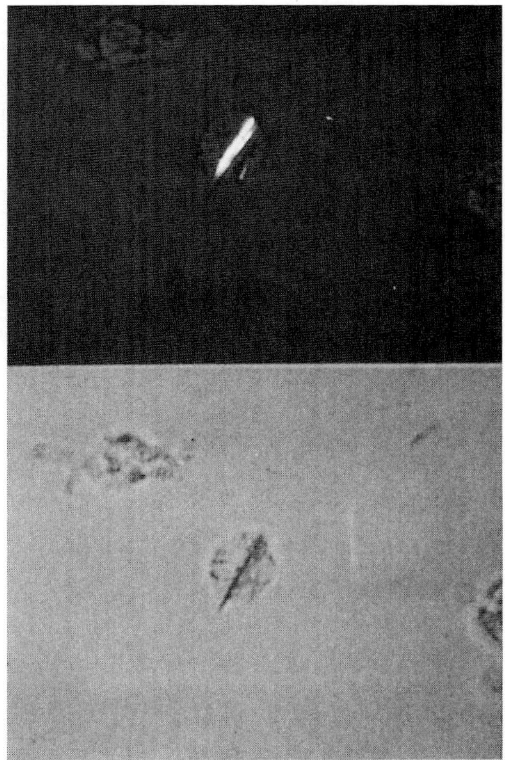

Figure 96–2. Monosodium urate crystals phagocytosed by a polymorphonuclear leukocyte in the joint fluid during an acute attack of gout. In the top section, compensated polarized light demonstrates two longer crystals (approximately 13 μm) and one shorter crystal (approximately 9 μm). The bottom section shows the same field under ordinary light. Here only one of the longer crystals is identifiable. This demonstrates the superiority of compensated polarized light over ordinary light microscopy when evaluating joint fluid for crystals. *(Reprinted from the Clinical Slide Collection on the Rheumatic Diseases. Copyright 1991. Used by permission of the American College of Rheumatology.)*

▶ Questions

Problem Identification

1. a. *Create a list of the patient's drug therapy problems.*
   b. *What information (symptoms, signs, laboratory values) indicates the presence or severity of an acute gouty attack?*
   c. *Could any of the patient's problems have been caused by drug therapy?*

Desired Outcome

2. *What are the goals of pharmacotherapy in this case?*

Therapeutic Alternatives

3. a. *What nondrug therapies might be useful for this patient?*
   b. *What feasible pharmacotherapeutic alternatives are available for treatment of the acute attack of gouty arthritis?*

Optimal Plan

4. *What drug, dosage form, dose, schedule, and duration of therapy are best for this patient?*

Outcome Evaluation

5. *What clinical and laboratory parameters are necessary to evaluate the therapy for achievement of the desired therapeutic outcome and to detect or prevent adverse effects?*

Patient Education

6. *What information should be provided to the patient to enhance adherence, ensure successful therapy, and minimize adverse effects?*

▶ Clinical Course

Mr. Jones responded completely to the initial therapy that you recommended, with total resolution of his joint pain in 5 days. Within 6 months after his initial presentation, he experienced two more episodes of acute gouty arthritis. Although his BP is adequately controlled on alternative therapy (an ACE inhibitor), he has not followed dietary guidelines, resulting in continued elevation of serum uric acid (> 10.5 mg/dL) and inability to lose weight. He has also not tolerated colchicine prophylactic therapy that was initiated after resolution of his acute gout attacks due to persistent diarrhea. Short-term courses of an NSAID (sulindac) were effective in controlling his second and third acute attacks. A 24-hour urine collection was obtained after 3 days on a purine-free diet. The results revealed a urine uric acid value of 750 mg.

▶ Follow-Up Questions

1. *Provide an interpretation of the urine uric acid value.*
2. *What recommendations do you have for further management of this patient?*

▶ Self-Study Assignments

1. Which uric acid lowering therapy would be most useful in a patient with chronic hyperuricemia and diminished renal function? Outline the rationale for your response, and prepare dosage regimens of the drug for patients with varying degrees of renal impairment.
2. Make a list of the NSAIDs that have FDA-approved labeling for the treatment of acute gouty attacks. Compare the dosage regimens used, and contact a local pharmacy to determine which agents provide the most economical therapy.
3. New, safer gout drugs, including febuxostat, anti IL-8, and Y-700, are on the horizon. What type of drug is each of these agents, what is their mechanism of action, how are they administered (dose, schedule, route), and what are their advantages?

▶ Clinical Pearl

Oral colchicine can cause serious diarrhea resulting in dehydration and electrolyte disturbances; although IV colchicine avoids these GI effects, it may result in local extravasation injury.

References

1. Anonymous. Effective management of gout often requires multiple medications. Drug Ther Perspect 2001; 17 (12): 8–12.
2. Schumacher HR Jr, Boice JA, Daikh DI, et al. Randomized double blind trial of etoricoxib and indomethacin in treatment of acute gouty arthritis. BMJ 2002; 324:1488–1492.

SECTION 13

Disorders of the Eyes, Ears, Nose, and Throat

97 GLAUCOMA

▶ Another Silent Disease (Level II)

Tien T. Kiat-Winarko, PharmD, BSc

▶ After completing this case study, students should be able to:

- Recognize the importance of regular eye examinations and the difference between glaucoma and ocular hypertension.
- List the risk factors for developing open-angle glaucoma.
- Select and recommend agents from different pharmacologic classes when indicated and provide the rationale for drug selection.
- Recommend conventional glaucoma therapy as well as new options in glaucoma management when indicated.
- Implement the basic ophthalmologic monitoring parameters used in glaucoma therapy.
- Educate patients on their medication regimen and proper ophthalmic administration technique.

PATIENT PRESENTATION

Chief Complaint

"My left eye is foggy, and I get blurred vision and headaches."

HPI

Lee Angeles is a pleasant 34 yo man with a history of advanced open-angle glaucoma who presents to his ophthalmologist with complaints of fogging and distortion of vision in the left eye lasting 6 to 12 hours. This occasionally progresses to tunnel vision, with chronic sensitivity to fluorescent lights and throbbing band-like squeezing headaches lasting for hours. He also complains of periodic distortion in the left eye for the past 3 months, sometimes associated with central area visual blurring.

He was in his usual state of health until he had a skydiving accident 9 years ago and fractured his thoracic spine at the level of T9–10. During that hospitalization, he complained of blurred vision. Ophthalmology consult was sought and he was ultimately diagnosed with advanced open-angle glaucoma. He was managed by a general ophthalmologist for several years, who prescribed Timoptic 0.5% ou BID, Propine 0.1% ou BID, and Ocusert Pilo-40 od and Ocusert Pilo-20 os Q week. He was subsequently referred to a glaucoma specialist because of worsening of his condition. He had undergone laser trabeculoplasty ou prior to his referral. The glaucoma specialist examined the patient, and a complete work-up was done on the initial visit.

Bilateral laser trabeculoplasty was performed 8 years ago with an initial decrease in IOP; however, IOP subsequently increased several months later. Filtering surgery was performed in Boston ou 7 years ago. Multiple prior brain MRIs revealed no abnormal findings. Other ocular history includes severe myopia since childhood, history of dry eyes, and history of contact lens wear.

PMH

Childhood asthma that resolved at puberty

Depression as a consequence of chronic open-angle glaucoma and worsening of vision after completion of his PhD program

S/P ultrasonic renal lithotripsy secondary to nephrolithiasis associated with acetazolamide use

S/P tonsillectomy as a child

FH

Father, mother, and sister have glaucoma. Father has HTN.

SH

PhD in molecular biology from Harvard. Single. No history of smoking. Drank 4 cans of beer per day for 3 years during postgraduate study. Currently drinks 2 to 3 cans of beer/week.

Meds

Betoptic 0.5% ou BID
Iopidine 0.5% os TID
Trusopt 2% os TID
FML 0.1% ou TID
Bion Tears ou BID
Nifedipine 10 mg po TID
Trental 400 mg po TID
Paxil 20 mg po once daily
Also performs eye massage ou QID
Past medications include pilocarpine 4%, Timoptic 0.5%, Propine, Diamox sequels 500 mg, and Pred-Forte 1%

All

NKDA

PE

VS

BP 120/82, P 70, R 18, T 98.3°F

Eyes

Visual acuity: OD—hand motion at 3 inches with correction spectacles; OS—20/30

Slit-lamp exam: Lid margins were without inflammation ou; conjunctiva without injection; normal tear break-up, did not stain with fluorescein; cornea clear and smooth; anterior chamber deep and quiet; lenses—clear ou; iris round without neovascularization or abnormality; no mass/nodules; filtering bleb is visible at 11 o'clock meridian.

Intraocular pressure: OD—14 mm Hg; OS—20 mm Hg

Vitreous examination: clear ou

Disks: OD—the disc appeared whitish, fully cupped and showed marked pallor; cup-to-disk (C/D) ratio = 1.0; OS—C/D ratio = 0.99 with only a narrow rim present (normal C/D ratio = < 0.33)

Color vision: OD—unable to see; OS—WNL

Visual fields: OD—unable to see the Amsler grid; can only see hand motion at 3 inches away; OS—several paracentral scotomata with the Amsler grid; 20/30. Diurnal curve of IOP revealed pressures between 10 mm Hg and 21 mm Hg.

CV

RRR without m/r/g; carotid pulses are brisk and equal bilaterally without bruits

Neuro

Smell and corneal sensation are intact bilaterally. Facial symmetry, tone, and sensation are intact bilaterally. Cranial nerves VIII through XII were intact. Gait was intact. Finger-to-nose and rapid alternating movement tests were normal. Reflexes were symmetric and normal. Sensation was intact and symmetric to pinprick, proprioception, and light touch. Motor strength of all extremities was 5/5.

Labs

Na 138 mEq/L	Bun 10 mg/dL
K 3.3 mEq/L	SCr 0.9 mg/dL
Cl 99 mEq/L	FBG 105 mg/dL
CO_2 25 mEq/L	

Assessment

High myopia with advanced chronic juvenile open-angle glaucoma
No evidence of macular edema
No cataracts
S/P filtering procedure ou
Depression associated with chronic open-angle glaucoma

Plan

Increase eye massage to 8 times/day
Follow-up in 6 weeks
Repeat filtering surgery/trabeculectomy with mitomycin C to further lower IOP
Switch nifedipine to nimodipine for better CNS/ophthalmic absorption to increase blood flow
Counsel with neuro-ophthalmologist, retina ophthalmologist, and neurologist

▶ Questions

Problem Identification

1. a. *Identify this patient's drug therapy problems.*
   b. *What risk factors for primary open-angle glaucoma (POAG) are present in this patient?*
   c. *What information (signs, symptoms) indicates the presence or severity of this patient's glaucoma?*

Desired Outcome

2. *What are the goals of pharmacotherapy in this case?*

Therapeutic Alternatives

3. a. *What nondrug therapies might be useful for this patient?*
   b. *What feasible pharmacotherapeutic alternatives are available for treatment of the patient's glaucoma?*

Optimal Plan

4. a. *Devise an optimal pharmacotherapeutic regimen for the treatment of this patient's glaucoma.*
   b. *What alternatives would be appropriate if the initial therapy fails or cannot be used?*

Outcome Evaluation

5. *What clinical and laboratory parameters are necessary to evaluate the therapy for achievement of the desired therapeutic outcome and to detect or prevent adverse effects?*

Patient Education

6. *What information should the patient receive about the disease of glaucoma, proper medication administration technique, and possible side effects of treatment?*

▶ Self-Study Assignments

1. Perform a literature search on the reason why antimetabolites such as mitomycin C and 5-FU are used in glaucoma surgery. What is the mechanism of action of these antimetabolites in trabeculectomy pressure-lowering surgery?
2. Perform a literature search and explain the rationale for using nimodipine and pentoxifylline in advanced open-angle glaucoma. How do these agents work to increase blood flow to the eye and retard the progression of nerve damage?
3. Under what circumstances should the product Ocusert-pilo be used? Compare the advantages and disadvantages of using this long-acting ocular insert.

References

1. Kane H, Gaasterland DE, Monsour M. Response of filtered eyes to digital ocular pressure. Ophthalmology 1997;104:202–206.
2. Liu JH. Circadian rhythm of intraocular pressure. J Glaucoma 1998;7:141–147.
3. Sacca SC, Rolando M, Marletta A, et al. Fluctuations of intraocular pressure during the day in open-angle glaucoma, normal-tension glaucoma and normal subjects. Ophthalmologica 1998; 212:115–119.
4. Brandt JD, VanDenburgh AM, Chen K, et al. Comparison of once- or twice-daily bimatoprost with twice-daily timolol in patients with elevated IOP: A 3-month clinical trial. Ophthalmology 2001;108:1023–1031.
5. Aung T, Chew PT, Yip CC, et al. A randomized double-masked crossover study comparing latanoprost 0.005% with unoprostone 0.12% in patients with primary open-angle glaucoma and ocular hypertension. Am J Ophthalmol 2001;131:636–642.
6. Katz LJ, Twelve-month evaluation of brimonidine-purite versus brimonidine in patients with glaucoma or ocular hypertension. J Glaucoma 2002;11:119–126.
7. Herbette LG, Mason PE, Sweeney KR, et al. Favorable amphiphilicity of nimodipine facilitates its interactions with brain membranes. Neuropharmacology 1994;33:241–249.
8. Mundorf T, Williams R, Whitcup S, et al. A 3-month comparison of efficacy and safety of brimonidine-purite 0.15% and brimonidine 0.2% in patients with glaucoma or ocular hypertension. J Ocul Pharmacol Ther 2003;19:37–44.

98 ALLERGIC RHINITIS

▶ Reining in Rhinitis (Level I)

W. Greg Leader, PharmD

▶ After completing this case study, students should be able to:

- Classify a patient's allergic rhinitis based on the signs and symptoms of the disease.
- Educate patients on appropriate measures to limit or avoid exposure to specific antigens.
- Compare and contrast available agents used to treat allergic rhinitis with respect to efficacy and safety.
- Develop a safe and effective therapeutic regimen for the management of allergic rhinitis based on disease severity.
- Educate patients with allergic rhinitis on appropriate medication use.

PATIENT PRESENTATION

Chief Complaint

As per the patient's mother: "She has bouts of sneezing, and then her nose clogs up or starts running. Her eyes are red, and she coughs a lot. She can't sleep at night because her mouth is dry and she can't breathe, and she is falling asleep at school."

HPI

Nicole Fontenot is a 7 yo girl who presents with her mother to her family practitioner with complaints of upper respiratory symptoms. The symptoms have been continuous for the last two months, occur to varying degrees year-round, worsen during the spring and summer, and return to baseline in the winter. Her mother indicates that she has not had fever or complained of throat pain, but she does have a chronic cough that gets worse at night. The cough is non-productive.

PMH

Otitis media × 2 (last 3 years ago)
Acute sinusitis × 4 (last 4 months ago)
Bronchitis × 3 (last 4 months ago)

FH

Father, age 27, with a history of persistent asthma; mother, age 25, with a history of allergic rhinitis and allergy to wasp venom, and brother, age 4, with persistent asthma.

SH

Lives in a three-bedroom home built on a concrete slab. Neither parent smokes, and there are no animals in the house. The family has a golden retriever that stays the back yard. Nicole plays spring and summer soccer and fall basketball.

Meds

Benadryl 25mg po at bedtime
EpiPen PRN Jr. (available for emergency use)
Flintstones Chewable vitamins

All

Penicillin—Hives
Bee venom

ROS

No wheezing, shortness of breath, chest pain, abdominal discomfort, bowel or bladder symptoms, dysuria, or focal weakness.

PE

Gen
The patient appears tired but is in NAD. She is breathing through her mouth, sniffing, and rubbing her nose and eyes. There are dark circles under her eyes. She appears younger than her stated age.

VS
BP 100/60, P 88, RR 21, T 37.3°C; Ht 47″ (25th percentile), Wt 23.2 kg (50th percentile)

HEENT
NC/AT; PERRLA; EOMI. Conjunctivae are pink. Periorbital edema and discoloration. TMs are intact. There is no epistaxis. Nasal mucous membranes and turbinates are swollen and pale in color. There is no tenderness over frontal and maxillary sinuses. Right central incisor is missing. There are no oropharyngeal lesions, and the throat is nonerythematous.

Neck
Supple; no lymphadenopathy

Chest
CTA bilaterally; no wheezes

Heart
RRR S_1 and S_2 normal, no murmurs

Abdomen
Soft, non-tender, (+) BS, no masses or HSM

Extremities
No CCE, abrasion below the right knee

Neuro
Alert and awake, DTRs 2+; 5/5 strength; CN I–XII intact

Labs
Phadiatop (+)

Assessment
This is a 7-year-old girl with nasal congestion most likely due to allergy.

Plan
Histex 5 mL po QID to treat nasal symptoms. Discontinue the diphenhydramine. The patient is to return in two weeks for follow-up.

Questions

Problem Identification

1. a. *Create a list of the patient's drug therapy problems.*
   b. *What information (signs, symptoms, laboratory values) indicates the presence or severity of allergic rhinitis?*
   c. *Could any of the patient's problems have been caused by drug therapy?*
   d. *What additional information from the patient history is needed to satisfactorily assess this patient?*

Desired Outcome

2. *What are the goals of pharmacotherapy in this case?*

Therapeutic Alternatives

3. a. *What nondrug therapies might be useful for this patient?*
   b. *What feasible pharmacotherapeutic alternatives are available for treatment of allergic rhinitis?*

Optimal Plan

4. a. *What drug, dosage form, dose, schedule, and duration of therapy are best for this patient?*
   b. *What alternatives would be available if the initial therapy fails?*

Outcome Evaluation

5. *What clinical and laboratory parameters are necessary to evaluate the therapy for achievement of the desired therapeutic outcome and to detect or prevent adverse effects?*

Patient Education

6. *What information should be provided to the patient to enhance compliance, ensure successful therapy, and minimize adverse effects?*

Self-Study Assignments

1. Outline a plan to treat this patient if she returns for follow-up with no change in nasal symptoms and increased ocular symptoms.
2. Search the literature on leukotrienes in the treatment of allergic rhinitis and prepare a table that summarizes the results of controlled clinical trials.
3. Make a recommendation as to a single first-generation antihistamine, second-generation antihistamine, and intranasal steroid to include on a hospital or HMO formulary. Support your recommendations with efficacy, safety, and economic data.
4. Outline a treatment plan for a pregnant patient with allergic rhinitis. Justify your selection of pharmacologic agents based on their efficacy and safety profiles.

Clinical Pearl

Up to 80% of patients with asthma have symptoms of allergic rhinitis. Intranasal corticosteroid treatment of allergic rhinitis improves both rhinitis and asthma symptoms, as well as decreases bronchial hyperresponsiveness.

References

1. Bosquet J, Van Cauwenberge P, Khaltaev N; Aria Workshop Group; World Health Organization. Allergic rhinitis and its impact on asthma. J Allergy Clin Immunol 2001;108(5 Suppl):S147–S334
2. Fornadley JA, Corey JP, Osguthorpe JD, et al. Allergic rhinitis: Clinical practice guideline. Committee on Practice Standards, American Academy of Otolaryngic Allergy. Otolaryngol Head Neck Surg 1996;115:115–122.
3. Bosquet J, Khaltaev N, Bond C, et al. The ARIA Workshop Group. The management of allergic rhinitis symptoms in the pharmacy. www.whiar.com/pharmguide/pharm.pdf: 1–25. Accessed August 10, 2004.
4. Casale TB, Blaiss MS, Gelfard E, et al. First do no harm: Managing antihistamine impairment in patients with allergic rhinitis. J Allergy Clin Immunol 2003; 111:S835–842.
5. Weiner JM, Abramson MJ, Puy RM. Intranasal corticosteroids versus oral H_1-receptor antagonists in allergic rhinitis: Systematic review of randomized controlled trials. BMJ 1998;317:1624–1629.
6. Scadding GK. Corticosteroids in the treatment of pediatric allergic rhinitis. J Allergy Clin Immunol 2001;108(1 Suppl):S59–S64.
7. Pedersen S. Assessing the effect of intranasal steroids on growth. J Allergy Clin Immunol 2001;108(1 Suppl):S40–S44.
8. Nathan RA. Pharmacotherapy for allergic rhinitis: A critical review of leukotriene receptor antagonists compared with other treatments. Ann Allergy Asthma Immunol 2003;90:182–190.
9. Pullerits T, Praks L, Ristioja V, et al. Comparison of a nasal glucocorticoid, antileukotriene, and a combination of antileukotriene and antihistamine in the treatment of seasonal allergic rhinitis. J Allergy Clin Immunol 2002;109: 949–955.
10. Wilson AM, Orr LC, Sims EJ, et al. Effects of monotherapy with intra-nasal corticosteroid or combined oral histamine and leukotriene receptor antagonists in seasonal allergic rhinitis. Clin Exp Allergy 2001;31:61–68.

SECTION 14

Dermatologic Disorders

99 ACNE VULGARIS

▶ The Graduate (Level II)

Rebecca M. Law, PharmD
Wayne P. Gulliver, MD, FRCPC

▶ After completing this case study, students should be able to:

- Understand risk factors and aggravating factors in the pathogenesis of acne vulgaris.
- Understand the treatment strategies for acne, including appropriate situations for using nonprescription and prescription medications and use of topical and systemic therapies.
- Educate patients with acne on systemic therapies.
- Monitor the safety and efficacy of selected systemic therapies.

PATIENT PRESENTATION

Chief Complaint

"I can't stand this acne!"

HPI

Elaine Morgan is an 18 yo young woman with a history of facial acne since age 15. One month ago she completed a 3-month course of minocycline in combination with Differin (adapalene). Her acne has flared up again and she has again presented to her family physician for treatment.

PMH

Has irregular menses as a result of polycystic ovarian disease diagnosed 3 years ago, which has not required medical treatment. However, it has resulted in an acne condition that was initially quite mild; she responded well to nonprescription topical products. In the past 2 years, the number of facial lesions has increased despite OTC, and later prescription, drug treatments. Initially, Benzamycin Gel was beneficial, but this had to be discontinued because of excessive drying. Differin was used next and it controlled her condition for about 6 months, then the acne worsened and oral antibiotics were added. Most recently, she has received two 3-month courses of minocycline over the past year. She has also noted some scarring and cysts in the past few months.

FH

Parents alive and well; two older brothers (ages 21 and 25). Father had acne with residual scarring.

SH

The patient is under some stress because she is graduating in a few weeks. She wants to do well in school so she will qualify for the best colleges. Both of her brothers graduated with honors. She is sexually active, and her boyfriend uses condoms.

Meds

None currently

All

NKDA

ROS

In addition to the complaints noted above, the patient has dysmenorrhea and mild hirsutism.

PE

Gen
Alert, moderately anxious teenager in NAD

VS
BP 110/70, RR 15, T 37°C, Ht 5′2″, Wt 45 kg

Skin
Comedones on forehead, nose, and chin. Papules and pustules on the nose and malar area. A few cysts on the chin. Scars on malar area. Increased facial hair.

HEENT
PERRLA, EOMI, fundi benign, TMs intact

Chest
CTA bilaterally

Cor
RRR without m/r/g, S_1 and S_2 normal

Abd
(+) BS, soft, non-tender, no masses

MS/Ext
No joint aches or pains; peripheral pulses present

Neuro
CN II–XII intact

Labs

Na 140 mEq/L	Hgb 13.0 g/dL	AST 21 IU/L	LDL-C 90 mg/dL
K 3.7 mEq/L	Hct 38%	ALT 39 IU/L	Trig 90 mg/dL
Cl 100 mEq/L	Plt 300 × 10^3/mm^3	LDH 105 IU/L	DHEAS 6 μmol/L
CO_2 25 mEq/L	WBC 7.0 × 10^3/mm^3	Alk phos 89 IU/L	Testosterone 2.0 ng/mL
BUN 12 mg/dL		T. bili 1.0 mg/dL	Prolactin 15 ng/mL
SCr 1.0 mg/dL		Alb 3.9 g/dL	FSH 150 mIU/mL
Glu 100 mg/dL		T. chol 170 mg/dL	LH 30 mIU/mL

▶ Questions

Problem Identification

1. a. *Create a drug therapy problem list for this patient.*
   b. *Which signs and symptoms consistent with acne does this patient demonstrate?*
   c. *How does polycystic ovarian disease contribute to this patient's acne and other physical findings?*

Desired Outcome

2. *What are the treatment goals for this patient?*

Therapeutic Alternatives

3. *What feasible therapeutic alternatives are available for management of this patient's acne and hyperandrogenism?*

Optimal Plan

4. *What treatment regimen is best suited for this patient?*

Outcome Evaluation

5. *How would you monitor the therapy you recommended for efficacy and adverse effects?*

Patient Education

6. *How would you educate the patient about this treatment regimen to enhance compliance and ensure successful therapy?*

▶ Clinical Course

Two months later, the patient has developed bloating, weight gain, and increased appetite, likely related to the therapy prescribed. She also reveals that her maternal grandmother and aunt both died of melanoma and a friend told her that she should not be using her new therapy.

▶ Follow-Up Question

1. *What is the most appropriate course of action?*

▶ Self-Study Assignments

1. Review the dysmorphic syndrome associated with acne.
2. Review the nonpharmacologic management of acne, including stress reduction and dietary changes.

▶ Clinical Pearl

In females with acne, scarring + cysts + two courses of oral antibiotics means hormonal therapy and "consider isotretinoin."

References

1. Law RM. The pharmacist's role in the treatment of acne. America's Pharmacist 2003;125(6):35–42.
2. Bastian H, for the Cochrane Collaboration Consumer Network. Hot Topic of the Month: January 2003. Common Acne. pp. 1–16.
3. Lehmann HP, Robinson KA, Andrews JS et al. Acne therapy: a methodologic review. J Am Acad Dermatol 2002;47:231–40.
4. Management of Acne. Summary, Evidence Report/Technology Assessment: Number 17. AHRQ Publication No. 01-E018, March 2001. Agency for Healthcare Research and Quality, Rockville, MD. http://www.ahrq.gov/clinic/epcsums/acnesum.htm. Accessed August 23, 2004.
5. Webster GF. Acne vulgaris. BMJ 2002;325:475–479.

6. Cheung AP, Chang RJ. Polycystic ovary syndrome. Clin Obstet Gynecol 1990;33:655–667.
7. Wooltorton E. Accutane (isotretinoin) and psychiatric adverse effects. CMAJ 2003;168(1):66.
8. Wooltorton E. Diane-35 (cyproterone acetate): safety concerns. CMAJ 2003; 168(4):455–456.
9. Berson DS, Shalita AR. The treatment of acne: The role of combination therapies. J Am Acad Dermatol 1995;32(5pt3):S31–S41.
10. Karagas MR, Stukel TA, Dykes J, et al. A pooled analysis of 10 case-control studies of melanoma and oral contraceptive use. Br J Cancer 2002;86:1085–1092.

100 PSORIASIS

▶ The Harried School Teacher (Level II)

Rebecca M. Law, PharmD
Wayne P. Gulliver, MD, FRCPC

▶ After completing this case study, students should be able to:

- Understand the pathophysiology of plaque psoriasis, including clinical presentation and skin changes.
- Understand the sequence of using topical, photochemical, and systemic treatment modalities for psoriasis.
- Compare the efficacy and adverse effects of systemic therapies for psoriasis including standard therapies (methotrexate, acitretin, cyclosporine, azathioprine, hydroxyurea, and sulfasalazine); newer agents (efalizumab and alefacept); and investigational agents (infliximab and gentanercept).
- Select appropriate therapeutic regimens for patients with plaque psoriasis.
- Educate patients with psoriasis about proper use of pharmacotherapeutic treatments, potential adverse effects, and necessary precautions.

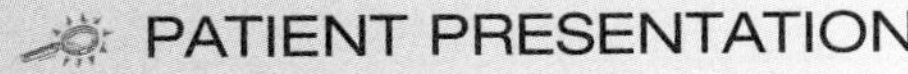

PATIENT PRESENTATION

Chief Complaint

"Nothing is helping my psoriasis."

HPI

Gerald Kent is a 50 yo man with a 25+ year history of psoriasis who presented to the outpatient dermatology clinic 2 days ago with another flare-up of his psoriasis. He was admitted to the inpatient dermatology service for a severe flare-up of plaque psoriasis involving his arms, legs, elbows, knees, palms, abdomen, back, and scalp (see Figure 100–1).

He was diagnosed with plaque psoriasis at age 23. He initially responded to topical therapy with medium-potency topical corticosteroids, later to calcipotriol. He subsequently required photochemotherapy using psoralens with UVA phototherapy (PUVA) to control his condition. PUVA eventually became ineffective, and 10 years ago he was started on oral methotrexate 5 mg once/week. Dosage escalations kept his condition under fairly good control for about 5 years. Flare-ups during that period were initially managed with SCAT (short-contact anthralin therapy), but they eventually became more frequent and lesions were more widespread despite increasing the methotrexate dose. A liver biopsy performed about five years ago showed no evidence of fibrosis, hepatitis, or cirrhosis.

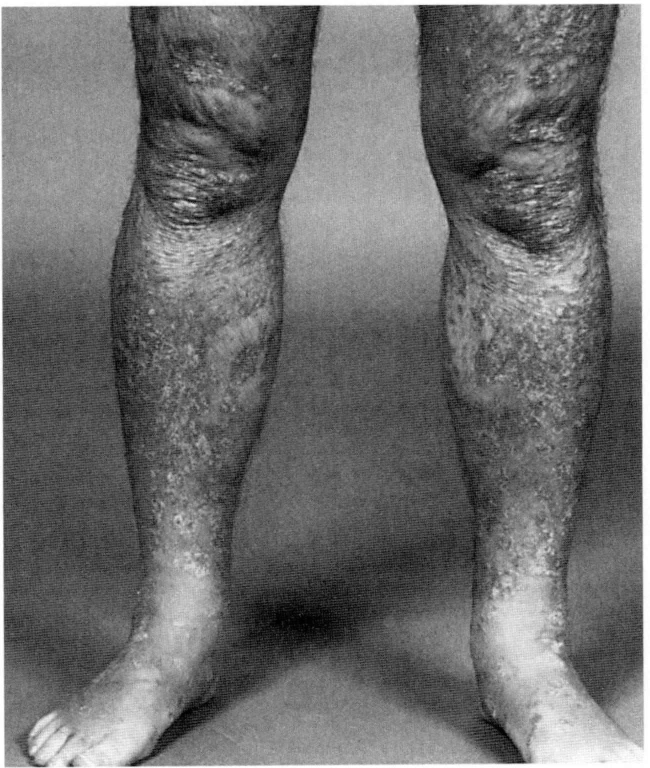

Figure 100–1. Example of severe plaque psoriasis involving the lower extremities in a male patient. *(Photo courtesy of Wayne P. Gulliver, MD.)*

After requiring two SCAT treatments in a 4-month period, along with methotrexate 25 mg/week po (given as two doses of 12.5 mg 12 hours apart), a change in therapy was considered necessary at that time. Because he was receiving maximum recommended methotrexate doses and had already reached a lifetime cumulative methotrexate dose of 2.2 g, he was changed to his current cyclic regimen of cyclosporine microemulsion (Neoral) 75 mg twice daily for 3 months, followed by acitretin (Soriatane) 25 mg once daily with dinner for 3 months, and repeat. Flare-ups became infrequent and were again successfully managed by SCAT. However, in the last 6 months he has already required two SCAT treatments for flare-ups. This is his third flare-up this year.

PMH

One episode of major depressive illness triggered by the death of his first wife, which occurred 16 years ago (age 34). He was treated by his family physician who prescribed fluoxetine for 6 months. He has had no recurrences. He has no other chronic medical conditions and no other acute or recent illnesses.

FH

Parents alive and well. Two sisters. No history of psoriasis, immune disorders, or malignancy. Father has HTN and type 2 diabetes.

SH

Patient is an elementary school teacher; non-smoker; social use of alcohol (glass of wine with dinner). He is married and has two children ages 10 and 12 with his second wife. There has been an increased workload for the past year because of layoffs at his school board.

Meds

Neoral 75 mg twice daily po; in one month, he is scheduled to change to acitretin 25 mg once daily for the following 3 months (cyclic therapy)

Acetaminophen for occasional headaches

All

NKDA

ROS

Skin feels very itchy despite using a non-medicated moisturizer TID. No joint aches or pains. No complaints of shortness of breath. Occasional nausea associated with a cyclosporine dose. Has been feeling jumpy and stressed because of tensions at work but does not feel depressed.

PE

Gen

Alert, mildly anxious 50 yo white man in NAD

VS

BP 139/86, P 88, T 37°C; Ht 5′9″, Wt 75 kg

Skin

Confluent plaque psoriasis with extensive lesions on abdomen, arms, legs, back, and scalp. Thick crusted lesions on elbows, knees, palms, and soles. Lesions are red to violet in color, with sharply demarcated borders except where confluent, and are loosely covered with silvery-white scales. There are no pustules or vesicles. There are excoriations on trunk and extremities consistent with scratching.

HEENT

PERRLA, EOMI, fundi benign, TMs intact; extensive scaly lesions on scalp as noted

Neck/LN

No lymphadenopathy; thyroid non-palpable

Chest

CTA bilaterally

CV

RRR without m/r/g; S_1 and S_2 normal

Abd

(+) BS, soft, non-tender, no masses; extensive scaly lesions and excoriations on skin as noted above

Genit

WNL

Rect

Deferred

MS/Ext

No joint swelling, increased warmth, or tenderness; skin lesions as noted above; no nail involvement; peripheral pulses 2+ throughout

Neuro

A & O × 3; CN II–XII intact; DTRs 2+ toes downgoing

Labs

Na 139 mEq/L	Hgb 13.5 g/dL	AST 22 IU/L
K 4.0 mEq/L	Hct 35.0%	ALT 38 IU/L
Cl 102 mEq/L	Plt 255 × 10^3/mm^3	LDH 107 IU/L
CO_2 25 mEq/L	WBC 6.0 × 10^3/mm^3	Alk phos 98 IU/L
BUN 14 mg/dL		T. bili 1.0 mg/dL
SCr 1.0 mg/dL		Alb 3.7 g/dL
Glu 98 mg/dL		Uric acid 4 mg/dL
		T. chol 180 mg/dL

Questions

Problem Identification

1. a. *Create a list of this patient's drug therapy problems.*
   b. *What signs and symptoms consistent with psoriasis does this patient demonstrate?*
   c. *What risk factors for a flare-up of psoriasis are present in this patient?*
   d. *Could the signs and symptoms be caused by any drug therapy he is receiving?*

Desired Outcome

2. *What are the goals of pharmacotherapy for psoriasis in this patient?*

Therapeutic Alternatives

3. a. *What nonpharmacologic alternatives are available for managing the patient's psoriasis and its related symptoms?*
   b. *What feasible pharmacotherapeutic alternatives are available for controlling the patient's disease and its related symptoms at this point?*

Optimal Plan

4. *What drug regimen is best suited for treating this flare of the patient's psoriasis and its related symptoms?*

Outcome Evaluation

5. *How should you monitor the therapy you recommended for efficacy and adverse effects?*

Patient Education

6. *What information should be provided to the patient to enhance compliance and ensure successful therapy?*

▶ Self-Study Assignments

1. Perform a literature search to identify potential future topical therapies for psoriasis, such as NSAIDs, protein kinase C inhibitors, methotrexate gel, and an implantable 5-fluorouracil formulation.
2. Perform a literature search to identify potential future systemic therapies for psoriasis, including glucosamine and immunomodulators such as monoclonal antibodies and cytokines.

▶ Clinical Pearl

The 3 "R"s of systemic therapy for psoriasis are Rotate Regimens Regularly.

References

1. Callen JP, Krueger GG, Lebwohl M, et al. AAD consensus statement on psoriasis therapies. J Am Acad Dermatol 2003;49:897–899.
2. Yamauchi PS, Rizk D, Kormeili T, et al. Current systemic therapies for psoriasis: Where are we now? J Am Acad Dermatol 2003;49(2 Suppl):S66–S77.
3. Gottlieb A. Immunobiologic agents for the treatment of psoriasis: Clinical research delivers new hope for patients with psoriasis. Arch Dermatol 2003;139: 791–793.
4. Gottlieb G, Casale TB, Frankel E, et al. CD4+ T-cell-directed antibody responses are maintained in patients with psoriasis receiving alefacept: Results of a randomized study. J Am Acad Dermatol 2003;49:816–825.
5. Piascik P. Alefacept, first biologic agent approved for treatment of psoriasis. J Am Pharm Assoc 2003;43:649–650.
6. Lebwohl M, Tyring SK, Hamilton TK, et al. Efalizumab Study Group. A novel targeted T-cell modulator, efalizumab, for plaque psoriasis. N Engl J Med 2003;349:2004–2013.
7. Gordon KB, Papp KA, Hamilton TK, et al. Efalizumab Study Group. Efalizumab for patients with moderate to severe plaque psoriasis: A randomized controlled trial. JAMA 2003;290:3073–3080.
8. Efalizumab (Raptiva) for treatment of psoriasis. Medical Lett 2003;45(1171): 97–98.
9. FDA approves Enbrel for psoriasis. National Psoriasis Foundation, May 3, 2004. Available at: http://www.psoriasis.org/news/news/2004/20040430_enbrelpsoriasis.php. Accessed August 20, 2004.
10. Leonardi CL, Powers JL, Matheson RT, et al. Etanercept as monotherapy in patients with psoriasis. N Engl J Med 2003;349:2014–2022.

101 ATOPIC DERMATITIS

▶ A Seasonal Itch (Level I)

Rebecca M. Law, PharmD
Poh Gin Kwa, MD, FRCPC

▶ After completing this case study, students should be able to:

- Understand risk factors and aggravating factors in the pathogenesis of atopic dermatitis.
- Understand the treatment strategies for atopic dermatitis, including nonpharmacologic management.
- Educate patients and/or their caregivers about management of atopic dermatitis.
- Monitor the safety and efficacy of selected pharmacologic therapies.

PATIENT PRESENTATION

Chief Complaint

"My son always has this reddish rash on his cheeks and chin."

HPI

Paul is an 8-month-old baby boy who has had a reddish skin rash on his cheeks and chin since age 2 months. His mother thought it was due to his drooling and teething. She has tried many different moisturizers with minimal benefit. This skin rash seemed to be getting worse for the past 2 months. Paul is always scratching his face and this has led to some bleeding. For the past week, the lesions on his face have become yellowish and crusty. The skin rash also seems to worsen in the winter months. However, it does not clear completely in the summer months.

PMH

The baby has been bottle-fed from birth; he was never breast-fed.

At 4 months of age, he had acute otitis media. When treated with ampicillin he developed a generalized maculopapular skin rash.

He has had no other major medical problems.

FH

Baby's paternal grandmother has a history of chronic eczema, and his paternal grandfather is allergic to strawberries (broke out with generalized hives). There is a strong family history of other atopic diseases (e.g., asthma, eczema, hay fever) on both sides of the family.

SH

Mother is single, receives social assistance, and lives in a poor section of the city. She is a heavy smoker and had no prenatal care. Mother says the baby is constantly irritable and wakes her up at night. She feels quite stressed and smokes more. The father died in a gang fight when she was 4 months pregnant with Paul. The grandparents are not supportive.

Meds

Paul is taking no medications

All

Paul is possibly allergic to ampicillin (broke out with a generalized maculopapular skin rash).

His skin lesions seem to worsen when eating baby food containing tomatoes, strawberries, or eggs.

ROS

Mother thinks that Paul must be very itchy since he is constantly scratching at his face, despite her application of a non-medicated moisturizer three times daily

PE

Gen

Alert, irritable baby. Not acutely ill-looking

VS

BP 90/50, P 120, T 37°C, Ht 72 cm, Wt 9 kg, Head circumference 45 cm

Skin

Generally dry. Likely pruritic, erythematous papules and vesicles on the face, chin, trunk, and extensor surfaces of the extremities. Due to subsequent scratching there are excoriations and exudates on the cheeks and chin, leading to yellow crusty lesions. There are no lesions on top of the nose.

The rest of the physical exam was normal.

Labs

		WBC Differential	
Na 139 mEq/L	Hgb 13.0 g/dL	Neutros 66%	IgE 15 IU/mL[a]
K 4 mEq/L	Hct 36%	Bands 3%	RAST elevated
Cl 100 mEq/L	Plt 200 × 10^3/mm^3	Eos 5%	
CO_2 25 mEq/L	WBC 9.0 × 10^3/mm^3	Lymphs 24%	
		Basos 1%	
		Monos 1%	

[a] Reference range of IgE at age 9 months = 0.76 – 7.31 IU/mL

Skin swab of cheek lesion

Gram stain

Numerous Gram (+) cocci in bunches

Culture

Staphylococcus aureus

Sensitivity

Cloxacillin – I
Ciprofloxacin – I
Vancomycin – S
TMP/SMX – R
Penicillin G – R

Questions

Problem Identification

1. a. *Create a drug therapy problem list for this patient.*
   b. *What signs and symptoms of disease does this patient demonstrate?*
   c. *What risk factors or aggravating factors may have contributed to the patient's medical condition?*
   d. *Could the patient's signs and symptoms be caused by a drug?*

Desired Outcome

2. *What are the treatment goals for this patient?*

Therapeutic Alternatives

3. *What feasible nonpharmacologic and pharmacologic alternatives are available for management of this patient's medical condition(s)?*

Optimal Plan

4. *What treatment regimen is best suited for this patient?*

Outcome Evaluation

5. *How would you monitor the management strategies you recommended for efficacy and adverse effects?*

Patient Education

6. *How would you inform the patient's caregiver about the treatment regimen to enhance compliance and ensure successful therapy?*

Self-Study Assignments

1. Review the use of phototherapy for atopic dermatitis.
2. Discuss how a 10-year old child with atopic dermatitis might differ from an 8-month old infant (with respect to clinical presentation and treatment strategies).

Clinical Pearl

In atopic dermatitis, eliminating triggers, appropriate skin care, and controlling the itch are as important as pharmacologic treatment.

References

1. Eichenfield LF, Hanifin JM, Luger TA, et al. Consensus conference on pediatric atopic dermatitis. J Am Acad Dermatol 2003;49:1088–1095.
2. Beltrani VS. The clinical spectrum of atopic dermatitis. J Allergy Clin Immunol 1999;104(3 Pt 2):S87–S98.

3. National Institute of Arthritis and Musculoskeletal and Skin Diseases. Handout on Health: Atopic Dermatitis. U.S. Department of Health and Human Services, revised April 2003. Available at: www.niams.nih.gov/hi/topics/dermatitis. Accessed August 27, 2004.
4. Koblenzer CS. Itching and the atopic skin. J Allergy Clin Immunol 1999;104(3 Pt 2):S109–S113.
5. Leiferman KM. A role for eosinophils in atopic dermatitis. J Am Acad Dermatol 2001;45(1 Suppl 1):S21–S24.
6. Reitamo S, Ansel JC, Luger TA. Itch in atopic dermatitis. J Am Acad Dermatol 2001;45(1 Suppl):S55–S56.
7. Hanifin JM, Cooper KD, Ho VC, et al. Guidelines of care for atopic dermatitis, developed in accordance with the American Academy of Dermatology (AAD)/American Academy of Dermatology Association "Administrative Regulations for Evidence-Based Clinical Practice Guidelines." J Am Acad Dermatol 2004;50:391–404.
8. Hanifin JM, Tofte SJ. Update on therapy of atopic dermatitis. J Allergy Clin Immunol 1999;104(2 Pt 2):S123–S125.
9. Lewis E. Atopic Dermatitis: Disease overview and the development of topical immunomodulators. Formulary 2002;37(Suppl 2):3–15.
10. Lever R. The role of food in atopic eczema. J Am Acad Dermatol 2001;45(1 Suppl):S57–S60.

102 CUTANEOUS REACTION TO DRUGS

▶ Where Did These Spots Come From? (Level I)

Rebecca M. Law, BS Pharm, PharmD
Wayne P. Gulliver, MD, FRCPC

▶ After completing this case study, students should be able to:

- Understand the approach to identifying or ruling out a suspected drug-induced skin reaction.
- Recognize the signs and symptoms of drug-induced vasculitis.
- Determine an appropriate course of action for a patient with a suspected drug-induced skin reaction.
- Educate patients with suspected drug-induced vasculitis about appropriate management and necessary precautions.

PATIENT PRESENTATION

Chief Complaint

"I have spots on my legs and I ache all over!"

HPI

Edward Powers is a 52 yo man who presented to his family physician with a 2-day history of fever, pain/burning upon urination, urinary frequency/urgency, and some abdominal discomfort. His physician diagnosed a urinary tract infection with possible prostatitis and prescribed ciprofloxacin 500 mg po BID for 14 days.

The patient adhered to the regimen; his temperature normalized the next day and his urinary tract symptoms and abdominal discomfort resolved within 2 to 3 days. He continued to take ciprofloxacin as directed. Nine days after starting therapy, he noticed red, pinpoint lesions on his feet that were associated with burning and discomfort. His legs became swollen, the number of lesions increased, and blisters began to form. He also noticed increasing discomfort, heaviness, and burning in his legs. The next morning his wife brought him to the ED and he was admitted.

PMH

Unremarkable.

FH

Parents A & W, no siblings.

SH

Married, lives with his wife and two sons. He is a nonsmoker and has an occasional beer with friends. No recent changes in diet or in his living environment.

Meds

Ciprofloxacin 500 mg po BID × 14 days, started 10 days PTA
No additional drugs taken including OTCs or herbals

All

NKDA

ROS

Patient complains of generalized muscle aches and joint pains in addition to complaints noted above.

PE

Gen

Fairly anxious 52 yo white man in NAD but in some discomfort

VS

BP 120/90, HR 80, RR 18, T 38.5°C

Skin

2-mm red, unblanchable lesions over feet and legs that are palpable and tender; 5-mm hemorrhagic blisters over feet and legs, most numerous around feet and ankles, ending at midthigh

HEENT

PERRLA, EOMI, fundi benign, TMs intact

Chest

CTA bilaterally

Cor

RRR without murmurs, rubs or gallops; S_1 and S_2 normal

Abd
(+) BS, soft, nontender, no masses

MS/Ext
Generalized muscle aches and pains, joint stiffness. Peripheral pulses present

Neuro
CN II–XII intact

Labs

Na 140 mEq/L	Hgb 14 g/dL	AST 15 IU/L	ESR 25 mm/h
K 4.0 mEq/L	Hct 44%	ALT 22 IU/L	RF negative
Cl 101 mEq/L	Plt 400 × 10^3/mm^3	LDH 120 IU/L	ANA (–)
CO_2 26 mEq/L	WBC 6.0 × 10^3/mm^3	HbsAg (–)	ASO titer (–)
BUN 9 mg/dL	65% PMNs	Anti-HbsAg (–)	Anti-ds DNA (–)
SCr 0.7 mg/dL	2% Bands	Anti-HCV (–)	anti-Sm Ab (–)
Glucose 95 mg/dL	2% Eos		Cryoglobulins (–)
	1% Basos		
	20% Lymphs		
	10% Monos		

▶ Questions

Problem Identification

1. a. *What current signs and symptoms of disease does this patient demonstrate?*
   b. *Considering the signs, symptoms, and laboratory values that are present, what evidence supports or refutes rheumatoid arthritis, systemic lupus erythematosus, hepatitis, or drug therapy as possible causes of his problems?*

Desired Outcome

2. *What are the treatment goals for this patient?*

Therapeutic Alternatives

3. a. *What nonpharmacologic alternatives are available for the treatment of this patient?*
   b. *What pharmacotherapeutic alternatives are available for the treatment of this patient?*

Optimal Plan

4. *Design an optimal pharmacotherapeutic plan for this patient.*

Outcome Evaluation

5. *How would you monitor this patient?*

Patient Education

6. *How would you inform this patient about his drug therapy?*

▶ Self-Study Assignments

1. Differentiate among the various manifestations of cutaneous drug reactions, including fixed drug reactions, photoallergic and phototoxic reactions, bullous reactions, morbilliform and urticarial reactions, pigmentation, lichenoid eruptions, Stevens–Johnson syndrome, hypersensitivity syndrome, and vasculitis.
2. Obtain information on common agents that have been known to cause vasculitis.

▶ Clinical Pearl

Drugs can cause any type of skin reaction. When a patient taking medication develops any skin reaction or lesion, consider all potential causes of the skin lesion including the possibility that it may be drug-related. Carefully evaluate the link as unlikely, possible, probable, or definitive.

References

1. Calabrese LH, Duna GF. Drug-induced vasculitis. Curr Opin Rheumatol 1996;8:34–40.
2. de Araujo TS, Kirsner RS. Vasculitis. Wounds 2001;13:99–110.
3. Lee A, Thomson J. Drug-induced skin reactions. Pharm J 1999;262:357–362.
4. Beuselinck B, Devuyst O. Ciprofloxacin-induced hypersensitivity vasculitis. Acta Clin Belg 1994;49(3–4):173–176.
5. Gamboa F, Rivera JM, Gomez Mateos JM, et al. Ciprofloxacin-induced Henoch–Schonlein purpura. Ann Pharmacother 1995;29:84.
6. Roujeau JC, Stern RS. Severe adverse cutaneous reactions to drugs. N Engl J Med 1994;331:1272–1285.
7. de Shazo RD, Kemp SF. Allergic reactions to drugs and biologic agents. JAMA 1997;278:1895–1906.
8. Wolkenstein P, Revuz J. Drug-induced severe skin reactions. Incidence, management, and prevention. Drug Saf 1995;13:56–68.

SECTION 15

Hematologic Disorders

103 IRON DEFICIENCY ANEMIA

▶ Sally's Belly Pain (Level I)

William J. Spruill, PharmD, FASHP
William E. Wade, PharmD, FASHP, FCCP

▶ After completing this case study, the student should be able to:

- Recognize that the consumption of selected OTC products may lead to the development of iron deficiency anemia.
- Recognize other common conditions that might predispose a patient to iron deficiency anemia.
- Recognize the signs, symptoms, and laboratory manifestations associated with iron deficiency anemia.
- Select appropriate iron therapy for the treatment of iron deficiency anemia.
- Inform patients of the potential adverse effects associated with iron therapy.
- Educate patients about the importance of adherence to their iron therapy regimen.

PATIENT PRESENTATION

Chief Complaint

"I have belly pain and feel tired all the time."

HPI

Sally Lowblood is a 47 yo woman who presents to your pharmacy with the above complaint. With further questioning, she relates the onset of her GI complaints at the time she initiated self-medication with Aleve for pain associated with "arthritis" in her right knee. The stomach pain has progressively gotten worse over the past 2 months. She describes this pain as a burning sensation that usually begins 30 minutes to 1 hour after meals and may or may not be relieved by antacid administration. Upon reviewing her medication profile, you note that she has a prescription for PRN ranitidine. Further questioning reveals a history of PUD approximately 4 years ago. When asked what OTC medications she is currently consuming and how long she has been taking them, she responds that she started taking Aleve 1 tablet twice daily 7 months ago for knee arthritis. Because of progressive arthritis pain and a loss of adequate relief, she increased the dose of Aleve to 2 tablets twice a day 2 months ago. You suggest that she discontinue the Aleve, begin acetaminophen for her "arthritis," and make a referral to her primary care physician for follow-up of her symptoms of fatigue and abdominal pain. Additionally, you faxed a brief referral note to the physician detailing this encounter and her recent medication history. You also recommend that she not consume OTC medications in the future without first consulting her pharmacist or physician and that she not take doses in excess of the manufacturer's recommended dose. A therapeutic trial of glucosamine is also discussed with Ms. Lowblood as possible adjunctive therapy for her osteoarthritis.

▶ Clinical Course

Three days later, she is evaluated by her family physician, which provides the following additional information.

PMH

Osteoarthritis diagnosed after a recent fall; self-medicates with naproxen (Aleve)
History of heavy menses
PUD 4 years ago

FH

Father died from MI 10 years ago; mother had a history of PUD. She has two sisters, both living with no known medical problems. Two daughters without medical problems.

SH

Occasionally consumes alcohol; denies tobacco or illicit drug use.

ROS

Burning pain in stomach after meals; denies heartburn, melena, vomiting BRB; good appetite, has one daily BM; no weight changes over past 5 years; (+) fatigue; tires easily; (–) paralysis, fainting, numbness, paresthesia, or tremor; headache once every 3 to 4 months; has myopic vision; (–) tinnitus or vertigo; has hay fever in spring; (–) cough, sputum production, or wheezing; denies chest pain, edema, dyspnea, or orthopnea; denies nocturia, hematuria, dysuria, or Hx of stones; P_2G_2; onset of menses at age 11; heavy flow for past 8 years; last Pap smear 6 months ago; unilateral joint pain in right knee of recent onset; frequent early morning stiffness in RLE.

Meds

Aleve 2 tablets po BID
Mylanta PRN
Ranitidine 150 mg po PRN

All

"Mycins" (upset stomach)
Aspirin (upset stomach)

PE

Gen

WDWN African American woman in NAD who appears her stated age

VS

BP 124/78, P 80, RR 12, T 37°C; Ht: 5′7″, Wt 60 kg

Skin

Without lesions, bruising, or discoloration; decreased turgor

HEENT

NC/AT; EOM intact; (–) nystagmus; PERRLA; slightly pale conjunctiva; normal funduscopic exam without retinopathy; TMs intact; deviated nasal septum; no sinus tenderness; several dental caries; native teeth present; oropharynx clear

Neck/LN

Supple without masses; normal thyroid; (–) JVD

Lungs/Thorax

Trachea midline; clear to A & P; breath sounds equal bilaterally

Breasts

Symmetric bilaterally; without masses or discharge; normal axilla

CV

RRR; PMI at 5th ICS, MCL; (–) bruits, murmurs, S_3 or S_4

Abd

Soft, but tender to palpation; no masses; normal peristalsis; without bruits

Genit/Rect

Normal external female genitalia, uterus, and adnexa; rectal exam (+) stool guaiac

MS/Ext

Spooning of finger nails; (–) CCE; joint enlargement and limited ROM of right knee, changes consistent with DJD

Neuro

DTR 2+; normal gait

Other

Peripheral blood smear: hypochromic, microcytic red blood cells (see Figure 103–1).

Labs

Na 140 mEq/L	Hgb 9.2 g/dL	WBC 6.5 × 10^3/mm^3	AST 12 IU/L	Ca 9.2 mg/dL
K 4.5 mEq/L	Hct 27.6%	81% Segs	ALT 15 IU/L	Iron 36 μg/dL
Cl 102 mEq/L	RBC 3.4 × 10^6/mm^3	Bands 2%	T. bili 0.2 mg/dL	TIBC 705 μg/dL
CO_2 20 mEq/L	MCV 72 μm^3	15% Lymphs	LDH 115 IU/L	Transferrin sat 5.1%
BUN 15 mg/dL	MCH 20 pg	1% Monos	T. prot 7.2 g/dL	Ferritin 9.8 ng/mL
SCr 0.7 mg/dL	MCHC 28 g/dL	1% Eos	Alb 4.5 g/dL	B_{12} 680 pg/mL
Glucose 105 mg/dL	RDW 16.1%		Chol 189 mg/dL	Folic acid 8.2 ng/mL

UA

pH 4.8, SG 1.030, protein (–), glucose (–), ketones (–), RBC 1/lpf, WBC 3/lpf; casts (–)

Assessment

1. Iron deficiency anemia possibly secondary to NSAID-induced gastropathy and heavy menses
2. OA of right knee

Plan

Refer to gastroenterologist

▶ Clinical Course

Two days later, the patient is seen by a gastroenterologist and undergoes EGD with biopsy. The findings include extensive gastritis with multiple bleeding lesions.

Final assessment: Iron deficiency anemia secondary to NSAID-induced gastritis.

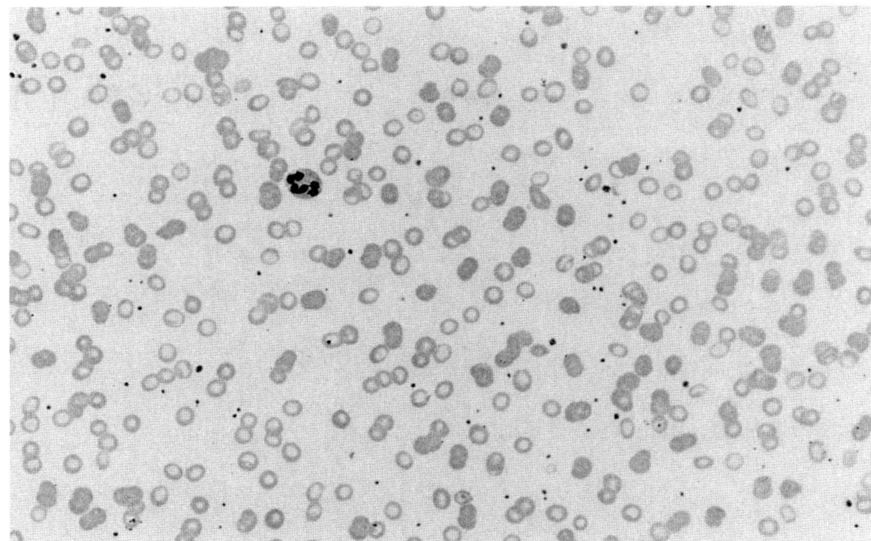

Figure 103–1. Blood smear with hypochromic, microcytic red blood cells. (Wright-Giemsa × 330). *(Photo courtesy of Lydia C. Contis, MD.)*

Questions

Problem Identification

1. a. *What potential drug therapy problems does this patient have?*
   b. *What signs, symptoms, and laboratory findings are consistent with the finding of iron deficiency anemia secondary to blood loss?*

Desired Outcome

2. *What are the goals of pharmacotherapy for this patient's anemia?*

Therapeutic Alternatives

3. a. *What nondrug therapy may be effective in managing this anemia?*
   b. *What pharmacotherapeutic alternatives could be used to treat this patient's anemia?*

Optimal Plan

4. *Outline an optimal pharmacotherapy plan for this patient.*

Outcome Evaluation

5. *What clinical and laboratory parameters are necessary to evaluate the therapy for achievement of the desired therapeutic outcome and to detect and prevent adverse effects?*

Patient Education

6. *What information should be provided to the patient to enhance compliance, ensure successful therapy, and minimize adverse effects?*

Clinical Course

In addition to the anemia therapy you recommended, Ms. Lowblood is given a prescription for omeprazole 20 mg po once daily. Upon her return to the clinic 1 month later for evaluation, she has no complaints of adverse effects from her medications. The patient indicates that she is fairly compliant with her iron therapy and is not experiencing any dose-limiting side effects. At that time, she is instructed to return in 3 months. Laboratory values continue to improve and her next follow-up visit is in 6 months. Laboratory values at 1, 3, and 6 months into therapy are as shown in Table 103–1.

At the 6-month follow-up visit, it was decided to discontinue the anemia treatment.

TABLE 103–1. Laboratory Test Values

Test (units)	1 Month	3 Months	6 Months
RBC count (× 10^6/mm^3)	3.6	4.0	4.3
Hgb (g/dL)	9.9	11.9	14.1
Hct (%)	29.9	35.9	42
MCV (μm^3)	78	86	90
MCH (pg)	24	29	31
MCHC (g/dL)	30	33	34
RDW (%)	15.8	14.9	12.8
Serum iron (μg/dL)	47	79	98
TIBC (μg/dL)	385	380	392
Transferrin sat (%)	12.2	20.8	25
Ferritin (ng/mL)	69	120	163
Stool guaiac	Negative	Negative	Negative

▶ Self-Study Assignments

1. Make a list of all potential medications that should be avoided within close proximity of iron administration.
2. Perform a literature search to determine the status of the efficacy of various iron formulations that have other "enhancing" ingredients added to them, such as ascorbic acid and stool softeners. When, if ever, are these products indicated?
3. What monitoring steps should be incorporated into your pharmaceutical care plan to:
   a. Check for recurrence of signs/symptoms of iron deficiency due to her history of heavy menses?
   b. Encourage the patient to avoid future NSAID therapy?
   c. Monitor for recurrence of signs and symptoms of gastropathy?
   d. Monitor for efficacy of new treatments (such as acetaminophen or glucosamine) for her osteoarthritis?

▶ Clinical Pearl

1. A transient increase in the reticulocyte count 7 to 10 days after beginning therapy can be used to confirm the correct diagnosis and treatment and to rule out other causes of anemia.
2. Therapeutic doses of iron must be given for 3 to 6 months to ensure repletion of all iron stores; the serum ferritin is the best parameter to monitor iron stores after correction of the hemoglobin and hematocrit.

References

1. Swain RA, Kaplan B, Montgomery E. Iron-deficiency anemia—When is parenteral therapy warranted? Postgrad Med 1996;100:181–185.
2. Sunder-Plassmann G, Horl WH. Safety aspects of parenteral iron in patients with end-stage renal disease. Drug Saf 1997;17:241–250.
3. Fishbane S, Ungureanu VD, Maesaka JK, et al. The safety of intravenous iron dextran in hemodialysis patients. Am J Kidney Dis 1996,28:529–534.
4. Faich G, Strobos J. Sodium ferric gluconate complex in sucrose: Safer intravenous iron therapy than iron dextrans. Am J Kidney Dis 1999,33:464–470.

104 VITAMIN B_{12} DEFICIENCY

▶ Treatment for Life (Level I)

Barbara J. Mason, PharmD
Beata Ineck, PharmD

▶ After completing this case study, students should be able to:

- Recognize the signs, symptoms, and laboratory abnormalities associated with B_{12} deficiency anemia.
- Select an appropriate dosage regimen for treatment of B_{12} deficiency anemia.
- Describe monitoring parameters for the initial and subsequent evaluations of patients with B_{12} deficiency anemia.
- Educate patients treated with vitamin B_{12} therapy.

PATIENT PRESENTATION

Chief Complaint

"I've been feeling terrible for a year and I can't remember anything."

HPI

Larry Wise is a 74 yo man who presents to the Veterans Affairs Medical Center (VAMC) for a routine check-up. Upon questioning he states that he has been feeling weak, lightheaded, and "terrible" for a year now, but has not had any weight loss.

PMH

Multiple DVT with resulting chronic venous insufficiency
Type 2 DM
HTN
Prostate cancer, s/p prostatectomy, past history of four weeks of pelvic XRT, two months ago.
S/P CVA
Hyperlipidemia
DJD
Type B chronic atrophic gastritis
(+) *Helicobacter pylori*

FH

Positive for DM; father died of stroke.

SH

Retired minister, single; no alcohol or tobacco use; lives near the VAMC and returns for frequent follow-up visits. Dietary—"tea and toast" intake due to financial limitations, poor dentition, and living alone.

ROS

(–) SOB, headache, chest pain, joint pain, polyuria, or polydipsia.

Meds

Docusate sodium 100 mg po BID
Omeprazole 20 mg po once daily before breakfast
Glipizide 20 mg po BID
Pravastatin 20 mg po at bedtime
Quinapril 15 mg po once daily
Pseudoephedrine 60 mg po once daily
Warfarin sodium 5 mg po once daily
Metformin 500 mg po BID

All

Codeine (rash)

PE

Gen

This is an elderly, pleasant, white man in NAD

VS

BP 141/95, P 84; Wt 73.9 kg, BMI 24.1, Ht 5′9″

Skin

Pale, turgor normal, (–) vitiligo

HEENT

Left eye almost blind, retinal detachment, PERRLA, EOMI, fundi showed no cotton wool exudates; (–) photophobia, (+) glossitis, poor dentition

Neck

Supple, no lymphadenopathy or thyromegaly

Lungs

Bilateral BS, no wheezes or crackles

CV

RRR; III/VI systolic murmur heard best at the right sternal border; no rubs

Abd

Soft, non-tender, no masses, (+) bowel sounds

Ext

No lower leg edema, no warmth or pain, (+) paresthesias

Rect

Good sphincter tone, guaiac (–) stool

Neuro

A & O × 3, CN right visual field intact, hearing intact, slight left facial weakness, sensory—decreased pinprick on right LE and UE, proprioception intact bilaterally, coordination intact, decreased vibratory sensation LE, (–) ataxia

Labs (all fasting)

Na 140 mEq/L	Hgb 11.3 g/dL	AST 19 IU/L	Iron 85 mcg/dL
K 4.2 mEq/L	Hct 33.5%	ALT 13 IU/L	Ferritin 48 ng/mL
Cl 106 mEq/L	RBC 3.95 × 10^6/mm^3	Alk Phos 77 IU/L	Transferrin 250 mg/dL
CO_2 24 mEq/L	Plt 221 × 10^3/mm^3	T. bili 2.0 mg/dL	Direct Coombs' (–)
BUN 13 mg/dL	WBC 5.8 × 10^3/mm^3	D. bili 1.0 mg/dL	EPO 26 IU/L
SCr 1.2 mg/dL	MCV 84.8 μm^3	T. Chol 201 mg/dL	B_{12} 177 pg/mL
Glu 238 mg/dL	MCH 28.6 pg	LDL-C 116 mg/dL	INR 3.5
	MCHC 33.8 g/dL	RBC folate 247 ng/mL	Homocysteine 20 μmol/L
	Retic (corr) 0.4%	TSH 2.93 mIU/L	HDL 45 mg/dL
		HbA1c 8.4%	Triglycerides 100 mg/dL

Peripheral Blood Smear

Anisocytosis, poikilocytosis, giant platelets, hypersegmented neutrophils, and macrocytic red blood cells with megaloblastic changes (see Figure 104–1).

Assessment

Cobalamin deficiency; mild hypoproliferative anemia secondary to pelvic XRT and/or prostate metastatic to marrow.

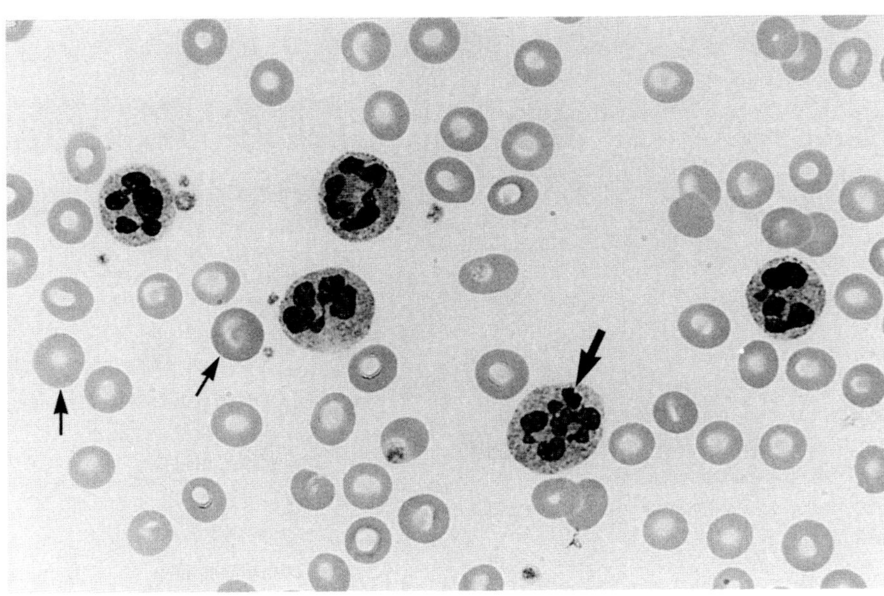

Figure 104–1. Blood smear with enlarged hypersegmented neutrophils, one with eight nuclear lobes *(large arrow);* and macrocytes *(small arrows)* (Wright-Giemsa ×1650). *(Photo courtesy of Lydia C. Contis, MD.)*

Questions

Problem Identification

1. a. *Create a drug therapy problem list for this patient.*
   b. *What information indicates the presence or severity of the B_{12} deficiency?*
   c. *Could the B_{12} deficiency have been caused by drug therapy?*
   d. *What additional information is needed to assess this patient's B_{12} deficiency?*

Desired Outcome

2. *What are the goals of pharmacotherapy in this case?*

Therapeutic Alternatives

3. a. *What nondrug therapies might be useful for this patient?*
   b. *What feasible pharmacotherapeutic alternatives are available for treatment of the B_{12} deficiency?*

Optimal Plan

4. *What drug, dosage form, dose, schedule, and duration of therapy are best for this patient?*

Outcome Evaluation

5. *What clinical and laboratory parameters are necessary to evaluate the therapy for achievement of the desired therapeutic outcome and to detect or prevent adverse effects?*

Patient Education

6. *What information should be provided to the patient to enhance compliance, ensure successful therapy, and minimize adverse effects?*

Follow-Up Question

1. *How would antibiotic treatment of a patient with Helicobacter pylori affect concurrent cobalamin deficiency?*

Self-Study Assignments

1. Defend the argument that universal screening of older patients for Vitamin B_{12} deficiency should be conducted. Have a debate with a classmate who defends the opposite point of view.
2. Describe the potential relationship between vitamin B_{12} deficiency, cardiovascular disease, and plasma homocysteine levels.
3. What is the rationale for screening for iron deficiency in patients with pernicious anemia?

Clinical Pearl

Patients with inconclusive evidence of B_{12} deficiency (e.g., low serum vitamin B_{12} levels, nonspecific symptoms, and normal hemoglobin) may merit treatment for a few months; a positive symptomatic response suggests that vitamin B_{12} deficiency was the underlying cause.

References

1. Wulffele M, Kooy A, Lehert P, et al. Effects of short-term treatment with metformin on serum concentrations of homocysteine, folate, and vitamin B_{12} in type 2 diabetes mellitus: A randomized, placebo-controlled trial. J Intern Med 2003;254:455–463.
2. Force RW, Meeker AD, Cady PS, et al. Increased vitamin B_{12} requirement associated with chronic acid suppression therapy. Ann Pharmacother 2003;37:490–493.
3. Dharmarajan TS, Adiga GU, Norkus EP. Vitamin B_{12} deficiency. Recognizing subtle symptoms in older adults. Geriatrics 2003;58(3):30–38.
4. Tefferi A. Anemia in adults: A contemporary approach to diagnosis. Mayo Clin Proc 2003;78:1275–1284.
5. Seshadri S, Beiser A, Selhub J, et al. Plasma homocysteine as a risk factor for dementia and Alzheimer's disease. N Engl J Med 2002;346:476–483.
6. Aronow WS. Homocysteine: The association with atherosclerotic vascular disease in older persons. Geriatrics 2003;58:22–28.
7. Kaptan K, Beyan C, Ural AU, et al. *Helicobacter pylori*—Is it a novel causative agent in vitamin B_{12} deficiency? Arch Intern Med 2000;160:1349–1353.
8. Toh BH, van Driel IR, Gleeson PA. Pernicious anemia. N Engl J Med 1997; 337:1441–1448.
9. Andres E, Godot B, Schlienger JL. Food–cobalamin malabsorption: A usual cause of vitamin B_{12} deficiency. Arch Intern Med 2000;160:2061–2062.
10. Lindren A., Lindstedt G, Kilander AF. Advantages of serum pepsinogen A combined with gastrin or pepsinogen C as first-line analytes in the evaluation of suspected cobalamin deficiency: A study in patients previously not subjected to gastrointestinal surgery. J Intern Med 1998;244:341–349.
11. Lane LA, Rojas-Fernandez. Treatment of vitamin B12-deficiency anemia: Oral versus parenteral therapy. Ann Pharmacother 2002;36:1268–1272.

105 FOLIC ACID DEFICIENCY

The Piano Man (Level I)

Beata Ineck, PharmD, BCPS
Barbara J. Mason, PharmD

After completing this case study, students should be able to:

- Identify the confounding factors that may contribute to the development of folic acid deficiency (e.g., medications, concurrent disease states, dietary habits).
- Recognize the signs, symptoms, and laboratory abnormalities associated with folic acid deficiency.
- Recommend an appropriate treatment regimen to rectify anemia resulting from folic acid deficiency.
- Describe appropriate monitoring parameters for initial and subsequent monitoring of folic acid deficiency.
- Educate patients with folic acid deficiency regarding pharmacologic and nonpharmacologic interventions used to correct folic acid deficiency.

PATIENT PRESENTATION

Chief Complaint

"I have been more irritable, tired, and restless lately."

HPI

Kenneth Johnson is a 73 yo man with a long history of bipolar disorder who presents to his retirement group meeting at the mental health clinic with the above complaints. He states that he has been waking up frequently at night, dreaming about the past. He also reports the presence of visual hallucinations and racing thoughts.

PMH

Bipolar disorder; on lithium in the past with lithium toxicity about 1 year ago
BPH; s/p TURP 11 years ago
Osteoarthritis
HTN
Mild memory loss
Questionable compliance with medications in the past

SH

Retired; lives with girlfriend; enjoys singing and playing the piano at senior centers; (+) alcohol, no tobacco.

Meds

Acetaminophen 325 mg, 2 po Q 6 H PRN
HCTZ 12.5 mg po once daily
Loratadine 10 mg po once daily
Docusate sodium 100 mg po BID
Tamsulosin 0.4 mg po once daily 30 minutes after dinner
Divalproex 500 mg po BID with food
Cholestyramine 4 g po BID

All

Terazosin—"it makes me dizzy and I fell once."

ROS

(+) Right knee pain; (–) paresthesias or muscle weakness

PE

Gen

Elderly Caucasian man, appears younger than stated age of 73, cooperative, oriented × 3, slight rambling speech, easily redirectable

VS

BP 165/82, P 59, RR 18, T 35.7°C

Skin

Seborrheic keratoses over back area, pale

HEENT

NC/AT; actinic keratoses on face, PERRLA, EOMI, probable immature cataract left eye, decreased hearing bilaterally, decreased movement through left nostril, dentures present, (–) glossitis

Neck

Normal motion of the neck; trachea midline; no thyromegaly; no bruit, masses, or other abnormalities

Thorax

Lungs normal to inspection and CTA

CV

RRR without murmur

Abd

NT/ND, bowel tones (+)

Ext

Enlarged ankles bilaterally; right knee enlarged with decreased ROM; (–) ataxia

Neuro

CN II–XII grossly intact; muscle strength in LE equal bilaterally; decreased muscle strength in LUE as compared to RUE; DTRs absent in LE bilaterally; vibratory sense intact

Labs

Na 142 mEq/L	Hgb 12.8 g/dL	RDW 12.8%	*Fasting Lipid Profile*
K 4.0 mEq/L	Hct 38.4%	AST 16 IU/L	T. chol 190 mg/dL
Cl 112 mEq/L	RBC 3.94 × 10^6/mm^3	ALT 7 IU/L	LDL 96 mg/dL
CO_2 27 mEq/L	Plt 216 × 10^3/mm^3	Alk Phos 87 IU/L	HDL 42 mg/dL
BUN 24 mg/dL	WBC 4.99 × 10^3/mm^3	T. bili 0.4 mg/dL	Trig 145 mg/dL
SCr 1.1 mg/dL	MCV 102.4 μm^3	Alb 3.3 g/dL	Iron 67 mcg/dL
Glu 93 mg/dL	MCH 35.6 pg	TSH 3.26 mIU/L	Folate 0.8 ng/mL
HbA1c 5.5%	MCHC 33.5 g/dL		B_{12} 331 pg/mL

Questions

Problem Identification

1. a. *What drug therapy problems exist in this patient?*
   b. *What signs, symptoms, and laboratory values indicate this patient has anemia secondary to folate deficiency?*
   c. *Could the patient's folate deficiency have been caused by drug therapy?*
   d. *What additional information is needed to satisfactorily assess this patient?*
   e. *Why is it important to differentiate folate deficiency from vitamin B_{12} deficiency, and how is this accomplished?*

Desired Outcome

2. *What are the goals of pharmacotherapy for this patient's anemia?*

Therapeutic Alternatives

3. a. *What nondrug therapies may be used to correct this patient's folic acid deficiency?*
   b. *What pharmacotherapeutic alternatives are available for the treatment of this patient's anemia?*

c. *What economic or psychosocial issues are applicable to this patient and how might they contribute to the development of folic acid deficiency?*

Optimal Plan

4. *What is the most appropriate drug, dosage form, dose, schedule, and duration of therapy for the resolution of this patient's anemia?*

Outcome Evaluation

5. *What parameters should be used to evaluate the efficacy and adverse effects of folic acid replacement therapy in this patient?*

Patient Education

6. *What information would you provide to this patient about his folic acid replacement therapy?*

▶ Self-Study Assignments

1. Why is periconceptional folic acid supplementation necessary? What might the consequence be if the folic acid requirements are not met?
2. What is the dual interaction between phenytoin and folic acid, and how should this interaction be managed?
3. How does folate deficiency relate to plasma homocysteine levels, and what role does this relationship have in the development of cardiovascular disease?

▶ Clinical Pearl

Impaired renal function is associated with higher levels of plasma homocysteine, and the strongest determinant of plasma homocysteine is the plasma folate level. Patients with end-stage renal disease often have homocysteine levels at least three times higher than the upper limit of normal.

References

1. Klee GG. Cobalamin and folate evaluation: Measurement of methylmalonic acid and homocysteine vs. vitamin B_{12} and folate. Clin Chem 2000;46(8 pt 2):1277–1283.
2. Snow CF. Laboratory diagnosis of vitamin B_{12} and folate deficiency: A guide for the primary care physician. Arch Intern Med 1999;159:1289–1298.
3. Rampersaud GC, Kauwell GP, Bailey LB. Folate: A key to optimizing health and reducing disease risk in the elderly. J Am Coll Nutr 2003;22:1–8.
4. Rader JI. Folic acid fortification, folate status and plasma homocysteine. J Nutr 2002;132(8 Suppl):2466S–2470S.
5. Swain RA, St. Clair L. The role of folic acid in deficiency states and prevention of disease. J Fam Pract 1997;44:138–144.
6. Mills JL. Fortification of foods with folic acid—How much is enough? N Engl J Med 2000;342:1442–1445.
7. Morris MS, Fava M, Jacques PR, et al. Depression and folate status in the US Population. Psycother Psychosom 2003;72(2):80–87.

106 SICKLE CELL ANEMIA

▶ A Crisis Situation (Level I)

Christine M. Walko, PharmD
R. Donald Harvey III, PharmD, BCPS, BCOP

▶ After completing this case study, students should be able to:

- Recognize the clinical characteristics associated with an acute sickle cell crisis.
- Discuss the presentation of acute chest syndrome and treatment options.
- Recommend optimal analgesic therapy based on patient-specific information.
- Identify optimal endpoints of pharmacotherapy in sickle cell anemia patients.
- Recommend treatment that may reduce the frequency of sickle cell crises.

PATIENT PRESENTATION

Chief Complaint

"I can't catch my breath and can't walk because my leg pain is unbearable."

HPI

John Davis is a 26-year-old African American man with sickle cell anemia who presents with a 2-day history of pain localized to his legs and lower back in addition to increasing shortness of breath and a dry cough that became productive yesterday. His pain has been unrelieved by two codeine 30 mg/ acetaminophen 300 mg tablets taken every 4 hours. Currently he rates his pain intensity at 8 to 9 out of 10. His last bowel movement was one day prior to admission.

PMH

Sickle cell anemia (SS disease) diagnosed shortly after birth with approximately 7 to 10 crises per year requiring hospitalization

Bilateral hip replacement at age 13 complicated by Salmonella osteomyelitis

One previous episode of acute chest syndrome 5 years ago

FH

Mother and father alive and well, both with sickle cell trait. One sister also with sickle cell trait.

SH

Currently in graduate school, lives with girlfriend of 3 years.

ROS

Denies nausea, vomiting, or diarrhea. No evidence of heart failure or cardiomegaly. Has had productive cough with yellow sputum for one day.

Meds

Folic acid 1 mg po daily

Hydroxyurea 1000 mg po once daily

Codeine 30 mg/acetaminophen 300 mg 1 to 2 tablets po Q 4 to 6 H PRN

All

Morphine (reported as hallucinations)

Sulfa (reported rash when very young)

PE

Gen

He is a thin, well-developed African-American man in moderate distress

VS

BP 125/70, P 102, RR 24, T 39.0°C; 65 kg, O_2 sat 93% on 4 L O_2

HEENT

PERRL, EOMI, oral mucosa soft and moist; normal sclerae and funduscopic exam

Skin

Normal turgor, no rashes or cellulitis noted

Neck

Supple, no lymphadenopathy or thyromegaly

CV

RRR, II/VI SEM, no rubs or gallops

Lungs

Crackles in both bases on auscultation, dullness to percussion

Abd

General tenderness upon palpation; mild distention; hypoactive bowel sounds; mild splenomegaly, no hepatomegaly or masses

Ext

Pulses 2+ bilaterally, no edema, local lower extremity tenderness, erythema and inflammation (L>R).

Neuro

A & O × 3; normal strength, reflexes intact

Labs

Na 132 mEq/L	Hgb 6.5 g/dL	AST 47 IU/L	Ca 8.6 mg/dL
K 4.0 mEq/L	Hct 18.3%	ALT 27 IU/L	Mg 1.8 mEq/L
Cl 99 mEq/L	Plt 654 × 10^3/mm^3	Alk Phos 77 IU/L	Phos 3.5 mg/dL
CO_2 30 mEq/L	WBC 19.4 × 10^3/mm^3	LDH 957 IU/L	(+) anti-E red cell antibody
BUN 28 mg/dL	89% Segs	T. bili 5.0 mg/dL	
SCr 0.5 mg/dL	1 % Bands	D. bili 0.8 mg/dL	
Glu 81 mg/dL	9% Lymphs	I. bili 4.2 mg/dL	
	1% Eos%	Alb 3.5 g/dL	
	MCV 80.3 μm^3		
	Retic 18.4%		

Other

Arterial Blood Gas

pH 7.49, pCO_2 38, O_2 72, Bicarb 30, O_2 Sat 93%

Hgb Electrophoresis

Hgb A_2 2%; Hgb F 8%; Hgb S 90%

Peripheral blood smear

Sickle forms present, Howell–Jolly bodies present (see Figure 106–1).

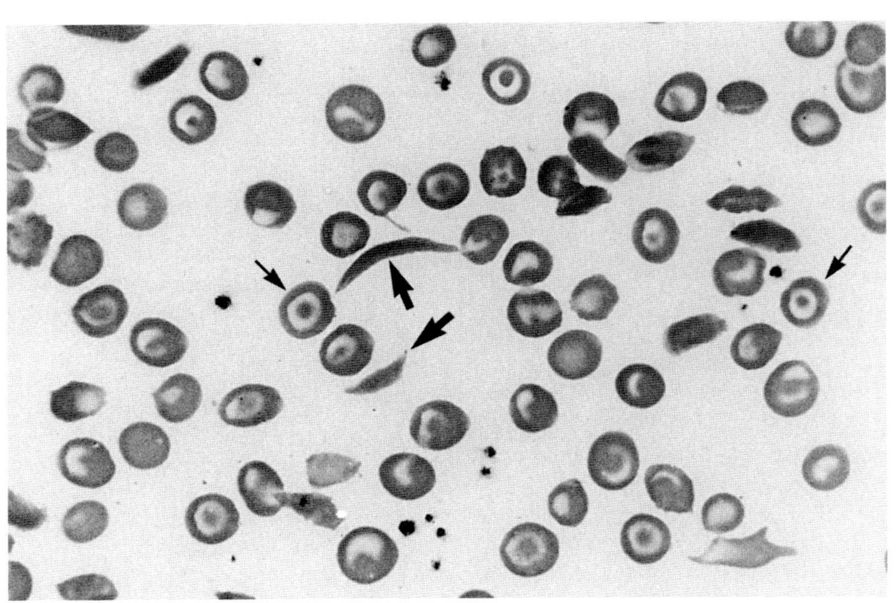

Figure 106–1. Peripheral blood with sickle cells *(large arrows)* and target cells *(small arrows)* (Wright-Giemsa × 1650). *(Photo courtesy of Lydia C. Contis, MD.)*

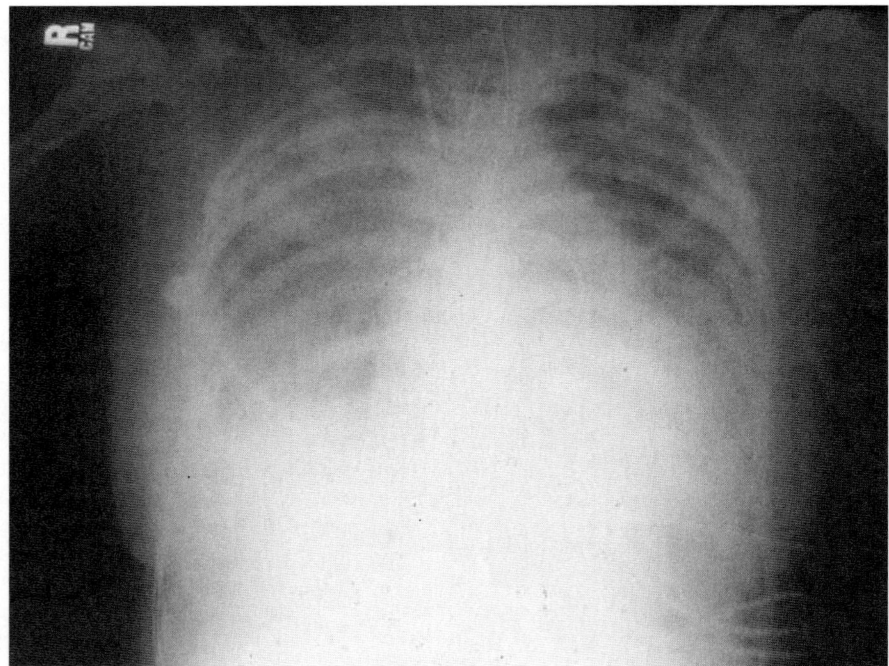

Figure 106–2. Lung radiograph of patient with acute chest syndrome secondary to sickle cell anemia. *(Photo courtesy of Kenneth I. Ataga, MD.)*

Chest X-Ray (see Figure 106–2)
This is a portable chest X-ray remarkable for diffuse interstitial infiltrates in both lung fields consistent with acute chest syndrome. There is notable cardiomegaly.

ECG
Normal sinus rhythm

Echocardiogram
Normal LV function

Assessment
A 26-year-old, African American man in sickle cell crisis with probable acute chest syndrome.

▶ Questions

Problem Identification

1. a. *Create a list of the patient's drug therapy problems.*
   b. *Which signs, symptoms, and laboratory values are consistent with an acute sickle cell crisis in this patient?*
   c. *Which signs, symptoms, and laboratory values support a diagnosis of acute chest syndrome in this patient?*
   d. *What additional information is needed to satisfactorily assess this patient?*

Desired Outcome

2. *What are the goals of pharmacotherapy in this case?*

Therapeutic Alternatives

3. a. *What nondrug therapies might be useful for this patient?*
   b. *What feasible pharmacotherapeutic alternatives are available for treatment of the patient's pain and constipation?*

Optimal Plan

4. *Outline a detailed therapeutic plan to treat all facets of this patient's acute sickle cell crisis and acute chest syndrome. For all drug therapies, include the dosage form, dose, schedule, and duration of therapy.*

Outcome Evaluation

5. a. *What clinical and laboratory parameters are necessary to evaluate therapy for achievement of the desired therapeutic outcome and to detect or prevent adverse effects?*

▶ Clinical Course

The plans you recommended have been initiated, and on the second day of hospitalization the patient's pain is markedly improved, oxygen saturation improved to 98% on 2L, and he is afebrile. He is still not moving his bowels and is having increased abdominal distention. Additionally, he mentions that he is frequently noncompliant with his home medications because of inability to afford the copayments.

b. *Considering this information, what changes (if any) in the pharmacotherapeutic plan are warranted while the patient is hospitalized?*

c. *What changes (if any) could be made to the patient's home medication regimen to decrease the number of hospitalizations for pain crisis in this patient?*

Patient Education

6. *What information should be provided to the patient to enhance compliance, ensure successful therapy, and minimize adverse effects?*

▶ Follow-Up Question

1. *What laboratory parameters may be followed to evaluate medication compliance and hematologic response while minimizing toxicity?*

▶ Self-Study Assignments

1. Determine the likelihood of the patient's offspring having sickle cell trait and/or disease if the father has:
   a. Normal hemoglobin
   b. Sickle cell trait
   c. Sickle cell disease
2. Describe the complications associated with frequent crises in each organ system.
3. Discuss the role of prophylactic antibiotics in the management of sickle cell anemia.

▶ Clinical Pearl

Allogeneic bone marrow transplantation has proven curative in pediatric sickle cell anemia patients. Approximately 20% of patients have a matched sibling donor, and matches may also be found through the National Marrow Donor Program.

References

1. Vichinsky EP, Neumayr LD, Earles AN, et al. Causes and outcomes of the acute chest syndrome in sickle cell disease. National Acute Chest Syndrome Study Group. N Engl J Med 2000; 342:1855–1865.
2. Vichinsky EP, Styles LA, Colangelo LH, et al. Acute chest syndrome in sickle cell disease: Clinical presentation and course. Cooperative Study of Sickle Cell Disease. Blood 1997; 89:1787–1792.
3. Steinberg MH. Management of sickle cell disease. N Engl J Med 1999; 340:1021–1030.
4. Bellet PS, Kalinyak KA, Shukla R, et al. Incentive spirometry to prevent acute pulmonary complications in sickle cell diseases. N Engl J Med 1995; 333:699–703.
5. Herndon CM, Jackson KC, Hallin PA. Management of opioid-induced gastrointestinal effects in patients receiving palliative care. Pharmacotherapy 2002; 22:240–250.
6. Steinberg MH, Barton F, Castro O, et al. Effect of hydroxyurea on mortality and morbidity in adult sickle cell anemia: Risks and benefits up to 9 years of treatment. JAMA 2003; 289:1645–1651.

SECTION 16

Infectious Diseases

107 USING LABORATORY TESTS IN INFECTIOUS DISEASES

► Bad Bug (Level III)

Steven J. Martin, PharmD, BCPS, FCCM
Eric G. Sahloff, PharmD

► After completing this case study, students should be able to:

- Outline the qualitative evaluation of the Gram-stain
- Discuss the use of urine antigen testing in the diagnosis of pneumonia
- Describe the proper method for blood collection for culture
- Discuss the proper means for identifying extended-spectrum β-lactamase production in clinical bacterial specimens
- Describe the appropriate serum sampling times for antibiotic concentration determination to individualize drug dosing

PATIENT PRESENTATION

Chief Complaint

Not obtainable; patient is obtunded.

HPI

Julian Donaldson is a 73 yo man who lives in the Crescent Village retirement facility, and he is seen in the ED of the University Medical Center after being found unresponsive in his bed this afternoon. He had a high fever (103.7°F) at the nursing home, and has developed labored breathing. Over the past several days the staff report that Julian has been coughing and seemed to have an upper respiratory tract infection. He has previously been in good health and is able to manage all activities of daily living.

PMH

Coronary artery disease
Hypercholesterolemia
Hypothyroidism
Osteoarthritis
Epilepsy

FH

Both parents are deceased (mother age 88 MI, father age 96 stroke). He is a bachelor with no children.

SH

Retired university professor of engineering; has lived in the retirement facility for 4 years; no alcohol, tobacco, or illicit drug use.

ROS

Unable to obtain due to patient's condition

Meds

Amlodipine 5 mg po once daily
Pravastatin 30 mg po at bedtime
Levothyroxine 100 mcg po once daily
Valproic acid 1000 mg po sustained-release at bedtime
Lamotrigine 25 mg po every other day
Celecoxib 100 mg po BID
Nitroglycerin 0.4 mg SL PRN

All

NKA

PE

Gen

The patient is an elderly man in considerable respiratory distress.

VS

BP 104/68, P 122, RR 42, T 41°C, Wt 160 lb., Ht 5′10″

Skin

Warm and diaphoretic

HEENT

NC/AT; PERRLA; conjunctivae pink; sclerae clear; EOMI; disk margins sharp; no arteriolar narrowing, A-V nicking, hemorrhages, or exudates; ear canals clear and drums negative; nares normal; teeth intact, tonsils intact and normal, pharynx negative

Neck/LN

Trachea midline; thyroid palpable, no nodes

Chest

Rhonchi bilaterally, dullness to percussion and diminished breath sounds in RLL

CV

Tachycardic, normal S_1 and S_2, no heaves, thrills, or bruits

Abd

Soft, non-distended; no masses or tenderness; liver, spleen, and kidneys not felt; no CVA tenderness

Genit/Rect

Not performed

MS/Ext

Deferred

Neuro

Does not respond to voice; responds to pain with withdrawal

Labs

Na 138 mEq/L	Hgb 12.7 g/dL	WBC 19.4×10^3/mm^3
K 4.1 mEq/L	Hct 38.4%	78% Neutros
Cl 104 mEq/L	RBC 4.7×10^6/mm^3	9% Bands
CO_2 22 mEq/L	Plt 155×10^3/mm^3	12% Lymphs
BUN 22 mg/dL	MCV 81.8 μm^3	1% Monos
SCr 1.5 mg/dL	MCH 27.1 pg	PT 11.6 sec
Glu 116 mg/dL	MCHC 33.1 g/dL	aPTT 28.1 sec
	RDW 15%	TSH 3.52 mIU/L

ABG

pH 7.50; pO_2 65 mm Hg; pCO_2 29 mm Hg; HCO_3 22 mEq/L
O_2 saturation 87% on FiO_2 1 L via non-rebreather mask

Chest X-Ray

Infiltrate in right lower lobe; bilateral pleural effusions

Assessment

RLL pneumonia with impending respiratory collapse
Respiratory alkalosis secondary to pneumonia and tachypnea

Plan

1. Emergent endotracheal intubation and mechanical ventilation
2. Following intubation, fiberoptic bronchoscopy with bronchoalveolar lavage for collection of distal pulmonary secretion samples for Gram stain, culture, and sensitivity
3. Collect two sets of blood cultures (anaerobic and aerobic) from two separate sites

---

▶ Questions

Problem Identification

1. a. *Create a list of this patient's drug therapy problems.*
   b. *What subjective and objective data indicate the presence of infection?*

Desired Outcome

2. a. *What are the desired treatment goals for this patient's current medical problems?*
   b. *Why are two sets of blood culture obtained?*

▶ Clinical Course

The patient is intubated and mechanically ventilated with 100% O_2. Bronchoscopy is performed and a sample of alveolar washing is sent to the microbiology laboratory for direct examination and culture. Gram stain reveals many WBC, 0 epithelial cells, many Gram-negative rods, few Gram positive cocci in clusters.

The patient is started on ceftazidime 1 gram IV Q 12 H, gentamicin 180 mg Q 24 H, and vancomycin 1 gram IV Q 24 H.

   c. *The microbiology laboratory performed a Gram stain on the pulmonary secretion sample. How should the microbiologist evaluate the sample quality, and how is the semi-quantitative analysis helpful in directing initial empiric therapy?*
   d. *In addition to the pulmonary secretion sample, describe how urinary antigen tests can assist in the identification of the pathogen responsible for this patient's pneumonia.*

Therapeutic Alternatives

3. a. *When should serum gentamicin and vancomycin concentrations be collected for individualization of drug dosing?*

TABLE 107–1. Preliminary Susceptibility Report

Antibiotic	Interpretation
Aztreonam	R
Amikacin	R
Ampicillin/sulbactam	R
Ceftazidime	R
Ceftriaxone	R
Cefotaxime	R
Ciprofloxacin	R
Imipenem	S
Gentamicin	R
Piperacillin/tazobactam	R
Tobramycin	R

▶ Clinical Course

The laboratory identifies *Enterobacter cloacae* as the predominant pathogen in the respiratory culture. The susceptibility profile is shown in Table 107–1.

b. The microbiology lab does not routinely test cefepime using automated methods. Because of its stability to many β-lactamases, cefepime may be a viable therapeutic option. What other testing methods are available to determine the activity of cefepime against this isolate?

c. Given the unusual resistance profile for this organism, what additional testing should be performed on this isolate to identify specific resistance mechanisms?

Optimal Plan

4. The microbiology laboratory provided both a minimum inhibitory concentration (MIC) and an interpretation of that MIC for each antimicrobial agent tested. How are the MIC and the interpretation correlated?

▶ Clinical Course

The patient's antibiotic regimen was switched to imipenem 500 mg IV Q 12 H, but the intensivist is concerned about the use of this drug in a patient with epilepsy and renal dysfunction. She has requested the laboratory test cefepime against the *Enterobacter* isolate. The cefepime MIC for this organism was 8 mcg/mL. The patient's antibiotic was again switched to cefepime 2 grams IV Q 12 H. The patient's fever abated, and his WBC count (day 3 of hospitalization) was $13.0 \times 10^3/mm^3$, with 77% neutros, 2% bands, 18% lymphs, 2% monos, and 1% eos.

Outcome Evaluation

5. a. Would the determination of the minimum bactericidal concentration (MBC) for this organism against cefepime, or the evaluation of the serum bactericidal titer (SBT) be helpful in the management of this infection?

b. Outline a follow-up plan for monitoring the efficacy of this therapeutic regimen.

▶ Self-Study Assignments

1. What is the expected turn-around time for the microbiology laboratory to provide a full organism identification and susceptibility profile for a sputum specimen?
2. How do the results of the disk-diffusion susceptibility test differ from the results of automated testing methods?
3. When would the use of nucleic acid amplification methods be necessary in making a diagnosis?

▶ Clinical Pearl

The data received from the clinical laboratory is limited in its precision by the quality of the specimen that was sent and the process that was used to collect it. Precisely labeling samples for culture, quantification, or other laboratory analysis, including site of collection, time and date of collection, and patient identifiers will improve the value of the data that is provided back to the clinician.

References

1. Al Balooshi N, Jamsheer A, Botta GA. Impact of introducing quality control/quality assurance (QC/QA) guidelines in respiratory specimen processing. Clin Microbiol Infect 2003; 9:810–815.
2. Tan MJ, Tan JS, File TM. Legionnaires disease with bacteremic coinfection. Clin Infect Dis 2002; 35:533–539.
3. Roson B, Fernandez-Sabe N, Carratala J, et al. Contribution of a urinary antigen assay (Binax NOW) to the early diagnosis of pneumococcal pneumonia. Clin Infect Dis 2004; 38:222–226.
4. National Committee for Clinical Laboratory Standards. Methods for Dilution Antimicrobial Susceptibility Tests for Bacteria that Grow Aerobically: Approved Standard–6th ed. NCCLS document M7-A5 (ISBN 1–56238–486–4). NCCLS, 940 West Valley Road, Suite 1400, Wayne, PA 19087–1898 USA, 2003.
5. Sahloff EG, Martin SJ. Extended-spectrum β-lactamase resistance in the ICU. J Pharm Pract 2002; 15:96–105.

108 BACTERIAL MENINGITIS

▶ Trouble on Day One (Level II)

Sherry Luedtke, PharmD

▶ After completing this case study, students should be able to:

- Identify risk factors and common presenting signs and symptoms of bacterial meningitis in infants.
- Differentiate common bacterial pathogens associated with bacterial meningitis in newborns versus older children.
- Recommend appropriate empiric antimicrobial therapy for bacterial meningitis in infants.
- Identify appropriate parameters for monitoring antimicrobial therapy for treatment of bacterial meningitis in infants.

PATIENT PRESENTATION

Chief Complaint

Unobtainable.

HPI

Jason is a 37-week gestation, 3,504-g infant male with respiratory distress. He was delivered via spontaneous vaginal delivery to a 25 yo G_1P_1 white woman. The delivery was uncomplicated with initial Apgar scores of 9/9. The infant was transferred to normal nursery with some mild grunting and retracting that required supplemental oxygen for the first 2 hours of life. He was later taken to the mother to nurse. Six hours later, he developed tachypnea, grunting, retracting, and became hypotensive. Two boluses of 10 mL/kg NS were administered with little improvement in perfusion. He was placed on dopamine, blood cultures were drawn, antibiotics were initiated, and he was transferred to a nearby neonatal intensive care unit.

Maternal History

Uncomplicated prenatal course and delivery. Premature rupture of the membranes for 41 hours prior to delivery. Rubella immune, HbsAg (–), GBS (+), RPR (–). Mother ran a low-grade fever for 12 hours prior to delivery and received a dose of ampicillin plus gentamicin for suspected chorioamnionitis at 3 and 1 hour prior to delivery. Maternal meds: prenatal vitamins, iron supplement. Mother denies alcohol use, tobacco, and use of illicit drugs.

Meds

Ampicillin 350 mg IV Q 12 H (200 mg/kg/day)
Cefotaxime 175 mg IV Q 12 H (50 mg/kg/dose)
Dopamine 5 mcg/kg/min

PE

Gen

Appears to be large, a well-developed male newborn, with dusky undertones and tachypnea on oxygen hood

VS

BP 85/37, HR 148, RR 77, T 36.8°C; Wt 3,504 g; length 53 cm; HC 34.7 cm

Skin

Grayish-pink color

HEENT

No nasal flaring, sutures overriding (*Note:* Open/bulging sutures or "pulsatile" sutures may be seen in some cases, which is indicative of elevated cerebrospinal fluid pressure.)

Neck/LN

Clavicles intact

Chest

Lungs clear bilaterally; chest wall rise is symmetric; there is grunting and mild intercostal retractions

CV

RRR, grade I/VI systolic murmur LLSB

Abd

Soft, distended, (+) BS, liver 1 cm below RCM, 3 vessel cord (*Note:* Two-vessel umbilical cords in neonates are associated with an increased incidence of other congenital anomalies, such as cleft palate and heart defects.)

Genit/Rect

Normal uncircumcised external genitalia, testes descended; rectal midline, patent anus

Ext

20 digits, brachial pulses palpable, capillary refill > 4 sec

Neuro

Mildly hypotonic, responds to stimuli

Labs

Na 138 mEq/L	Hgb 18.7 g/dL	*CBG*
K 3.9 mEq/L	Hct 54.7%	pH 7.26
Cl 109 mEq/L	Plt 297 × 10^3/mm^3	pO_2 57.3 mm Hg
CO_2 21 mEq/L	WBC 3.2 × 10^3/mm^3	PCO_2 29.6 mm Hg
SCr 1.3 mg/dL	8% Neutros	HCO_3 25.2 mEq/L
Glu 103 mg/dL	13% Bands	BE –2.9 mEq/L
	76% Lymphs	T. bili 2.2 mg/dL
	1% Eos	Ca 8.3 mg/dL
	2% Basos	CRP 14.3 mg/L

Other

Urine and CSF serology: *Haemophilus influenzae* type B (–), *Streptococcus pneumoniae* (–), Group B Streptococcus (+), *Neisseria meningitis* (–), *N. meningitis B/Escherichia coli* (–)

CSF chemistry/cell count: color/appearance hazy, glucose 40 mg/dL, protein 281 mg/dL, WBC 306/mm^3 (5% Lymphs, 62% Monos, 33% Neutros), RBC 16/mm^3

Cultures

Blood, urine, CSF pending

Chest X-Ray

Minimal interstitial prominence suggesting retained lung fluid

Assessment

1. Group B Streptococcus meningitis
2. Hypoperfusion and metabolic acidosis
3. Neutropenia

▶ Questions

Problem Identification

1. a. *What drug therapy problems does this infant have?*
   b. *What risk factors does this patient have for bacterial meningitis?*
   c. *What clinical and laboratory findings indicate the presence of meningitis and its severity?*
   d. *Describe strategies for preventing Group B Streptococcus (GBS) infections in newborns.*

Desired Outcome

2. *What are the goals of drug therapy in this situation?*

Therapeutic Alternatives

3. a. *What nondrug therapies might be useful for managing this patient?*
   b. *Describe the antimicrobial alternatives available for the management of meningitis in this patient.*
   c. *What are the implications of intrapartum antibiotic use on the management of symptomatic and asymptomatic newborns at risk for GBS infections?*
   d. *Discuss adjuvant drug therapy options in newborns with severe neutropenia and sepsis.*
   e. *What supportive therapies may be used to manage the patient's hypoperfusion and resulting metabolic acidosis?*

▶ Clinical Course

Blood cultures returned positive for group B Streptococcus. CSF cultures (drawn after antibiotics were initiated) were negative and urine cultures were positive for group B Streptococcus. Sensitivity studies revealed an MIC < 0.12 mcg/mL to ampicillin. Repeat CRP at 24 hours of life was 7.8 mg/L and the repeat CBC at that time revealed: Hgb 19.4 g/dL, Hct 58.1%, Plt 230 $\times 10^3$/mm^3, WBC 7.9 $\times 10^3$/mm^3 (15% segs, 17% bands, 67% lymphs, 1% basos).

Optimal Plan

4. *Given this new information, what therapy would you recommend for the management of this infant?*

Outcome Evaluation

5. *Describe the monitoring parameters necessary to evaluate the efficacy and safety of the therapy.*

▶ Clinical Course

The infant was treated with the regimen you recommended, and his perfusion, muscle tone, respiratory distress, and metabolic acidosis improved within the first 24 hours of treatment. Supplemental oxygen was removed at that time. Seventy-two hours after initiation of antibiotic therapy, a repeat CBC showed completed resolution of the infant's leukopenia. A repeat lumbar puncture performed on day 5 of therapy was clear, at which time gentamicin was discontinued. The patient was discharged on day 7 of therapy to receive an additional 7 days of IV ampicillin as home therapy. Audiometry testing performed after completion of antibiotic therapy was normal. The child had no evidence of neurologic impairment as a consequence of the infection at follow-up evaluations.

▶ Self-Study Assignments

1. Evaluate the use of extended-interval dosing of gentamicin in the management of newborns.
2. Discuss the role of adjunctive cytokine measurements in the evaluation of sepsis and meningitis in infants.
3. Describe the properties of antimicrobial agents that allow them to penetrate the CNS during meningitis.

▶ Clinical Pearl

Infants may become colonized and/or infected with group B Streptococcus despite negative maternal group B streptococcal cultures.

References

1. Polin, RA, Harris MC. Neonatal bacterial meningitis. Semin Neonatol 2001;6:157–172.
2. Centers for Disease Control and Prevention. Prevention of perinatal group B streptococcal disease: Revised guidelines from the CDC. MMWR 2002;51:RR-11:1–22.
3. Hengst JM. The role of C-reactive protein in the evaluation and management of infants with suspected sepsis. Adv Neonatal Care 2003;3(1):3–13.
4. Taketomo CK, Hodding JH, Kraus DM. Pediatric Dosage Handbook, 9th ed. Hudsen, OH, Lexi-Comp, 2002.

109 PEDIATRIC COUGH ILLNESS/ACUTE BRONCHITIS

▶ Cassidy's Cough Continues (Level II)

Justin J. Sherman, PharmD
W. Greg Leader, PharmD

▶ After completing this case study, students should be able to:

- Evaluate signs and symptoms of cough illness/acute bronchitis in children, the duration of symptoms, and relevant laboratory values in order to rule out more serious illness, especially pneumonia.
- Discuss why sputum cultures and gram stains are not useful in evaluating and treating children with cough illness/acute bronchitis.
- Select alternatives to antibiotic treatment of cough illness/acute bronchitis, discuss why routine antibiotics are not indicated, and identify other medications that have no value in this disorder.
- Identify nonpharmacologic and pharmacologic treatment alternatives for relief of symptoms.

PATIENT PRESENTATION

Chief Complaint

"What do you mean the medication the doctor prescribed is not an antibiotic? My son has been coughing up phlegm for five days now and has been running a fever, too."

HPI

Monique Comeaux presents a prescription for zanamivir to the pharmacist for her 3 yo son, Cassidy, several days after the New Year holiday. She is outraged that her family practitioner (the second physician she has taken her son to within five days) did not write a prescription for an antibiotic. She brought her son to a pediatrician with complaints of a 2-day history of productive, purulent cough and a fever of 103°F. After obtaining a blood sample for labs, the pediatrician told her that it was "just a viral infection" and did not prescribe anything for it. Cassidy also had complained of runny nose, pain in his head and legs, and a "funny feeling all over". Disgusted with the physician's "lack of help," she brought her son to their family physician 3 days later. By this time, all of the other symptoms had resolved by themselves with the exception of the productive cough. The second physician gave Mrs. Comeaux a prescription for the neuraminidase inhibitor and suggested that she bring the child back in if the cough continued over the next 2 or 3 weeks. He did not explain to the mother at the time why he was prescribing that particular medication. The unresolved cough combined with the initial spike in fever troubled the boy's mother, and she has sought the community pharmacist's advice for any other options.

Upon questioning the child, Cassidy confirms that he is "feeling better" except for the cough. His mother denies that Cassidy has been tired, wheezing, coughing at night, or coughing as he plays in the yard. However, she states that she has heard Cassidy cough in the morning; she suggests that it could be from his "nose draining" throughout the night.

PMH

Healthy, 4.5 kg infant at birth

Has been fully immunized, including a 7-valent pneumococcal vaccination (Prevnar)

No other health problems to date

FH

Mother and father are both in good health. Father is 35 years old, a middle-manager for a very successful shrimp boat company. Mother is a former high school teacher who now stays at home with Cassidy. No siblings. Neither parent has been vaccinated for influenza this past winter, but both have been vaccinated previously for pneumonia.

SH

Parents have been married for 7 years with one child. The mother is a homemaker and devotes her full time and attention to Cassidy. Although Cassidy does not spend time in a formal daycare center, his mother organizes several "play groups" with other stay-at-home mothers several times per week; she admitted that a few children were coughing at the last play group. She also takes him to "mother's day out" once a month. She admits to occasional EtOH use when entertaining and has a 10 pack-year smoking history (1 pack/day for 10 years). Her husband has a 30 pack-year smoking history (2 packs/day for 15 years), but his wife states that he smokes "mostly at work."

Meds

Acetaminophen PRN for the first 2 days of illness

Also, the patient's mother presents a prescription for Zanamivir 10 mg (2 inhalations) BID × 5 days

All

NKDA

ROS

No malaise, wheezing, or nocturnal coughing; no nausea, vomiting, or diarrhea.

Limited PE

Gen

Well-developed male child in NAD. Patient has a productive cough and seems to be very attentive to the conversation between the adults.

VS

BP 110/65, P 105, RR 30, T 37.8°C (auditory canal measurement); Ht 100 cm, Wt 17 kg

Mrs. Comeaux stated that Cassidy had a chest x-ray that was normal; she also brought the following labs and sputum culture results with her from the pediatrician's office:

	WBC Differential
Hgb 12 g/dL	Segs 51%
Hct 36%	Bands 2%
RBC 4.9 × 10^6/mm^3	Lymphs 37%
WBC 6.5 × 10^3/mm^3	Monos 6%
	Eos 3%
	Basos 1%

Sputum culture: No pathogen isolated

Assessment

A 3 yo male child with presumed cough illness/acute bronchitis that is likely viral in origin.

Questions

Problem Identification

1. a. *Create a list of the patient's drug therapy problems.*
   b. *What information (signs, symptoms, laboratory values) indicates the presence or severity of acute bronchitis?*
   c. *Could any of the patient's problems have been caused by undiagnosed bronchial hyperreactivity?*
   d. *What additional information must be considered prior to completing the assessment of this patient?*

Desired Outcome

2. *What are the goals of pharmacotherapy in this case?*

Therapeutic Alternatives

3. a. *What nondrug therapies might be useful for this patient?*
   b. *What feasible pharmacotherapeutic alternatives are available for treatment of cough illness/acute bronchitis that has not lasted beyond ten days after onset of symptoms?*
   c. *What psychosocial considerations are applicable to this patient?*

Optimal Plan

4. *What drugs, dosage form, dose, schedule, and duration of therapy are best to alleviate this patient's symptoms?*

Outcome Evaluation

5. *What clinical and laboratory parameters are necessary to evaluate the therapy for achievement of the desired outcome and to detect or prevent adverse effects?*

Patient Education

6. *What information should be provided to the patient and his mother to enhance compliance, ensure successful therapy, and minimize adverse effects?*

► Self-Study Assignments

1. Compare and contrast the treatment guidelines for acute bronchitis of viral origin in children and adults.[1,2]
2. Prepare an education pamphlet on cough illness/acute bronchitis directed at both parents and general practice physicians. Be sure to address why antibiotics are not usually first-line therapy.
3. Perform a literature search to obtain recent peer-reviewed publications on the use of antibiotics in uncomplicated bronchitis. Review these articles and draw your own conclusions.

► Clinical Pearl

Educating parents about the inappropriate use of antibiotics for pediatric cough illness/acute bronchitis is effective. In one study, the percentage of parents who brought their child to a second physician because an antibiotic was not prescribed by the first significantly decreased after an educational intervention.[11]

References

1. O'Brien KL, Dowell SF, Schwartz B, et al. Cough illness/bronchitis–principles of judicious use of antimicrobial use. Pediatrics 1998;101(1 Suppl):178–181.
2. Gonzales R, Bartlett JG, Besser RE, et al. Principles of appropriate antibiotic use for treatment of uncomplicated acute bronchitis: Background. Ann Intern Med 2001;134:521–529.
3. Gadomski AM. Potential interventions for preventing pneumonia among young children: lack of effect of antibiotic treatment for upper respiratory infections. Pediatr Infect Dis J 1993;12:115–120.
4. Vinson DC, Lutz LJ. The effect of parental expectations on treatment of children with a cough: a report from ASPN. J Fam Pract 1993;37:23–27.
5. Smucny J, Flynn C, Becker L, et al. Beta2-agonists for acute bronchitis (Cochrane Review). In: The Cochrane Library 2004;1:AB001726. Available on the Internet at: www.cochrane.org/cochrane/revabstr/AB001726.htm. Accessed July 19, 2004.
6. Schroeder K, Fahey T. Should we advise parents to administer over the counter medicines for acute cough? Systematic review of randomized controlled trials. Arch Dis Child 2002;86:170–175.
7. Gonzales R, Bartlett JG, Besser RE, et al. Principles of appropriate antibiotic use for treatment of uncomplicated acute bronchitis: background. Ann Intern Med 2001;134:521–529.
8. Finkelstein JA, Stille C, Nordin J, et al. Reduction in antibiotic use among US children, 1996–2000. Pediatrics 2003;112(3 Pt 1):620–627.
9. Mainous AG, Hueston WJ, Davis MP, et al. Trends in antimicrobial prescribing for bronchitis and upper respiratory infections among adults and children. Am J Pub Health 2003;93:1910–1914.
10. Mangione-Smith R, McGlynn EA, Elliott MN, et al. The relationship between perceived parental expectations and pediatrician antimicrobial prescribing behavior. Pediatrics 1999;103(4 Pt 1):711–718.
11. Trepka MJ, Belongia EA, Chyou PH, et al. The effect of a community intervention trial on parental knowledge and awareness of antibiotic resistance and appropriate antibiotic use in children. Pediatrics 2001;107(1):50–57.

110 PREVENTION AND TREATMENT OF INFLUENZA

► A Shot of Prevention (Level II)

Christina E. Schober, PharmD
Meredith L. Rose, PharmD

► After completing this case study, students should be able to:

- Identify appropriate target populations for vaccination against influenza.
- Discuss the available options for preventing influenza.
- Recognize influenza-related complications.
- Develop an individualized plan for treating influenza.
- Define strategies to control community outbreaks of influenza.

PATIENT PRESENTATION

Chief Complaint

"I'm here for my shots."

HPI

Stephanie Sullivan is a 77-year-old woman who recently moved into a personal care home. Over the past year, she has become increasingly dependent on the assistance of others for her activities of daily living. Additionally, because her gait is unsteady, she has a fear of falling. She presents today for a six-month follow-up appointment and for her yearly vaccination.

PMH
Chronic atrial fibrillation
CAD (s/p MI in 1994)
HF (NYHA class II–III)
Hyperlipidemia
COPD

FH
Her parents and sister are deceased; she is unable to provide the causes of death.

SH
Widowed × 20 years; (–) tobacco (quit 10 years ago); (–) EtOH

Meds
Warfarin 2.5 mg po daily
Digoxin 0.125 mg po daily
Ramipril 5 mg po daily
Atenolol 25 mg po daily
Furosemide 40 mg po daily
Spironolactone 25 mg po daily
Pravastatin 40 mg po HS
Potassium chloride 10 mEq po daily
Ipratropium bromide 2 puffs QID
Oxygen 2 liters per NC

All
Diltiazem (exfoliative dermatitis); PCN (hives)

ROS
Patient is without acute complaints. (–) visual changes, dizziness, hearing loss; (+) occasional epistaxis; (+) SOB (walking up stairs); (–) CP, PND, (+) stable 2 pillow orthopnea, mild bilateral leg edema; (–) N/V/D, constipation, BRBPR, hematuria, melena, polyuria, or dysuria.

PE

Gen
Elderly female, A & O × 3

VS
BP 106/68; P 72, irregularly irregular; RR 18; T 37.2°C; Ht 5′2″, Wt 138 lb.

Skin
Warm and dry, normal turgor, no lesions/tumors/moles

HEENT
PERRLA; EOMI; (+) dry nasal mucosa; (+) dentures

Neck
(–) bruits, thyromegaly, adenopathy, JVD

Lungs
CTA

Cardiac
Normal S_1 and S_2; (+) S_3; (–) murmur

Abdomen
Normal BS; (–) hepatosplenomegaly, bruits, masses, ascites

Genit/Rect
(–) guaiac

Extremities
Chronic venous stasis changes on left leg of the medial surface; (+) bilateral 1–2+ LE edema (stable)

Labs

Na 140 mEq/L	Hgb 14.4 g/dL	T Chol 174 mg/dL
K 5.4 mEq/L	Hct 43.2%	LDL 96 mg/dL
Cl 94 mEq/L	Plt 191 × 10^3/mm^3	HDL 48 mg/dL
CO_2 34 mEq/L	RBC 4.23 × 10^6/mm^3	Trig 112 mg/dL
BUN 17 mg/dL	RDW 13.5	TSH 1.464 mIU/L
SCr 1.2 mg/dL		INR 2.6
Glu 84 mg/dL		aPTT 31.6 sec

Diagnostic Tests
DXA scan: Hip T-score: –2.21
Pulse oximetry 96% on 2 L O_2

Vaccine history

Vaccine Type	Date Last Dose Received
Tetanus, Diphtheria (Td)	7 years ago (11/1997)
Influenza	11/03
Pneumococcal (polysaccharide)	09/03
Hepatitis B	Never
Hepatitis A	Never
Measles, Mumps, Rubella (MMR)	Unknown
Varicella	Acquired as a child (1924)
Meningococcal (polysaccharide)	Never

Assessment
Elderly woman with multiple medical conditions that put her at risk for complications of influenza

Questions

Problem Identification

1. a. *Develop a list of the patient's drug therapy problems.*
   b. *What indications does this patient have for administration of the influenza vaccine?*
   c. *What are the contraindications to receiving the influenza vaccine? Does this patient have any of these contraindications?*
   d. *If vaccination is desirable, what is the optimal timeframe for this patient to receive the influenza vaccine?*

Desired Outcomes

2. *What are the goals of influenza vaccination in this patient?*

Therapeutic Alternatives

3. a. *What influenza vaccine formulations are available for use with this patient?*
   b. *List alternative preventive measures that can be used for patients who are unable or unwilling to receive the influenza vaccine.*

Optimal Plan

4. a. *Provide your individualized treatment recommendations for protecting this patient against influenza virus infection.*
   b. *Outline your plans for managing each of the patient's other drug therapy problems.*

Outcome Evaluation

5. *What clinical indicators of effectiveness should be monitored after administration of the influenza vaccine?*

Patient Education

6. a. *If Mrs. Sullivan expressed concern over receiving the vaccine due to fear of contracting the flu, how would you respond?*
   b. *What information related to the adverse effects of the influenza vaccine should you provide the patient?*

► Clinical Course

In December of the following year, Mrs. Sullivan returns to the doctor's office with complaints of a one-day history of fever (38.5°C), muscle aches, headache, and dry cough. Her care giver reports that there has been an outbreak of influenza at her personal care home. Mrs. Sullivan was not scheduled for a follow-up visit with her PCP for two more weeks, and she has not yet received the influenza vaccine this season. Based on the patient's recent exposure and clinical presentation, she was diagnosed with influenza.

► Follow-Up Questions

1. *Describe the typical presentation of influenza-related illness. What specific symptoms are suggestive of influenza in this patient?*
2. *What influenza-related complications is this patient at risk for developing?*
3. *List available options for treating influenza in this patient. Include the drug name, dose, dosage form, route, frequency, and treatment duration.*
4. *Provide recommendations for controlling the influenza outbreak at the personal care home.*

► Self-Study Assignments

Given the expanded role of pharmacists as immunization providers in many states, you decide to start a pharmacy-based immunization program in your community pharmacy.

1. Develop a collaborative practice agreement with a physician to support the immunization program and handle emergency situations.
2. Create a sample letter to patients who may need the influenza vaccine to assist in marketing your service.
3. Investigate the reimbursement options for providing vaccination services in your area.

► Clinical Pearl

Antiviral therapy for influenza should not be administered for two weeks after administration of the live attenuated influenza vaccine because these drugs reduce the replication of influenza viruses and may reduce the efficacy of the LAIV.[1] Likewise, the vaccine should not be administered until 48 hours after cessation of influenza antiviral therapy.

References

1. Center for Disease Control and Prevention. Prevention and control of influenza: Recommendations of the Advisory Committee on Immunization Practices (ACIP). MMWR 2004;53(RR–6):1–40.
2. Lasky T, Terracciano GJ, Magder L, et al. The Guillain-Barre syndrome and the 1992–1993 and 1993–1994 influenza vaccines. N Engl J Med 1998;339:1797–1802.
3. Drinka PJ. Influenza vaccination and antiviral therapy: Is there a role for concurrent administration in the institutionalised elderly? Drugs Aging 2003;20(3):165–174.
4. Rothberg MB, Bellantonio S, Rose DN. Management of influenza in adults older than 65 years of age: Cost-effectiveness of rapid testing and antiviral therapy. Ann Intern Med 2003;139(5 Pt 1):321–329.
5. Stohr K. Preventing and treating influenza. BMJ 2003;326:1223–1224.
6. Cooper NJ, Sutton AJ, Abrams KR, et al. Effectiveness of neuraminidase inhibitors in treatment and prevention of influenza A and B: Systematic review and meta-analyses of randomized controlled trials. BMJ 2003;326:1–7.

111 COMMUNITY-ACQUIRED PNEUMONIA

► Linda's Labored Breathing (Level I)

Patrick P. Gleason, PharmD, BCPS

► After completing this case study, students should be able to:

- Recognize the common signs and symptoms of community-acquired pneumonia (CAP).
- Establish the goals of pharmacotherapy and monitoring parameters for a patient with CAP.
- Know which pathogens are commonly associated with CAP.
- Recommend an effective and economical antimicrobial regimen for CAP including specific antimicrobial agent(s), route of administration, and dose(s).
- Identify the patient parameters associated with clinical stability in order to convert from IV to oral antimicrobial therapy.

PATIENT PRESENTATION

Chief Complaint

"My mother is confused and sick."

HPI

Linda Tyler is a 72 yo woman who is widowed and a resort owner. She presents to clinic accompanied by her son, who lives with her. He reports that she has become confused in the past 24 hours. He states that the "flu" has been circulating through the household, and about 3 days ago Ms. Tyler came down with the flu. It began with chills and a cough that have gradually become worse and she now has difficulty catching her breath and staying warm. Her sputum is clear to white and she has reportedly been afebrile.

PMH

Nicotine dependence × 60 years
COPD for approximately 10 years
Osteoarthritis × 12 years

FH

Positive for HTN and breast cancer. Negative for CAD, hypercholesterolemia, asthma, and DM.

SH

Lives with son and his family. Smokes ½ ppd. Denies having received a blood transfusion. Usually has 1 to 2 EtOH drinks a day.

ROS

Difficult to conduct secondary to Ms. Tyler's mental state (mild obtundation). In addition to the findings reported in the HPI, her son states she had difficulty sleeping and was up much of last night coughing and with chills, which she confirms. He has not observed any episodes of emesis but reports that she has had a decreased appetite. He reports she has had increasing weakness but no dysphagia, dysarthria, or ataxia.

Meds

Prempro 0.625mg/2.5mg po once daily
Aspirin 325 mg 2 to 3 po QID
Combivent MDI 2 puffs QID (son reports she rarely uses)
Albuterol MDI 2 puffs QID PRN

All

Sulfa (unknown what specific reaction was)

PE

Gen

This is a mildly obtunded frail, thin, woman lying on the examination table with two blankets on her; she is tachypneic, tachycardic, appears uncomfortable, and has to be supported when sitting up. She is oriented to place only

VS

BP 100/60, P 112, RR 28, T 37.0°C, Wt 52 kg, Ht 5′5″, O_2 sat 82% on room air

Skin

Warm, clammy

HEENT

NC/AT; EOMI; PERRLA; grossly intact bilaterally. Nose is without discharge. Oropharynx is benign with no obvious mucosal lesions, although the tongue does deviate slightly to the right

Neck/LN

Neck is supple and without adenopathy or thyromegaly; no JVD

Lungs/Thorax

Breathing labored with tachypnea. The right side is CTA with diminished breath sounds throughout. The LUL is CTA with severely diminished breath sounds. She was unable to cooperate with E-to-A assessment. However, the LLL has the absence of breath sounds and dullness to percussion

CV

Tachycardic with regular rhythm; normal S_1, S_2; (–) S_3 or S_4

Abd

Normoactive BS; soft; NT

Genit/Rect

Deferred

MS/Ext

No CCE; strength is 4/5 throughout and symmetric. Pulses are 1+ bilaterally

Neuro

A & O × 1; oriented to place only. Responds to name. CNs II–XII intact. DTRs 2+; Babinski normal

Labs

Na 142 mEq/mL	Hgb 13.0 g/dL	Ca 8.2 mEq/L
K 3.5 mEq/mL	Hct 32%	Mg 1.3 mEq/L
Cl 99 mEq/ml	WBC 7.7 × 10^3/mm^3	Phos 2.7 mg/dL
CO_2 40 mEq/L	55% Neutros	CPK 36 IU/L
BUN 20 mg/dL	5% Bands	
SCr 1.3 mg/dL	34% Lymphs	
Glu 86 mg/dL	6% Monos	

UA

Hazy; SG 1.018, pH 6.0, glucose (–), protein (–), ketones (–), blood (–), bilirubin (–), nitrite (–), leukocyte esterase (–), occasional WBC/hpf, (–) RBC/hpf, (–) bacteria.

Chest X-Ray

Consolidation of the inferior segments of the LLL as well as the superior segment of the LLL. Remainder of the lungs are clear. Heart size is WNL.

Sputum Gram Stain

Very small quantity of sputum obtained with difficulty. Few WBC, many epithelial cells, few Gram (+) cocci in chains and pairs

Sputum and Blood Cultures

Pending

Assessment

Probable LLL pneumonia, etiology unknown.
Hypoxemia.

▶ Questions

Problem Identification

1. a. *Create a list of the patient's drug therapy problems.*
   b. *What information (signs, symptoms, laboratory and other diagnostic tests) indicates the presence of community-acquired pneumonia (CAP)?*
   c. *What are the common "typical" and "atypical" pathogens that can cause pneumonia?*
   d. *What signs and symptoms indicate the severity of CAP in this patient?*
   e. *What additional information is needed to satisfactorily assess this patient?*

Desired Outcome

2. *What are the goals of pharmacotherapy in this case?*

Therapeutic Alternatives

3. *What feasible pharmacotherapeutic alternatives are available for treatment of CAP?*

Optimal Plan

4. a. *What drug, dosage form, dose, schedule, and duration of therapy are best for this patient?*

▶ Clinical Course

The patient was immediately given O_2 by nasal cannula and admitted to the hospital. She was treated with the antimicrobial regimen you recommended. Her hypoxemia, tachypnea, tachycardia and mental status improved with oxygen therapy and supportive care during the 48 hours after treatment was initiated. However, her weakness and chills remain. Laboratory result changes include a WBC of $11.0 \times 10^3/mm^3$ and 2 of 3 blood cultures grew Gram-positive cocci in pairs and chains (*Streptococcus pneumoniae*). Repeat chest radiograph showed further consolidation of LLL pneumonia.

   b. *Given this new information, what changes in the antimicrobial therapy would you recommend?*

Outcome Evaluation

5. a. *What clinical and laboratory parameters are necessary to evaluate the therapy for achievement of the desired therapeutic outcome and to detect or prevent adverse events?*
   b. *At what point is it suitable to change from IV to oral therapy?*

▶ Clinical Course

The patient improved after the changes in therapy you recommended were implemented. On the ninth hospital day, she was discharged on gatifloxacin 400 mg po once daily for 14 days to be completed as an outpatient.

Patient Education

6. *What information should be provided to the patient about gatifloxacin to enhance compliance, ensure successful therapy, and minimize adverse events?*

▶ Self-Study Assignments

1. Compare and contrast the three most recent guidelines for treatment of community-acquired pneumonia from the Infectious Diseases Society of America (IDSA), the Centers for Disease Control and Prevention, and the American Thoracic Society (ATS).[2–4]
2. Determine appropriate pharmacotherapy recommendations for empiric outpatient treatment of community-acquired pneumonia.[2–4]
3. Identify how long it takes for the symptoms of pneumonia (e.g., cough, dyspnea, and fatigue) to resolve.[5]
4. What is the role of short-course treatment of community-acquired pneumonia?

▶ Clinical Pearl

Most community-acquired pneumonia trials excluded patients with HIV infection or presentation from a nursing home. These patients are likely to present with different signs and symptoms as well as pneumonia microbiologic etiology due to their underlying illness(es). With limited clinical trial information, much of the recommendations for these patients are based on expert opinion only.

References

1. Halm EA, Teirstein AS. Management of community-acquired pneumonia. N Engl J Med 2002;347:2039–2045.
2. Mandell LA, Bartlett JG, Dowell SF, et al. Update of practice guidelines for the management of community-acquired pneumonia in immunocompetent adults. Infectious Diseases Society of America. Clin Infect Dis 2003;37:1405–1433.
3. Heffelfinger JD, Dowell SF, Jorgensen JH, et al. Management of community-acquired pneumonia in the era of pneumococcal resistance: A report from the Drug-Resistant Streptococcus pneumoniae Therapeutic Working Group. Arch Intern Med 2000;160:1399–1408.
4. Niederman MS, Mandell LA, Anzueto A, et al. Guidelines for the management of adults with community-acquired pneumonia. Diagnosis, assessment of severity, antimicrobial therapy, and prevention. Am J Respir Crit Care Med 2001;163:1730–1754.
5. Fine MJ, Stone RA, Singer DE, et al. Process and outcomes of care for patients with community-acquired pneumonia: Results from the Pneumonia Patient Outcomes Research Team (PORT) cohort study. Arch Intern Med 1999;159:970–980.
6. Mandell LA, File TM. Short-course treatment of community-acquired pneumonia. Clin Infect Dis 2003;37:761–763.

112 OTITIS MEDIA

▶ Sophie's Sick Ear (Level II)

Patrick P. Gleason, PharmD, BCPS
Steven V. Johnson, PharmD, BCPS

▶ After completing this case study, students should be able to:

- Identify the signs and symptoms of acute otitis media (AOM).
- Identify risk factors associated with an increased incidence of AOM.
- Identify the pathogens most commonly causing AOM.
- Recommend an effective and economical antibiotic regimen including specific agent(s), route of administration, and dose(s).
- Recognize the role of delaying antibiotic therapy for AOM.
- Educate parents about recommended drug therapy using appropriate non-technical terminology.

PATIENT PRESENTATION

Chief Complaint
"My ear is sick and hurts."

HPI
Sophie Pittenger is a 3 yo girl who is brought to her pediatrician in early February with a 1-day history of right ear pain and crying, and a 2-day history of decreased appetite and difficulty sleeping. Mom states that her temperature last night was normal by electronic axial thermometer (37.0°C). Last night Sophie was given acetaminophen, but the pain was not improved and none has been given today. When Sophie is asked if anything hurts, she points to her right ear and says "my ear is sick and hurts".

PMH
Former 41-week, 3.5-kg healthy infant at birth.

Immunizations are up-to-date, including 7-valent pneumococcal vaccination (Prevnar).

First episode of AOM at age 9 months. Recurrent AOM × 1 over the past 12 months; most recent episode 7 months ago treated successfully with Augmentin. The only adverse effect was significant diarrhea with Augmentin.

Sophie was seen approximately 1 month ago for a persistent nonproductive cough of 1-week duration. A diagnosis of bronchitis was made and a trial of albuterol nebulization did not improve the condition. Per parents, the cough improved after installation of a humidifier in Sophie's room.

FH
Parents both in good health. One sibling, 6 years old, in good health.

SH
Sophie lives at home with her parents, who are both employed. She attends day care. Parents are non-smokers. There is a pet cat in the home.

Meds
Acetaminophen PRN for the last 24 hours (none in the past 12 hours)

All
NKDA

PE

Gen
WDWN white female, now crying

VS
BP 110/60, HR 132, RR 36, T 37.8°C; Wt 15.8 kg, Ht 90 cm

HEENT
Both TMs erythematous (with R > L); right TM non-bulging, and mobile with slight purulent fluid behind TM; both TMs landmarks appear normal including the pars flaccida, the malleus, and the light reflex below the umbo. However, the Left TM landmarks are more clear then the right landmarks. Throat is erythematous; nares patent

Neck
Supple

Chest
Some crackles at bases bilaterally, but improved since last visit (1 month ago).

CV
RRR

Abd
Soft, non-tender

Genit
Tanner stage I

Ext
No c/c/e; moves all extremities well; warm, pink, no rashes

Neuro
Responsive to stimulation, DTR 2+ no clonus, CNs intact

Assessment
Possible Right Ear AOM

▶ Questions

Problem Identification

1. a. *Create a drug therapy problem list for this patient.*
   b. *What subjective and objective data support the diagnosis of acute otitis media (AOM), and is the diagnosis certain or uncertain in this case?*
   c. *How is the severity of otitis media determined?*
   d. *What risk factors for AOM are present in this child?*

Desired Outcome

2. *What are the goals of pharmacotherapy for AOM in this child?*

Therapeutic Alternatives

3. a. *What bacterial organisms typically cause AOM?*
   b. *What pharmacotherapeutic alternatives are available for treatment of AOM in this patient?*
   c. *Should this patient receive antibiotic therapy at this time, or should watchful waiting (observation) be the course of action? Defend your answer.*

Optimal Plan

4. *If antibiotics are indicated, which of the alternatives would you recommend to treat this child's AOM? Include the dose, duration of therapy, and rationale for your selection.*

Outcome Evaluation

5. *How should the therapy you recommended be monitored for efficacy and adverse effects?*

Patient Education

6. *How would you provide important information about this therapy to the child's mother and/or father?*

▶ Self-Study Assignments

1. Describe a scenario in which it would be appropriate to use azithromycin to treat AOM.
2. Review the literature for evidence supporting antibiotic prophylaxis therapy in children with frequent ear infections.

▶ Clinical Pearl

Middle-ear fluid is present for one month after resolution of AOM in 50% of children, regardless of whether they received antibiotic therapy or placebo. Fluid clears by 3 months in 90% of children whether or not they receive antibiotics.

References

1. American Academy of Pediatrics Subcommittee on Management of Acute Otitis Media. Diagnosis and management of acute otitis media. Pediatrics 2004;113:1451–1465. http://www.aap.org/policy/paramtoc.html (Accessed July 27, 2004).
2. Rothman R, Owens T, Simel DL. Does this child have acute otitis media? JAMA 2003;290:1633–1640.
3. Hendley JO. Otitis Media. N Engl J Med 2002;347:1169–1174.
4. Siegel RM, Kiely M, Bien JP, et al. Treatment of otitis media with observation and a safety-net antibiotic prescription. Pediatrics 2003;112(3 Pt 1):527–531.
5. O'Neill P. Clinical evidence: Acute otitis media. BMJ 1999;319:833–835.
6. New York Regional Otitis Project. Observation option toolkit for acute otitis media. State of New York, Department of Health, Publication #4894, March 2002. www.health.state.ny.us/nysdoh/antibiotic/antibiotic.htm (Accessed July 21, 2004)

113 STREPTOCOCCAL PHARYNGITIS

▶ It's Not Just a Sore Throat (Level I)

Denise L. Howrie, PharmD
Elaine McGhee, MD

▶ After completing this case study, students should be able to:

- Identify patient-specific information including signs and symptoms, medical history, and findings on physical examination that support the diagnosis of Group A β-hemolytic streptococcal (GABHS) pharyngitis.
- Describe appropriate diagnostic tools for evaluating infectious pharyngitis.
- Compare commonly prescribed antibacterial agents with regard to spectrum, efficacy, and appropriateness of selection for GABHS pharyngitis.
- List common causes of anti-infective treatment failure in GABHS pharyngitis and recommend appropriate management strategies.

PATIENT PRESENTATION

Chief Complaint

"My throat hurts."

HPI

Katie Smith is a 5 yo girl who has been ill for 2 days with sore throat and fever of 38.2°C (axillary). Her appetite has been decreased for solid foods, but fluid intake has been adequate; she has also complained that her head hurts and she feels hot. There have been no vomiting or cold symptoms. No one else in the family is ill at the present time, although her mother states that "there's strep in the school."

PMH

Katie was the 8-lb, 7-oz product of a full-term pregnancy who was breast-fed and supplemented with formula
Hospitalizations: age 2 months for dacryocystitis
Development: normal for age
Three episodes of otitis media (last episode 10 months ago)

One episode of pneumonia at age 9 months
One episode of "strep throat" 3 months ago
Immunizations: up to date

FH
Noncontributory

ROS
Negative except for complaints noted in the HPI

Meds
None

All
NKDA

PE

VS
BP 92/50, HR 124, RR 20, T 37.°C (oral); Wt 49.5 lb.

Gen
Child is alert and oriented but irritable and uncooperative

Skin
No rashes

HEENT
Tonsils 3+, bright red, with white exudate; soft palate erythematous; tongue with strawberry appearance; TMs translucent

Neck/LN
Several small mobile anterior lymph nodes

Chest
CTA

CV
RRR, S_1 and S_2 normal, no murmurs

Abd
Soft, normal bowel sounds, no HSM

MS
Muscle strength and tone 5/5

CNS
CN II–XII intact, DTRs 2+

Labs
Rapid streptococcal antigen test positive

Assessment
A 5-year-old female with her second episode of GABHS pharyngitis.

▶ Questions

Problem Identification

1. a. *Create a list of the patient's drug therapy problem(s).*
   b. *What information indicates the presence or severity of pharyngitis?*
   c. *How can the diagnosis of streptococcal pharyngitis best be made in a timely manner?*

Desired Outcome

2. *State the goals of treatment of GABHS pharyngitis in this case.*

Therapeutic Alternatives

3. a. *What nondrug therapies may be helpful in this child?*
   b. *What therapeutic alternatives are available for treatment of pharyngitis?*

Optimal Plan

4. a. *What drug, dosage form, dose, schedule, and duration of therapy are best for this patient?*
   b. *What alternatives would be appropriate if the initial therapy cannot be used?*
   c. *If the child's symptoms recur after completion of the prescribed regimen, what options are then available?*

Outcome Evaluation

5. *What clinical and laboratory parameters are necessary to evaluate the therapy for achievement of the desired outcome and to detect or prevent adverse effects?*

Patient Education

6. *What information should be provided to the patient's parents to enhance compliance, ensure success of therapy, and minimize adverse effects?*

▶ Self-Study Assignments

1. Select five antibacterial agents that may be prescribed for treatment of GABHS pharyngitis in this child. Calculate and compare costs of therapy based upon recommended doses, available liquid formulations, and available units (i.e., suspension volumes/bottle).
2. Interview 10 parents about recent use of antibiotics in his/her child, including indications for use, use with/without diagnostic tests including bacterial cultures, whether antibiotics are routinely requested and why. Comment on your survey results and your conclusions regarding the appropriate or inappropriate use of antibiotics in these families.

▶ Clinical Pearl

Symptoms resolve within several days in the majority of patients with GABHS pharyngitis, regardless of whether antibiotics are prescribed.

References

1. Bisno AL. Acute pharyngitis. N Engl J Med 2001;344:205–211.
2. Bisno AL. Gerber MA, Gwaltney JM, et al. Practice guidelines for the diagnosis and management of group A streptococcal pharyngitis. Infectious Diseases Society of America. Clin Infect Dis 2002;35:113–125.
3. McIsaac WJ, Kellner JD, Aufricht P, et al. Empirical validation of guidelines for the management of pharyngitis in children and adults. JAMA 2004:291:1587–1595.
4. Curtin-Wirt C, Casey JR, Murray PC, et al. Efficacy of penicillin vs. amoxicillin in children with group A beta hemolytic streptococcal tonsillopharyngitis. Clin Pediatr 2003;42:219–225.
5. Tan JS. Treatment recommendations for acute pharyngitis. Curr Treat Options Infect Dis 2003;5:143–150.
6. Casey JR, Pichichero ME. Meta-analysis of cephalosporin versus penicillin treatment of group A streptococcal tonsillopharyngitis in children. Pediatrics 2004;113:866–882.
7. Shulman ST, Gerber MA. So what's wrong with penicillin for strep throat? Pediatrics 2004;113:1816–1819.
8. Casey JR, Pichichero ME. Meta-analysis of cephalosporins versus penicillin for treatment of group A streptococcal tonsillopharyngitis in adults. Clin Infect Dis 2004;38:1526–1534.
9. Bisno AL. Are cephalosporins superior to penicillin for treatment of acute streptococcal pharyngitis? Clin Infect Dis 2004;38:1535–1537.

114 RHINOSINUSITIS

▶ Head Case (Level II)

Steven V. Johnson PharmD, BCPS
Patrick P. Gleason PharmD, BCPS

▶ After completing this case study, students should be able to:

- Recognize the differences in clinical features between acute bacterial, acute viral, and inflammatory rhinosinusitis.
- Identify the most common organisms that cause acute bacterial rhinosinusitis.
- Identify the role of antibiotic therapy for acute bacterial rhinosinusitis.
- Identify the signs and symptoms of severe infection that necessitate prompt antibiotic therapy.

PATIENT PRESENTATION

Chief Complaint

"I have had a cold for about a month that does not seem to go away and now a headache that has lasted for at least a week."

HPI

Marlene Schuele is a 31 yo woman who presents to her PCP with purulent rhinorrhea from the L nostril, pus in the nasal cavity, and a constant headache of moderate severity that began 7 days ago. The headache is not consistent with her typical migraines. It is most often in the left temporal region but sometimes occurs bilaterally with forehead involvement. She states that it feels as though her head is in a vice grip when she bends over, such as when she ties her shoes. She says it all started about a month ago and was typical of a common cold that she gets three or four times a year. She had nasal congestion, sneezing, runny nose, and fatigue. Her sneezing stopped, but she says that her nasal congestion continues and has actually worsened. She said she went to the emergency department 2 weeks ago and was told she had sinusitis and was given a prescription for a "Z-pack". She now reports a thick yellow-green discharge that continually drains and is not relieved by Sudafed. She developed a fever 4 days ago and also has a dry cough that worsens during the night. She says she thinks she got better on the antibiotic but is not really sure.

PMH

Migraine headaches, 1 to 2 per month

FH

Father with HTN
Mother with IDDM × 30 years

SH

Denies smoking and IVDU. Has 3 to 4 glasses of wine a week with dinner. She is married and has a 5-year-old son.

Meds

Ortho-Novum 1/35–28
Tylenol ES PRN headaches
Tylenol PM to help sleep
Zomig 5 mg PRN for migraine (1 to 2 times/month)

All

PCN → rash

PE

Gen

Tired looking white female in NAD

VS

BP 110/72, HR 81, RR 16, T 38.3°C; Wt 61 kg, Ht 5′

HEENT

PERRLA; funduscopy normal. Tortuous, injected conjunctivae; anicteric sclerae. Mild nasal crusting and mucosal hypertrophy (L > R) without evidence of polyp formation. Thick purulent mucus-filled postnasal discharge; no oral lesions; tympanic membranes intact. No periorbital swelling. Ears non-erythematous and non-bulging; throat is erythematous

Neck

Supple, no JVD or lymphadenopathy

Chest

CTA; equal air entry bilaterally; no crackles or wheezing

CV

S_1, S_2 normal; no S_3 or S_4; regular rate and rhythm

Abd

Soft, non-tender, bowel sounds present

Ext

No C/C/E

Neuro

Oriented to person, place, and time. Deep sensation and visual fields intact. CN II–XII intact

Labs

None drawn

Questions

Problem Identification

1. a. *Create a drug therapy problem list for this patient.*
   b. *What subjective and objective data support the diagnosis of acute bacterial sinusitis vs. viral vs. inflammatory rhinosinusitis?*
   c. *Is this patient considered to have a severe infection?*

Desired Outcome

2. *What are the goals of pharmacotherapy in this patient?*

Therapeutic Alternatives

3. a. *What are the most likely causative organisms in this patient?*
   b. *What antibiotics and dosage regimens are alternatives for this patient?*
   c. *What are the most likely reasons why this patient has an infection despite receiving previous antibiotic therapy?*

Optimal Plan

4. a. *Based on the patient's presentation, what antibiotic would you recommend for therapy? Include drug name, dosage form, schedule, and duration of therapy.*
   b. *What adjunctive measures can be employed to optimize this patient's medical therapy?*

Outcome Evaluation

5. *How should the therapy you recommend be monitored for efficacy and adverse effects?*

Patient Education

6. *How would you inform the patient about her therapeutic regimen?*

► Follow-Up Question

1. *For questions related to the use of Echinacea for the treatment of upper respiratory tract infections, please see Section 20 of this Casebook.*

► Self-Study Assignments

1. What is considered to be the "gold standard" for diagnosing acute bacterial rhinosinusitis and why is it rarely done in clinical practice?
2. What is the incidence of cross reactivity of cephalosporin allergy in patients with a documented penicillin allergy?
3. Is a change in mucus color from clear to yellow or green an indication of a bacterial infection, or is that the natural course of a viral infection?

Clinical Pearl

Most cases of acute sinusitis are caused by a viral infection, but an antibiotic is prescribed in 85% to 98% of cases. The illness often resolves in otherwise-healthy patients without antibiotic treatment, even if it is bacterial in origin. Only 0.2% to 2% of viral upper respiratory tract infections in adults are complicated by bacterial rhinosinusitis.

References

1. Agency for Health Care Policy and Research. Evidence Report/Technology Assessment Number 9. Diagnosis and treatment of acute bacterial rhinosinusitis. AHCPR Publication No. 99-E016. 1999. Summary available on the Internet at www.ahcpr.gov/clinic/epcsums/sinussum.htm. Accessed July 23, 2004.
2. Sinus and Allergy Health Partnership. Antimicrobial treatment guidelines for acute bacterial rhinosinusitis. Otolaryngol Head Neck Surg 2004;130(1):1–45.
3. Snow V, Mottur-Pilson C, Hickner JM. Principles of appropriate antibiotic use for acute sinusitis in adults. Ann Intern Med 2001;134:495–497.
4. Hickner JM, Bartlett JG, Besser RE, et al. Principles of appropriate antibiotic use for acute rhinosinusitis in adults: Background. Ann Intern Med 2001;134:498–505.
5. Williams JW Jr, Aguilar C, Cornell J, et al. Antibiotics for acute maxillary sinusitis (Cochrane Review). In: The Cochrane Library, Issue 3, 2004. Available on the Internet at: www.update-software.com/abstracts/AB000243.htm. Accessed July 23, 2004.

115 PRESSURE SORES

► When Life Gets You Down (Level III)

Richard S. Rhodes, PharmD
Catherine A. Heyneman, PharmD, MS
Christopher T. Owens, PharmD

► After completing this case study, students should be able to:

- Comprehend the etiology and pathophysiology of pressure sores (decubitus ulcers).

- Understand pressure ulcer risk assessment and classification.
- Identify conditions or risk factors that predispose individuals to pressure ulceration.
- Recommend different options for treating decubitus ulcers.
- Define goals, strategies, and interventions for prevention of decubitus ulcers.

PATIENT PRESENTATION

Chief Complaint

"I have raw places on my back and rear that really hurt."

HPI

William Anderson is an 84 y/o man who was just admitted to the Hill Side Nursing Home complaining of constant pain and tenderness on his lower back and buttock. The pain started approximately 4 weeks ago and has gotten progressively worse. His wife noticed that he had several sores that started as areas of redness and have evolved to open wounds displaying small amounts of drainage.

PMH

COPD × 11 years
Urinary overflow incontinence × 10 years
Depression × 2 years
DJD; hip fracture 7 years ago
Trace heme (+) stool → (–) × 3 in the last year

FH

Father and brother were mine workers and died at ages 68 and 62 from complications of silicosis. Mother died of "old age" at 88 years of age.

SH

Retired at age 65 after 45 years as a mine worker; completed high school. 60+ year h/o cigarette use which continues; heavy EtOH abuse × 50+ years. Married for 52 years; wife is 75 yo and in relatively good health but is unable to provide adequate care for her husband at home; one son. Patient has spent all of his time in bed for the past 9 months because of chronic illnesses (depression, DJD, COPD). His wife is physically unable to assist with his ambulation.

Meds

Nortriptyline 50 mg po once daily
Ipratropium bromide MDI 2 puffs QID
Baclofen 10 mg po once daily
Lorazepam 0.5 mg po TID
Acetaminophen 325 mg po Q 4–6 H PRN
Alkanna Root applied topically to sores BID

All

NKDA

ROS

In addition to complaints noted above, he also has pain in his joints that hurt too much to get out of bed. Because the pain occurs with any physical activity and because of his difficulty breathing on exertion he wants to "just stay in bed." He reports trouble sleeping and also feels sad and depressed most of the time. Patient admits wetting himself at least 5 times a week due to an inability to "make it to the bathroom on time" to urinate. He states he doesn't belong in a nursing home and feels he was admitted because no one wanted him.

PE

Gen

Ill-appearing, frail, elderly man; pale, weak, slightly overweight, rigid in appearance, slightly confused; responds to questions slowly, in apparent discomfort

VS

BP 152/76, P 85, RR 28, T 37°C; Wt 95.3 kg, Ht 5′10″

Skin

Overall fair to poor skin turgor, diffuse macular rash on the ischial and sacral area. The sacral area revealed 2 areas of denuded skin above and on either side of the anal opening, measuring 1 cm × 2 cm (right buttock) and 3 cm × 3 cm (left buttock) surrounded by 2 cm of erythema around the outer edges, with creamy, yellowish, sloughing of necrotic tissue with some drainage. These shallow craters involving the epidermis are characteristic of stage II decubitus ulcers (see Figure 115–1) and do not appear to be clinically infected at this time. Immediately over and covering the coccyx is a stage I decubitus ulcer displaying a small 1 cm × 1 cm erythematous area of tender, intact skin.

HEENT

PERRLA, EOMI; TMs intact, oropharynx clear, funduscopic exam normal; tongue and mucous membranes slightly dry, nares and throat clear

Lungs/Thorax

Breath sounds decreased bilaterally, chest is resonant on percussion, diffuse breath sounds on auscultation, wheezes present bilaterally on inspiration and expiration, slight rhonchi without rales

CV

Normal heart sounds, RRR, no m/r/g

Abd

Soft, NT/ND, normal BS, no masses

Genit/Rect

Normal male genitalia, slightly enlarged prostate, normal sphincter tone, guaiac (–)

MS/Ext

No CCE, normal appearing musculature for patient's age, stiffness in hands and knees consistent with DJD, peripheral pulses palpable (PPP) bilaterally. Hand stiffness bilaterally, slight swelling of MCPs and PIPs of right hand. Knee stiffness, but no visible swelling or inflammation of either knee; ↓ ROM. Wrists, elbows, shoulders, and ankles have normal ROM, without swelling

Neuro

A and O × 2, slightly confused, memory intact, diminished DTRs (L > R), no motor or sensory deficits, CNs intact

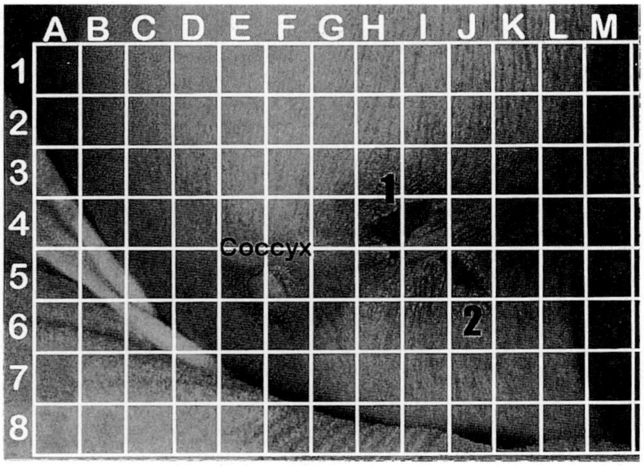

Figure 115–1. Photograph of a patient with 2 small stage II decubitus ulcers on the right and left buttock below the coccyx (marked 1 and 2). *(Reprinted with permission from: Rhodes RS, Heyneman CA, Culbertson VL, et al. Topical phenytoin treatment of stage II decubitus ulcers in the elderly. Ann Pharmacother 2001;35(6):675–681.)*

Labs

Sodium 139 mEq/L	Hgb 13.2 g/dL	AST 52 IU/L	T. chol 218 mg/dL
Potassium 5.2 mEq/L	Hct 43.0%	ALT 44 IU/L	Trig 60 mg/dL
Chloride 101 mEq/L	Plt 276 × 10^3/mm^3	Alk Phos 68 IU/L	Uric acid 4.0 mg/dL
CO_2 24 mEq/L	WBC 11.0 × 10^3/mm^3	GGT 22 IU/L	Iron 88 μg/dL
BUN 11 mg/dL	63% Neutros	LDH 208 IU/L	T_4 5.9 μg/dL
SCr 1.4 mg/dL	25% Lymphs	T. bili 1.1 mg/dL	TSH 1.8 mIU/L
Glu 122 mg/dL	10% Monos	T. prot 6.0 g/dL	
Ca 8.5 mg/dL	1% Eos	Alb 3.1 g/dL	
Phos 2.7 mg/dL	1% Basos	Glob 2.5 g/dL	

UA

Color yellow, appearance clear; glucose (–), ketones (–), bilirubin (–), SG 1.02, blood (–), pH 5.5, urobilinogen 0.2 mg/dL, nitrite (–), leukocyte esterases (–)

ABG

pH 7.37, po_2 71 mm Hg, pco_2 44 mm Hg, HCO_3 26 mEq/L, BE –1 mEq/L, O_2 sat 92%, +O_2 16.0 vol %, tHgb 14.3 g/dL, CO-Hgb 6%

Questions

Problem Identification

1. a. *Create a list of the patient's drug therapy problems.*
   b. *Which of the patient's medical problems contribute to the development of pressure sores?*
   c. *List other risk factors (whether or not they are present in this patient) that predispose individuals to the development of pressure sores.*

Desired Outcome

2. *What are the goals of treatment for this patient's pressure sores?*

Therapeutic Alternatives

3. a. *What therapeutic interventions are available for treatment of the patient's pressure sores?*
   b. *What economic issues should be considered when making plans to prevent or treat pressure sores?*

Optimal Plan

4. a. *What drug dosage form, dose, schedule, and duration of therapy are best for this patient?*
   b. *What alternatives would be appropriate if the initial therapy fails or cannot be used?*

Outcome Evaluation

5. *Which clinical and laboratory parameters are necessary to evaluate the therapy for achievement of the desired therapeutic outcome and to detect or prevent adverse effects?*

Patient Education

6. *What information should be provided to the patient to enhance compliance, ensure successful therapy, and minimize adverse effects?*

Clinical Course

After the treatment you recommended was initiated, the sacral ulcer above and on the left side of the anal opening was completely healed on the twelfth day of therapy. The ulcer on the right was healed after 22 days of treatment. The stage I pressure sore on the coccyx evolved to a stage II decubitus ulcer and was healed after 4 weeks using the same treatment as the others. Nortriptyline was discontinued and sertraline was started at 50 mg po at bedtime, baclofen was increased to 10 mg po TID, albuterol MDI 2 puffs QID PRN was added, acetaminophen 1 g po QID was given on a regular schedule, and the herbal preparation was discontinued. These changes decreased sedation, increased mobility, improved breathing, and controlled the patient's incontinence. Osteoarthritis, difficulty sleeping, and anxiety all improved with better control of the patient's disease states.

Self-Study Assignments

1. Describe the phases of wound healing and the etiology and pathophysiology of pressure sores.
2. Perform a search of the most recent literature and develop institutional policies and procedures for the prevention and treatment of pressure sores.
3. Concerning the prevention and treatment of pressure sores, describe in your own words how you would educate a patient and/or family

on each of the following: risk factors; signs and symptoms of infection; pressure relief; body positioning; incontinence care; nutrition support; skin care; and dressing changes.

4. Describe the classification and staging of decubitus ulcers.

Clinical Pearl

The Agency for Healthcare Research and Quality publishes guidelines for clinicians and consumers on the prevention and treatment of pressure sores (www.ahcpr.gov).

References

1. Livesley NJ, Chow AW. Infected pressure ulcers in elderly individuals. Clin Infect Dis 2002;35:1390–1396.
2. Rhodes RS, Heyneman CA, Culbertson VL, et al. Topical phenytoin treatment of stage II decubitus ulcers in the elderly. Ann Pharmacother 2001;35(6):675–681.
3. Bello YM, Phillips TJ. Recent advances in wound healing. JAMA 2000;283:716–718.

116 DIABETIC FOOT INFECTION

Watch Your Step (Level II)

Renee-Claude Mercier, PharmD
A. Christie Graham, PharmD

After completing this case study, students should be able to:

- Recognize the signs and symptoms of diabetic foot infections and identify the risk factors and the most likely pathogens associated with these infections.
- Recommend appropriate antimicrobial regimens for diabetic foot infections, including for patients with drug allergies or renal insufficiency.
- Recommend appropriate home IV therapy and proper education to patients.
- Outline monitoring parameters for achievement of the desired pharmacotherapeutic outcome and prevention of adverse effects.
- Educate diabetic patients about adequate blood glucose control as part of an overall plan for good foot health.

PATIENT PRESENTATION

Chief Complaint

As per the patient's daughter: "She stepped on a piece of metal and now her foot is swollen."

HPI

Mary Littlehorse is a 65 yo Native-American woman, Navajo-speaking only, who presents to the ED complaining of a sore and swollen foot. A few days ago she stepped on a piece of metal and later noticed redness and soreness in the area which increased over the next several days. History is per translation by patient's daughter. Primary care physician is Dr. Kinder, Shiprock Indian Health Service.

PMH

Type 2 DM × 18 years
Hospitalized 6 months ago for diabetic ketoacidosis
Hypertension
Obesity
Chronic renal insufficiency
Depression

FH

Father is deceased (56 yo) secondary to MI, DM type 2, HTN
Mother is deceased secondary to breast cancer (41 yo)
One daughter, alive and well, 28 yo

SH

The patient lives with her 28 yo daughter in Shiprock, NM. She has been widowed × 2 years and has been significantly depressed since her husband's death. She denies tobacco, alcohol, and illicit drug use. She admits to non-adherence with her medications and glucometer.

Meds

Novolin 70/30 60 units Q AM and Q PM
Lisinopril 20 mg po once daily
Citalopram 20 mg po once daily
Glucotrol XL 10 mg po once daily
Trazodone 50 mg po at bedtime

All

NKDA

ROS

Negative except as noted above.

PE

Gen

The patient is an obese Native-American woman with a dull affect but in NAD

VS

BP 148/81, P 92, RR 20, T 37.4°C; Ht 5′1″, Wt 95 kg

Skin

Warm, coarse, and very dry

HEENT

PERRLA; EOMI; funduscopic exam is normal with absence of hemorrhages or exudates. TMs are clouded bilaterally but with no erythema or bulging. Oropharynx shows poor dentition but is otherwise unremarkable.

Neck/LN

Neck is supple; normal thyroid; no JVD; no lymphadenopathy

Chest

CTA

Heart

RRR, normal S_1 and S_2 with a grade I/VI systolic murmur at right sternal border

Abd

Distended, (+) BS, no guarding, no hepatosplenomegaly or masses felt

Ext

2+ edema with markedly diminished sensation of the right foot. Area of redness and induration 4 to 5 cm from portal of entry. Pedal pulses present. Pulses 2+ throughout. Normal range of motion. Poor nail care with some fungus and overgrown toenails.

Neuro

A & O × 3. CN II–XII intact. Motor system intact (overall muscle strength 4–5/5). Sensory system exam showed a decreased sensation to light touch of the lower extremities (both feet); intact upper body sensation.

Labs

Na 136 mEq/L	Hgb 12.6 g/dL
K 3.6 mEq/L	Hct 37.8%
Cl 98 mEq/L	Plt 390 × $10^3/mm^3$
CO_2 24 mEq/L	WBC 16.4 × $10^3/mm^3$
BUN 30 mg/dL	71% PMNs
SCr 1.5 mg/dL	8% Bands
Glu 181 mg/dL	15% Lymphs
HbA_{1c} 11.8%	6% Monos
ESR 18 sec	

X-Ray

Right foot: There is a metallic foreign body approximately 2 cm in length in the soft tissue inferior to the third metatarsal. No evidence of adjacent periosteal reactions or erosions to suggest radiographic evidence of osteomyelitis. No definite subcutaneous air is evident. Presence of vascular calcifications.

► Clinical Course

On the day of admission, the patient went to surgery for an I & D and removal of the foreign body. Blood and tissue specimens were sent for culture and sensitivity testing.

► Questions

Problem Identification

1. a. *Create a list of the patient's drug therapy problems.*
   b. *What signs, symptoms, or laboratory values indicate the presence of an infection?*
   c. *What risk factors for infection does the patient have?*
   d. *What organisms are most likely involved in this infection?*

Desired Outcome

2. *What are the therapeutic goals for this patient?*

Therapeutic Alternatives

3. a. *What nondrug therapies might be useful for this patient?*
   b. *What feasible pharmacotherapeutic alternatives are available for the empiric treatment of the foot infection?*
   c. *What economic and social considerations are applicable to this patient?*

Optimal Plan

4. *Outline a drug regimen that would provide optimal initial empiric therapy for the infection.*

Outcome Evaluation

5. a. *What clinical and laboratory parameters are necessary to evaluate your therapy for achievement of the desired therapeutic outcomes and monitoring for adverse effects?*

► Clinical Course

Ms. Littlehorse received the empiric therapy you recommended until the tissue cultures were reported positive for methicillin-resistant *Staphylococcus aureus (MRSA)*. The blood cultures were all found to have no growth. The patient remained hospitalized for an additional 2 weeks and received a more directed antimicrobial regimen and multiple surgical debridements of the wound. The cellulitis slowly improved over this time and multiple X-rays did not suggest osteomyelitis. She was then discharged to complete her antimicrobial regimen on an outpatient basis. Over the next 2 weeks, she received wound care at home and showed significant but slow progress in healing of the wound.

   b. *What therapeutic alternatives are available for treating this patient after results of cultures are known to contain MRSA?*
   c. *Design an optimal drug treatment plan for treating the MRSA infection during her hospitalization.*
   d. *Design an optimal pharmacotherapeutic plan for completion of her treatment after she is discharged from the hospital.*

Patient Education

6. *What information should be provided to the patient to enhance compliance, ensure successful therapy, and minimize adverse effects with IV vancomycin?*

► Self-Study Assignments

1. Review in more detail different therapeutic options available for home IV therapy, including the antimicrobial agents suitable for use, types of IV lines available, and contraindications to home IV therapy.

2. Outline the patient education you would provide for successful home IV therapy.
3. Describe how you would educate this diabetic patient about proper foot care to prevent further skin or tissue breakdown.

▶ Clinical Pearl

Treatment of diabetic foot infections with antimicrobial agents alone is often inadequate; local wound care (incision, drainage, debridement and amputation), good glycemic control, and immobilization of the limb are often required.

References

1. Levin ME. Management of the diabetic foot: Preventing amputation. South Med J 2002;95(1):10–20.
2. Lipsky BA, Pecoraro RE, Wheat LJ. The diabetic foot: Soft tissue and bone infection. Infect Dis Clin North Am 1990:4:409–432.
3. Lipsky BA, Pecoraro RE, Larson SA, et al. Outpatient management of uncomplicated lower-extremity infections in diabetic patients. Arch Intern Med 1990; 150:790–797.
4. Lipsky BA, Baker PD, Landon GC, et al. Antibiotic therapy for diabetic foot infections: Comparison of two parenteral-to-oral regimens. Clin Infect Dis 1997; 24:643–648.

117 INFECTIVE ENDOCARDITIS

▶ Don't Let Yourself Vegetate (Level II)

Manjunath P. Pai, PharmD
Renata Smith, PharmD
Keith A. Rodvold, PharmD, FCCP, BCPS

▶ After completing this case study, students should be able to:

- Identify the signs and symptoms of infective endocarditis.
- Select appropriate antimicrobial therapy based on a particular organism and the patient's drug allergies.
- Develop a penicillin desensitization protocol for patients allergic to penicillin.
- Recognize common adverse reactions of the chosen drug therapy and establish monitoring parameters.
- Identify candidates for outpatient antimicrobial therapy (OPAT) of infective endocarditis.
- Educate inpatients who are being discharged on OPAT for completion of infective endocarditis therapy.

PATIENT PRESENTATION

Chief Complaint

"I have been having fevers all week long"

HPI

Maya Corazo is a 33 yo woman who presents to the ED with complaints of fever, chills, nausea, vomiting, and anorexia. These symptoms developed approximately 2 weeks ago. The patient had her tooth extracted a month earlier and does not recall receiving any antibiotics either prior to or after that procedure.

PMH

Endocarditis diagnosed 4 years ago
Mitral valve replacement 4 years ago (porcine)
Hepatitis C diagnosed 6 years ago

FH

Noncontributory

SH

h/o IVDA (heroin and cocaine) for 10 years with last use 3 days PTA; denies EtOH use, smokes 1 pack/day and has a 10 pack-year tobacco history.

Meds

Tylenol 650 mg po Q 4–6 H PRN headaches
Warfarin 3 mg po once daily

All

Penicillin

ROS

Noncontributory except for complaints noted above.

PE

Gen
Patient is a cachectic woman in mild distress

VS
BP 81/54, P 118, RR 24, T 38.9°C; Ht 5′4″, Wt 48 kg (Wt 56 kg 4 months ago)

Skin/Nails
No evidence of petechiae, Janeway lesions, Osler nodes, or splinter hemorrhages. Multiple tattoos, numerous "track" marks

HEENT
Anicteric sclerae, PERRLA, pink conjunctivae, dry oral mucosa, no Roth spots; poor dentition.

Neck
No lymphadenopathy, JVD, or thyromegaly

CV
RRR, normal S_1 and S_2, S_3 present, II–III/VI SEM at LLSB

Lungs
Crackles in RLL; no wheezing

Abd
Soft with mild diffuse tenderness, no hepatomegaly, no splenomegaly

Genit/Rect
Normal; guaiac negative stool

Ext
Reflexes bilaterally 4/5 UE, 3/5 LE, Babinski decreased; no edema

Neuro
Non-focal; A & O × 3, (–) asterixis

Labs

Na 133 mEq/dL	Hgb 11.1 g/dL	WBC 25.4 × 10^3/mm^3
K 3.6 mEq/dL	Hct 32.6%	78% Neutros
Cl 91 mEq/dL	Plt 80 × 10^3/mm^3	8% Bands
CO_2 21 mEq/L	RDW 17.3%	12% Lymphs
BUN 45 mg/dL	MCV 81.1 μm^3	2% Monos
SCr 1.7 mg/dL	MCH 26.3 pg/cell	Alb 2.6 g/dL
Glu 145 mg/dL	MCHC 34 g/dL	INR 2.6
		ESR 93 mm/h

Urine Toxicology Screen
(+) Opiates, (–) barbiturates, (+) cocaine, (+) THC

ECG
Non-specific T-wave changes; increased QTc interval

Two-Dimensional Echocardiogram (Transthoracic)
2-cm pedunculated vegetation on the tricuspid valve with severe tricuspid regurgitation. Moderate left ventricular hypertrophy (see Figure 117–1 for location of heart valves and other cardiac structures).

Blood Cultures
3 of 3 sets (+) for *Staphylococcus aureus* (collection times: 13:40, 15:20, 16:15).

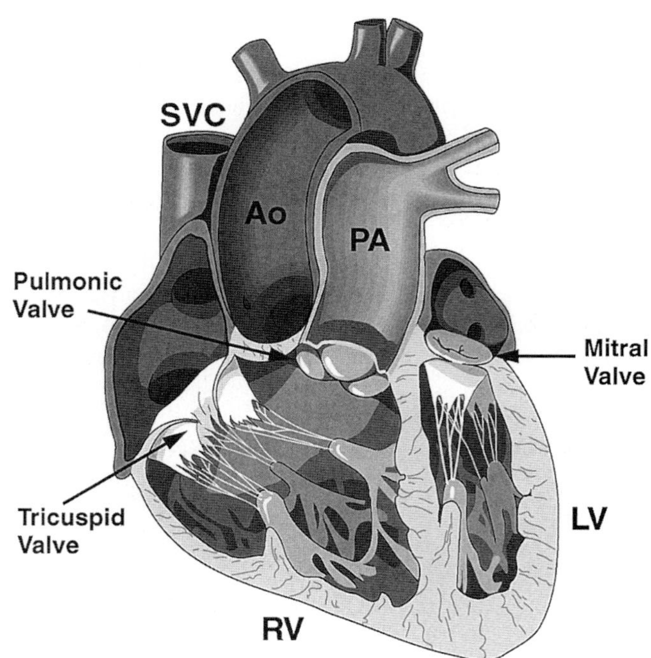

Figure 117–1. Diagram illustrating the location of the tricuspid, pulmonic, and mitral valves. SVC, superior vena cava, Ao, aorta; PA, pulmonary artery, RV, right ventricle, LV, left ventricle.

▶ Questions

Problem Identification

1. a. *Identify all of the drug therapy problems of this patient.*
   b. *What signs, symptoms, and other information indicate the presence of endocarditis in this patient?*
   c. *What risk factors does this patient have for developing endocarditis?*
   d. *Based on this patient's risk factors and location of the vegetation, does this patient have right-sided or left-sided endocarditis?*
   e. *What additional information (laboratory tests or patient information) is needed to satisfactorily assess this patient?*

Desired Outcome

2. *What are the goals of pharmacotherapy for infective endocarditis?*

▶ Clinical Course

The patient was started on empiric vancomycin with doses adjusted for her decreased renal function until susceptibilities for the *S. aureus* isolate became available. Susceptibility testing subsequently showed the organism to be sensitive to oxacillin, vancomycin, gentamicin, trimethoprim-sulfamethoxazole, cefazolin, linezolid, quinupristin/dalfopristin, and daptomycin. The organism was resistant to penicillin. When questioned about her penicillin allergy, the patient reported that she developed a bad rash, had shortness of breath, and "swelled up."

Therapeutic Alternatives

3. a. *What nondrug therapies might be used to treat this patient's endocarditis?*
   b. *Identify the therapeutic alternatives for the treatment of* S. aureus *endocarditis based on the organism's susceptibilities. Include the drug names, doses, dosage forms, schedules, and durations of therapy in your answer.*

Optimal Plan

4. a. *What is the most appropriate treatment plan for this patient (give drug name, dose, dosage form, schedule, and duration of therapy).*

▶ Clinical Course

After 8 days of IV vancomycin therapy, the patient's blood cultures are still positive. The organism continues to have the same susceptibilities.

b. *Given this new information, what is an appropriate, nonsurgical, therapeutic alternative for this patient?*

c. *Explain how you would desensitize this patient to penicillin, and provide your new treatment recommendations assuming that desensitization is successful.*

Outcome Evaluation

5. a. *What clinical and laboratory parameters should be monitored to evaluate the efficacy of therapy and to prevent adverse reactions?*

► Clinical Course

The patient has been treated for 8 days with vancomycin followed by 2 weeks of the therapy chosen in question 4.c. Blood cultures became negative 4 days after the new regimen was instituted. She is now afebrile (T_{max} 36.3°C), her white count is normalizing (WBC $10.4 \times 10^3/mm^3$ with no bands), her ESR is now 33 mm/h, she is feeling much better, and she wishes to leave the hospital now.

b. *Based on your assessment of this patient's response and her past history, what alternatives are available for completing her course of therapy?*

Patient Education

6. *If this patient is discharged home to complete her regimen on oral antibiotics, what information should be provided to her to enhance adherence and ensure successful therapy?*

► Self-Study Assignments

1. Compare the clinical data supporting the role of β-lactams versus glycopeptides for the management of methicillin-susceptible *Staphylococcus aureus* infective endocarditis.
2. Determine potential dosing regimens for patients with no drug allergies who have right-sided *S. aureus* endocarditis and who are on hemodialysis.
3. Evaluate clinical data supporting the role of rifampin as an adjunctive therapy for the management of prosthetic valve infective endocarditis

► Clinical Pearl

A recurrence of fever during the third and fourth week of therapy for infective endocarditis is more often related to hypersensitivity to β-lactam antibiotics than to treatment failure.

References

1. Dajani AS, Taubert KA, Wilson W, et al. Prevention of bacterial endocarditis: Recommendation by the American Heart Association. JAMA 1997;277:1794–1801.
2. Mylonakis E, Calderwood SB. Infective endocarditis in adults. N Engl J Med 2001;345:1318–1330.
3. Olaison L, Pettersson G. Current best practices and guidelines indications for surgical intervention in infective endocarditis. Infect Dis Clin North Am 2002;16:453–475.
4. Wilson WR, Karchmer AW, Dajani AS, et al. Antibiotic treatment of adults with infective endocarditis due to streptococci, enterococci, staphylococci, and HACEK microorganisms. JAMA 1995;274:1706–1713.
5. Fortun J, Navas E, Martinez-Beltran J, et al. Short-course therapy for right-side endocarditis due to *Staphylococcus aureus* in drug abusers: Cloxacillin versus glycopeptides in combination with gentamicin. Clin Infect Dis 2001;33:120–125.
6. DiNubile MJ. Short-course antibiotic therapy for right-sided endocarditis caused by *Staphylococcus aureus* in injection drug users. Ann Intern Med 1994;121:873–876.
7. Pryka RD, Rodvold KA, Erdman SM. An updated comparison of drug dosing methods. Part IV: Vancomycin. Clin Pharmacokinet 1991;20:463–476.
8. Andrews MM, von Reyn CF. Patient selection criteria and management guidelines for outpatient parenteral antibiotic therapy for native valve infective endocarditis. Clin Infect Dis 2001;33:203–209.
9. Heldman AW, Hartert TV, Ray SC, et al. Oral antibiotic treatment of right-sided staphylococcal endocarditis in injection drug users: Prospective randomized comparison with parenteral therapy. Am J Med 1996;101:68–76.
10. Lawlor MT, Sullivan MC, Levitz RE, et al. Treatment of prosthetic valve endocarditis due to methicillin-resistant *Staphylococcus aureus* with minocycline. J Infect Dis 1990;161:812–814.

118 PULMONARY TUBERCULOSIS

► Don't Breathe the Air Here (Level I)

Tina Penick Brock, MS
Dennis M. Williams, PharmD, FASHP, FCCP, FAPhA, BCPS

► After completing this case study, students should be able to:

- Recognize the signs and symptoms of active tuberculosis (TB).
- Recommend initial empiric drug therapy for a patient with active TB.
- Describe appropriate monitoring parameters to assess the effectiveness and toxicity of anti-TB drug therapies.
- Recognize common adverse events of drugs used to treat TB.
- Identify treatment options for patients with drug-resistant organisms.

PATIENT PRESENTATION

Chief Complaint

"I have been coughing for about a month and it seems like it's getting worse. Sometimes it's so bad that I don't have any energy."

HPI

Carl Stevens is a 48 year old man who presents to the Medicine Clinic complaining of a 1-month history of a persistent cough that has become more productive over the past 2 weeks. He also reports malaise, fever, night sweats, and a 12-kg weight loss over the past 2 months that he attributes to his current problem.

PMH

Seizure disorder since age 10 years
HTN for 5 years

FH

Mother died at age 52 from breast cancer and father died at age 59 from lung cancer. One brother, age 37, is HIV (+) and lives with the patient. One sister, age 55, is alive and has no known medical problems.

SH

Single, no children. He works as an aide in a local nursing home. He denies smoking or IV drug use. He had a 20-year history of alcohol abuse but has been sober for 10 years. His brother's HIV infection, attributed to IV drug abuse, is in the early stages with a CD4 count of 280 and a low viral load.

Meds

Phenytoin 300 mg po at bedtime
Hydrochlorothiazide 25 mg po once daily

Patient reports that he tries to be compliant with his therapies and takes them regularly except when he is unable to get his refills; over the past 2 months, he has gone 3 or 4 days without medication.

All

NKDA

ROS

Unremarkable except for complaints of recurrent headaches and intermittent abdominal pain. No seizures for 8 months.

PE

Gen

African American man who appears older than stated age. Appears fatigued, but otherwise in NAD.

VS

BP 138/88, P 84, RR 16, Temp 38.3°C; Wt 74 kg

Skin

Cool to touch; multiple bruises on extremities; moles on trunk

HEENT

PERRLA; EOMI; funduscopic exam with grade 2, mild arterial narrowing, no hemorrhages or exudates; TMs occluded bilaterally with wax. Pharynx shiny, no exudates

Neck

Supple; no lymphadenopathy, bruits, or JVD; no thyromegaly

Chest

Diffuse rhonchi in upper lobes, cavernous breath sounds in right upper lobe

CV

RRR; no m/r/g

Abd

(+) BS; non-tender; no masses; liver edge palpable

Genit/Rect

No masses or discharge; rectal tone decreased, prostate slightly enlarged; heme (+) stool

MS/Ext

No CCE; muscle strength 3–4/5 throughout; peripheral pulses present

Neuro

Sluggish, but A & O × 3; no focal abnormalities; CN II–XII intact; DTRs 2+; Babinski downgoing bilaterally

Labs

Na 138 mEq/L	Hgb 13 g/dL	WBC 4.5 × 10^3/mm^3	AST 72 IU/L
K 3.8 mEq/L	Hct 39%	62% PMNs	ALT 56 IU/L
Cl 96 mEq/L	RBC 4.1 × 10^6/mm^3	34% Lymphs	Alk Phos 120 IU/L
CO_2 23 mEq/L	MCV 98 μm^3	4% Monos	GGT 60 IU/L
BUN 30 mg/dL	MCH 32 pg		T. bili 1.0 mg/dL
SCr 1.3 mg/dL	Retic 0.4%		PT 14 sec
Glu 126 mg/dL			

Other

Consent for HIV testing obtained.

Chest X-Ray

Right upper lobe infiltrate with large cavitation, bases spared. (see Figure 118–1).

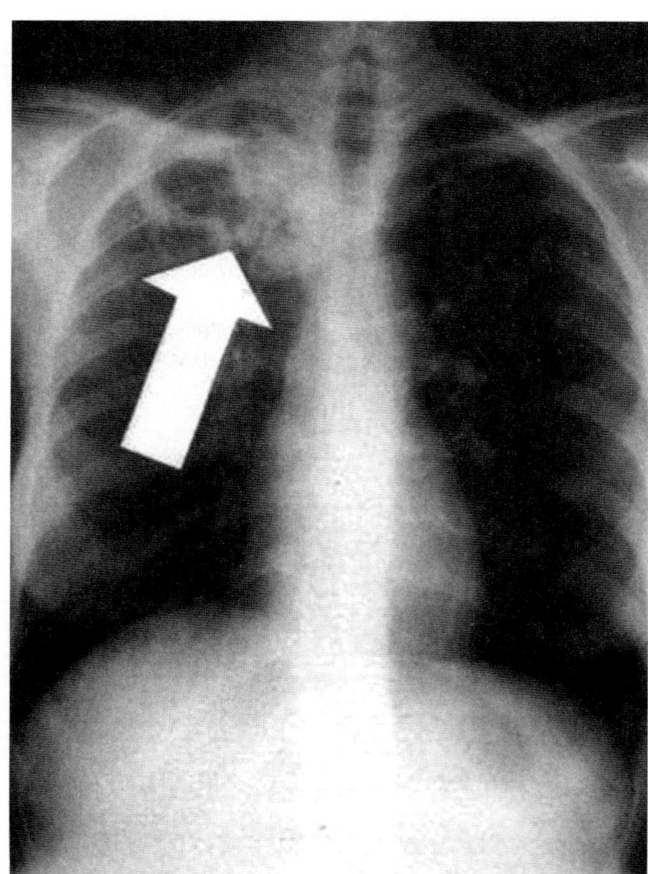

Figure 118–1. Chest radiograph. Arrow points to cavitation in patient's upper right lobe.

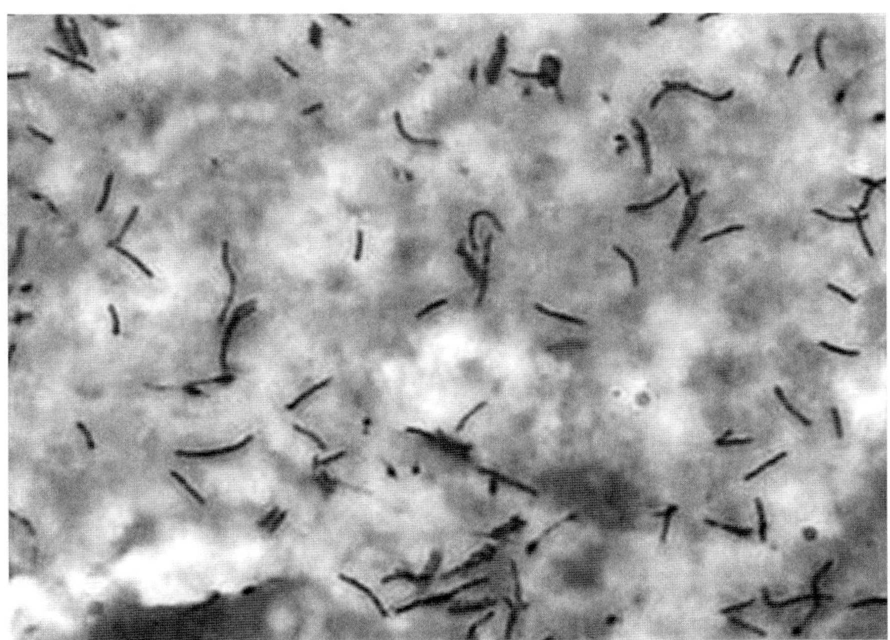

Figure 118–2. Acid-Fast Bacilli (AFB) smear. Acid-fast bacilli (shown as thin rods) are tubercle bacilli.

CT Chest

Small posterior peritracheal and hilar nodes. Cavity (3–4 cm) in right posterior segment, no air fluid level.

▶ Clinical Course

The patient was admitted and placed on respiratory isolation. Three separate sputum Gram stain specimens were reported to contain 3+ AFB (see Figure 118–2). An intermediate-strength PPD tuberculin skin test (Mantoux method) 5-TU was placed. Candida and mumps were used as controls. Sputum samples were cultured for AFB, fungi, and bacteria. After 48 hours, the PPD skin test was read as a 12-mm area of induration.

Assessment

Active pulmonary tuberculosis.

▶ Questions

Problem Identification

1. a. *Create a list of the patient's drug therapy problems.*
   b. *What signs, symptoms, and other findings are consistent with active TB infection?*
   c. *What factors place this patient at increased risk for acquiring TB?*

Desired Outcome

2. *What are the goals of therapy for this patient with active TB?*

Therapeutic Alternatives

3. a. *What nondrug therapies might be useful in this patient?*
   b. *What drug therapies are available for the treatment of active TB?*
   c. *What economic and social considerations are applicable to this patient?*

Optimal Plan

4. a. *What drug, dosage form, dose, schedule, and duration of therapy are best for this patient?*
   b. *What alternatives to daily administration of medicines exist?*

Outcome Evaluation

5. *What clinical and laboratory parameters are necessary to evaluate the therapy for achievement of the desired therapeutic outcome and to detect or prevent adverse effects?*

Patient Education

6. *What information should be provided to the patient to enhance compliance, ensure successful therapy, and minimize adverse effects?*

▶ Clinical Course

The patient is treated with the regimen you recommended under respiratory isolation in the hospital. The results of his HIV test were negative. After 10 days, his presenting symptoms have improved, and three consecutive sputum specimens have been negative for AFB. Because he had three negative smears, he was removed from respiratory isolation and subsequently discharged to home. After 6 weeks, the results of his initial cultures are available. *Mycobacterium tuberculosis* is present, and the sensitivity report indicates sensitivity to all first-line agents. A follow-up sputum culture at 2 months is negative for mycobacterium.

▶ Follow-Up Questions

1. *How should the sensitivity report influence the drug therapy?*
2. *After 3 months of therapy, an increase in the patient's AST and ALT are noted (AST 160 IU/L; ALT 190 IU/L). Other liver enzymes and total bilirubin are normal. The patient reports no new complaints. What changes would you make to the current therapy and monitoring plan?*
3. *What potential drug interactions should be evaluated? How should they be managed?*
4. *How should other close contacts of the patient, including the brother, be evaluated and treated?*

▶ Self-Study Assignments

1. How would therapy be different if the patient was HIV positive? A child or adolescent? A pregnant woman?
2. Discuss how the treatment would have been different if the patient had multidrug resistant organisms.
3. How does the treatment of extrapulmonary TB differ from the treatment of pulmonary TB?
4. What are the BCG vaccines? In what situations would BCG be recommended?

▶ Clinical Pearl

All patients receiving treatment for active TB should be considered for directly observed therapy (DOT).

With adequate drug therapy for TB, nearly all patients with drug-susceptible organisms become bacteriologically negative, recover, and remain well.

References

1. Targeted tuberculin testing and treatment of latent tuberculosis infection. American Thoracic Society. MMWR Morb Mortal Wkly Rep 2000;49(RR-6):1–51.
2. American Thoracic Society/Centers for Disease Control and Prevention/Infectious Diseases Society of America. Treatment of tuberculosis. MMWR Morb Mortal Wkly Rep 2003;52(RR11);1–77. Also published in: Am J Resp Crit Care Med 2003;167: 603–662.
3. Small PM, Fujiwara PI. Management of tuberculosis in the United States. N Engl J Med 2001;345:189–200.
4. Update: Fatal and severe liver injuries associated with rifampin and pyrazinamide for latent tuberculosis infection, and revisions in American Thoracic Society/CDC recommendations—United States 2001. MMWR Morb Mortal Wkly Rep 2001;50(34):33–35.

119 *CLOSTRIDIUM DIFFICILE*-ASSOCIATED DIARRHEA

▶ *C. difficile* Made Easy (Level I)

Eric G. Sahloff, PharmD
Steven J. Martin, PharmD, BCPS

▶ After completing this case study, students should be able to:

- Identify antibiotics commonly associated with the development of *Clostridium difficile*-associated diarrhea (CDAD) and the proposed mechanisms of this effect.
- Identify the signs and symptoms of CDAD.
- Interpret diagnostic tests for determining the presence of CDAD.
- Recommend optimal pharmacotherapy for the treatment of initial and recurrent cases of CDAD and monitor for efficacy of these treatments.
- Educate patients about drug therapy and adverse effects upon discharge.

PATIENT PRESENTATION

Chief Complaint

"Doc, you have to help me. I think I'm going to soil my pants!!"

HPI

A 43 yo man with a 4-year history of multiple knee surgeries due to a motorcycle accident is seen at your clinic for hospital follow-up. He was recently discharged from the hospital after a bout of osteomyelitis in his knee requiring IV antibiotics. During the previous admission, the patient initially received 4 days of cefazolin pending culture and susceptibility results from an intraoperative culture of the knee. Methicillin-resistant *Staphylococcus aureus* (MRSA) was reported and the antibiotic was switched to IV vancomycin 1 gram every 12 hours. The patient was subsequently sent home on vancomycin 2 grams IV daily and requested to follow up in your clinic. After the start of vancomycin therapy, the patient began having abdominal pain, tenderness, distention, cramping, and numerous episodes of diarrhea, peaking at more than 12 stools per day for the last several days.

PMH

Multiple surgeries due to motorcycle accident 4 years ago.

FH

Noncontributory

SH

Drinks "couple days a week, especially on weekends";1 pack cigarettes/day, no illicit drug use.

ROS

Occasional fevers; no chills, weight loss, or headaches. He denies rhinorrhea, cough, sore throat, chest pain, shortness of breath, or palpitations. No urinary urgency or hesitancy. He reports cramping and abdominal tenderness that is relieved by bowel movements. Greenish, watery diarrhea (> 10 stools daily) without hematochezia or melena started upon returning home.

Meds

Cefazolin 1 g IV Q 8 H × 4 days
Vancomycin 2 g Q 24 H (started 8 days ago)
Multivitamin 1 tab po daily
OxyContin 40 mg po Q 12 H
Percocet 1–2 tabs po Q 4–6 H PRN

All

PCN (hives)

PE

Gen

Patient is distressed because of excessive bowel movements and occasional knee pain; thirsty; no other complaints

VS

BP 128/75, P 86, RR 23, T (oral) 38.7°C; Ht 5′10″, Wt 85 kg

Skin

Dry, decreased skin turgor, otherwise normal appearing

HEENT

PERRLA; EOMI; mucus membranes dry, sunken eyes

Neck/LN

Supple with no JVD, bruits, or lymphadenopathy; normal thyroid

Chest

CTA

CV

RRR; normal S_1, S_2

Abd

Mildly distended with diffuse tenderness; (+) guarding; hyperactive BS × 4 quadrants

Genit/Rect

Rectal exam not performed

MS/Ext

Some right knee pain, decreased range of motion; strength 5/5 in both upper extremities and LLE, 2/5 RLE

Neuro

Alert and oriented × 3

Labs

Na 138 mEq/L	WBC 13.6 × 10^3/mm^3
K 4.2 mEq/L	51% Neutros
Cl 98 mEq/L	30% Bands
CO_2 31 mEq/L	13% Lymphs
BUN 38 mg/dL	6% Monos
SCr 1.0 mg/dL	
Glu 113 mg/dL	

Chest X-Ray

Clear

EKG

NSR; no acute ST wave changes, and no change from previous EKG.

UA

WNL

Intraoperative Cultures (Knee)

Gram (+) cocci in clusters; methicillin-resistant *Staphylococcus aureus*

C. difficile Toxin Enzyme Immunoassay (EIA) Test

Pending

Fecal Leukocytes

Not done

Assessment

1. Diarrhea—consider obtaining *C. difficile* culture
2. Osteomyelitis
3. Dehydration

▶ Clinical Course

The patient was started on metronidazole 250 mg po Q 8 H. Fluid supplementation was initiated. The stool *C. difficile* toxin was subsequently reported as positive.

▶ Questions

Problem Identification

1. a. *Create a list of the patient's drug therapy problems.*
   b. *The patient is confused about the cause of the diarrhea. Explain some of the possible causes of diarrhea and discuss the signs, symptoms, and laboratory values that are consistent with* C. difficile*-associated diarrhea (CDAD) in this patient.*
   c. *Which antibiotics are most likely to cause CDAD?*
   d. *If the* C. difficile *toxin test had been reported negative, would this have ruled out CDAD?*
   e. *What are some of the other procedures or tests that are used to diagnose CDAD?*

Desired Outcome

2. *What are the goals of pharmacotherapy in this case?*

Therapeutic Alternatives

3. a. *What nonpharmacologic treatments may be recommended in this case?*
   b. *What pharmacologic alternatives are available for CDAD?*

Optimal Plan

4. a. *The orthopedic surgeon states that that he would like the patient to receive 4 to 6 weeks of IV vancomycin because the patient has had prior problems with infection. Would this be adequate treatment for the CDAD?*
   b. *The resident wants to start the patient on loperamide to slow the diarrhea. Is this advisable?*
   c. *Was the patient's initial regimen of oral metronidazole 250 mg TID appropriate therapy?*
   d. *After a week of therapy the patient still has diarrhea, and a repeat toxin assay is positive. What are the possible causes of treatment failure?*
   e. *Given this new information, what therapeutic alternatives are available to treat this patient?*

Outcome Evaluation

5. *What clinical and laboratory parameters are necessary to evaluate the therapy for achievement of the desired therapeutic outcomes and to detect or prevent adverse effects?*

Patient Education

6. *What information should be provided to the patient to enhance compliance, ensure successful therapy, and minimize adverse effects?*

► Follow-Up Question

1. *Treatment was successful and the patient discontinued therapy for CDAD. Two weeks later, the diarrhea and similar signs and symptoms returned. How should the patient be treated?*

► Clinical Pearl

Infection control measures have proven effective in the prevention and reduction of risk for CDAD. Barrier methods such as glove use, hand washing and isolation rooms have been successful in decreasing horizontal transmission. Restriction of antimicrobial use may be the most appropriate method of decreasing CDAD.[5]

References

1. Landry ML, Topal J Ferguson D, et al. Evaluation of Biosite Triage *Clostridium difficile* Panel for rapid detection of *Clostridium difficile* in stool samples. J Clin Microbiol 2001;39:1855–1858.
2. Lozniewski A, Rabaud C, Dotto E, et al. Laboratory diagnosis of *Clostridium difficile*-associated diarrhea and colitis: Usefulness of Premier Cytoclane AB enzyme immunoassay for combined detection of stool toxins and toxigenic *C. difficile* strains. J Clin Microbiol 2001;39:1996–1998.
3. Centers for Disease Control and Prevention. Preventing the spread of vancomycin resistance—A report from the hospital infection control practices advisory committee. Fed Reg 1994;59:25758–25763.
4. Fekety R. Guidelines for the diagnosis and management of *Clostridium-difficile*-associated diarrhea and colitis. Am J Gastroenterol 1997;92:739–750.
5. Gerding DN, Johnson S, Peterson LR, Mulligan ME, Silva J. Clostridium difficile-associated diarrhea and colitis: SHEA position paper. Infect Control Hosp Epidimiol 1995;16:459–77.

120 INTRA-ABDOMINAL INFECTION

► Like Mother, Like Son (Level II)

Renee-Claude Mercier, PharmD
A. Christie Graham, PharmD

► After completing this case study, students should be able to:

- Recognize the signs and symptoms of bacterial peritonitis.
- Identify the bacteria commonly found in the different parts of the GI tract.
- Recommend appropriate empiric therapy for primary bacterial peritonitis.
- Establish a long-term plan for the patient regarding alcohol abuse and hepatitis C, including monitoring parameters and education.

PATIENT PRESENTATION

Chief Complaint

"My belly hurts so bad I can barely move."

HPI

John Chavez is a 67 yo Hispanic man who was brought to the ED by his wife. She stated that he has been suffering from nausea, vomiting, severe abdominal pain, and has been acting "goofy" for the last 2 to 3 days. His intake of food and fluids has been minimal over the past several days. He is a well-known patient of the ED who often presents with alcohol intoxication and severe hepatic encephalopathy.

PMH

Cirrhosis with ascites for the last 3 years
Hepatic encephalopathy
GERD
HTN
Cholecystectomy 10 years ago
Hepatitis C (+) × 4 years

FH

Mother was alcoholic; died 10 years ago in car accident. Father's history unknown.

SH

Retired construction worker; EtOH abuse with 10 to 12 cans of beer per day × 20 years; denies use of tobacco or illicit drugs; poor compliance with medications and dietary restrictions.

Meds

Lactulose 30 mL po QID PRN
Procardia XL 60 mg po once daily
Atenolol 50 mg po once daily
Spironolactone 100 mg po once daily
Famotidine 20 mg po BID
Maalox 30 mL po QID PRN

All

NKDA

ROS

As noted above.

PE

Gen

Elderly man who appears older than his stated age and is in severe pain

VS

BP 154/82, P 102, RR 32, T 39.4°C; current Wt 92 kg, IBW 68 kg

Skin

Jaundiced, warm, coarse, and very dry. Facial spider angiomata present.

HEENT

Yellow sclera; PERRLA; EOMI; funduscopic exam is normal. Tympanic membranes are clouded bilaterally, but with no erythema or bulging. Oropharynx showed poor dentition but was otherwise unremarkable.

Neck

Supple; normal size thyroid; no JVD or palpable lymph nodes

Chest

Lungs are CTA; shallow and frequent breathing

Heart

Tachycardia, normal S_1 and S_2 with no S_3 or S_4

Abd

Distended; pain upon pressure or movements; pain is sharp and diffuse throughout abdomen; (+) guarding. Unable to palpate liver or spleen. Decreased bowel sounds.

Ext

Unremarkable

Genit/Rect

Prostate normal size; guaiac (–) stool

Neuro

Oriented × 2 (time and person); lethargic and apathetic, slumped posture, slowed movements. CN II–XII intact. Motor system intact; overall muscle strength equal to 4–5/5; poor coordination and gait. Sensory system intact. Reflexes 3+

Labs

Na 142 mEq/L	Hgb 14.1 g/dL	AST 290 IU/L
K 3.9 mEq/L	Hct 42.6%	ALT 320 IU/L
Cl 96 mEq/L	Plt 250 × 10^3/mm^3	Alk Phos 350 IU/L
CO_2 20 mEq/L	WBC 18.25 × 10^3/mm^3	T. bili 3.2 mg/dL
BUN 44 mg/dL	73% Neutros	D. bili 1.4 mg/dL
SCr 1.2 mg/dL	9% Bands	NH_3 104 mcg/dL
Glu 101 mg/dL	13% Lymphs	
	5% Monos	

Abdominal X-Ray

No evidence of free air.

Chest X-Ray

No infiltrates; heart normal size and shape.

Blood Cultures

Pending × 2

Paracentesis

Ascitic fluid: leukocytes 720/mm^3, protein 2.5 g/dL, pH 7.28, lactate 30 mg/dL. Gram-stain: numerous PMNs, no organisms.

Assessment

Primary bacterial peritonitis.

▶ Clinical Course

Because of the recent low intake of food and fluids and the high BUN-to-creatinine ratio, the patient was thought to be dehydrated and was given 1 L/h of 0.9% NaCl in the ED. His breathing became progressively worse, and he had to be intubated and transferred to the intensive care unit.

▶ Questions

Problem Identification

1. a. *Create a list of the patient's drug therapy problems.*
   b. *What signs, symptoms, and laboratory values indicate the presence of primary bacterial peritonitis?*
   c. *What risk factors for infection are present in this patient?*
   d. *Which organisms are the most likely cause of this infection?*

Desired Outcome

2. *What are the therapeutic goals for this patient?*

Therapeutic Alternatives

3. a. *What nondrug therapies might be useful for this patient?*
   b. *What feasible pharmacotherapeutic alternatives are available for the treatment of the primary bacterial peritonitis?*

Optimal Plan

4. a. *Given this patient's condition, which drug regimens would provide optimal therapy for the infection?*
   b. *In addition to antimicrobial therapy, what other drug-related interventions are required for this patient?*

Outcome Evaluation

5. *What clinical and laboratory parameters are necessary to evaluate the therapy for achievement of the desired therapeutic outcome and to detect or prevent adverse effects?*

Patient Education

6. *What information should be provided to the patient to enhance compliance, ensure successful therapy, and minimize adverse effects?*

▶ Clinical Course

After 48 hours of IV antibiotics, Mr. Chavez was extubated. The blood cultures were reported positive for *Streptococcus pneumoniae,* resistant to penicillin G, sulfamethoxazole/ trimethoprim, and erythromycin; sensitive to cefotaxime, vancomycin, and levofloxacin. The ascitic fluid culture grew *Streptococcus pneumoniae* as well. He received cefotaxime 2 g IV Q 8 H for a total of 10 days. After 3 days of antimicrobial treatment, repeat blood cultures were negative. He rapidly improved, and upon discharge his mental status had returned to baseline.

▶ Self-Study Assignments

1. What are the primary differences (clinical manifestations, pathogens involved, diagnosis methods, and treatment) between primary and secondary bacterial peritonitis?
2. What are risk factors, clinical signs and symptoms, modes of transmission, diagnostic methods, prognosis, and therapeutic options associated with hepatitis C?

▶ Clinical Pearl

Bacteremia is present in up to 75% of patients with primary peritonitis caused by aerobic bacteria but is rarely found in those with peritonitis caused by anaerobes.

References

1. Such, J, Runyon BA. Spontaneous bacterial peritonitis. Clin Infect Dis 1998; 27:669–676.
2. Felisart J, Rimola A, Arroyo V, et al. Cefotaxime is more effective than is ampicillin-tobramycin in cirrhotics with severe infections. Hepatology 1985; 5:457–462.
3. Bohnen JM, Solomkin JS, Dellinger EP, et al. Guidelines for clinical care: Anti-infective agents for intra-abdominal infection. A Surgical Infection Society policy statement. Arch Surg 1992;127:83–89.

121 LOWER URINARY TRACT INFECTION

▶ Yearning and Burning (Level I)

Kelly A. Sprandel, PharmD
Christine A. Lesch, PharmD
Keith A. Rodvold, PharmD, FCCP, BCPS

▶ After completing this case study, students should be able to:

- Recognize the usual symptoms of an uncomplicated urinary tract infection (UTI) in females.
- Select specific drug therapy for the treatment of an uncomplicated UTI after consideration of patient symptoms, objective findings, and expected clinical response.
- Describe monitoring parameters to ensure efficacy and prevent toxicity during treatment.
- Educate patients about how to take the regimen, noting relationship with meals, proper storage, and potential side effects.

PATIENT PRESENTATION

Chief Complaint

"It still hurts when I urinate."

HPI

Sarah Ramsey is a 26 yo woman who presents to a Family Practice Clinic in Seattle with continuing complaints of dysuria, frequency of urination, and urgency to urinate. She was seen in the clinic 3 days ago with the same complaints and started on trimethoprim-sulfamethoxazole DS 1 tablet twice daily.

PMH

Diagnosed with 3 UTIs over the past year, treated with TMP-SMX.
H/O gonorrhea (2 years ago)

FH

Mother has DM; remainder of FH is noncontributory.

SH

Denies smoking; admits to occasional marijuana use; social EtOH use; sexually active (multiple partners), uses spermicide-coated condoms.

ROS

Denies having any vaginal discharge or bleeding, fevers, or chills. Reports having mild low back pain and pain during urination.

Meds

Ortho-Novum 7/7/7 1 po daily
MVI po daily

All

No known allergies

PE

Gen
Cooperative woman in no acute distress

VS
BP 110/60, P 68, R 18, T 36.8°C; Wt 57 kg, Ht 5′5″

Skin
Mild facial acne

HEENT
PERRLA, EOMI, fundi benign, TMs intact

Back
No CVA tenderness

Chest
CTA

CV
RRR

Abd
Soft, (+) bowel sounds, no organomegaly or tenderness

Pelvic
No vaginal discharge or lesions; LMP 2 weeks ago; mild suprapubic tenderness

Ext
Pulses 2+ throughout; full ROM

Neuro
A & O × 3; CN II–XII intact; reflexes 2+, sensory and motor levels intact

Labs
Not obtained

UA (from clinic visit 3 days ago)
Yellow, cloudy, pH 5.0, WBC 10–15 cells/hpf, RBC 1–5 cells/hpf, protein 10 mg/dL, trace blood, glucose (–), leukoesterase (+), many bacteria, nitrite positive (see Figure 121–1).

Urine Culture
Not performed

Assessment
Acute cystitis (see Figure 121–2).

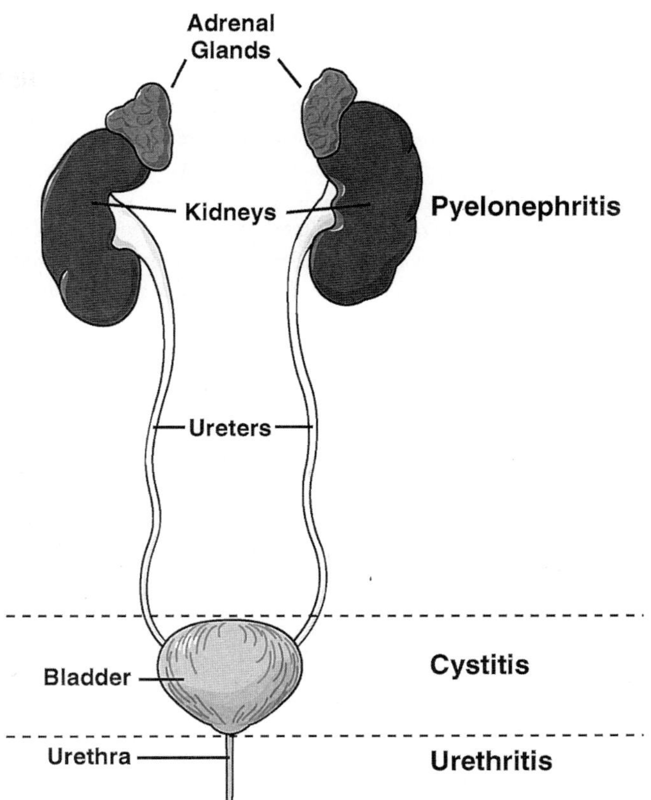

Figure 121–2. Anatomy and associated infections of the urinary tract.

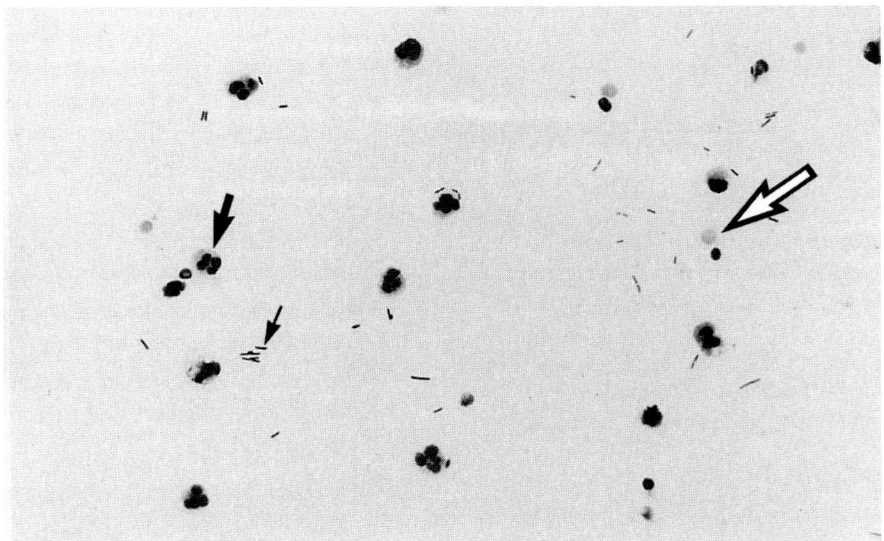

Figure 121–1. Urine sediment with neutrophils *(solid arrow),* bacteria *(small arrow),* and occasional red blood cells *(open arrow)* (Wright-Giemsa ×1650). *(Photo courtesy of Lydia C. Contis, MD.)*

▶ Questions

Problem Identification

1. a. *What clinical and laboratory features are consistent with the diagnosis of an acute uncomplicated lower UTI (cystitis) in this patient?*
   b. *How does one differentiate cystitis from urethritis (caused by* Chlamydia trachomatis, Neisseria gonorrhoeae, *or herpes simplex virus) or vaginitis (caused by Candida or Trichomonas species)?*
   c. *How should a patient experiencing her fourth episode of cystitis and not responding to treatment be managed? Should a urine culture and sensitivity test be performed?*
   d. *What are the most likely pathogens and frequency of occurrence causing this patient's infection?*
   e. *What factors can increase the risk of developing a UTI?*
   f. *List potential reasons that this patient may not be responding to treatment.*
   g. *Because this is her fourth episode of an uncomplicated UTI this year, should she receive prophylactic antibiotics to prevent further episodes?*

Desired Outcome

2. *What are the goals of pharmacotherapy in this case?*

Therapeutic Alternatives

3. a. *What are the desirable characteristics of an anti-infective agent selected for the treatment of this uncomplicated UTI?*
   b. *What feasible pharmacotherapeutic alternatives are available for empiric first-line and second-line treatment of an uncomplicated UTI?*
   c. *What nonpharmacologic therapies may be useful in preventing uncomplicated UTIs?*

Optimal Plan

4. *What drug, dosage form, dose, schedule, and duration of therapy are best for this patient?*

Outcome Evaluation

5. *What clinical and laboratory parameters are necessary to evaluate the therapy for achievement of the desired therapeutic outcome and to detect or prevent adverse effects?*

Patient Education

6. *What information should be provided to the patient to enhance compliance, ensure successful therapy, and minimize adverse effects?*

▶ Self-Study Assignments

1. Review the safety and efficacy of single-dose, 3-day, and 7-day antimicrobial therapy for the treatment of acute uncomplicated bacterial cystitis.
2. Perform a literature search to obtain information on the rates of resistance of *E. coli* to TMP-SMX and fluoroquinolone antibiotics. How do these rates compare to those reported at your institution?
3. Provide your assessment and recommendation on the role of phenazopyridine in treatment of UTIs.

▶ Clinical Pearl

UTIs occur rarely in young males except when there is an underlying structural abnormality or instrumentation of the urinary tract.

References

1. Hooton, TM. The current management strategies for community-acquired urinary tract infection. Infect Dis Clin N Am 2003;17:303–332.
2. Fihn SD. Acute uncomplicated urinary tract infection in women. N Engl J Med 2003;349:259–266.
3. Gupta K, Sahm DF, Mayfield D, et al. Antimicrobial resistance among uropathogens that cause community-acquired urinary tract infections in women: A nationwide analysis. Clin Infect Dis 2001;33:89–94.
4. Sahm DF, Thornsberry C, Mayfield DC, et al. Multidrug-resistant urinary tract isolates of Escherichia coli: Prevalence and patient demographics in the United States in 2000. Antimicrob Agents Chemother 2001;45:1402–1406.
5. Warren JW, Abrutyn E, Hebel JR, et al. Guidelines for antimicrobial treatment of uncomplicated acute bacterial cystitis and acute pyelonephritis in women. Infectious Diseases Society of America (IDSA). Clin Infect Dis 1999;29:745–758.
6. Wright SW, Wrenn KD, Haynes ML. Trimethoprim-sulfamethoxazole resistance among urinary coliform isolates. J Gen Intern Med 1999;14:606–609.
7. Gupta K, Scholes D, Stamm WE. Increasing prevalence of antimicrobial resistance among uropathogens causing acute uncomplicated cystitis in women. JAMA 1999;281:736–738.
8. Hooton TM. Recurrent urinary tract infection in women. Int J Antimicrob Agents 2001;17:259–268.

122 ACUTE PYELONEPHRITIS

▶ Outflanked (Level II)

Brian A. Potoski, PharmD

▶ After completing this case study, students should be able to:

- Differentiate the signs, symptoms, and laboratory findings associated with pyelonephritis from those seen in lower urinary tract infections.
- Recognize patient risk factors that predispose to development of pyelonephritis.
- Recommend appropriate empiric antimicrobial and symptomatic pharmacotherapy for a patient with suspected pyelonephritis.
- Make appropriate adjustments in pharmacotherapy based on patient response and culture results.
- Design a monitoring plan for a patient with pyelonephritis that allows objective assessment of the response to therapy.

PATIENT PRESENTATION

Chief Complaint

"There's pain in my stomach and back."

HPI

Terry Mitch is a 53 yo woman with a history of asthma, GERD, HTN, and CVA. She reports that she has had pain in her left flank region over the last three days, as well as pain in her abdomen. She complains of some nausea and reports four episodes of vomiting over the past 3 days. She has recently skipped several meals as a result. The patient reports urinary burning and frequency. She states that she often feels feverish and at times has chills. She reports no substernal chest pain, shortness of breath, cough, or sputum production. She denies any diarrhea. She reports no change in hemiparesis but states that she feels "weak and worn down."

PMH

HTN (duration unknown); BP averages 142/84 mm Hg on medication
GERD (duration unknown)
Asthma (duration unknown)
S/P stroke with right hemiparesis approximately 2 years ago

FH

Father died at age 72 with lung cancer; Mother is 75 yo and alive with CAD and CHF. One sister with diabetes, no other siblings.

SH

Non-smoker, no IVDA, occasional alcohol use. Divorced. Currently lives with her two sons from the previous marriage. She is employed at the local post office.

ROS

Reports recently taking naproxen sodium OTC PRN for her back and abdominal pain which doesn't seem to help. She has had one UTI in the past year but cannot remember others since.

Meds

Warfarin 5 mg po once daily
Hydrochlorothiazide 25 mg po once daily
Ranitidine 150 mg po BID
Captopril 12.5 mg po TID
Naproxen sodium 220 mg po TID

All

Penicillin—Develops an itchy rash

PE

Gen

Conscious, alert and oriented, middle-aged African-American woman in mild distress

VS

BP 142/84, P 80, RR 21, T 38.2°C; O_2 sat 97% room air; Ht 5′3″, Wt 59.6 kg (IBW 52.4 kg)

HEENT

NCAT, EOMI; funduscopic exam with no evidence of exudates or cotton wool spots; pharynx clear and dry

Skin

No tenting; dry

Neck

Supple, flat JVP

Chest

CTA

CV

RRR, normal S_1 and S_2; no S_3 or S_4

Abd

Mildly obese; active bowel sounds; soft with suprapubic tenderness to deep palpation. No rebound or guarding; no hepatosplenomegaly or masses.

Back

(+) CVAT; no paraspinal or spinal tenderness.

Genit/Rect

Normal female genitalia; no abnormal vaginal discharge; normal sphincter tone. LMP 3 months ago.

Ext

No CCE; dry flaky skin on lower legs bilaterally; pulses 2+ bilaterally.

Neuro

A & O × 3, CN II–XII intact; sensory and perception intact; old weakness noted on right side from previous CVA.

Labs and UA on Admission

See Table 122–1 and Figure 122–1.

TABLE 122–1. Laboratory Tests and Urinalyses on Days 1 Through 3 of Hospitalization

Parameter (units)	Day 1	Day 2	Day 3
Serum Chemistry			
Na (mEq/L)	134	136	138
K (mEq/L)	3.1	3.2	3.6
Cl (mEq/L)	99	101	105
CO_2 (mEq/L)	27	28	28
BUN (mg/dL)	45	32	17
SCr (mg/dL)	1.5	1.2	1.0
Glucose (mg/dL)	181	119	110
Hematology			
Hgb (g/dL)	10.3	9.5	8.8
Hct (%)	34.8	29.2	25.9
Plt (× 10^3/mm^3)	119	76	46
WBC (× 10^3/mm^3)	20.2	18.5	15.6
PMN/B/L/M[a] (%)	82/10/8/0	85/9/3/3	80/5/13/2
Urinalysis			
Appearance	Hazy		
Color	Amber		
pH	5.0		
Specific Gravity	1.017		
Blood	2+		
Ketones	Negative		
Leukocyte esterase	3+		
Nitrites	2+		
Urine protein, qualitative	Trace		
Urine glucose, qualitative	Trace		
WBC/hpf	487		
RBC/hpf	102		
Bacteria	Many		
WBC casts	2+		

[a] PMN, polymorphonuclear leukocytes; B, bands; L, lymphocytes; M, monocytes.

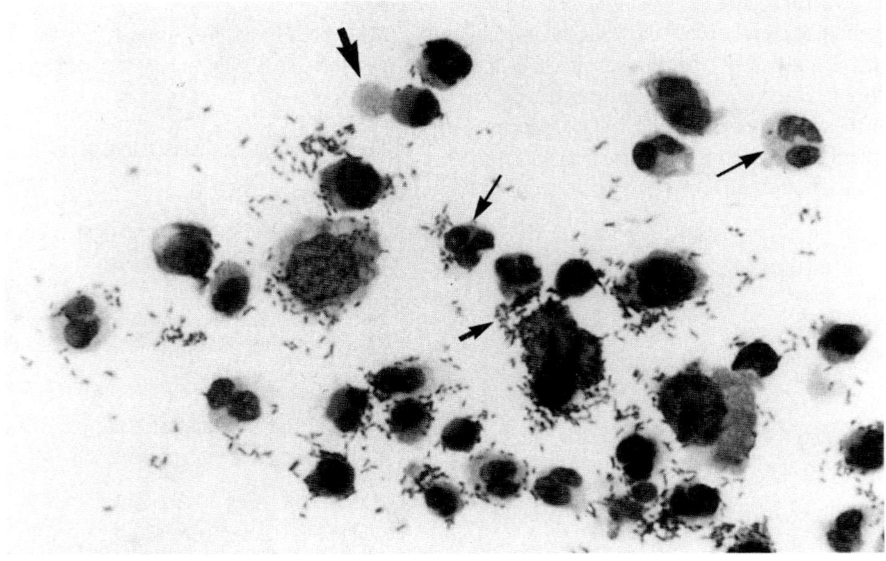

Figure 122–1. Urine sediment with red blood cells *(large arrow),* numerous neutrophils *(line arrows),* and bacteria *(small arrow)* (Wright × 1650). *(Photo courtesy of Lydia C. Contis, MD.)*

Chest X-Ray

Unremarkable; no infiltrates or consolidation.

CT Abdomen with Contrast

Findings: Liver, gallbladder, pancreas, spleen, and adrenals are unremarkable. No evidence of pneumoperitoneum or hemoperitoneum. No evidence of ascites or focal areas of fluid collection. The right kidney is unremarkable. A hypoattenuating lesion is seen involving the left kidney from mid-pole to lower-pole.

Impression: Hypoattenuating lesion in left kidney consistent with pyelonephritis; correlate with clinical picture.

Abdominal Ultrasound

Findings: No hydrocephalus of the kidneys bilaterally. There is a hypoechoic region within the lateral cortex of the left kidney that does not display through transmission.

Impression: Focal cortical thickening with decreased echogenicity involving the mid-left renal cortex, similar to the recent CT scan, most likely representing focal pyelonephritis. No renal abscess identified. No hydronephrosis.

Urine Gram Stain

Many Gram negative rods

Assessment

1. Pyelonephritis
2. Volume depletion
3. HTN

Questions

Problem Identification

1. a. *Create a list of the patient's drug therapy problems.*
   b. *What information (signs, symptoms, laboratory tests) indicates the presence and severity of pyelonephritis in this patient?*
   c. *List any potential contributing factors, including drug therapy, that may have predisposed this patient to developing pyelonephritis (see Figure 122–2).*
   d. *What additional information is needed to fully assess the patient?*

Desired Outcome

2. *What are the goals of pharmacotherapy in this patient?*

Therapeutic Alternatives

3. a. *What nondrug therapies might be useful for this patient?*
   b. *What organisms are commonly associated with pyelonephritis?*
   c. *What feasible pharmacotherapeutic alternatives are available for the empiric treatment of pyelonephritis?*

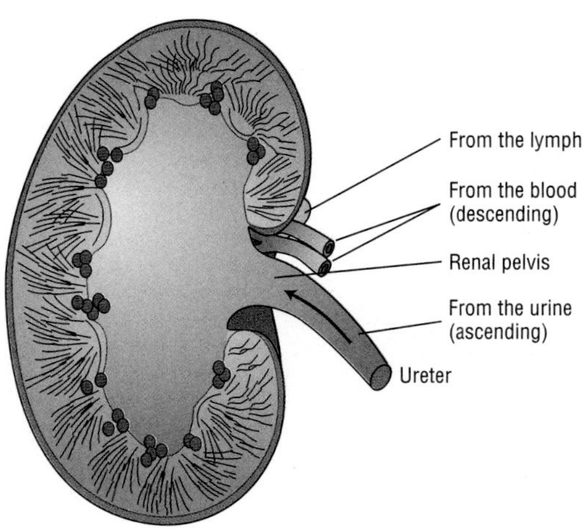

Figure 122–2. Routes of infection for pyelonephritis.

TABLE 122–2. Culture Results of Blood and Urine Samples Taken on Day 1 and Reported on Day 3.

Urine Culture
Result: >100,000 cfu/mL *Escherichia coli*

Antibiotic	Kirby-Bauer Interpretation
Ampicillin/Sulbactam	Intermediate
Ampicillin	Resistant
Cefazolin	Intermediate
Cefuroxime	Sensitive
Ceftriaxone	Sensitive
Levofloxacin	Sensitive
Piperacillin/tazobactam	Sensitive
Tobramycin	Sensitive
TMP–SMX	Sensitive

Blood Culture × 2 sets
Final Report: No growth × 5 days

Optimal Plan

4. *Outline an antimicrobial regimen that will provide appropriate empiric therapy for pyelonephritis in this patient.*

Outcome Evaluation

5. a. *What clinical and laboratory parameters are necessary to evaluate the antibiotic therapy for achievement of the desired therapeutic outcomes and to detect or prevent adverse effects?*

► Clinical Course

The patient was started on the empiric antimicrobial regimen you recommended. She required acetaminophen Q 6 H for back and abdominal pain, as well as occasional oxycodone 5 mg po Q 8 H PRN. Her fevers subsided with the initiation of acetaminophen. On day 3 of hospitalization, she was much improved and had begun to eat a normal diet. Laboratory tests for days 2 and 3 are included in Table 122–1. Culture results from admission were finalized on day 3 (late in the day), and are shown in Table 122–2.

b. *What recommendations, if any, do you have for changes in the initial drug regimen?*

Patient Education

6. *What information should be provided to the patient upon discharge to enhance adherence, ensure successful therapy, and minimize adverse effects?*

► Self-Study Assignments

1. Develop a protocol for switching patients from IV to oral therapy when treating pyelonephritis.
2. Perform a literature search to find clinical trials comparing drug therapy in pyelonephritis and compare inclusion criteria, drug regimens, outcomes, and costs of therapy.
3. Develop a clinical pathway that could be used for the management of suspected pyelonephritis.

► Clinical Pearl

Pyelonephritis can be managed with many different drugs. Choose agents that are bactericidal and cleared in the active form by the kidney. Drugs suitable for once-daily therapy help to reduce treatment costs.

References

1. Jinnah F, Islam MS, Rumi MA, et al. Drug sensitivity pattern of *E. coli* causing urinary tract infection in diabetic and non-diabetic patients. J Int Med Res 1996;24:296–301.
2. Warren JW, Abrutyn E, Hebel JR, et al. Guidelines for antimicrobial treatment of uncomplicated acute bacterial cystitis and acute pyelonephritis in women. Infectious Diseases Society of America (IDSA). Clin Infect Dis 1999;29:745–758.
3. Hooton TM, Stamm WE. Diagnosis and treatment of uncomplicated urinary tract infection. Infect Dis Clin North Am 1997;11:551–581.
4. Bailey RR, Begg EJ, Smith AH, et al. Prospective, randomized controlled study comparing two dosing regimens of gentamicin/oral ciprofloxacin switch therapy for acute pyelonephritis. Clin Nephrol 1996;46:183–186.
5. Pinson AG, Philbrick JT, Lindbeck GH, et al. ED management of acute pyelonephritis in women: a cohort study. Am J Emerg Med 1994;12:271–278.
6. Talan DA, Stamm WE, Hooton TM et al. Comparison of ciprofloxacin (7 days) and trimethoprim-sulfamethoxazole (14 days) for acute uncomplicated pyelonephritis in women. A randomized trial. JAMA 2000;283:1583–1590.

123 PELVIC INFLAMMATORY DISEASE AND OTHER SEXUALLY TRANSMITTED DISEASES

▶ Frankie and Jenny Were Lovers (Level II)

Denise L. Howrie, PharmD
Pamela J. Murray, MD, MHP

▶ After completing this case study, students should be able to:

- Identify relevant information from patient history, physical examination, and laboratory data suggestive of the diagnosis of a sexually transmitted disease (STD).
- List major complications of STDs and appropriate strategies for prevention and/or treatment.
- Discuss other health issues that may be present in patients referred for treatment of STDs.
- Provide appropriate treatment plans for patients with STDs, including drug(s), doses, and monitoring.
- Develop patient education strategies regarding drug treatment and possible adverse effects.

PATIENT PRESENTATION

Chief Complaint
"My lady and I don't feel good."

HPI
Frankie Mason is a 28 yo man who presents to a health clinic with complaints of 5 days of painful urination and increasing amounts of discolored urethral discharge. Today he noted four painful blisters on the penis. He is single, sexually active with two to three concurrent partners, and admits to unprotected sex "at least once" in the past 2 weeks. He does not know the sexual histories of his current or past sexual partners or their sexual partners. He denies IV drug use, is heterosexual, and has no active medical problems. He denies oral or rectal intercourse. He admits to over 15 lifetime sexual partners.

PMH
History of genital herpes 2 years ago, otherwise negative. He has not undergone testing for HIV and has not been immunized against hepatitis B. He is unaware of hepatitis C as an infectious disease asking, "Do you get that from sex or restaurant food?"

FH
Non-contributory.

SH
Denies cigarette use; has two to four beers "on weekends"; may be unreliable in keeping follow-up appointments because he states, "I don't like doctors."

ROS
Occasional headaches; denies stomach pain, constipation, vision problems, night sweats, weight loss, fatigue, or allergies

Meds
None

All
NKDA

PE

Gen
Patient is a well-developed male in NAD, very talkative

VS
BP 104/80, HR 72, RR 12, T 37.6°C; Wt 78 kg

Skin
No rashes or other lesions seen

HEENT
No erythema of pharynx or oral ulcers

Neck/LN
No lymphadenopathy, neck supple

Chest
Normal breath sounds, good air entry

CV
RRR, no murmurs

Abd
No tenderness or rebound, no HSM

Genit/Rect
Tanner Stage V, testes descended, non-tender, without erythema. Thick gray-white urethral discharge; four small erupting vesicles on penile tip and glans; negative rectal exam; no scrotal tenderness or swelling.

MS/Ext
No inguinal or other lymphadenopathy; no lesions or rashes; muscle strength and tone normal

Neuro
CN II–XII intact, DTRs 2+ bilaterally and symmetric

Urethral Smear
15 WBC/hpf, Gram stain (+) for intracellular gram-negative diplococci (see Figure 123–1); rare flagellated organisms by saline prep microscopy

Assessment
1. Urethritis caused by gonococcal and Trichomonas infections
2. Recurrent genital herpes

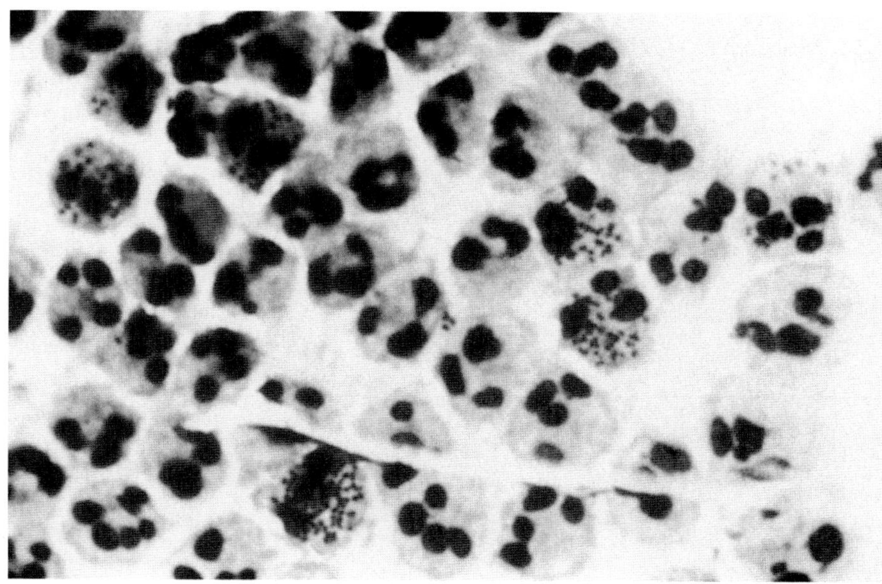

Figure 123–1. Gram-negative intracellular diplococci *(Neisseria gonorrhoeae).*

PATIENT PRESENTATION

Chief Complaint

"I feel sick to my stomach."

HPI

Jenny Klein is a 22 yo female sexual partner of Frankie who reports a 1-day history of increasingly severe dysuria, lower abdominal pain, fever, nausea, emesis × 2, and vaginal discharge. She is sexually active with "only Frankie," has no previous history of urinary or genital infection, and denies IV drug use. She is unaware of Frankie's multiple sexual partners. Her last menses ended 10 days ago and last intercourse was 7 days ago without use of a condom. She noted the vaginal discharge yesterday, which she describes as thick and yellow. She denies oral or rectal intercourse. She admits to three lifetime sexual partners.

PMH

Negative with no pregnancies

FH

HTN in maternal grandmother; history of depression.

SH

Denies nicotine or recreational drug use; occasional one to two glasses of wine; does not use hormonal or other contraception, reports occasional use of condoms; no routine medical care.

ROS

Occasional painful menses self-treated with acetaminophen.

Meds

None

All

NKDA

PE

Gen

Well-developed woman in moderate-to-severe abdominal discomfort

VS

BP 110/76, HR 120, RR 16, T 39.2°C; Wt 52 kg

Skin

No rashes seen

HEENT

No erythema of pharynx or oral ulcers

Neck/LN

No lymphadenopathy, neck supple

Chest

Normal breath sounds, good air entry; breasts Tanner Stage V

CV

RRR, no murmurs

Abd

Guarding of right and mid-lower quadrants with palpation

Genit/Rect

Pubic hair Tanner Stage V. Vulva with no ulcers visible; moderate erythema with mild excoriations. Vagina with large amount of thick yellow-white discharge and mild erythema. Cervix shows erythema and extensive yellow-white discharge from the os; no masses on bimanual exam; cervical motion tenderness; adnexal tenderness and fullness.

MS/Ext

No adenopathy, lesions or rashes; no arthritis or tenosynovitis

Neuro

CN II–XII Intact, DTRs 2+ and symmetric bilaterally

Labs

Na 138 mEq/L	Hgb 12.2 g/dL	WBC $12.75 \times 10^3/mm^3$
K 4.2 mEq/L	Hct 37%	66% Neutros
Cl 102 mEq/L	Plt $250 \times 10^3/mm^3$	12% Bands
BUN 22 mg/dL		10% Lymphs
SCr 0.9 mg/dL		12% Monos
Glu 106 mg/dL		

Other

Examination of vaginal discharge: pH 6.0, no yeast or hyphae seen; KOH prep negative, whiff test negative; flagellated organisms and increased WBC seen by saline prepared microscopy; negative for clue cells.

UA

Rare WBC/hpf, protein 100 mg/dL, Gram stain (–)

Assessment

1. PID
2. Infection of the genital tract: cervicitis, vaginitis, and urethritis

▶ Questions

Problem Identification

1. a. *For each patient, create a list of drug therapy problems.*
   b. *What information indicates the presence or severity of each STD in each patient?*
   c. *Should any additional tests be performed in these patients?*
   d. *What complications of infection can be reduced or avoided with appropriate therapy for each patient?*

Desired Outcome

2. *State the goals of treatment for each patient.*

Therapeutic Alternatives

3. *What therapeutic options are available for treatment of each patient?*

Optimal Plan

4. a. *What treatment regimen (drug, dosage form, dose, schedule, and duration) is appropriate for these patients?*
   b. *What alternatives would be appropriate if the initial therapy cannot be used?*

Outcome Evaluation

5. a. *What clinical and laboratory parameters are necessary to evaluate the therapy for achievement of the desired outcome and to detect or prevent adverse effects?*

▶ Clinical Course

Two days later, the following test results are received.

Frankie: *Chlamydia* PCR positive, urethral discharge culture positive for *Neisseria gonorrhoeae*.

Jenny: *Chlamydia* PCR positive, vaginal discharge culture positive for *Neisseria gonorrhoeae*.

b. *What changes, if any, in antibacterial therapy are required?*

Patient Education

6. *What information should be provided to Frankie to enhance compliance, ensure success of therapy, and minimize adverse effects?*

▶ Self-Study Assignments

1. Calculate patient costs of two regimens each for treatment of herpes genitalis, chlamydial urethritis, and gonococcal urethritis. How do cost and convenience compare for the various regimens?
2. Sexually active adolescents are a high-risk group for development of STDs. Identify biologic, social, and psychological factors that affect this risk. How can the clinician address adolescent risks?

▶ Clinical Pearl

The incidence of STDs is higher than reported, despite improved methods for diagnosis and treatment. Adolescents constitute a high-risk group for all STDs, including PID, who require specialized interventions and education to reduce disease prevalence.

References

1. Centers for Disease Control and Prevention. Sexually transmitted diseases treatment guidelines—2002. Morb Mortal Wkly Rep MMWR 2002;51 (RR-06):1–80.
2. Burstein GR, Murray PJ. Diagnosis and management of sexually transmitted disease pathogens among adolescents. Pediatr Rev 2003;24:75–82.
3. Burstein GR, Murray PJ. Diagnosis and management of sexually transmitted diseases among adolescents. Pediatr Rev 2003;24:119–127.
4. Burstein GR, Workowski KA. Sexually transmitted diseases treatment guidelines. Curr Opin Pediatr 2003:15:391–397.
5. Berg AO. Screening for chlamydial infection: Recommendations and rationale. Am J Prev Med 2001;20(3 Suppl):90–94.

124 SYPHILIS

▶ Hitting Below the Belt (Level I)

Alex K. McDonald, PharmD
Dennis M. Williams, PharmD, FASHP, FCCP, BCPS

▶ After completing this case study, students should be able to:

- Identify activities or behaviors that put an individual at risk for contracting a sexually transmitted disease (STD).
- Discuss the tests used to diagnose syphilis and evaluate treatment.
- Recommend appropriate therapies for the treatment of syphilis.
- Educate patients receiving treatment for an STD.
- Discuss the association between syphilis and HIV infection.
- Describe appropriate monitoring of syphilis infection in a pregnant patient.

PATIENT PRESENTATION

Chief Complaint
"I'm here for a follow-up visit because I am pregnant."

HPI
Mabel Connors is a 27 yo woman who presents for prenatal care. Her last normal menstrual period was 14 weeks ago. She is a divorced mother of two children.

PMH
Unremarkable. This is her third pregnancy (G_3P_2). She has delivered two other healthy babies who are now 10 and 6 years old.

FH
She has been divorced for 5 years. The father of her two children is no longer in the area, and she doesn't know how to contact him. Her parents live in another state. Father is in good health. Mother has HTN and DM.

SH
Single woman who has been living with her brother and his family in a trailer for 4 years; works at a textile mill. She reports being sexually active since age 14 with numerous sexual partners. She states that she has been involved in a monogamous relationship with her current boyfriend for one year. She does not use oral contraceptives due to previous problems with migraine headaches. Patient states that her partner uses condoms most of the time. Denies use of tobacco or alcohol.

ROS
Complaints of nasal congestion, heartburn, and episodes of N/V on most mornings for past 3 weeks. Patient denies previous skin lesions, rashes, or alopecia.

Meds
None

All
NKDA

PE

Gen
WDWN pregnant Caucasian woman who appears anxious but in NAD

VS
BP 130/70, P 90, RR 18, T 37°C; Wt 62.7 kg (baseline 60 kg)

Skin
Warm, dry, non-jaundiced; without bruising or lesions; hair quantity, distribution, and texture unremarkable

HEENT
NC/AT; TMs pearly gray revealing good cone of light bilaterally; PERRLA; EOMI; optic disk margins appropriately sharp; nasal mucous membranes moist; no oropharyngeal lesions

Neck
Supple; no lymphadenopathy, bruits, JVD, or thyromegaly

Chest
CTA bilaterally

Breast
No masses or dimples; no axillary lymphadenopathy

CV
RRR; no m/r/g

Abd
(+) BS; non-tender; no masses or organomegaly; 15-week fundal height with (+) fetal heart sounds (rate 140 bpm)

Neuro
A & O × 3; no focal abnormalities; CN II–XII intact.

Labs

Na 141 mEq/L	Hgb 14.3 g/dL
K 4.6 mEq/L	Hct 36.0%
Cl 101 mEq/L	WBC $5.5 \times 10^3/mm^3$
CO_2 28 mEq/L	Plt $225 \times 10^3/mm^3$
BUN 13 mg/dL	
SCr 0.9 mg/dL	
Glu 87 mg/dL	

Assessment
27 yo woman who is 14 weeks pregnant. As per CDC guidelines, will screen serologically for syphilis during the early stages of this pregnancy.

▶ Clinical Course

A positive RPR titer of 1:16 is reported the afternoon of the physical examination. This result is confirmed 2 days later with a positive TP–PA (Treponema Pallidum–Particle Agglutination) test. HBsAg (–), *Chlamydia* (–), GC culture (–), Pap smear (–). There are no signs/symptoms of syphilis and the patient doesn't recall any lesions or symptoms in the past.

▶ Questions

Problem Identification

1. a. *What information (signs, symptoms, laboratory values) indicates the presence or stage of syphilis?*
   b. *What is the role of the various laboratory tests used in the diagnosis of syphilis?*

Desired Outcome

2. *What are the goals of pharmacotherapy in this case?*

Therapeutic Alternatives

3. a. *What nondrug measures should be implemented in this case?*
   b. *What pharmacotherapeutic alternatives are available for this patient?*

Optimal Plan

4. a. *What is the recommended treatment (drug, dose, and duration) for this patient?*
   b. *What alternatives would you recommend if this patient were allergic to your first suggestion?*

Outcome Evaluation

5. *What clinical and laboratory parameters are necessary to evaluate the therapy for achievement of the desired therapeutic outcome and to detect or prevent adverse effects?*

Patient Education

6. a. *What information should be provided to the patient to enhance compliance, ensure successful therapy, and minimize adverse effects?*
   b. *What information should be provided to the patient to prevent a future sexually-transmitted disease?*

▶ Clinical Course

The patient subsequently delivered a uterine pregnancy at 41 weeks. At delivery, her RPR titer was 1:4 and a TP–PA was reactive. The infant's RPR was nonreactive.

▶ Follow-Up Questions

1. *What are potential explanations for these findings?*
2. *What further assessment and treatment should be considered for the patient?*
3. *What assessment and treatment should be considered for the infant?*

▶ Self-Study Assignments

1. What other therapies are currently being investigated as treatment for syphilis?
2. What tests or procedures are indicated to diagnose neurosyphilis?
3. How would the presence of neurosyphilis alter the recommended treatment regimen?

▶ Clinical Pearl

In pregnant patients with syphilis and penicillin allergy, desensitization to penicillin is recommended because there are no acceptable treatment alternatives.

Reference

1. Centers for Disease Control and Prevention. Syphilis. Sexually transmitted diseases treatment guidelines 2002. MMWR Morbid Mortal Wkly Rep 2002;51(RR-06):18–30. Available on the Internet at www.cdc.gov. Accessed July 24, 2004.

125 GENITAL HERPES AND CHLAMYDIAL INFECTIONS

▶ Double Trouble (Level II)

Suellyn J. Sorensen, PharmD, BCPS

▶ After completing this case study, students should be able to:

- Identify subjective and objective data consistent with genital herpes and *Chlamydia.*
- Recommend appropriate therapies for the treatment of genital herpes and *Chlamydia.*
- Provide effective and comprehensive counseling for patients with genital herpes and *Chlamydia.*
- Identify drug interactions of clinical significance and provide recommendations for managing them.

PATIENT PRESENTATION

Chief Complaint

"I have painful blisters in my genital area and I have terrible headaches and muscle aches."

HPI

Lisa Flint is a 20 yo nulligravida woman who presents to the county health STD clinic for evaluation of genital lesions that have been present for 3 days. She has also noticed a white non-odorous vaginal discharge that has lasted 14 days. She admits to anal and vaginal intercourse with two regular partners in the last 60 days. It has been 5 days since her last sexual encounter.

PMH

Recurrent UTIs; most recent 3 months ago
Vaginal candidiasis; most recent 6 months ago
Gonorrhea 5 years ago
Trichomonas vaginalis 2 years ago

FH

Mother with type 2 DM; father died at age 50 of an acute MI.

SH

Lives with her boyfriend and works at a Mexican restaurant. She admits to occasional use of alcohol and marijuana.

Meds

Loestrin-21 1 tablet po daily
Multivitamin with iron 1 tablet po daily
Ibuprofen 200 mg po PRN
Ciprofloxacin 250 mg po once daily

All

Penicillin (hives and tongue swelling)

ROS

(–) Cough, night sweats, weight loss, dysuria, or urinary frequency; (+) diarrhea and anorectal pain; LMP 6 weeks ago

PE

Gen

Thin young woman in NAD

VS

BP 136/71, P 78, RR 17, T 37.8°C; Wt. 51 kg, Ht 5′5″

Skin

Dry, no lesions, normal color and temperature

HEENT

PERRLA, EOMI without nystagmus

Neck

Supple; no adenopathy, JVD, or thyromegaly

Chest

Air entry equal; no crepitations or wheezing

CV

RRR, normal S_1 and S_2; no S_3 or S_4; no murmurs or rubs

Abd

Soft, mild tenderness to palpation in RLQ, (+) bowel sounds, no HSM

Genit/Rect

Tender inguinal adenopathy. External exam clear for nits and lice, several extensive shallow small painful vesicular lesions over vulva and labia, swollen and red. Vagina red, rugated, moderate amounts of creamy white discharge. Cervix pink, covered with above discharge, non-tender, ~3 cm. Corpus non-tender, no palpable masses. Adnexa with no palpable masses or tenderness. Rectum with no external lesions; (+) diffuse inflammation and friability internally, no masses.

Ext

Peripheral pulses 2+ bilaterally, DTRs 2+, no joint swelling or tenderness

Neuro

Alert and oriented, CN II–XII intact

Labs

Na 135 mEq/L	Hgb 12.9 g/dL	WBC 6.3 × 10^3/mm^3	RPR non-reactive
K 4.0 mEq/L	Hct 37.3%	64% PMNs	Preg test: hCG pending
Cl 102 mEq/L	Plt 255 × 10^3/mm^3	2% Bands	HIV serology: ELISA pending
CO_2 27 mEq/L		1% Eos	
BUN 11 mg/dL		24% Lymphs	
SCr 0.9 mg/dL		9% Monos	
Glu 72 mg/dL			

Other

Vaginal discharge-whiff test (–); pH < 4.5; wet mount *Trichomonas* (–), clue cells (–), monilia (+)

▶ Clinical Course

The following results were reported 5 days later.

- Viral culture of genital vesicular fluid: HSV-2 isolated
- Vulval swab DFA monoclonal stain: HSV-2 isolated
- Rectal and cervical bacterial cultures: *Neisseria gonorrhoeae* (–)
- Rectal and cervical cultures: *Chlamydia trachomatis* (+)

▶ Questions

Problem Identification

1. a. *Create a list of the patient's drug therapy problems.*
   b. *What subjective and objective clinical data are consistent with a primary genital herpes infection?*
   c. *Could any of the patient's problems have been caused by drug therapy?*

Desired Outcome

2. *What are the goals of pharmacotherapy in this case?*

Therapeutic Alternatives

3. a. *What nondrug therapies might be useful for this patient?*
   b. *What feasible pharmacotherapeutic alternatives are available for treatment of genital herpes and* Chlamydia*?*

Optimal Plan

4. *What drug, dosage form, dose, schedule, and duration of therapy are best for treating this patient's genital herpes and chlamydial infections?*

Outcome Evaluation

5. *What clinical and laboratory parameters are necessary to evaluate the therapy for achievement of the desired therapeutic outcome and to detect or prevent adverse effects?*

Patient Education

6. *What information should be provided to the patient to enhance compliance, ensure successful therapy, and minimize adverse effects?*

► Follow-Up Questions

1. *Six months later Lisa calls the STD clinic complaining of genital lesions that look and feel the same as the lesions she had 6 months earlier when seen and treated in the clinic. Should this episode of recurrent genital herpes be treated? If so, what therapies would be appropriate?*
2. *Is daily suppressive therapy indicated because she had a recurrent episode?*
3. *When is Herpes treatment indicated for sexual partners?*
4. *When is Chlamydia treatment indicated for sexual partners?*
5. *What additional pharmacotherapeutic interventions should be made to address the drug therapy problems that were identified in question 1.a.?*

► Self-Study Assignments

1. Determine whether there is a role for vaccines in the future management of herpes simplex disease.
2. Recommend alternative agents for the treatment of acyclovir-resistant herpes.
3. Explain the relationship between herpes simplex and HIV infections.
4. Describe herpes simplex complications that may require hospitalization, and recommend an appropriate treatment regimen.

► Clinical Pearl

- Most genital herpes infections are transmitted by persons who have asymptomatic viral shedding and are unaware that they have the infection.
- Systemic antiviral drugs control the signs and symptoms of genital herpes infection, but they do not eradicate latent virus.

References

1. Centers for Disease Control and Prevention. Genital herpes simplex (HSV) infection; Chlamydial infection. Sexually transmitted diseases treatment guidelines 2002. MMWR Morb Mortal Wkly Rep 2002;51(RR06):1–80. Available on the Internet at www.cdc.gov (Accessed July 24, 2004).
2. Anonymous. Drugs for sexually transmitted infections. Med Lett 1999;41:85–90.
3. Valtrex caplets package insert. Research Triangle Park, NC, GlaxoSmithKline, August 2003.
4. Famvir tablets package insert. Barcelona, Spain, Novartis Farmaceutica S.A. for Novartis Pharmaceuticals Corporation, East Hanover, NJ, February 2002.
5. CDC sexually transmitted diseases treatment guidelines. Clin Infect Dis 2002;35(Suppl 2):S135–S210.

126 OSTEOMYELITIS AND SEPTIC ARTHRITIS

► My Brother's Kicker (Level I)

Edward P. Armstrong, PharmD, BCPS, FASHP
Leslie L. Barton, MD

► After completing this case study, students should be able to:

- Recognize the most common presenting signs and symptoms of acute osteomyelitis and septic arthritis.
- Recommend alternative treatment approaches for acute osteomyelitis and septic arthritis in pediatric patients.
- Outline a treatment plan for empiric therapy of acute osteomyelitis and septic arthritis.
- Outline monitoring parameters for antibacterial treatment of osteomyelitis and septic arthritis, including efficacy and toxicity of therapy.

PATIENT PRESENTATION

Chief Complaint

"My knee still hurts."

HPI

John Grant is an 8 yo boy referred to the Infectious Disease Clinic because of persistent right knee pain 1 month after being kicked in the right knee by his brother. The day after the incident, he was seen in urgent care because of right knee pain and was sent home with symptomatic therapy. He returned to urgent care 1 week later (3 weeks ago) because of persistent tenderness in that knee.

He was again sent home only to be seen 1 week later (2 weeks ago), at which time physical examination suggested and x-rays confirmed the diagnosis of osteomyelitis of the distal right femur (see Figure 126–1). He had a WBC count of $8.0 \times 10^3/mm^3$, ESR of 21 mm/h, and tenderness over the right lateral femoral condyle. He underwent aspiration of the lesion, which revealed no pus. He was started on home IV therapy with cefazolin 500 mg IV Q 6 H. He had continued to play soccer during the first 2 weeks after his injury.

He was seen 1 week ago because of increasing knee pain after 1 week of antibiotic therapy. He denied any systemic symptoms and was afebrile. His ESR had risen to 48 mm/h; x-rays showed an increased size of the femoral lytic lesion. Aspiration of the knee joint revealed purulent fluid. The bone culture and the knee aspirate revealed no growth. Arthroscopic surgery of the knee was performed and cefazolin was continued.

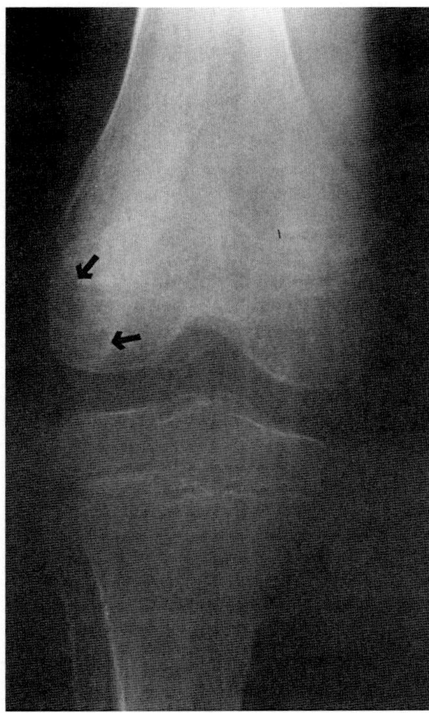

Figure 126–1. Lytic lesion of the distal right femur indicating osteomyelitis.

Three days ago at an office visit with the orthopedic surgeon, his mother reported mild improvement of the pain. She related that his pain had diminished during the preceding 3 days; he could now sleep through the night. He was still unable to bear weight on his right leg and was only able to ambulate with crutches. His ESR was 56 mm/h.

PMH

No prior history of serious diseases or infections
Immunizations are up-to-date

FH

No family history of early childhood deaths secondary to severe infection.

SH

Mother and father live in the household and are well, as are three siblings. There are three dogs in the home.

ROS

No positive findings with regard to head, eyes, ears, nose, throat, cardiorespiratory systems, skin lesions, or recent illness. No recent travel. No other significant trauma.

Meds

Cefazolin 500 mg IV Q 6 H

All

NKA

PE

Gen

His general appearance is that of a thin, apprehensive boy in no distress unless his right knee is flexed, extended, or palpated

VS

BP 93/50, P 104, RR 22, T 36.0°C; Wt 26.6 kg, Ht 4′4″

Skin

No lesions

HEENT

Eyes without corneal lesions, normal fundi; throat and pharynx without exudate; nose without discharge or congestion

Neck/LN

No lymphadenopathy or thyromegaly

Lungs/Thorax

Chest is clear to percussion and auscultation

CV

Normal S_1 and S_2; no murmurs present

Abd

Soft without hepatosplenomegaly

Genit/Rect

Genitalia are normal; circumcised male

MS/Ext

Swollen, slightly tender right knee held in flexion with marked decreased ROM. He has developed some tightness around the joint and is unable to bear weight on standing and preferred use of a posterior splint

Neuro

Reflexes 2+; plantar reflexes downgoing; no cerebellar or sensorial abnormalities; normal strength and tone except where not measurable at the right knee

Assessment

Continued distal femoral osteomyelitis and adjacent septic arthritis of the right knee, secondary to delayed and partial treatment of the staphylococcal infection. The persistently elevated ESR and slow resolution of knee symptoms are of concern.

▶ Questions

Problem Identification

1. a. *Create a list of the patient's drug therapy problems.*
   b. *What information (signs, symptoms, laboratory values) indicates the presence or severity of acute osteomyelitis?*
   c. *What information (signs, symptoms, laboratory values) indicates the presence of septic arthritis?*

Desired Outcome

2. *What are the goals of pharmacotherapy in this case?*

Therapeutic Alternatives

3. a. *What nondrug therapies might be useful for this patient?*
   b. *What feasible pharmacotherapeutic alternatives are available for the empiric treatment of acute osteomyelitis?*

Optimal Plan

4. *What drug, dosage form, dose, schedule, and duration of therapy are best for this patient?*

▶ Clinical Course

An x-ray taken after low-dose antibiotic treatment showed a persistent lesion (see Figure 126–2). The I.D. consultant continued the cefazolin but changed the regimen to 100 mg/kg/24 h given in 3 divided doses. She recommended clinical reevaluation with repeat WBC and ESR in 1 week. If his ESR is the same, or (preferably) lower, cefazolin is to be discontinued and oral cephalexin 100 mg/kg/day in 4 divided doses is to be initiated. Reevaluation of the patient after 1 week of oral therapy was planned.

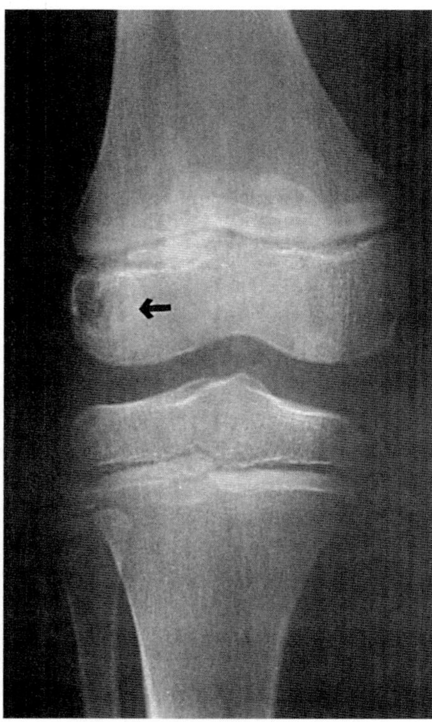

Figure 126–2. Persistent lesion of the distal right femur after low-dose antibiotic treatment.

Ten days later, the patient was again seen in the Pediatric Infectious Disease Clinic where clinical evaluation revealed no additional findings. The patient continued to be afebrile and his ESR was 12 mm/h. He was still on crutches, but he had recently removed the right posterior leg splint. His mother had been helping him perform some passive range-of-motion exercises. His right leg was still maintained in a flexed position at the knee. He had full range of motion at the right hip but decreased flexion and extension at the right knee. The gastrocnemius circumference was slightly diminished on the right side, but strength on both plantar flexion and dorsiflexion of the right foot was normal. He had been tolerating the oral antibiotic regimen without apparent abdominal discomfort, diarrhea, or rash. Oral cephalexin was to be continued for at least three additional weeks at the same dose of 100 mg/kg/day.

Outcome Evaluation

5. *What clinical and laboratory parameters are necessary to evaluate the therapy for achievement of the desired therapeutic outcome and to detect or prevent adverse effects?*

Patient Education

6. *What information should be provided to the patient's caregiver to enhance compliance, ensure successful therapy, and minimize adverse effects?*

▶ Self-Study Assignments

1. Plan alternative IV and oral treatment regimens in the event that the patient could not tolerate the antibiotic initially used.
2. Compare optimal oral treatment strategies for osteomyelitis in adults with those in children.

▶ Clinical Pearl

The ultimate prognosis of acute osteomyelitis and septic arthritis is based on the speed of diagnosis, prompt initiation of appropriate antimicrobial therapy, and surgical drainage, if needed.

References

1. Martinez-Aguilar G, Hammerman WA, Mason EO, et al. Clindamycin treatment of invasive infections caused by community-acquired, methicillin-resistant and methicillin-susceptible Staphylococcus aureus in children. Pediatr Infect Dis J 2003;22:593–598.
2. Karwowska A, Davies HD, Jadavji T. Epidemiology and outcome of osteomyelitis in the era of sequential intravenous-oral therapy. Pediatr Infect Dis J 1998;17:1021–1026.
3. Burnett MW, Bass JW, Cook BA. Etiology of osteomyelitis complicating sickle cell disease. Pediatrics 1998;101:296–297.

4. Nelson JD. Skeletal infections in children. Adv Pediatr Infect Dis 1991;6:59–78.
5. Unkila-Kallio L, Kallio MJ, Eskola J, et al. Serum C-reactive protein, erythrocyte sedimentation rate, and white blood cell count in acute hematogenous osteomyelitis of children. Pediatrics 1994;93:59–62.
6. Dagan R. Management of acute hematogenous osteomyelitis and septic arthritis in the pediatric patient. Pediatr Infect Dis J 1993;12:88–92.
7. Lew DP, Waldvogel FA. Osteomyelitis. N Engl J Med 1997;336:999–1007.
8. Kaplan SL, Deville JG, Yogev R, et al. Linezolid Pediatric Study Group. Linezolid versus vancomycin for treatment of resistant Gram-positive infections in children. Pediatr Infect Dis J 2003;22:677–686.

127 GRAM-NEGATIVE SEPSIS

▶ Not by Antibiotics Alone

Steven J. Martin, PharmD, BCPS, FCCM
Sandy J. Close, PharmD, BCPS

▶ After completing this case study the student should be able to:

- Utilize current consensus guidelines to identify sepsis and severe sepsis at the bedside.
- Evaluate the hemodynamic status of a patient with sepsis, given specific patient data, and design an initial pharmacotherapeutic plan.
- Discuss the suspected pathogens in Gram-negative sepsis, and outline an initial empiric treatment strategy.
- Identify the patient in whom drotrecogin alfa (activated) would be appropriate, including consideration of relative and absolute contraindications.

PATIENT PRESENTATION

Chief Complaint
Not available

HPI
John Jacobson is a 68 yo man admitted to the hospital 2 weeks ago for CAP and COPD exacerbation. After a complicated hospital course, he developed hypotension and respiratory distress on day 15 of his hospital stay.

PMH
COPD

FH
Noncontributory

SH
(+) Tobacco 1 ppd × 40 years

ROS
Not available

Meds
Combivent 2 puffs Q 6 H
Albuterol nebulizer Q 6 H and PRN
Docusate Sodium 100 mg ng BID
Multivitamin 1 tablet daily
Metoprolol 5 mg IV PRN for systolic BP >150 mm Hg

All
PCN (rash—10 years ago)

PE

Gen
Elderly man, confused and in respiratory distress

VS
BP 90/60, P 100, RR 22, T 39°C; Ht 5′11″, Wt 67 kg

HEENT
PERRLA, TMs intact, oropharynx clear, no exudates or masses

Neck
Supple; no adenopathy, JVD

Lungs
LUL is CTA with diminished breath sounds; the LLL has the absence of breath sounds

CV
Tachycardic, no murmurs

Abd
Soft, non-tender, non-distended; (–) BS

Genit/Rect
Normal

Ext
Good pulses, skin warm, no stigmata of endocarditis

Neuro
A & O × 1 (person); no focal findings

Labs

Na 131 mEq/L	Hgb 11.8 g/dL	Ca 9.1 mg/dL
K 4.4 mEq/L	Hct 33%	Mg 1.8 mEq/L
Cl 95 mEq/L	Plt 97 × 10^3/mm^3	Phos 4.3 mg/dL
CO_2 23 mEq/L	WBC 14.2 × 10^3/mm^3	Alb 2.7 g/dL
BUN 67 mg/dL	65% Polys	PT 17.5 sec
SCr 2.3 mg/dL	10% Bands	INR 2.0
Glu 169 mg/dL	20% Lymphs	
	5% Monos	

CXR
Extensive LUL infiltrate; remainder of the lungs are clear

Assessment
Respiratory distress, hypotension and nosocomial pneumonia; R/O sepsis

Plan
Stabilize the patient and transfer to the MICU

▶ Clinical Course

The patient was intubated and transferred to the MICU. One liter of normal saline was given for hypotension. The patient's pressure remained 88/60 mm Hg after infusion of the normal saline.

▶ Questions

Problem Identification

1. a. *Devise a drug therapy problem list for this patient.*
   b. *What signs and symptoms must be present to diagnose sepsis in this patient?*
   c. *How is sepsis differentiated from severe sepsis?*

Desired Outcome

2. a. *What are the short-term goals of therapy for this patient?*
   b. *What are the long-term goals in the management of sepsis?*

Therapeutic Alternatives

3. a. *What alternatives are available to treat hypotension in sepsis patients?*
   b. *When should vasoactive agents be started?*
   c. *When should inotropic therapy be considered, and which agents are appropriate?*
   d. *When are corticosteroids used to treat sepsis?*

▶ Clinical Course—ICU Day 1

After the patient was admitted to the MICU, medications initiated by the ICU team included (in addition to the agents recommended previously by you):

Famotidine 20 mg IV Q 12 H
Enoxaparin 40 mg subQ once daily
The Tmax (maximum temperature) in the last 24 hours is 40°C, and the patient is still hypotensive even though fluids and vasopressors have been maximized.

Microbiology
Sputum: Many gram-negative rods
Urine/Blood: No growth

Optimal Plan

4. a. *Provide an empiric antibiotic regimen for the treatment of nosocomial pneumonia in this patient.*
   b. *The medical team wishes to start drotrecogin alfa (activated) in this patient. Is this patient an appropriate candidate for the drug?*
   c. *How should drotrecogin alfa (activated) therapy be administered and monitored?*
   d. *What other drug-related aspects of care should be considered for patients with critical illness?*

▶ Clinical Course—ICU Day 3

The patient's BP has ranged from 90–110/72–84 in the last 24 hours. Tmax was 39.8°C and is currently 39.0°C. On physical exam, mild edema is noted at the site of the peripherally-inserted central catheter (PICC). Labs are essentially unchanged with the following exceptions:

Hgb 9.1 g/dL	Plt 39 × 10³/mm³
Hct 28.2%	PT 13.9
WBC 2.9 × 10³/mm³	INR 1.3

Microbiology

Sputum Culture:
Pseudomonas aeruginosa heavy growth

Sensitivities	
Aztreonam	R
Ciprofloxacin	R
Pipercillin	R
Pipercillin/tazobactam	R
Gentamicin	R
Tobramycin	S
Cefuroxime	R
Cefepime	S
Imipenem/cilastatin	S

   e. *Based on this new information, what changes in antimicrobial therapy would you recommend?*
   f. *How long should antimicrobial therapy be continued in this patient?*

▶ Clinical Course—ICU Day 4

Drotrecogin alfa therapy is discontinued. The patient no longer requires vasopressor therapy and is extubated.

Outcome Evaluation

5. *What parameters should be monitored to evaluate the efficacy and toxicity of this patient's treatment?*

► Clinical Course—ICU Day 6

The patient has been discharged to the floor. Preparations are being made for the patient to continue necessary medications at home.

Patient Education

6. *What information should be provided to this patient about his antimicrobial therapy and other medications upon discharge from the medical floor?*

► Self Study Assignments

1. Review hemodynamic monitoring parameters and their correlation with various shock states.
2. Review literature reference #3 below regarding drotrecogin alfa (activated) and describe the characteristics of patients in whom this drug would be most beneficial.
3. Review mechanisms of antimicrobial resistance by organism and drug class. Create a list of antimicrobial agents to which organisms are more likely to develop resistance.

► Clinical Pearl

The systemic inflammatory response syndrome (SIRS) resulting from an infection defines sepsis. The causative pathogen may be easily eradicated (such as *E. coli* in the urine), but the SIRS may worsen and ultimately be the demise of the patient. Treatment of this infection (i.e., sepsis) requires much more than simply appropriate antibiotics.

References

1. Levy MM, Fink MP, Marshall JC, et al. 2001 SCCM/ESICM/ACCP/ATS/SIS International Sepsis Definitions Conference. Crit Care Med 2003; 31:1250–1256.
2. Rivers E, Nguyen B, Havstad S, et al. Early goal-directed therapy in the treatment of severe sepsis and septic shock. N Engl J Med 2001;345:1368–1377.
3. Delinger RP, Carlet JM, Masur H, et al. Surviving Sepsis Campaign guidelines for management of severe sepsis and septic shock. Crit Care Med 2004;32: 858–873.
4. Hollenber SM, Ahrens TS, Carpati CM, et al. Practice parameters for hemodynamic support of sepsis in adult patients. Crit Care med 1999;27: 639–660.
5. Annane D, Sebille V, Charpentier C, et al. Effect of treatment with low doses of hydrocortisone and fludrocortisone on mortality in patients with septic shock. JAMA 2002;288:862–871.
6. Paul M, Benuri-Silbiger I, Soares-Weiser K, et al. Beta-lactam monotherapy versus beta-lactam-aminoglycoside combination therapy for sepsis in immunocompetent patients: Systematic review and meta-analysis of randomized trials. BMJ 328(7441):668. Epub 2004 Mar 02.
7. Wunderink RG, Rello J, Cammarata SK, et al. Linezolid vs vancomycin: Analysis of two double-blind studies of patients with methicillin-resistant *Staphylococcus aureus* nosocomial pneumonia. JAMA 2003;124:1789–1797.
8. Bernard GR, Vincent JL, Laterre PF, et al. Efficacy and safety of recombinant human activated protein C for severe sepsis. N Engl J Med 2001;344:699–709.
9. van den Berghe G, Wouters P, Weekers F, et al. Intensive insulin therapy in critically ill patients. N Eng J Med 2001;345:1359–1367.
10. Chastre J, Wolff M, Fagon JY, et al. Comparison of 8 vs 15 days of antibiotic therapy for ventilator-associated pneumonia in adults: A randomized trial. JAMA 2003;290:2588–2598.

128 DERMATOPHYTOSIS

► Walking the Lecture Circuit (Level II)

Robert L. Maher Jr., PharmD

► After completing this case study, students should be able to:

- Identify the risk factors for tinea pedis and onychomycosis.
- Know the pathogens associated with tinea pedis and onychomycosis.
- Discuss the risks and benefits of the therapeutic alternatives available for the treatment of tinea pedis and onychomycosis.
- Develop a patient-specific therapeutic plan for the management of tinea pedis and onychomycosis.
- Understand the managed-care issues related to onychomycosis.

PATIENT PRESENTATION

Chief Complaint

"My feet are killing me. White flakes are appearing on my feet again. Why are my toenails brittle and yellow?"

HPI

Harold White is a 67 yo man who presents to the dermatology clinic for evaluation of his feet. He is a former law professor who now is a frequent speaker at law conferences and meetings. Two months ago when he was out of town attending a conference, he experienced mild itching and redness on his feet. He went to the gift shop in his hotel and bought 0.5% hydrocortisone cream, which gave him some relief. However, 1 week after the conference, white flakes appeared on both of his feet, and he realized that it was a recurrence of his athlete's foot.

Today, he complains that the itching still bothers him and is not relieved by tolnaftate and hydrocortisone creams. He also complains that his toenails have turned yellow and brittle. He states that he tried not to miss his daily walks, even though it has been raining for the past 2 weeks. However in the last week, he has had to miss his daily walk because of pain in his toenails. He wants a cure as soon as possible because he has to travel again next week for another lecture series.

PMH

Athlete's foot 6 months ago
Osteoarthritis of both knees × 2 years
CAD
Hx of MI, s/p CABG 2001
Mild CHF
Hypercholesterolemia × 3 years
HTN × 5 years
GERD with recurrent symptoms
S/P cholecystectomy 4 years ago

FH

Father died at age 73 of CHF; mother is alive with HTN.

SH

Professor in criminal law; has been an avid runner in the past, jogging at least 2 miles/day for 30 years; changed to walking several years ago because of OA of the knees and heart disease. Drinks one glass of wine with dinner; likes traveling and gourmet dining.

ROS

Denies fever, chills, fatigue, numbness and tingling in extremities, or recent trauma to his feet. Complains of brittle and yellow toenails and dry, scaling, and itchy feet; decreased ambulation due to pain in toenails.

Meds

Aspirin 81 mg po daily × 1 year
Pravastatin 20 mg po daily × 1 year
Coreg 6.25 mg po BID
Digoxin 0.25 mg po daily
Lisinopril 10 mg po daily
Ranitidine 150 mg po at bedtime
Hydrocortisone 0.5% cream applied TID PRN to itchy feet
Tolnaftate cream applied BID PRN to itchy feet
Ibuprofen 200 mg po Q 4 H PRN knee pain
Multiple vitamins 1 tablet po daily
Glucosamine 500 mg po TID

All

Citrus foods and juices (upset stomach)

PE

Gen

Pleasant, talkative, anxious man who is wearing a suit and a pair of old, foul-smelling tennis shoes

VS

BP 145/89, P 95, RR 18, T 37.0°C, Ht 5′6″, Wt 78 kg

Skin

Moist and soft

HEENT

PEERLA, EOMI, oropharynx clear, moist mucous membranes, normal fundi

Neck/LN

Neck supple, normal lymph nodes and thyroid gland, no JVD

Lungs/Chest

Normal breath sounds, chest CTA

CV

RRR; normal S_1 and S_2; no murmur

Abd

Soft and nontender, no guarding or HSM

Genit/Rect

Normal male genitalia, rectal exam not performed

MS/Ext

Mild erythematous skin; fine silvery white flakes on the plantar surfaces of both feet; dry scales and hyperkeratotic skin covering the soles of both feet. Yellow-brown discoloration and thickening of the first, second, and third toenails of both feet; brittle toenails. Patellar crepitus of both knees; no synovial thickening or inflammation; normal range of motion; 2+ pulses throughout

Neuro

Intact, A & O × 3, normal DTRs, CNs intact, normal plantar flexion

Labs (one month ago)

			Fasting Lipid Panel
Na 145 mEq/L	Hgb 13.8 g/dL	AST 20 IU/L	T. chol 220 mg/dL
K 4.1 mEq/L	Hct 41 4%	ALT 30 IU/L	LDL 136 mg/dL
Cl 110 mEq/L	Plt 160 × 10^3/mm^3	Alk phos 78 IU/L	HDL 54 mg/dL
CO_2 25 mEq/L	WBC 9.8 × 10^3/mm^3	GGT 89 IU/L	Trig 150 mg/dL
BUN 22 mg/dL		T. bili 1.2 mg/dL	
SCr 1.1 mg/dL			
Glu 98 mg/dL			

Other

Microscopy of toenail debris—KOH preparation viewed with dark-field illumination reveals branching and filamentous hyphae consistent with dermatophyte infection.
Fungal culture of toenail debris—pending.

Assessment

67 yo man with tinea pedis and onychomycosis.

▶ Questions

Problem Identification

1. a. *Create a list of the patient's drug therapy problems.*
   b. *What are the subjective and objective signs and symptoms of tinea pedis and onychomycosis in this patient?*
   c. *What are the differential diagnoses for these conditions?*
   d. *What are the common pathogens associated with tinea pedis and onychomycosis?*
   e. *What are the risk factors for tinea pedis and onychomycosis in this patient?*

Desired Outcome

2. *What are the goals of treatment for tinea pedis and onychomycosis in this patient?*

Therapeutic Alternatives

3. a. *What nondrug therapies might be useful for this patient?*
   b. *What feasible pharmacotherapeutic alternatives are available for treatment of the tinea pedis and onychomycosis?*

Optimal Plan

4. *What drug, dosage form, dose, schedule, and duration of therapy are best for this patient?*

Outcome Evaluation

5. *Which clinical and laboratory parameters are necessary to evaluate the therapy for achievement of the desired therapeutic outcome and to detect or prevent adverse effects?*

Patient Education

6. *What information should be provided to the patient to enhance compliance, ensure successful therapy, and minimize adverse effects?*

▶ Clinical Course

The patient's symptoms of athlete's foot slowly resolved over 4 weeks, and appearance of his toenails improved after 3 months of therapy.

▶ Follow-Up Questions

1. *What are the cardiovascular risk factors in this patient?*
2. *How does his risk factor status affect your management of his hypercholesterolemia?*

▶ Self-Study Assignments

1. What is the role of oral azole therapy in the treatment of tinea pedis?
2. Discuss the advantages and disadvantages of using itraconazole or terbinafine for the management of onychomycosis.
3. What medical necessity documentation is needed to ensure payment by a managed care company for oral therapy of onychomycosis?
4. What are the potential benefits of using a topical cream instead of a topical gel for the management of tinea pedis?

▶ Clinical Pearl

Tinea pedis is a risk factor for onychomycosis. Management of onychomycosis requires long-term treatment and is associated with high rates of relapse.

References

1. Goldsmith H. Practice management and managed care issues in onychomycosis. J Am Podiatr Med Soc 1997;87:532–539.
2. Meis JF, Verweij PE. Current management of fungal infections. Drugs 2001; 61(Suppl 1):13–25.
3. Sigurgeirsson B, Olafsson JH, Steinsson JB, et al. Long-term effectiveness of treatment with terbinafine vs itraconazole in onychomycosis: A 5-year blinded prospective follow-up study. Arch Dermatol 2002;138:353–357.
4. Tosti A, Piraccini BM, Stinchi C, et al. Treatment of dermatophyte nail infections: An open randomized study comparing intermittent terbinafine therapy with continuous terbinafine treatment and intermittent itraconazole therapy. J Am Acad Dermatol 1996;34:595–600.
5. Bootman JL. Cost-effectiveness of two new treatments for onychomycosis: An analysis of two comparative clinical trials. J Am Acad Dermatol 1998;38(5 Pt 3):S69–S72.

129 BACTERIAL VAGINOSIS

▶ Competition Among Bacteria (Level I)

Charles D. Ponte, PharmD, BC-ADM, BCPS, CDE, FAPhA, FASHP, FCCP

▶ After completing this case study, students should be able to:

- Identify predisposing factors associated with bacterial vaginosis.
- List the common clinical and diagnostic findings associated with bacterial vaginosis.
- Develop a therapeutic plan for the management of bacterial vaginosis.
- Describe the role of the pharmacist in the overall management of infectious vaginitis.

PATIENT PRESENTATION

Chief Complaint

"I'm here for a follow-up visit."

HPI

Brenda Singer is a 20 yo woman who comes to the University Health Service for a rescheduled follow-up visit for cervicitis. She missed her initial follow-up appointment 3 weeks ago. She was diagnosed 1 month ago and started on doxycycline 100 mg po BID × 7 days. At that time, a test for *Chlamydia* was non-reactive. She states that she has completed her course of doxycycline despite some mild nausea attributed to the drug. Her sexual partners had been informed and were scheduled for treatment. She has resumed sexual activity since finishing the doxycycline and mentions that her period is late. She also complains of some mild vaginal discomfort and a "funny" odor. Her last period was approximately 6 weeks ago. She admits to inconsistent use of a diaphragm for contraception.

PMH

Noncontributory

FH

Noncontributory

SH

Is a student in the College of Business and Economics. Has multiple sexual partners; partners rarely use condoms. Has smoked one-half pack of cigarettes per day since age 16. Alcohol use is mostly beer, mixed drinks on occasion.

ROS
Noncontributory except that she has noticed a small amount of thin white mucus on her underclothing.

Meds
Doxycycline 100 mg po BID × 7 days (completed with no problems except some mild nausea)
Multivitamins 1 po QD

All
Dogs → itchy eyes and sneezing; house dust → watery eyes, sneezing; sulfas → measles-like pruritic rash

PE
Limited because of follow-up of specific gynecologic complaint.

Gen
Patient is a healthy appearing 20 yo woman in NAD

VS
BP 100/70, P 80, RR 16, T 37°C; Ht 5′6″, Wt 51.3 kg

Genit/Rect
External genitalia WNL; vagina with a small amount of thin white mucus; positive whiff test; pH 5.0. Cervix—not completely visualized; appears clear with a small amount of mucoid discharge from the os. Uterus is slightly enlarged, non-tender, anteverted, no cervical motion tenderness. Adnexa without tenderness or masses

Labs
Microscopic examination of vaginal secretions: 20–25 WBC/hpf; 10–15 clue cells/hpf; 0 Lactobacilli/hpf; 15–20 squamous epithelial cells/hpf
Serum pregnancy test - positive

Assessment
Resolving cervicitis
Bacterial vaginosis
Early pregnancy

Questions

Problem Identification

1. a. *Create a list of the patient's drug therapy problems.*
   b. *What clinical or laboratory information indicates the presence of bacterial vaginosis (see Table 129–1)?*
   c. *What is the pathophysiologic basis for the development of bacterial vaginosis?*
   d. *Could the patient's problem have been caused by drug therapy?*

Desired Outcome

2. *What are the goals of pharmacotherapy in this case?*

Therapeutic Alternatives

3. a. *What feasible pharmacotherapeutic alternatives are available for the treatment of bacterial vaginosis?*
   b. *What economic, psychosocial, and ethical considerations are applicable to this patient?*

Optimal Plan

4. a. *What drug, dosage form, dose, schedule, and duration of therapy are best for this patient?*
   b. *What alternatives would be appropriate if the initial therapy fails or cannot be used?*

Outcome Evaluation

5. *What clinical and laboratory parameters are necessary to evaluate the therapy for achievement of the desired therapeutic outcome and to detect or prevent adverse effects?*

Patient Education

6. *What information should be provided to the patient to enhance adherence, ensure successful therapy, and minimize adverse effects?*

TABLE 129–1. Characteristics of Different Types of Vaginitis

Characteristic	*Candida*	Bacterial	*Trichomonas*	Chemical
Pruritus	++	+/–	+/–	++
Erythema	+	+/–	+/–	+
Abnormal discharge	+	+	+/–	–
Viscosity	Thick	Thin	Thick/thin	–
Color	White	Gray	White, yellow, green-gray	–
Odor	None	Foul, "fishy"	Malodorous	–
Description	Curd-like	Homogeneous	Frothy	–
pH	3.8–5.0	> 4.5	5.0–7.5	–
Diagnostic tests	KOH prep. shows long, thread-like fibers of mycelia microscopically	+ "whiff test," "clue cells"	Pear-shaped protozoa, cervical "strawberry" spots	–

▶ Clinical Course

After completion of the treatment you recommended, the patient returns to the clinic for follow-up. She voices no complaints except that she has been experiencing some vaginal itching and painful intercourse. Physical examination reveals whitish cottage-cheese-like material adherent to the vaginal mucosa. The vulva also appears erythematous. Microscopic analysis of vaginal secretions revealed hyphae and budding yeast. No white cells are noted. Vaginal pH is normal. The patient is diagnosed with vaginal candidiasis.

▶ Follow-Up Questions

1. *What is the most likely cause of this patient's vaginal candidiasis?*
2. *What other issues should be addressed with the patient during this follow-up visit?*
3. *What is the role of the pharmacist in the management of patients with infectious vaginitis?*

▶ Self-Study Assignments

1. Discuss the management of a patient who fails a specific course of treatment for bacterial vaginosis.
2. Discuss the pros and cons of screening asymptomatic pregnant women for the presence of bacterial vaginosis.
3. Describe the best therapeutic approach for a woman diagnosed with bacterial vaginosis who is breast-feeding her infant.
4. Discuss the role of sexual transmission in the pathogenesis of bacterial vaginosis.

▶ Clinical Pearl

Avoid condom or diaphragm use with clindamycin 2% vaginal cream. The vehicle is petroleum-based (mineral oil) and will weaken the integrity of latex products, increasing the risk of pregnancy.

References

1. Joesoef MR, Schmid GP, Hillier SL. Bacterial vaginosis: Review of treatment options and potential clinical indications for therapy. Clin Infect Dis 1999; 28(Suppl 1):S57–S65.
2. Tam MT, Yungbluth M, Myles T. Gram stain method shows better sensitivity than clinical criteria for detection of bacterial vaginosis in surveillance of pregnant, low-income women in a clinical setting. Infect Dis Obstet Gynecol 1998; 6:204–208.
3. Burstein GR, Murray PJ. Diagnosis and management of sexually transmitted disease pathogens among adolescents. Pediatr Rev 2003; 24(3):75–82.
4. Nasraty S. Infections of the female genital tract. Prim Care 2003;30(1): 193–203.
5. Centers for Disease Control and Prevention. Diseases characterized by vaginal discharge. 2002 Guidelines for treatment of sexually transmitted diseases. MMWR Morb Mortal Wkly Rep 2002;51(RR-06):42–44. Available on the Internet at www.cdc.gov.
6. Sobel JD. Bacterial vaginosis. Ann Rev Med 2000; 51:349–56.
7. Monif GRG. Bacterial vaginosis: A new perspective. Infect Med 2001;18:25–26.

130 CANDIDA VAGINITIS

▶ When OTC Beats Rx (Level II)

Rebecca M. Law, PharmD

▶ After completing this case study, students should be able to:

- Distinguish *Candida* vaginitis from other types of vaginitis.
- Know when to refer a patient with symptoms of vaginitis to a physician for further evaluation and treatment.
- Choose an appropriate product for the patient with *Candida* vaginitis.
- Educate patients with vaginitis about proper use of pharmacotherapeutic treatments and nonpharmacologic management strategies.

PATIENT PRESENTATION

Chief Complaint

"I'm having the same problem I had 2 weeks ago and my doctor is away until next Monday. Can you give me some more of these suppositories?"

HPI

Sophie Kim is a 32 yo woman who presents to your pharmacy with the above complaint. Upon further questioning, you find that she was diagnosed 3 weeks ago by her physician as having a vaginal *Candida* infection. She was prescribed nystatin suppositories 100,000 units intravaginally for 14 nights. She stated that she had finished the prescription a week ago and had felt better then. However, 3 days ago she began to notice mild vaginal itching again. She thought it was her new control-top panty hose and stopped wearing them, but the itching got worse and became fairly severe with a burning sensation. There was also a white, dry, curd-like vaginal discharge that was non-odorous. This seemed to be identical to what she had experienced 3 weeks ago. Her physician is away until next week, and she wondered if the pharmacy can give her some more suppositories.

PMH

Diabetes Type 1 since age 11. Her blood glucose is well controlled with careful monitoring due to her pregnancy.

Recurrent leg ulcers and foot infections for which she has been prescribed antibiotics on a frequent basis. Currently there are no ulcers or infections and she is not on antibiotics.

Last month she began using tights (with an adjustable waist) to help prevent varicose veins.

SH

Nonsmoker; drinks alcohol in moderate amounts (one to two drinks maximum) at social functions. She is married and is 71/2 months pregnant.

Meds

Lente insulin 20 units subQ Q AM for past year

Insulin Lispro 6 units subQ 15 minutes prior to breakfast, 8 units 15 minutes prior to lunch, and 10 units 15 minutes prior to dinner, for past 4 months

Materna 1 po Q AM

ROS

Not performed

PE

Wt 70 kg, Ht 5′5″ BP 120/78

No further assessments performed.

Labs

Not available

▶ Questions

Problem Identification

1. a. *What signs and symptoms indicate the presence and severity of Candida vaginitis (see Table 130–1)?*
   b. *What predisposing factors for Candida vaginitis might exist in this patient?*

Desired Outcome

2. *What are the goals of therapy for this patient?*

Therapeutic Alternatives

3. *What pharmacotherapeutic alternatives are available for the treatment of Candida vaginitis?*

Optimal Plan

4. *Design a pharmacotherapeutic plan for this patient.*

Outcome Evaluation

5. *What parameters should be monitored to assess the efficacy of the treatment and to detect adverse effects?*

Patient Education

6. *What information should the patient receive about her treatment?*

▶ Self-Study Assignments

1. Obtain information on tests used to diagnose different types of vaginitis.
2. Compare the retail cost of nonprescription vaginitis treatments in your area.
3. Outline your plan for communicating your treatment recommendations to the patient's physician.

▶ Clinical Pearl

Patients with symptoms suggestive of bacterial vaginitis or sexually transmitted disease (fever, abdominal or back pain, foul-smelling discharge) should be referred to a physician for further evaluation and treatment.

References

1. Young GL, Jewell D. Topical treatment for vaginal candidiasis (thrush) in pregnancy (Cochrane Review). In: The Cochrane Library, 4; 2003. Chichester, UK: John Wiley & Sons, Ltd. Abstract available at: http://www.cochrane.de/cochrane/revabstr/ab000225.htm. Accessed July 28, 2004.
2. Pappas PG, Rex JH, Sobel JD, et al. Guidelines for treatment of candidiasis. Clin Infect Dis 2004;38:161–189.
3. Briggs, GG, Freeman RK, Yaffe SJ. Drugs in Pregnancy and Lactation, 6th ed. Baltimore, MD, Williams and Wilkins, 2002.
4. Black RA, Hill DA. Over-the-counter medications in pregnancy. Am Fam Physician 2003;67:2517–2524.

TABLE 130–1. Characteristics of Different Types of Vaginitis

Characteristic	*Candida*	Bacterial	*Trichomonas*	Chemical
Pruritus	++	+/–	+/–	++
Erythema	+	+/–	+/–	+
Abnormal discharge	+	+	+/–	–
Viscosity	Thick	Thin	Thick/thin	–
Color	White	Gray	White, yellow, green-gray	–
Odor	None	Foul, "fishy"	Malodorous	–
Description	Curd-like	Homogeneous	Frothy	–
pH	3.8–5.0	> 4.5	5.0–7.5	–
Diagnostic tests	KOH prep. shows long, thread-like fibers of mycelia microscopically	+ "whiff test," "clue cells"	Pear-shaped protozoa, cervical "strawberry" spots	–

5. Press N. Sexually transmitted diseases. In: Gray J, ed. Therapeutic Choices, 4th ed. Canadian Pharmacists Association, 2003:1012–1027.
6. U.S. Food and Drug Administration. FDA updates safety information for miconazole vaginal cream and suppositories. FDA Talk paper. March 5, 2001. Available at: www.fda.gov/bbs/topics/ANSWERS/2001/ANS01071.html. Accessed August 27, 2004.
7. Watson MC, Grimshaw JM, Bond CM, et al. Oral versus intra-vaginal imidazole and triazole anti-fungal treatment of uncomplicated vulvovaginal candidiasis (thrush). Cochrane Review. In: The Cochrane Library, 4, 2003. Chichester, UK: John Wiley & Sons, Ltd. Abstract available at: http://www.cochrane.org/cochrane/revabstr/AB002845.htm. Accessed July 28, 2004.
8. Sanchez JM, Moya G. Fluconazole teratogenicity. Prenat Diagn 1998;18:862–863.
9. Jick SS. Pregnancy outcomes after maternal exposure to fluconazole. Pharmacotherapy 1999;19:221–22.
10. Pirotta M, Gunn J, Chondros, P, et al. Effect of lactobacillus in preventing post-antibiotic vulvovaginal candidiasis: A randomized controlled trial. BMJ 2004;329:548. E pub 2004 Aug 27.

131 SYSTEMIC FUNGAL INFECTION

► Solving a Budding Problem (Level III)

Travis W. Cooper, PharmD, BCPS
Anya Rockwell, PharmD

► After completing this case study, students should be able to:

- Describe the pathogenesis and potential sequelae of hematogenous fungal infections in hospitalized patients.
- Given a case scenario, identify risk factors that predispose a patient to systemic fungal infection.
- Discuss the clinical utility of antifungal prophylaxis in non-neutropenic, critically ill patients in intensive care units.
- Differentiate fungal colonization from invasion/dissemination.
- Recommend empiric antifungal therapy based upon patient history/clinical condition, site of infection, and antifungal resistance patterns.
- List specific monitoring parameters for antifungal use in critically ill patients.

PATIENT PRESENTATION

Chief Complaint

"My chest feels so tight, and I just can't seem to breathe anymore."

HPI

Wanda Stevenson is a 57 yo woman admitted with a COPD exacerbation. She became progressively more short of breath with increased wheezing, severe tachypnea, and accessory muscle use over the week preceding her admission. After failing both BIPAP and CPAP trials after hospitalization, she was sedated with etomidate and midazolam, and orotracheally intubated. Seven days into her hospital stay, she became harder to oxygenate and began to produce thick, purulent sputum. A chest x-ray revealed diffuse bilateral infiltrates, and empiric antibiotic therapy was initiated for treatment of ventilator-associated pneumonia. A nasogastric tube was placed for enteral feedings and 2 days later the patient produced 600 mL of dark, reddish-black aspirate that was guaiac positive. On day 18, the patient developed diminished bowel sounds with a distended abdomen and mild RUQ tenderness. She also exhibited intermittent episodes of delirium and a hypoventilation syndrome of unknown origin. Gastric residual was 75 mL at last check. A right internal jugular (IJ) line and urinary catheter were placed 10 and 14 days ago, respectively.

PMH

COPD
Diabetes mellitus
Depression
Hypercholesterolemia
HTN

PSH

Noncontributory

FH

Mother alive with hypothyroidism ~25 years; father alive with hypertension ~30 years.

SH

Denies alcohol and IVDU; 45 pack-year smoker. Lives alone.

Meds

Heparin 5,000 units subQ Q 8 H
KCl 20 mEq NG once daily
Metoclopramide 10 mg IV Q 6 H
Furosemide 20 mg IV Q 6 H
Methylprednisolone 60 mg IV Q 6 H
Ipratropium 500 mcg nebulized Q 6 H
Albuterol 2.5 mg nebulized Q 6 H
Terazosin 5 mg NG BID
Simvastatin 20 mg NG once daily
Lorazepam continuous IV infusion titrated to a Riker sedation agitation score of 3 to 4
Morphine sulfate 2 mg IV Q 2 H
Piperacillin/tazobactam 4.5 g IV Q 8 H
Tobramycin 600 mg IV Q 24 H
Enteral feeding (Pulmocare) at 30 mL/h

All

Iodinated compounds → maculopapular rash
Meperidine → hypotension with rash
Metronidazole → peripheral neuropathies

PE

Gen
Morbidly obese white woman with vitiligo of extremities. APACHE II = 12

VS
BP 115/75, HR 122, RR 26–30 (preintubation), T 38.7°C; Wt 128 kg, Ht 5′9″

Skin
Slight monilial overgrowth on skin folds lateral to vaginal area

HEENT
PERRLA; funduscopy reveals clear disk margins without exudates. Patient orotracheally intubated; ocular lubricant applied bilaterally

Neck
Supple without stiffness or lymphadenopathy; mild JVD

Chest
Resolving diffuse bilateral infiltrates; diminished breath sounds with wheezes bilaterally

CV
S_1, S_2 normal with regular rate and rhythm; no S_3, S_4, or murmurs

Abd
Absent bowel sounds; (+) RUQ tenderness; mild abdominal wall tenderness (without rebound)

Ext
1+ pitting edema of extremities; no clubbing or cyanosis. Significant atonia of left arm; grip strength 1/5 in both upper extremities

Neuro
Plantar reflexes downgoing. DTRs depressed bilaterally. Patient is moderately sedated, responds to noxious stimuli.

Labs

Na 139 mEq/L	Hgb 14.5 g/dL	WBC $21.1 \times 10^3/mm^3$	Ca 8.8 mEq/L
K 3.5 mEq/L	Hct 42.5%	89% Neutros	Mg 2.5 mEq/L
Cl 98 mEq/L	Plt $239 \times 10^3/mm^3$	5% Lymphs	Phos 5.2 mg/dL
CO_2 32 mEq/L		3% Monos	Alb 2.5 g/dL
BUN 43 mg/dL		0% Eos	LDH 1229 IU/L
SCr 1.3 mg/dL		3% Basos	CK 209 IU/L
Glu 267 mg/dL			

UA
Yellow, hazy, SG 1.022, pH 5.5; no protein, bilirubin, albumin, glucose, or ketones; nitrite and leukocyte esterase negative; few bacteria; 10–25 RBC/hpf; 0–2 WBC/hpf, 0–1 squamous epithelial cells/hpf

Tracheal Aspirate
Purulent

Non-bronchoscopic BAL
30,000 cfu Enterobacter cloacae
5,000 cfu yeast

ABG
pH 7.39, Pco_2 52 mm Hg, Po_2 87 mm Hg, HCO_3 31 mEq/L, Sao_2 88% (60% Fio_2, tidal volume 650 mL, PEEP 5 cm H_2O, assist control 14 breaths/min)

Abdominal Flat Plate
Colonic dilatation; right colonic/ileal air–fluid level; no pneumoperitoneum.

CT Head
Right maxillary sinusitis.

▶ Questions

Problem Identification

1. a. *Identify the patient's initial drug therapy problems and provide recommendations for managing each of them.*

▶ Clinical Course

The patient continues to have low-grade fevers, and her WBC increases to $42.0 \times 10^3/mm^3$ with 80% PMNs, 10% bands, 5% lymphs, 3% monos, 1% eos, and 1% basos. An abdominal CT is performed that reveals no abscesses. She is evaluated by the gastroenterology and surgical services, both of which agree to an exploratory laparotomy. Subsequently, she is found to have a perforated cecum, and a right hemicolectomy is performed. Enteral feedings are temporarily discontinued and TPN is initiated. Five days after the operation, the patient's SCr increases to 1.9 mg/dL, her WBC increases from 23 to $32 \times 10^3/mm^3$, and she develops moderate hypotension. Microscopic analysis of the patient's urine reveals 60–80 WBCs, light bacteria, and the presence of > 10^5 CFU/mL *Candida* ("germ tube" negative) on 2 successive cultures (See Figure 131–1). One set of blood cultures taken on the day of surgery is now positive (1 of 2 tubes) for *Staphylococcus epidermidis*.

b. *What risk factors for disseminated fungal infection are present in this patient?*

c. *Should prophylactic antifungal therapy be used in patients with multiple risk factors for invasive candidiasis?*

d. *Does this patient meet the criteria for colonization or invasive/disseminated fungal infection?*

Desired Outcome

2. *What are the goals of pharmacotherapy for this patient's infection?*

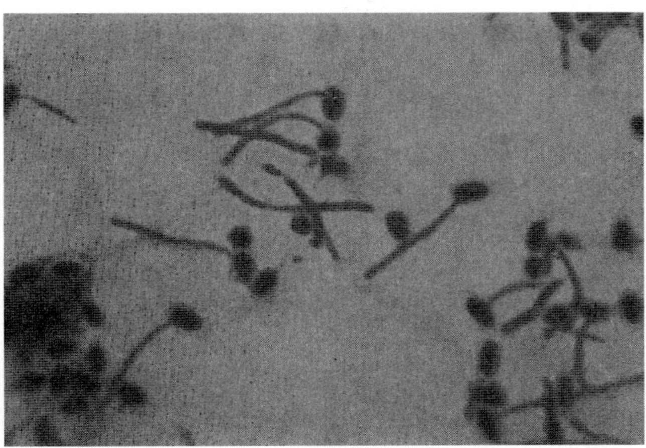

Figure 131–1. Germ tubes of *Candida albicans.* A germ tube-negative culture, as isolated in this patient, is indicative of non-*albicans Candida species.* Given the variable susceptibility profile of such pathogens, identification to the species level and diligent patient evaluation are important to ensure that the correct antifungal therapy has been employed. *(Reproduced with permission from Beneke ES, Rippon JW, Rogers AL. Human Mycoses: A Scope Publication. Upjohn, 1986.)*

Therapeutic Alternatives

3. a. *What nondrug measures would you recommend for treatment of this fungal infection?*

▶ Clinical Course

The patient's right IJ catheter is removed, the catheter tip is sent for culture, and a new central line is placed in the left IJ. Four days later, 1 set of blood cultures (right IJ) is positive (1 of 2 tubes) for *S. epidermidis* and the most recent cultures (left IJ) are positive for yeast ("germ tube" negative). The patient is started on fluconazole 400 mg IV once daily.

b. *What are the most likely causative pathogens in this patient?*

▶ Clinical Course

The patient continues to be hypotensive, and the previous catheter-tip culture reveals 6 CFU of *S. epidermidis.* The latest blood, urine, and sputum cultures are positive for *Candida glabrata.*

c. *What pharmacotherapeutic agents are available for the acute therapy of this infection?*

d. *What is the significance of the catheter-tip cultures, the continued positive blood and urine cultures, and the positive sputum cultures?*

Optimal Plan

4. *What drug therapy (including dose and route of administration) would you recommend for this patient?*

Outcome Evaluation

5. *How should the antifungal regimen be monitored for efficacy and adverse effects?*

▶ Clinical Course

The patient responds well to the antifungal therapy with resolution of the hypotension, fevers, leukocytosis, and candidemia.

▶ Follow-Up Questions

1. *What are appropriate indications for the use of liposomal formulations of Amphotericin B?*
2. *How much longer should therapy be continued?*

▶ Self-Study Assignments

1. Conduct a literature search on candiduria as an early marker of disseminated fungal infection.
2. Compare the types of fungal pathogens that would be expected in patients with candidemia caused by hematologic malignancy versus patients with solid tumors or non-oncologic illnesses.
3. Develop an algorithm for the management of patients with candidemia using the practice guidelines for the treatment of candidiasis. Incorporate newer available antifungals into this algorithm.

▶ Clinical Pearl

A reduction in the incidence of amphotericin B nephrotoxicity may be achieved by administering saline boluses before and after the infusion. Patients receiving extended-spectrum penicillins such as ticarcillin (5.2 mEq sodium/g), mezlocillin (1.85 mEq sodium/g), and piperacillin (1.98 mEq sodium/g) may not require as much additional saline to minimize nephrotoxicity.

References

1. Blumberg HM, Jarvis WR, Soucie JM, et al. Risk factors for candidal bloodstream infections in surgical intensive care unit patients: The NEMIS prospective multicenter study. Clin Infect Dis 2001;33:177–186.
2. Rex JH, Walsh TJ, Sobel JD, et al. Practice guidelines for the treatment of candidiasis. Infectious Diseases Society of America. Clin Infect Dis 2000;30:662–678.
3. Chastre J, Wolff M, Fagon JY, et al. Comparison of 8 vs 15 days of antibiotic therapy for ventilator-associated pneumonia in adults: A randomized trial. JAMA. 2003; 290:2588–2598.
4. Kontoyiannis DP, Bodey GP, Mantzoros CS. Fluconazole vs. amphotericin B for the management of candidemia in adults: A meta-analysis. Mycoses 2001;44: 125–135.
5. Pappas PG, Rex JH, Lee J, et al. A prospective observational study of candidemia: Epidemiology, therapy, and influences on mortality in hospitalized adult and pediatric patients. Clin Infect Dis 2003;37:634–643.
6. Mora-Duarte J, Betts R, Rotstein C, et al. Comparison of caspofungin and amphotericin B for invasive candidiasis. N Engl J Med 2002;347:2020–2029.
7. Mermel LA, Farr BM, Sherertz RJ, et al. Guidelines for the management of intravascular catheter-related infections. Clin Infect Dis 2001;32:1249–1272.

8. Rex JH, Pappas PG, Karchmer AW, et al. A randomized and blinded multicenter trial of high-dose fluconazole plus placebo versus fluconazole plus amphotericin B as therapy for candidemia and its consequences in non-neutropenic subjects. Clin Infect Dis 2003;36:1221–1228.

132 INFECTIONS IN IMMUNOCOMPROMISED PATIENTS

► Bottomed Out (Level II)

Douglas Slain, PharmD, BCPS

► After completing this case study, students should be able to:

- Construct a prudent empiric antibiotic regimen for a febrile neutropenic patient.
- Determine appropriate situations to use vancomycin in empiric antimicrobial regimens for the treatment of febrile neutropenic episodes.
- Differentiate between traditional dosing and high-peak, extended-interval dosing of aminoglycosides in the treatment of neutropenic patients with fever.
- Explain the role of various antifungal agents in the treatment of neutropenic patients with fever.

PATIENT PRESENTATION

Chief Complaint

"Just didn't feel right, and had a fever"

HPI

Anne Binlow is a 58 yo woman who is being evaluated on the inpatient oncology unit for fever "spikes" while neutropenic. She was admitted to the hospital to receive post-remission or "consolidation" chemotherapy with cytarabine for AML 12 days ago. She was diagnosed with AML about 3 months ago and received induction chemotherapy with cytarabine and idarubicin. The AML appeared to be in remission after the induction therapy. She tolerated the induction course well but experienced neutropenia, thrombocytopenia, hair loss, nausea, mucositis and some vomiting. She did spike a fever after the induction chemotherapy course for which she received 12 days of ceftazidime and gentamicin. No pathogen or site of infection was identified during that episode. Her consolidation chemotherapy was administered via a Hickman catheter. She was started on fluoroquinolone prophylaxis for this neutropenic cycle.

PMH

GERD
HTN
Osteoarthritis
S/P partial hysterectomy 10 years ago.

FH

Mother died of colon cancer, aunt died of breast cancer.

SH

Dietician at suburban hospital. Married with 3 children. Denies smoking or ethanol use.

ROS

(+) Diarrhea, (+) mucositis, (+) nausea; denies vomiting, cough, fever, or chills.

Home Meds

Naproxen 500 mg po twice daily
Premarin 0.625 mg po once daily
Ciprofloxacin 500 mg po Q 12 H
Omeprazole 20 mg po once daily
Metoprolol extended-release 50 mg once daily
Acetaminophen 650 mg Q 4 H PRN

All

Ibuprofen → extreme stomach upset and exacerbates GERD

PE

Gen

Patient is 58 yo Caucasian woman who appears to be somewhat anxious and uncomfortable.

VS

BP 110/75, P 90, RR 20, T 38.2°C; Ht 5′7″, Wt 155 lb.

Skin

Warm and dry. Area around Hickman exit site is tender and indurated

HEENT

PEERLA, EOMI, nares patent, mild mucositis

Neck/Lymph Nodes

Neck supple; no lymphadenopathy

Lungs/Thorax

CTA

Breasts

No rashes or palpable masses

Heart

RRR, no murmurs, rubs, or gallops

Abd

Soft, NT, no masses palpable

Genit/Rect

Grossly normal, no dysuria or hematuria, stool guaiac negative

MS/Ext

No deformity, mild weakness

Neuro

A & O × 3; CN II–XII grossly intact

Labs

Na 135 mEq/L	Hgb 9.0 g/dL	WBC 1.2×10^3/mm^3	AST 22 IU/L
K 3.9 mEq/L	Hct 24.8%	PMNs 15%	ALT 27 IU/L
Cl 106 mEq/L	RBC 3.5×10^6/mm^3	Bands 5%	Alk Phos 140 IU/L
CO_2 24 mEq/L	Plt 85×10^3/mm^3	Lymphs 65 %	LDH 240 IU/L
BUN 28 mg/dL		Monos 15%	T. Bili 2.1 mg/dL
SCr 1.2 mg/dL			Mg 1.8 mg/dL
Glu 98 mg/dL			

UA

Color yellow, opacity clear, protein (–), glucose (–), ketones (–), pH 7.1, RBC 1/hpf, WBC 1/hpf, bacteria none, leukocyte esterase (–), Nitrite (–)

Blood Cultures Drawn on Previous Day

Left peripheral catheter: No growth at 24 hours
Right peripheral catheter: No growth at 24 hours
Hickman port: No growth at 24 hours

Chest X-Ray

Unremarkable

Assessment

1. AML—received a post-remission consolidation cycle of chemotherapy.
2. Febrile episode in neutropenic patient.
3. Thrombocytopenia.
4. Elevated SCr; decreased renal function.

Plan

1. Continue next chemotherapy cycle after resolution of neutropenia and thrombocytopenia.
2. Draw another set of blood cultures and begin empiric antimicrobials:
   Ceftazidime 2 g IV Q 8 H (infused over 30 min)
   Gentamicin 80 mg IV Q 12 H (infused over 30 min)
   Vancomycin 1 g IV Q 12 H (infused over 60 min)
3. Monitor platelets. Avoid invasive procedures.
4. Monitor renal function and hydrate with IV fluids. D/C naproxen and use oxycodone/acetaminophen PRN for arthritic pain.

► Questions

Problem Identification

1. a. *Create a list of the patient's drug therapy problems:*
   b. *What information (signs, symptoms, laboratory values) indicates the presence or severity of each of the drug therapy problems?*

Desired Outcome

2. *What are the goals of pharmacotherapy for this patient's drug therapy problems?*

Therapeutic Alternatives

3. a. *What nondrug therapies might be useful for this patient ?*
   b. *What feasible pharmacotherapeutic alternatives are available for treating this febrile neutropenic episode?*

Optimal Plan

4. *What drug regimen is best for the empiric treatment of febrile neutropenia in this patient?*

Outcome Evaluation

5. *What clinical and laboratory parameters are necessary to evaluate the therapy for achievement of the desired therapeutic outcome and to detect or prevent adverse effects?*

Patient Education

6. *What information should be provided to the patient to enhance compliance, ensure successful therapy, and minimize adverse effects?*

► Clinical Course

Three days after the initiation of the empiric antibiotic regimen, the patient is still febrile and the following laboratory results are reported: SCr 1.8 mg/dL, ANC 0.350 x 10^3/mm^3, platelets 95×10^3/mm^3

Serum gentamicin concentrations

Peak: 5.0 mg/L (collected at: 9:00 AM)
Trough: 2.1 mg/L (collected at 7:30 AM)
Dose 80 mg Q 12 H (time of dose 8:00 AM)

Blood Cultures

Left peripheral catheter: No growth
Right peripheral catheter: (+) for yeast
Hickman port: (+) for yeast and coagulase-negative Staphylococci (few)

The team decided to add liposomal amphotericin B (AmBisome) 3 mg/kg once daily and to stop gentamicin. The patient also had her Hickman catheter removed. The final identification of the yeast in the blood and catheter was *Candida albicans*. The patient became afebrile two days after the Ambisome was started. All subsequent blood and urine cultures were negative for microbial growth. Ms. Binlow's neutropenia resolved 3 days after becoming afebrile. Therapy with vancomycin and ceftazidime was continued for 5 days after becoming afebrile. On the day that vancomycin and ceftazidime therapy stopped, her SCr was 0.9 mg/dL. The patient continued therapy with Ambisome for a total of 15 days. She is now being evaluated for a second course of consolidation chemotherapy.

► Follow-Up Questions

1. *What other antifungal therapies could have been used for the treatment of Mrs. Binlow's candidemia?*
2. *If the patient develops febrile neutropenia after another course of*

consolidation chemotherapy, what anti-infective regimens would be advisable?

▶ Self-Study Assignments

1. How do the different types of lipid-based amphotericin B (liposomal, lipid-complex, colloidal dispersion) formulations and amphotericin B deoxycholate compare in terms of efficacy and safety?
2. Identify situations where use of colony-stimulating factors, such as filgrastim or sargramostim, should be advocated in the therapy of neutropenia.

▶ Clinical Pearl

The addition of amphotericin B should be considered in neutropenic patients who remain febrile despite 3 to 5 days of broad-spectrum antibacterial therapy.

References

1. Klastersky J. Science and pragmatism in the treatment and prevention of neutropenic infection. J Antimicrob Chemother 1998;41(Suppl D):13–24.
2. Hughes WT, Armstrong D, Bodey GP, et al. 2002 guidelines for the use of antimicrobial agents in neutropenic patients with cancer. Clin Infect Dis 2002;34:730–51.
3. Mermel LA, Farr BM, Sherertz RJ, et al. Guidelines for the management of intravascular catheter-related infections. Clin Infect Dis 2001;32:1249–1272.
4. The International Antimicrobial Therapy Cooperative Group of the European Organization for Research and Treatment of Cancer. Efficacy and toxicity of single daily doses of amikacin and ceftriaxone versus multiple daily doses of amikacin and ceftazidime for infection in patients with cancer and granulocytopenia. Ann Intern Med 1993;119(7 Pt 1):584–593.
5. Walsh TJ, Finberg RW, Arndt C, et al. Liposomal amphotericin B for empirical therapy in patients with persistent fever and neutropenia. N Engl J Med 1999;340:764–771.
6. Rubin ZA, Somani J. New options for the treatment of invasive fungal infections. Semin Oncol 2004;31 (2 Suppl 4):91–98.

133 ANTIMICROBIAL PROPHYLAXIS FOR SURGERY

▶ To Be Able to Walk Down the Aisle (Level II)

Susan J. Skledar, RPh, MPH
Paige Robbins Gross, RPh

▶ After completing this case study, students should be able to:

- Describe the risk factors that may predispose a patient to surgical wound infection.
- List the major causative organisms for surgical wound infection for most surgical procedures.
- Recommend appropriate antimicrobial regimens for prophylaxis of surgical wound infection.
- Outline monitoring parameters for postoperative surgical wound infection.
- Discuss the importance of optimal timing of presurgical antimicrobial doses in relation to incidence of postoperative surgical wound infection.

PATIENT PRESENTATION

Chief Complaint

"My left knee is getting more painful, and it is starting to affect my daily activities. Before I could get by with taking my pain pills, but now the pills don't work anymore and I feel like I am getting more and more crippled."

HPI

Holly Robertson is a 68 yo woman who presents for preoperative assessment and preparation for a left total knee replacement for osteoarthritis. Previously, her osteoarthritis was controlled with a narcotic/non-narcotic combination agent and NSAIDs as needed. Her pain is increasingly intolerable, and her mobility has decreased.

PMH

Osteoarthritis × 10 years

Asthma × 10 years, which she attributes to her exposure to chemicals while being a hairdresser. Her asthmatic episodes have never required hospitalization but did require brief corticosteroid treatment about 1 year ago. Asthma is currently well controlled on her present regimen

Postmenopausal

Seasonal allergies

Hysterectomy 1976

Cystocele 1993

Arthroscopy of left knee 4 years ago, complicated 1 week later by an invasive staphylococcal infection for which she received 6 weeks of IV vancomycin therapy

FH

She has one child who is alive and well. Her mother died in her 80s from stroke and diabetes. Her father died at age 60 from an acute MI.

SH

She does not smoke or drink. She is widowed and is presently engaged.

ROS

She denies any pain or discomfort in her right knee. No headaches, visual blurring, or history of thyroid problems, GI or GU difficulties, HTN, DM, heart disease, PUD, DVT, or PE. Patient receives regular mammograms, which have been WNL.

Meds

Serevent inhaler 2 puffs QID

AeroBid inhaler 2 puffs QID

Claritin 10 mg po once daily
Ambien 10 mg po at bedtime
Voltaren 75 mg po once daily
Vicodin 1 to 2 tablets po Q 4–6 H PRN

All
Penicillin and cephalexin (severe hives); sulfa (confusion)

PE

Gen
WDWN woman in NAD; appears younger than her stated age

VS
BP 110/70; P 80, regular; RR 16; T 36.7°C

HEENT
NC/AT; EOMI; PERRLA; ENT all WNL

Neck
Supple; no enlargement or nodal involvement; no bruits; thyroid normal

Thorax
CTA & P

Breasts
Exam deferred

CV
RRR; S_1 and S_2 normal without m/r/g

Abd
Soft, NT/ND; (+) BS; no bruits or organomegaly

Ext
The left knee incision from prior arthroscopy is well healed and is slightly warm; no edema or pus. Sensation not impaired

Neuro
A & O × 3; CN II–XII intact. Strength is equal throughout

Labs

Na 140 mEq/L	Hgb 11.8 g/dL	WBC 8.0 × 10^3/mm^3
K 4.0 mEq/L	Hct 34.7%	77% Polys
Cl 100 mEq/L	Plt 250 × 10^3/mm^3	15% Lymphs
CO_2 23 mEq/L		5% Monos
BUN 18 mg/dL		3% Eos
SCr 0.8 mg/dL		
Glu 95 mg/dL		

ECG
NSR; no abnormalities noted

Assessment
A recent aspiration and biopsy of her left knee shows no evidence of recurrent staphylococcal infection. Because of increasing pain and decreasing mobility, the patient is a candidate for a left total-knee replacement. Her asthma is well controlled on her current regimen, which will be maintained. She is also at low risk for cardiovascular complications. Therefore, the patient is a suitable candidate to undergo this procedure.

▶ Questions

Problem Identification

1. a. *Prepare a complete drug therapy problem list for the patient.*
   b. *What are the risk factors for surgical wound infection (SWI) in patients undergoing surgical procedures?*
   c. *What organisms are the most likely causes of infection in orthopedic surgery patients?*
   d. *What recent event in this patient's PMH should be a caution for close monitoring of this patient for postoperative SWI?*

Desired Outcome

2. *What are the therapeutic goals for this patient?*

Therapeutic Alternatives

3. a. *What nonpharmacologic interventions should be considered in this patient pre- and postsurgery?*
   b. *What pharmacotherapeutic alternatives are available to minimize postoperative wound infection in this type of surgery?*
   c. *What pharmacotherapeutic alternatives are available to manage postoperative pain for this patient?*

Optimal Plan

4. *What antimicrobial drugs, dosage form, schedule, and duration of therapy are best for this patient?*

Outcome Evaluation

5. *Which clinical and laboratory parameters are necessary to evaluate therapy for achievement of desired outcomes and to detect and prevent adverse drug reactions?*

▶ Clinical Course

The patient tolerated surgery well, and drains were inserted prior to closure without complication. She did not show signs of infection postoperatively. She received the antimicrobial regimen you recommended for 2 days after surgery, and her postoperative pain was adequately controlled with the IV and then oral treatment you suggested. She was discharged on postoperative day 4 with a normal temperature and normal WBC and differential. Her discharge pain prescription was for Vicodin one tablet every four hours for mild to moderate pain and two tablets every four hours for severe pain. She was told to follow up in 1 week with her orthopedic surgeon. Because she has no cardiovascular risks, diabetes, or history of DVT/PE, she was not discharged on an anticoagulant.

Patient Education

6. *What information should be provided to the patient to enhance compliance, ensure successful therapy, and minimize adverse events?*

▶ Self-Study Assignments

1. Describe the sequence of pain management for this patient from PCA to oral pain medications.
2. Review recommendations for surgical prophylaxis for other types of surgical procedures.
3. Review the typical length of stay and expected course of recovery for a patient undergoing a total joint replacement, focusing on the difference between joint replacements and hip fractures.

▶ Clinical Pearl

Patients who receive antimicrobials within 3 hours after incision have a surgical wound infection rate almost three times that of patients who receive the first dose within 60 minutes before incision.

References

1. Classen DC, Evans RS, Pestotnik SL, et al. The timing of prophylactic administration of antibiotics and the risk of surgical-wound infection. N Engl J Med 1992;326:281–286.
2. Lizan-Garcia M, Garcia-Caballero J, Asensio-Vegas A. Risk factors for surgical-wound infection in general surgery: A prospective study. Infect Control Hosp Epidemiol 1997;18:310–315.
3. Mangram AJ, Horan TC, Pearson ML, et al. Guideline for prevention of surgical site infection, 1999. Centers for Disease Control and Prevention (CDC) Hospital Infection Control Practices Advisory Committee. Am J Infect Control 1999:27: 96–120.
4. ASHP therapeutic guidelines on antimicrobial prophylaxis in surgery. American Society of Health-System Pharmacists. Am J Health-Syst Pharm 1999; 56:1839–1888.
5. Culver DH, Horan TC, Gaynes RP, et al. Surgical wound infection rates by wound class, operative procedure, and patient risk index. National Nosocomial Infections Surveillance System. Am J Med 1991;91:(3B): 152S–157S.
6. Anonymous. Antimicrobial prophylaxis in surgery. Med Lett 2001;43 (1116–1117):92–98.
7. Deacon JM, Pagliaro AJ, Zelicof SB, et al. Prophylactic use of antibiotics for procedures after total joint replacement. J Bone Joint Surg 1996;78:1755–1770.
8. National Surgical Infection Prevention Project. Centers for Medicare and Medicaid Services (CMS) and the Centers for Disease Control and Prevention (CDC). Available on the Internet at: www.surgicalinfectionprevention.org. Accessed July 28, 2004.

134 PEDIATRIC IMMUNIZATION

▶ Ensuring a Healthy Start (Level II)

John D. Grabenstein, RPh, PhD, FASHP, FAPhA
Daniel T. Casto, PharmD, FCCP

▶ After completing this case study, students should be able to:

- Develop a plan for administering any needed vaccines, when given a patient's age, immunization history, and medical history.
- Recognize the differences in *Haemophilus influenzae* type b (Hib)-conjugate vaccines currently in use in the United States.
- Explain why the use of DTaP is preferred over DTwP and IPV is preferred over OPV.
- Describe appropriate use of hepatitis B and varicella vaccines.
- Educate a child's parents on the benefits and risks associated with pediatric vaccines and ways to minimize adverse effects.
- Recognize *inappropriate* reasons for deferring immunization.
- Identify objective sources of information about public concerns involving vaccine safety.

PATIENT PRESENTATION

Chief Complaint

"My daughter was in the hospital because of seizures, and they told me to come here today to have her checked."

HPI

Jennifer Thomas is a 6.5-month-old girl who is being seen in the General Pediatrics Clinic for the first time, in follow-up to a recent hospitalization for an episode of convulsions. Three weeks ago the child experienced a 10-minute tonic-clonic seizure after waking up from a nap. She was seen in the ED with a temperature of 39.1°C. On physical exam, the only abnormality noted was that both TMs were red and bulging. A sepsis work-up was performed because of persistent lethargy, and the patient was hospitalized for evaluation. All cultures were negative; neurologic exam failed to identify an obvious cause of the seizures. The infant was discharged after 2 days with the diagnoses of febrile seizures and bilateral otitis media, for which she was prescribed a 10-day course of amoxicillin.

PMH

Minimal prenatal care, but delivered at 36 weeks gestation via uncomplicated vaginal delivery; birth weight 3,300 g; discharged with mother on day 3 of life. Mother states that her child has had only one or two "colds," no other illnesses, and has not required any medical care. No contact with the medical system until the ED visit and hospitalization 3 weeks ago. No previous immunizations, except hepatitis B vaccine given at birth.

FH

No history of seizures among immediate family members. Maternal grandmother has diabetes mellitus and a seizure disorder secondary to head trauma sustained in an automobile accident. No history of CHD or cancer in family members.

SH

Mother age 19, father age 20, brother age 26 months. Mother stays at home, father works intermittently for a temporary agency as a laborer. They live in a government-subsidized, 2-bedroom apartment. Also living with them are maternal grandparents, mother's 20 y/o sister, and the sister's 17-month-old child. No recent illness among household contacts. No pets at home, and one smoker in house (grandfather). The family receives food stamps but is not enrolled in the Women-Infants-Children (WIC) program. Jennifer's diet consists of whole milk, cereal, and some table foods.

Meds

None
Amoxicillin course was completed about a week and a half ago
No recent OTC medication use

All

NKDA

ROS

Negative

PE

Gen

Alert, happy, relatively small, appropriately developed 6-month-old infant in NAD. Wt 6.4 kg (< 25th percentile), length 24.5 in (50th percentile), FOC 43 cm (50th percentile)

VS

BP 110/66, P 130, RR 28, T 36.8°C (axillary)

HEENT

AF open, flat; PERRL; funduscopic exam not performed; ears clear; normal looking TMs, landmarks visualized, no effusion present; nose clear; throat normal

Cor

RRR, no murmurs

Lungs

Clear bilaterally

Abd

Soft, non-tender, no masses or organomegaly

Genit

Normal external genitalia

GI

Normal bowel sounds; rectal exam deferred, no fissures noted

Ext

Pale nail beds, skin dry and cool; capillary refill < 2 seconds

Neuro

Alert; normal DTRs bilaterally

Labs

Hgb 10.1 g/dL, Hct 32.4%; no other labs obtained

Assessment

Normal-appearing infant, with resolved otitis media, 3 weeks s/p febrile convulsion, in need of immunizations and social service assistance.

▶ Questions

Problem Identification

1. *Create a list of the patient's drug therapy problems.*

Desired Outcome

2. *What immediate and long-term goals are reasonable in this case?*

Therapeutic Alternatives

3. *What vaccines should be administered to this child today? (Helpful hint: The following Web sites may be useful in answering this and other questions: www.cdc.gov/nip and www.aap.org).*

Optimal Plan

4. a. *What immunization schedule should be followed for this patient?*
   b. *In addition to vaccination, what additional therapy is warranted in this case, considering the patient's dietary history and laboratory values?*

Outcome Evaluation

5. *How should the response to the pharmacotherapeutic plan be assessed?*

Patient Education

6. *What important information about vaccination needs to be explained to this infant's mother?*

▶ Follow-Up Question

1. *The mother says, "I've heard people say that vaccines are dangerous. Is that true?" How should you respond?*

▶ Self-Study Assignments

1. The routine schedule for immunizing infants and children in the United States is updated by the American Academy of Pediatrics and the Centers for Disease Control and Prevention (CDC) each year in January, in their respective official publications. Review the most current recommendations and provide a summary of how your recommendations for this case would be different if a 6.5-month-old previously vaccinated patient in need of more immunizations came into your clinic today.
2. Surf the Internet for immunization-related Web sites; then use www.immunofacts.com to find the National Immunization Program's home page, and review at least two Vaccine Information Statements (VISs).
3. Develop a list of diseases and medications that should be considered contraindications to administration of live virus vaccines.

▶ Clinical Pearl

There is no need to restart an immunization series (e.g., DTaP) if the interval between doses is longer than that recommended in the routine schedule for immunizing infants and children. Instead of starting over, merely count the doses administered (provided that they were given at an appropriate age and with an acceptable minimum interval) and complete the series.

References

1. American Academy of Pediatrics. Active and passive immunization. In: Red Book—Report of the Committee on Infectious Diseases, 26th ed. Elk Grove Village, IL, American Academy of Pediatrics, 2003:1–81.
2. Advisory Committee on Immunization Practices. Recommended childhood and adolescent immunization schedule—United States, July to December 2004. MMWR Morb Mortal Wkly Rep 2004;53(16):Q1–Q4 (updated annually at www.cdc.gov/nip/recs/child-schedule.pdf).

135 ADULT IMMUNIZATION

▶ It's Not Just For Kids Anymore (Level II)

Pat S. Rafferty, PharmD, BCPS, CDE

▶ After completing this case study, students should be able to:

- Develop a plan for administering any needed vaccines when given a patient's age, immunization history, and medical history.
- Recognize the usual regimen recommended to maintain an adult's immunizations "up-to-date."
- Explain why certain vaccines are given more than once and must be administered at various intervals during a patient's life.
- Educate patients concerning the risks associated with vaccines they may be given and ways to minimize adverse effects.

PATIENT PRESENTATION

Chief Complaint
"My sister just got out of the hospital."

HPI
Gloria Martinez is a 35 yo Spanish-speaking woman who presents to your clinic with her brother for a hospitalization follow-up in November. She came to the United States from Mexico 2 months ago to live with her brother and his family. She was recently discharged from a hospital stay for uncontrolled diabetes. Before moving to the U.S., she had been treating her diabetes with an herbal preparation that was recommended by a neighbor. Gloria's sister-in-law operates a daycare facility out of the home and has two pre-school age children of her own. Gloria has had only occasional health care for most of her life and does not have any medical records available for this visit. When asked about her previous immunizations, she states "I had a shot when I cut my foot years ago, but I don't remember any others." Gloria has been caring for her elderly mother in Mexico who passed away. Her family was very poor and she doesn't recall seeing the doctor very often as a child. She doesn't recall if she ever had chicken pox as a child. "You'd have to ask my mom, she's the one that remembers all that stuff."

PMH
Type 2 diabetes × 5 years; just discharged from hospital for nonketotic hyperosmolar syndrome

FH
Father died of injuries sustained in farming accident at age 50; mother recently passed away at age 60 as a consequence of CVA. One brother as noted.

SH
Not married, not sexually active. No previous pregnancies. For most of her adult life she has been caring for her mother. Denies alcohol use or smoking.

Meds
ASA 81 mg daily
Lovastatin 40 mg once daily
Metformin 1000 mg BID
Lisinopril 10 mg once daily

All
NKDA

ROS
Still fatigued from hospital stay, but previous hyperosmolar symptoms resolved. No dizziness, chest pain, polyuria, polydipsia. No signs of hypoglycemia.

PE

Gen
Obese Spanish speaking woman in NAD

VS
BP 128/78 (R arm, seated), P 80, RR 20, T 37.0°C Wt 90 Kg, Ht 5′4″

HEENT
NCAT, PERRLA, EOMI, TMs intact

Neck/LN
No lymphadenopathy or masses; no JVD

Cor
No murmurs or rubs

Lungs
Clear to auscultation

Abd
NT/ND, no HSM; normal BS

Genit
Deferred

Ext
No CCE

Neuro
Alert; CN II–XII intact; normal DTRs bilaterally

Labs

Na 140 mEq/L	Hgb 14.3 g/dL	CO_2 25 mEq/L	Plt 180 × 10^3/mm^3
K 3.8 mEq/L	Hct 39.5%	BUN 20 mg/dL	Urine pregnancy test (–)
Cl 104 mEq/L	WBC 5.8 × 10^3/mm^3	SCr 1.2 mg/dL	
		Glu (fasting) 190 mg/dL	

Assessment

35 yo woman with poorly controlled diabetes, recently hospitalized with nonketotic hyperosmolar syndrome; has recently started medication for diabetes. Recent immigrant from Mexico in need of immunizations, which appear to have been neglected for years. No record of childhood immunizations or diseases.

▶ Questions

Problem Identification

1. *Create a list of the patient's drug therapy problems.*

Desired Outcome

2. a. *What immediate immunization goals are appropriate in this case?*
   b. *Provide the rationale for giving each of the vaccines to this patient.*
   c. *What long-term goals are appropriate for comprehensive management of this patient?*

Therapeutic Alternatives

3. *Identify the therapeutic alternatives for addressing this patient's immunization needs.*

Optimal Plan

4. *What immunization schedule should be followed for this patient?*

Outcome Evaluation

5. *How should the response to the pharmacotherapeutic plan be assessed?*

Patient Education

6. *What important information about vaccination needs to be explained to this patient?*

▶ Self-Study Assignments

1. Immunization schedules are constantly under study and often undergo revision. Surf the Internet for immunization-related Web sites; then use www.immunofacts.com to determine which adult immunizations are currently recommended.
2. Describe the type of information that can be found at www.immunize.org.
3. Develop a list of diseases and medications that should serve as indicators that patients are candidates for vaccination.
4. What activities or characteristics would make this patient eligible for the Hepatitis A vaccine? The Hepatitis B vaccine?
5. Locate the most current recommendations for immunization of health care workers. Using these recommendations as a guide, assess the immunization status of five of your classmates.
6. Many patients do not have adequate immunizations due to misconceptions about the potential for side effects and the risk of contracting disease. What information is available from the CDC or other organizations that addresses patients' concerns? How could you use this information to address an individual or group that had questions about immunizations?

▶ Clinical Pearl

It is important that all residents of long-term care facilities be immunized against influenza to avoid outbreaks within the facility and to reduce unnecessary influenza-related hospitalizations and deaths. The most effective strategy is to immunize both patients and staff at these facilities, because employees can transmit the virus to patients before there is any clinical evidence of infection.

References

1. Centers for Disease Control and Prevention. Prevention and control of influenza: Recommendations of the Advisory Committee on Immunization Practices (ACIP). MMWR Morb Mortal Wkly Rep 2003;52(RR-8):1–36.
2. Centers for Disease Control and Prevention. General recommendations on immunization: Recommendations of the Advisory Committee on Immunization Practices (ACIP) and the American Academy of Family Physicians. MMWR Morb Mortal Wkly Rep 2002;51(RR-2):1–36.
3. Centers for Disease Control and Prevention. Recommended adult immunization schedule—United States, 2003–2004. MMWR Morb Mortal Wkly Rep 2003; 52(40):965–969.
4. Centers for Disease Control and Prevention. Prevention of varicella. Updated recommendations of the Advisory Committee on Immunization Practices (ACIP). MMWR Morb Mortal Wkly Rep 1999;48(RR-6):1–5.
5. American Diabetes Association. Standards of medical care for patients with diabetes mellitus. Diabetes Care 2003;26:S33–S50.
6. Centers for Disease Control and Prevention. Using live, attenuated influenza vac-

cine for prevention and control of influenza. MMWR Morb Mortal Wkly Rep 2003;52(RR-13):1–8.
7. Couch RB. Prevention and treatment of influenza. N Engl J Med 2000;343: 1778–1787.

136 CYTOMEGALOVIRUS (CMV) RETINITIS

▶ The Eyes and HAART (Level II)

Patty Fan-Havard, PharmD

▶ After completing this case study, students should be able to:

- Discuss the prevalence of CMV retinitis in the era of highly active antiretroviral therapy (HAART).
- Identify the predisposing risk factors for relapse and the common signs and symptoms of CMV retinitis.
- Discuss the risks and benefits of the therapeutic alternatives used for the treatment of progressive CMV retinitis.
- Develop a patient-specific therapeutic plan for the management of CMV retinitis.
- Provide pertinent patient education information about the medications that are commonly used to manage CMV retinitis.

PATIENT PRESENTATION

Chief Complaint

"I have blurry vision in the right eye which has worsened over the past week."

HPI

Antonio Rodriguez is a 32 yo Hispanic homosexual male with advanced AIDS and CMV retinitis who presents to the ID Service with a 1-week history of fever, worsening of blurry vision and photophobia in the right eye. The present illness began 1 week prior to admission when he noticed fever and difficulty in reading newspaper print. His visual symptoms progressively worsened. He was diagnosed with CMV retinitis in zone 2 of the left eye 14 months ago. At that time, he received induction therapy with IV ganciclovir twice daily for 21 days followed by IV ganciclovir maintenance therapy for 3 months with subsequent placement of an intraocular implant in the left eye. He had a CD4+ count of 16 cells/mm^3 and viral load of 320,590 copies/mL at the HIV Clinic outpatient visit 2 months ago. Mr. Rodriguez declined starting highly active antiretroviral therapy (HAART) because he felt his CMV retinitis was stable.

PMH

- AIDS × 2 years
- CMV retinitis diagnosed 14 months ago; discontinuation of IV ganciclovir maintenance therapy secondary to recurrent catheter-line sepsis
- Ganciclovir implant in the left eye
- Oral candidiasis
- Catheter-line sepsis × 3

FH

Noncontributory

SH

Homosexual; partner died 3 years ago of AIDS. He has since lived with his mother who is well. Currently, he is unemployed and receiving government disability.

ROS

No nausea, vomiting, diarrhea, chills, night sweats, or weight loss.

Meds

- Ganciclovir implant (initially placed in the left eye 10 months earlier with a replacement 3 months prior to admission)
- Ganciclovir 1 g po TID
- Trimethoprim-sulfamethoxazole 1 DS tablet po once daily
- Azithromycin 1,200 mg po once weekly
- Vitamins

All

NKDA

PE

Gen

Thin, cachectic male in NAD

VS

BP 128/72; P 72; RR 20; T 38.3°C; Wt 64 kg; Ht 5′9″

Skin

Soft, intact, warm, and dry. No evidence of rash, lesions, ecchymosis, petechiae, or cyanosis

HEENT

PERRLA; EOMI; funduscopic exam of the right eye reveals fluffy, white retinal patches with focal hemorrhages and vascular cuffing extending into zone 1, consistent with CMV retinitis; the left eye reveals no new lesions

Neck/LN

Supple, no masses, normal thyroid, no bruits

Lungs/Chest

Normal breath sounds, chest CTA

CV

RRR, normal S_1 and S_2 without murmurs, rubs, or gallops

Abd

Soft, non-tender, no hepatosplenomegaly, bowel sounds present

Genit/Rect

Normal male genitalia; rectal exam normal, (–) occult blood in stool

MS/Ext

Neuromuscular intact, distal pulses 1–2+, no edema, full ROM

Neuro

A & O × 3, CN II–XII intact, normal DTRs

Labs on admission

Na 139 mEq/L	Hgb 12.2 g/dL	AST 33 IU/L
K 3.7 mEq/L	Hct 30.7%	ALT 20 IU/L
Cl 100 mEq/L	Plt 150 × 10^3/mm^3	Alk phos 59 IU/L
CO_2 23 mEq/L	WBC 2.2 × 10^3/mm^3	GGT 102 IU/L
BUN 10 mg/dL	76% polys	T. bili 0.7 mg/dL
SCr 2.0 mg/dL	13% lymphs	
Glu 102 mg/dL	8% monos	
	3% eos	

Viral blood serology

CMV antibody (+); CMV antigen (–)

Blood culture × 4

Pending

CXR

No infiltrates or effusions

ECG

Normal sinus rhythm

Surrogate markers for HIV infection from 14 months ago

	Months Prior to Admission			
Surrogate HIV Markers	**14**	**10**	**6**	**2**
CD4 count (cells/mm^3)	43	39	26	16
HIV RNA (copies/mL)	120,400	157,280	219,854	320,590
HIV RNA by RT-PCR assay[a]	Non-detectable (< 50 copies/mL)			

[a] RT-PCR = Reverse transcriptase polymerase chain reaction

Assessment

32 yo HIV-infected man, antiretroviral-naive, with advanced AIDS, relapse of CMV retinitis, renal insufficiency.

▶ Questions

Problem Identification

1. a. *Create a list of this patient's drug therapy problems.*
   b. *What information (signs, symptoms, and laboratory findings) is consistent with relapse of CMV retinitis in this patient?*
   c. *What are the risk factors for relapse of CMV retinitis in this patient?*

Desired Outcome

2. *What are the goals of therapy for this patient?*

Therapeutic Alternatives

3. *What feasible pharmacotherapeutic alternatives are available for treatment of CMV retinitis in this patient?*

Optimal Plan

4. *Based on your current assessment of the patient's disease severity, recommend an appropriate treatment regimen.*

Outcome Evaluation

5. *Which clinical and laboratory parameters are necessary to evaluate the therapy for the desired therapeutic outcome and prevention of adverse effects?*

Patient Education

6. *What information should be provided to the patient to ensure successful therapy?*

▶ Follow-Up Questions

1. *Based on this patient's present illness, will Mr. Rodriguez benefit from the HAART regimen? Why or why not?*
2. *What intraocular complications may occur after initiation of HAART? How should the complications be managed?*
3. *What is the current guideline for discontinuing prophylactic therapy for AIDS-associated opportunistic infections?*

▶ Self-Study Assignments

1. Perform a literature search on the treatment options of progressive non-drug-resistant and drug-resistant CMV retinitis in patients with AIDS.
2. Discuss the mechanisms of resistance to ganciclovir, foscarnet, and cidofovir.
3. Review the current USPHS/IDSA guidelines for the prevention of opportunistic infections in HIV-infected individuals.

▶ Clinical Pearl

Relapse of CMV retinitis is common in AIDS patients not on antiretroviral therapy and necessitates frequent re-induction therapy. The development of drug-resistant CMV disease is inevitable with prolonged therapy. The immune recovery associated with HAART might allow successful discontinuation of anti-CMV maintenance therapy in some patients. However, intraocular inflammatory reactions, presumably immunologically mediated and not CMV-associated, may occur in HAART responders with inactive CMV retinitis.

References

1. Musch DC, Martin DF, Gordon JF, et al. Treatment of cytomegalovirus retinitis with a sustained-release ganciclovir implant. The Ganciclovir Implant Study Group. N Engl J Med 1997;337:83–90.
2. Holland GN, Buhles WC Jr, Mastre B, et al. A controlled retrospective study of ganciclovir treatment for cytomegalovirus retinopathy. Use of a standardized system for the assessment of disease outcome. UCLA CMV Retinopathy Study Group. Arch Ophthalmol 1989;107:1759–1766.
3. Jacobson MA. Treatment of cytomegalovirus retinitis in patients with the acquired immunodeficiency syndrome. N Engl J Med 1997;337:105–114.
4. Mortality in patients with the acquired immunodeficiency syndrome treated with either foscarnet or ganciclovir for cytomegalovirus retinitis. Studies of Ocular Complications of AIDS Research Group, in collaboration with the AIDS Clinical Trials Group. N Engl J Med 1992;326:213–220.
5. Drew WL, Ives D, Lalezari JP, et al. Oral ganciclovir as maintenance treatment for cytomegalovirus retinitis in patients with AIDS. N Engl J Med 1995;333: 615–620.
6. Martin DF, Kupperman BD, Wolitz RA et al. Oral ganciclovir for patients with cytomegalovirus retinitis treated with a ganciclovir implant. Roche Ganciclovir Study Group. N Engl J Med 1999;340:1063–1070.
7. Jung D, Dorr A. Single-dose pharmacokinetics of valganciclovir in HIV- and CMV-seropositive subjects. J Clin Pharmacol 1999;39:800–804.
8. Parenteral cidofovir for cytomegalovirus retinitis in patients with AIDS: The HPMPC peripheral cytomegalovirus retinitis trial. A randomized, controlled trial. Studies of Ocular Complications of AIDS Research Group in Collaboration with the AIDS Clinical Trials Group. Ann Intern Med 1997;126:264–274.
9. Zegans ME, Walton RC, Holland GN, et al. Transient vitreous inflammatory reactions associated with combination antiretroviral therapy in patients with AIDS and cytomegalovirus retinitis. Am J Ophthalmol 1998;125:292–300.
10. 2001 USPHS/IDSA guidelines for the prevention of opportunistic infections in persons infected with human immunodeficiency virus. U.S. Public Health Service (USPHS) and Infectious Diseases Society of America (IDSA); November 28, 2001. Available on the Internet at: www.aidsinfo.nih.gov. Accessed April 1, 2004.

137 HIV INFECTION

The Antiretroviral-naive Patient (Level II)

Susan Chuck, PharmD, BCPS
Kinnari S. Khorana, PharmD
Keith A. Rodvold, PharmD, FCCP, BCPS

► After completing this case study, students should be able to:

- Describe situations in which antiretroviral therapy should be initiated in patients with HIV infection and determine the desired outcome of such therapy.
- Recommend appropriate first-line antiretroviral therapies for the antiretroviral-naive person.
- Provide patient counseling on the proper dose, administration, and adverse effects of antiretroviral agents.

PATIENT PRESENTATION

Chief Complaint
"I think I'm ready to start HIV meds."

HPI
Raymond Washington is a 32 yo man who was diagnosed with HIV 1 year ago while hospitalized for treatment of *Pneumocystis carinii* pneumonia. At that time, he was actively using heroin and admitted himself to a drug rehabilitation center upon discharged from the hospital. He successfully completed his 28-day rehabilitation program and is now stabilized on methadone and followed at an outpatient methadone clinic. He comes to the HIV Clinic at regular 2- to 3-month intervals for routine follow-up, most recently 2 weeks ago. At that time, we had a lengthy discussion about starting antiretroviral therapy. He had been reluctant to start antiretrovirals until he was able to stabilize social and economic aspects of his life. Blood was drawn for baseline surrogate markers.

PMH
HIV infection diagnosed 1 year ago while hospitalized; HIV risk factor—men having sex with men (MSM)
Pneumocystis jiroveci pneumonia diagnosed 1 year ago; treated with IV TMP–SMX and prednisone taper
History of thrush; treated with po fluconazole

FH
Noncontributory

SH
History of IVDU; now stable on methadone. Lives in an apartment with his male partner. Works at a pizzeria as a busboy.

ROS
The patient voices no complaints. He has had no recent weight loss, fever, night sweats, cough, nausea, vomiting, or diarrhea.

Meds
Bactrim DS 1 tablet po daily
Methadone 60 mg po daily

All
PCN → rash

PE

Gen
Well-developed Caucasian man in NAD

VS
BP 112/76, P 80, RR 16, T 36.6°C; Wt 72 kg, Ht 5′11″

Skin
Warm and dry without lesions

HEENT
Oral cavity without thrush/erythema; sinuses non-tender; PERRLA; ears and nose clear; funduscopic exam deferred

Neck/LN
Generalized lymphadenopathy

Chest
Clear, normal breath sounds; no rales or rhonchi

CV
RRR; normal S_1 and S_2 without murmurs

Abd
(+) BS, soft without HSM; no pain or tenderness

Genit/Rect
Deferred

MS/Ext
No wasting, full ROM

Neuro
A & O × 3, no cranial nerve abnormalities noted

Baseline Labs
RPR nonreactive; toxoplasma IgG (–); hepatitis serology (–)

Other Labs
See Table 137–1.

Assessment
HIV-infected man, antiretroviral-naive.

TABLE 137–1. Laboratory Values for the Previous Visit and for Subsequent Visits

Parameter (units)	2 Weeks Ago	This Visit	1 Month Later	3 Months Later
General				
Weight (kg)	110	107	110	115
Hematology				
Hgb (g/dL)	12.2	12.9	12.4	12.6
Hct (%)	37.9	39.0	38.5	38.4
Plt (× 10^3/mm^3)	220	114	145	161
WBC (× 10^3/mm^3)	2.4	3.3	3.1	3.3
Lymphs (%)	34.6	40.5	40.8	46.1
Monos (%)	21.6	13.0	12.4	16.5
Eos (%)	11.6	8.8	6.5	4.2
Basos (%)	0.7	0.9	1.3	1.0
Neutros (%)	31.5	36.8	39.0	32.2
ANC (× 10^3/mm^3)	1.0	1.2	1.2	1.1
Chemistry				
BUN (mg/dL)	14	17	16	10
SCr (mg/dL)	0.9	1.1	1.1	1.0
T. bili (mg/dL)	—	0.6	—	0.6
Alb (g/dL)	—	4.4	—	4.4
LDH (IU/L)	206	210	186	347
AST (IU/L)	31	34	29	34
ALT (IU/L)	19	20	18	32
Surrogate Markers				
CD4 (%)	12	—	13	15
CD4 (cells/mm^3)	156	—	173	249
CD8 (%)	54	—	52	51
HIV RNA (RT-PCR)[a] (copies/mL)	256,958	—	20,568	3,472

[a] Reverse transcriptase polymerase chain reaction assay.

Questions

Problem Identification

1. a. *What information (signs, symptoms, laboratory values) indicates the severity of HIV disease? Assess this patient's HIV disease at this visit and determine whether he has AIDS.*
   b. *Is it rational to begin antiretroviral therapy in this patient?*
   c. *Is prophylactic therapy for any HIV-associated opportunistic pathogen indicated in this patient?*

Desired Outcome

2. *What are the goals of pharmacotherapy in this case?*

Therapeutic Alternatives

3. a. *What therapeutic options are available for treating this antiretroviral-naive man?*
   b. *What economic, psychosocial, racial, and ethical considerations are applicable to this patient?*

Optimal Plan

4. a. *Design an individualized antiretroviral regimen for this man. State the drug name, dosage form, dose, schedule, and duration of therapy for the regimen you choose.*
   b. *Design an antiretroviral regimen that would be appropriate if the patient informs you that he has difficulty swallowing large pills.*
   c. *Design an antiretroviral regimen that would be appropriate if the patient states that medicines often upset his bowels, and he prefers to avoid anything that may cause him trouble.*
   d. *Explain the role of HIV resistance testing in designing a regimen for the antiretroviral-naïve patient.*

Outcome Evaluation

5. *What parameters should you select to monitor the clinical efficacy and toxicity of the pharmacotherapeutic regimen? Specify the frequency with which you would monitor these parameters. For laboratory parameters, state the range of values or significant change in values (i.e., log change, x-fold change, and specific HIV RNA values) that would indicate that the desired therapeutic outcome has been achieved.*

Patient Education

6. a. *What important information would you provide to this patient about his therapy?*
   b. *Explain in non-technical terms the surrogate markers and their use in monitoring HIV disease.*
   c. *If this man changed his mind about starting antiretrovirals, what questions would you ask him? Explain in non-technical terms when therapy is indicated and what the potential benefits are.*

Clinical Course

Your recommendations on the antiretroviral regimen were accepted. The patient returns to the HIV clinic for his 1-month and 4-month follow-up visits. After each visit the laboratory results are faxed to you.

Parameter	1 Month Later	3 Months Later
Duration of HIV infection	1 year+	1¼ years
HIV RNA (RT-PCR)	20,568 copies/mL	3,472 copies/mL
CD4 lymphocyte count	173 cells/mm^3	249 cells/mm^3
Symptoms of HIV infection	Asymptomatic	Asymptomatic

Follow-Up Questions

1. *Considering this new information, provide an assessment of the patient's HIV disease status at each of the two visits.*
2. *Provide an assessment of the antiretroviral regimen efficacy at each follow-up visit.*

Self-Study Assignments

1. Review the current literature regarding recommended therapy for the antiretroviral-naive and treatment-experienced individuals. What is the recommended first-line therapy, and what are the indications to change to alternative therapy? What is known about therapy of HIV and survival?
2. Review the current literature regarding the development of HIV resistance to antiretroviral agents and strategies for the prevention and management of resistance.

Clinical Pearl

According to current Department of Health and Human Services (DHHS) and International AIDS Society (IAS) guidelines, antiretroviral therapy is indicated in two groups of HIV-infected individuals: (1) all persons with HIV-related symptoms; and (2) a CD4 lymphocyte count below 200 cells/mm^3 with any HIV RNA value. DHHS guidelines recommend offering antiretroviral therapy in HIV-infected individuals with CD4 lymphocyte counts between 200 and 350 cells/mm^3 although this may be considered controversial. IAS guidelines also suggest considering antiretroviral therapy for CD4 lymphocyte counts between 200 and 350 cells/ mm^3; this recommendation is strengthened when the HIV RNA is > 50,000 copies/mL or the CD4 lymphocyte count declines by more than 100 cells/ mm^3 per year. DHHS guidelines note that experts disagree on whether patients with HIV RNA >55,000 (RT-PCR or bDNA) copies/mL with CD4 lymphocyte count > 350 cells/mm^3 should be offered therapy.

References

1. Centers for Disease Control. 1993 AIDS surveillance case definition for adolescents and adults. MMWR 1992;41(RR-17):1–9.
2. Centers for Disease Control. Appendix: Revised surveillance case definition of HIV infection. MMWR 1999;48(RR-13);29–31.
3. Guidelines for the use of antiretroviral agents in HIV-infected adults and adolescents. Department of Health and Human Services (DHHS) Panel on Clinical

Practices for Treatment of HIV Infection. March 23, 2004. Available on the Internet at www.aidsinfo.nih.gov.

4. Yeni PG, Hammer SM, Hirsch MS, et al. Treatment for adult HIV infection: 2004 recommendations of the International AIDS Society-USA Panel. JAMA 2004;292:251–265.
5. US Public Health Service (USPHS) and Infectious Diseases Society of America (IDSA). 2001 USPHS/IDSA guidelines for the prevention of opportunistic infections in persons infected with human immunodeficiency virus. Accessed at www.aidsinfo.nih.gov.
6. Hirsch MS, Brun-Vezinet F, Clotet B, et al. Antiretroviral drug resistance testing in adults infected with human immunodeficiency virus type 1: 2003 recommendations of an International AIDS Society-USA Panel. Clin Infect Dis 2003:37: 113–128.

138 HIV AND HEPATITIS C COINFECTION

► Viral Invasion (Level III)

Jennifer J. Kiser, PharmD
Peter L. Anderson, PharmD
Courtney V. Fletcher, PharmD

► After completing this case study, students should be able to:

- Identify when changes in antiretroviral therapy are warranted.
- Identify important considerations for choosing alternative antiretroviral therapies.
- Understand the concept of HIV genotyping.
- Identify pharmacologic interactions between antiretrovirals and medications used to treat Hepatitis C.
- Utilize the primary and secondary literature to provide pharmacotherapy recommendations for conditions without definitive treatment guidelines.

PATIENT PRESENTATION

Chief Complaint
"I am here to find out if I need to switch my HIV meds."

HPI
John James is a 49 yo man with HIV and hepatitis C virus (genotype 3a) coinfection. He has been taking stavudine, lamivudine, and efavirenz to treat HIV for approximately 3 years. Nine weeks ago he began treatment with peginterferon alfa-2a and ribavirin for hepatitis C. Although his HIV viral load was undetectable when he began treatment for hepatitis C (HIV RNA < 20 copies/mL, CD4 283 cells/mm^3), it has been elevated at his last two clinic visits. Complete hematology profile, fasting lipids, CMP, and HIV genotype were obtained one week ago and the results have returned.

PMH
Pneumocystis jiroveci pneumonia 5 years ago
HIV infection diagnosed 13 years ago
Hepatitis B and C infections—precise duration unknown

FH
Non-contributory

SH
Single, recently moved in with ill, elderly mother. Works part-time at a restaurant. IV drug use approximately 8 years ago. Smokes 1 pack of cigarettes per day. Recovering alcoholic, last drink 1 year ago.

Meds
Bactrim DS 1 po daily
Stavudine 40 mg po BID
Lamivudine 150 mg po BID
Efavirenz 600 mg po at bedtime
Peginterferon alfa-2a 180 mcg subQ every Friday
Ribavirin 400 mg po BID

All
NKDA
Immunizations
Influenza annually
Pneumococcal vaccine 5 years ago

ROS
Persistent fatigue/weakness, occasional flu-like symptoms from interferon injections, long-standing mild numbness and tingling in lower extremities bilaterally

PE

Gen
Thin, somnolent man in NAD

VS
BP 121/69, P 68, RR 18, T 36.8°C, Wt 63 kg, Ht 5′7″

Skin
No visible lesions

HEENT
PERRLA; no papilledema; fundi normal; ears and nose clear; oral cavity without inflammation, exudate, or lesions

Neck/LN
Supple; good range of motion; no fat accumulation on upper back/neck

Lungs/Thorax
CTA

CV
NSR, normal S_1 and S_2; no rubs, murmurs, or gallops

Abd
No pain or tenderness, no hepatosplenomegaly, BS (+), no notable accumulation of fat in abdominal area

Genit/Rect
Guaiac (–) stool; no visible genital or anal lesions; prostate exam not performed

MS/Ext
Pedal pulses 2+, no edema, nails normal, normal ROM, no cyanosis, no clubbing

Neuro
A & O × 3; Babinski (–); CN II–XII intact; normal strength, coordination, and gait; depressed ankle reflexes; decreased sensation and response to painful stimuli in lower extremities bilaterally; prior nerve conduction studies reveal slightly slowed nerve conduction velocity in lower extremities bilaterally

Labs
See Table 138–1.

Liver biopsy findings approximately 1 year ago
Grade 2 inflammation and stage 3–4 fibrous portal extension

TABLE 138–1. Serial Laboratory Values Beginning One Year Prior to the Present Visit

Parameter (units)	1 Year Ago	6 Months Ago	9 Weeks Ago (Start IFN/RBV)	5 Weeks Ago	1 Week Ago
Liver Panel					
Albumin (g/dL)	3.2	3.5	3.4	3.3	3.1
AST (IU/L)	280	47	46	51	38
ALT (IU/L)	527	75	85	64	42
Alk phos (IU/L)	85	77	72	86	121
T. bili (mg/dL)	0.6	0.6	0.8	0.7	0.6
INR (sec)	–	1.12	–	–	–
Chemistry					
Na (mEq/L)	137	136	138	139	140
K (mEq/L)	3.7	3.5	4.3	3.9	4.2
Cl (mEq/L)	99	102	104	103	106
CO_2 (mEq/L)	26	25	24	26	25
BUN (mg/dL)	15	11	8	10	14
SCr (mg/dL)	1.2	0.9	0.9	1.0	0.8
Glu (mg/dL)	115	89	91	98	102
Ca (mg/dL)	9.5	8.9	8.2	8.9	9.7
Fasting Lipids					
Cholesterol (mg/dL)	176	–	–	163	–
Triglycerides (mg/dL)	184	–	–	172	–
Thyroid Function					
TSH (mIU/L)	3.3	–	3.1	–	3.3
Hematology					
RBC ($\times 10^6/mm^3$)	4.39	4.68	3.88	3.32	2.95
Hgb (g/dL)	14.9	15.2	14.8	12.3	11.4
Hct (%)	44.7	45.6	44.4	36.9	34.2
Plt ($\times 10^3/mm^3$)	170	162	160	152	148
MCV (μm^3)	106	104	105	106	109
WBC count ($\times 10^3/mm^3$)	9.4	7.8	6.8	4.2	4.0
Lymphs (%)	26.3	34.4	64.2	44.9	40.9
Monos (%)	7.5	10.8	10.9	10.2	10.3
Eos (%)	0.6	0.8	0.2	0.4	0.1
Basos (%)	0.0	0.2	0.2	0.0	1.3
Neutros (%)	65.6	53.8	24.6	44.5	47.3
Virology					
CD4 (cells/mm^3)	276		283		272
HIV RNA (copies/mL) by RT-PCR method	<20	143	<20	566	4,324
HCV RNA (copies/mL)	>500,000				<60

HIV genotype

K103N, no other significant mutations

Assessment

1. Failure to suppress plasma HIV RNA levels to "below detection" (i.e., persistent HIV viremia)
2. Hepatitis C responding to peginterferon alfa-2a and ribavirin treatment
3. Anemia
4. Peripheral neuropathy

▶ Questions

Problem Identification

1. a. *Create a list of the patient's drug therapy problems.*
   b. *What information (signs, symptoms, laboratory values) indicates the presence or severity of the patient's drug therapy problems?*
   c. *What additional information is needed to satisfactorily assess this patient?*

Desired Outcome

2. *What are the desired goals of pharmacotherapy in this case?*

Therapeutic Alternatives

3. *What nondrug and pharmacologic treatments are available for this patient's drug therapy problems?*

Optimal Plan

4. *What drug(s), dose(s), and schedule(s) should be used to treat the HIV infection in this patient?*

Outcome Evaluation

5. *What clinical and laboratory parameters are necessary to evaluate each of the patient's drug regimens for achievement of the desired therapeutic outcomes and to detect or prevent adverse effects?*

Patient Education

6. *What information should be provided to the patient to enhance compliance, ensure successful therapy, and minimize adverse effects?*

▶ Clinical Course

The patient returns to clinic 12 weeks after his last visit. His anemia has improved with the treatment you recommended. He continues to receive peginterferon alfa-2a and ribavirin for hepatitis C. The patient wishes to remain on lamivudine 150 mg and stavudine 40 mg po Q12 H. Lopinavir/ritonavir 400/100 mg po Q12 H was substituted for efavirenz. He has had two undetectable HIV viral loads (HIV RNA <20 copies/mL) since switching to this antiretroviral regimen. However, he reports feeling very weak and short of breath recently. The patient also describes constant heartburn, feeling bloated, and having no appetite. He has tender hepatomegaly on physical exam. Abnormal laboratory findings include: AST 139 IU/L, ALT 211 IU/L, CO_2 17 mEq/L, anion gap 22 mEq/L, lactate 5.3 mEq/L (repeated and confirmed), arterial pH 7.43, pO2 87 mm Hg, pCO2 30 mm Hg.

▶ Follow-Up Questions

1. *Which medications may have contributed to the development of hyperlactatemia in this patient?*
2. *What pharmacotherapeutic interventions would you make at this time?*

▶ Self-Study Assignments

1. Review the current literature on treatment of hepatitis C in patients coinfected with HIV.
2. Review the current literature regarding the use of combination antiretroviral therapy, with special regard to new agents, potential drug interactions, and the use of ritonavir to increase plasma exposures of other concomitant protease inhibitors.
3. Review the literature regarding resistance testing for patients with HIV disease.
4. Review the current guidelines for treating opportunistic infections including when to initiate and withdraw primary and secondary prophylaxis.
5. Review the symptoms and management of nucleoside analog-related mitochondrial toxicities.

▶ Clinical Pearl

Approximately 25% of patients infected with HIV are also infected with hepatitis C virus. Although data regarding optimal treatment of patients coinfected with HIV and HCV are incomplete, the threat of liver disease is too great to delay treatment. Clinicians must be vigilant in identifying and managing the additive toxicities of concomitant HIV and HCV therapy.

References

1. Guidelines for the prevention of opportunistic infections in persons infected with HIV—November 28, 2001. Available on the Internet at www.aidsinfo.nih.gov/guidelines.
2. Soriano V, Sulkowski M, Bergin C, et al. Care of patients with chronic hepatitis C and HIV coinfection: Recommendations from the HIV-HCV International Panel. AIDS 2002;16:813–828.
3. Luciano CA, Pardo CA, McArthur JC. Recent Developments in the HIV neuropathies. Curr Opin Neurol 2003;16:403–409.

4. Guidelines for the use of antiretroviral agents in HIV-infected adults and adolescents—March 23, 2004. Available on the Internet at www.aids info.nih.gov/guidelines.
5. Fried MW. Side effects of therapy of hepatitis C and their management. Hepatology 2002;36(5 Suppl 1):S237–244.
6. Torriani FJ, Rodriguez-Torres M, Rockstroh JK, et al. APRICOT Study Group. Peginterferon alfa-2a plus ribavirin for chronic hepatitis C virus infection in HIV-infected patients. N Engl J Med 2004;351:438–450.
7. Dieterich DT, Spivak JL. Hematological disorders associated with hepatitis C virus infection and their management. Clin Infect Dis 2003:37;533–541.
8. Brau N. Update on chronic hepatitis C in HIV/HCV-coinfected patients: Viral interactions and therapy. AIDS 2003;17:2279–2290.
9. Schambelan M, Benson C, Carr A, et al. Management of metabolic complications associated with antiretroviral therapy for HIV-1 infection: Recommendations of an International AIDS Society—USA Panel. J Acquir Immune Defic Syndr 2002;31:257–275.

SECTION 17

Oncologic Disorders

139 BREAST CANCER

▶ The Role of Neoadjuvant Chemotherapy (Level II)

Laura Boehnke Michaud, PharmD

▶ After completing this case study, students should be able to:

- Explain the importance of regular breast self-examinations, screening mammograms, and professional breast exams for women.
- Design appropriate monitoring parameters to detect and prevent adverse effects associated with the chemotherapy regimens used for breast cancer.
- Educate patients on the most likely adverse effects of chemotherapy and the actions they should take if they occur.
- Provide patient education on the proper dosing, administration, and adverse effects of letrozole therapy.

PATIENT PRESENTATION

Chief Complaint

"I have pain in my breast and under my arm."

HPI

Sara Gleason is a 69 yo woman whose history dates back to 3 to 4 weeks ago when she noted a painful lump in the upper outer quadrant of her left breast, including the axillary area. A mammogram was done that was suggestive of malignancy. She had not had regular mammograms previously.

PMH

CAD; s/p angioplasty 5 or 6 years ago; denies any chest pain since
HTN; does not remember how long; she states "for years"
S/P cholecystectomy
TAH/BSO at age 45
S/P appendicitis

FH

No known family history of cancer.

SH

Previous smoker, quit 8 years ago. She denies tobacco or drug use.

Endocrine Hx

Menarche age 12; menopause age 45 (surgical); first child age 17; $G_5P_5A_0$. Last Pap smear 10 years ago. HRT stopped 3 to 4 weeks ago when she found the lump.

Meds

Procardia XL 90 mg po once daily
Zestril 20 mg po once daily
Paxil 30 mg po once daily
Tylenol #3, 2 tablets po once daily PRN back pain

All

None

ROS

Negative except for complaints noted above.

PE

Gen

Moderately obese 69 yo African-American woman who appears her stated age. Awake, alert, in NAD

VS

BP 130/84, P 74, RR 88, T 37.1°C; Ht 5′6″, Wt 78 kg

HEENT

NC/AT; PERRLA; EOMI; ears, nose, and throat are clear

Neck/LN

Supple. No lymphadenopathy, thyromegaly, or masses. No supraclavicular or infraclavicular adenopathy.

Breasts

Left: skin retraction with arms elevated; no nipple retraction or discharge expressible; edema of the skin in left upper outer quadrant without associated erythema; hard 5 × 5 cm mass in upper outer quadrant, not fixed to skin, no ulceration; 2 cm, firm, tender palpable mass in axilla.

Right: without mass or lymphadenopathy.

Lungs

CTA and percussion

CV

RRR; no murmurs, rubs, or gallops

Abd

Moderately obese; soft, non-distended, non-tender; no HSM; bowel sounds normal. Cholecystectomy scar noted.

Spine

No tenderness to percussion

Ext

No CCE

Neuro

No deficits noted

Labs

Na 137 mEq/L	Hgb 10.8 g/dL	WBC 7.0 × 10^3/mm^3	AST 37 IU/L
K 4.2 mEq/L	Hct 31.8%	34% Neutros	Alk Phos 97 IU/L
Cl 96 mEq/L	RBC 3.42 × 10^6/mm^3	42% Lymphs	LDH 547 IU/L
CO_2 24 mEq/L	Plt 313 × 10^3/mm^3	10% Monos	T. bili 0.3 mg/dL
BUN 8 mg/dL	PT 11.4 sec	14% Eos	CA 27.29 21.5 U/mL
SCr 1.4 mg/dL	INR 0.9		CEA 2.4 ng/mL
Glu 90 mg/dL	aPTT 23.5 sec		

Chest X-Ray

Lungs are clear

Other

Diagnostic bilateral mammogram (see Figure 139–1):

1. American College of Radiology Category V report highly suspicious for malignancy in left breast with evidence for advanced carcinoma with associated diffuse skin thickening, skin retraction. Spiculated mass with extensive infiltration of the surrounding fatty tissue. Overlying skin looks retracted and there is diffuse skin thickening both laterally and medially when compared to the other side. Associated lymphadenopathy with an enlarged lymph node approximately 2 cm in diameter that is suspicious for a metastatic node.
2. Size of the malignancy in left breast measures approximately 8 × 9 × 7 cm. Associated with interductal calcifications extending toward the nipple, indicating that at least a portion of this has a ductal cell origin. There may be extension to the pectoral muscle. The right breast shows no abnormality.

Unilateral ultrasound left breast and left axilla with biopsy:

1. Solid-appearing mass favoring malignancy in left upper outer quadrant. Ill-defined mass that is hypoechoic and has abnormal vascularity demonstrated by color Doppler ultrasound and with cystic shadowing. This mass measures 4.3 × 2.8 × 2 cm in dimension. There is skin thickening and some suggestion of soft tissue edema associated with it. Fine-needle aspiration (FNA) was performed with two passes with preliminary cytologic evaluation suggestive of malignancy.
2. Abnormal axillary adenopathy. Within the left axilla are at least three lymph nodes that are abnormal in appearance. The node that measures 1.1 × 1.0 × 0.8 cm was sampled with FNA using a 20-gauge needle with two passes without complication. Preliminary cytologic evaluation suggested malignancy.

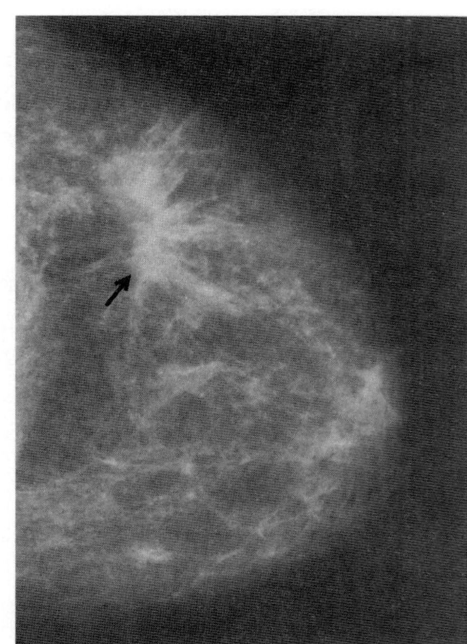

Figure 139–1. Mammogram of left breast. Arrow indicates area of abnormality highly suspicious for malignancy.

Fine-needle aspiration of left breast mass and left axillary mass:

1. Left breast 2 o'clock: breast carcinoma, ductal type, modified Black's nuclear grade III (poorly differentiated), ER 54 fm, PR 34 fm.
2. Left axillary lymph node: metastatic adenocarcinoma; the cytomorphology of the malignant cells in the lymph node aspiration is similar to that seen in the breast aspiration material.

Core needle biopsy of left breast mass:

1. Infiltrating ductal carcinoma, modified Black's nuclear grade III (poorly differentiated), Her2/neu overexpression 1+ (negative).

Ultrasound liver:

1. No lesions suggestive of metastases were identified in the liver. A 0.6 × 0.7 cm faintly visible hyperechoic area was suspected to the left side and slightly cephalad aspect of the ligamentum venosum. The appearance is more compatible with hemangioma than with metastases.

Bone scan:

1. No definite evidence of active osseous metastases.
2. Significant degenerative changes involving the lower lumbar spine and multiple peripheral joints. Increased tracer uptake in the lower lumbar spine, moderate increased uptake in the shoulders, elbows, wrists, knees, and small joints of both feet is noted. These findings are consistent with degenerative joint disease.

▶ Questions

Problem Identification

1. a. *Identify all of the patient's drug therapy problems.*
   b. *Given the above clinical information, what is this patient's current clinical stage of cancer?*

Desired Outcome

2. a. *What is the goal of cancer therapy for this patient?*
   b. *What is the prognosis for this patient based on tumor size and nodal status?*
   c. *In addition to stage of disease, what other factors may be helpful in determining the prognosis for breast cancer?*

Therapeutic Alternatives

3. *List the general types of treatment options that are available for the patient at this time, and briefly discuss their advantages and limitations.*

Optimal Plan

4. *Outline the optimal treatment plan for this patient that includes both pharmacologic and nonpharmacologic measures. If antineoplastic chemotherapy is part of your plan, identify the specific regimen you would use and provide your rationale.*

▶ Clinical Course

The patient does well with the standard therapeutic plan you outlined. Six months after completion of chemotherapy, she returns to the clinic complaining of bone pain in her lower back and left hip. She is still taking anastrozole. Restaging is performed that includes a bone scan, chest x-ray, CT scan of the abdomen, and additional laboratory tests. The bone scan reveals metastases to the lumbar spine and left acetabulum, without impending fracture or spinal cord compression. The chest x-ray shows two small nodules in the lower lobe of the left lung. The physician's assessment is that she has developed bone and lung metastases. The plan is to begin chemotherapy with capecitabine and discontinue the anastrozole.

Outcome Evaluation

5. a. *What adverse effects can be anticipated with this regimen?*
   b. *What information is needed before calculating an appropriate dose of capecitabine for this patient? What dose would you recommend for this patient?*

Patient Education

6. *What information should the patient be given about the general effects she should expect to experience after this treatment?*

▶ Clinical Course

Ms. Gleason responds well to the capecitabine therapy and has received six courses. Her lung nodules are no longer detectable. She has palmar plantar erythrodysesthesia and is unable to walk long distances due to the pain in her feet. Her hands are also affected and have peeled and are cracked. The physician decides to stop chemotherapy and observe the patient off therapy.

Eighteen months later, the patient complains of new pain in the right hip and left rib cage. A staging work-up reveals bone metastases in the right hip and left sixth and seventh ribs posteriorly. Laboratory values were within normal limits with the exception of the following: LDH 932 IU/L, Hgb 9.0 g/dL, Hct 28.0%, MCV 78 μm^3. The patient has been taking acetaminophen 1,000 mg every 4 hours with little relief of her pain and is experiencing a great deal of fatigue.

▶ Follow-Up Questions

1. *What are the patient's drug therapy problems at this time?*
2. *What are the treatment goals at this time?*
3. *What pharmacotherapeutic alternatives are available for each of the patient's current problems?*

▶ Clinical Course

The physician decided to start the patient on fulvestrant therapy for her metastatic breast cancer.

▶ Follow-Up Question

4. *What important information would you provide to the patient about her new therapy for breast cancer?*

▶ Self-Study Assignments

1. Perform a literature search to obtain recent information on clinical trials with trastuzumab as a single agent and in combination with chemotherapy, focusing on efficacy and tolerability (e.g., cardiotoxicity, infusion-related, and pulmonary reactions).
2. Perform a literature search to obtain recent information on clinical trials demonstrating the benefits of the hormonal therapies anastrozole, letrozole, and exemestane, and the role they play in treating breast cancer.
3. Develop a treatment plan for hand/foot syndrome (palmar plantar erythrodysesthesia) associated with chemotherapy.
4. Develop a treatment plan for chemotherapy-associated anemia.

▶ Clinical Pearl

Breast cancer in its early stages is a very curable cancer (Stage I has 70% to 90% 5-year disease-free survival), but in advanced stages the spread of disease virtually eliminates the possibility of cure (in Stage IV, up to 10% survive 5 years with minimal disease but are rarely "cured"). This is very strong evidence supporting routine screening and patient education efforts.

References

1. Bonadonna G, Valagussa P. Primary chemotherapy in operable breast cancer. Semin Oncol 1996;23:464–474.
2. Green M and Hortobagyi G. Neoadjuvant chemotherapy for operable breast cancer. Oncology 2002;16:871–890.
3. Early Breast Cancer Trialists' Collaborative Group. Tamoxifen for early breast cancer: An overview of the randomized trials. Lancet 1998;351:1451–1467.
4. Baum M, Buzdar A, Cuzick J, et al. Anastrozole alone or in combination with tamoxifen versus tamoxifen alone for adjuvant treatment of postmenopausal women with early-stage breast cancer: Results of the ATAC (Arimidex, Tamoxifen Alone or in Combination) trial efficacy and safety update analyses. Cancer 2003;98:1802–1810.
5. Blum JL, Jones SE, Buzdar AU, et al. Multicenter phase II study of capecitabine in paclitaxel-refractory metastatic breast cancer. J Clin Oncol 1999;17:485–493.

140 NON-SMALL CELL LUNG CANCER

▶ Remember the Surgeon General's Warning (Level II)

Courtney F. Smith, PharmD, BCOP
Jane M. Pruemer, PharmD, BCOP, FASHP

▶ After completing this case study, students should be able to:

- Recognize the most common symptoms of non-small cell lung cancer (NSCLC).
- Monitor carboplatin and paclitaxel therapy.
- Educate patients on the anticipated side effects of carboplatin, paclitaxel, and radiation therapy.
- Identify potential complications associated with NSCLC.
- Design a pharmacotherapeutic plan for the treatment of hypercalcemia.
- Recommend potential second-line chemotherapy agents for treating refractory NSCLC.
- Describe appropriate treatment strategies for brain metastases.

PATIENT PRESENTATION

Chief Complaint

"I have been coughing up blood."

HPI

This 58 yo woman presents to the ED with complaints of a dry, nonproductive cough for 2 months, dyspnea on exertion; and hemoptysis for 1 week.

PMH

HTN
Hyperlipidemia
Anemia of unknown etiology × 1 year
Aortic insufficiency
Hysterectomy
PPD (−)

FH

No history of cancer, heart disease, or stroke.

SH

Divorced, lives with daughter; 40 pack-year cigarette smoking history (approximately 1 ppd × 40 years); no EtOH use; no known recent exposure to TB.

Meds

Folic acid 1 mg po daily
Ferrous sulfate 325 mg po TID
Diltiazem CD 240 mg po daily
Hydrochlorothiazide 25 mg po daily
Simvastatin 20 mg po daily
Nizatidine 150 mg po BID

All

NKDA

ROS

(+) For pulmonary symptoms as in noted in HPI; no headaches, dizziness, or blurred vision

PE

Gen

Mildly overweight African American woman in slight distress

VS

BP 120/65, P 90, RR 30, T 37.2°C; Ht 5′3″, Wt 69.9 kg

Skin

Patches of dry skin; no lesions

HEENT

PERRLA; EOMI; fundi benign; TMs intact

Neck/LN

No lymphadenopathy; neck supple

Breasts

No masses, no discharge

Lungs

Wheezing in RUL; remainder of lung fields are clear

Heart

RRR; slight systolic murmur on left lateral side; normal S_1, S_2

Abd

Soft, non-tender; no splenomegaly or hepatomegaly

Genit/Rect

Normal female genitalia; guaiac (–) stool

Neuro

A & O × 3; sensory and motor intact, 5/5 upper, 4/5 lower; CN II–XII intact; (–) Babinski

Labs

Na 138 mEq/L	Hgb 11.9 g/dL	Ca 8.7 mg/dL
K 3.1 mEq/L	Hct 36.8%	Mg 2.0 mg/dL
Cl 99 mEq/L	Plt 267 × $10^3/mm^3$	
CO_2 23 mEq/L	WBC 9.4 × $10^3/mm^3$	
BUN 13 mg/dL		
SCr 1.0 mg/dL		
Glu 118 mg/dL		

Chest X-Ray

PA and lateral views reveal a possible mass in right upper lobe (see Figure 140–1).

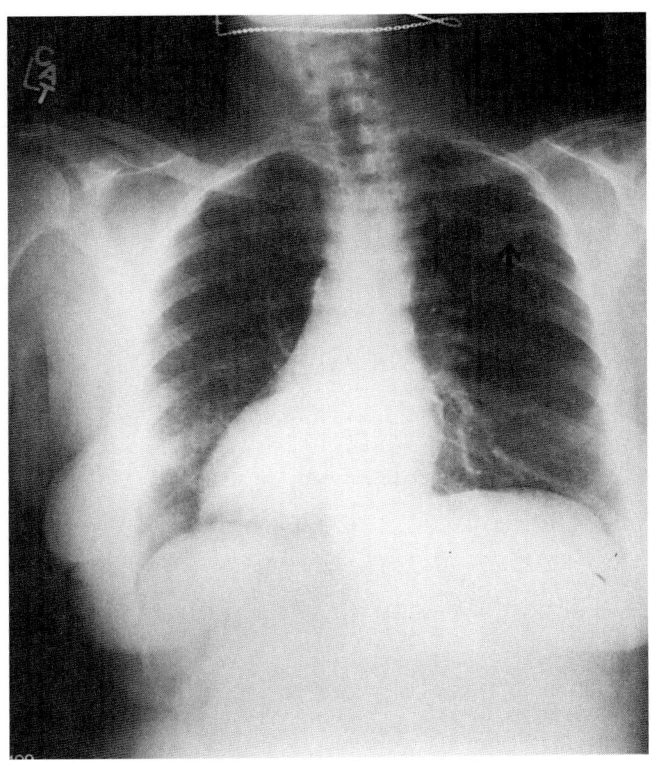

A

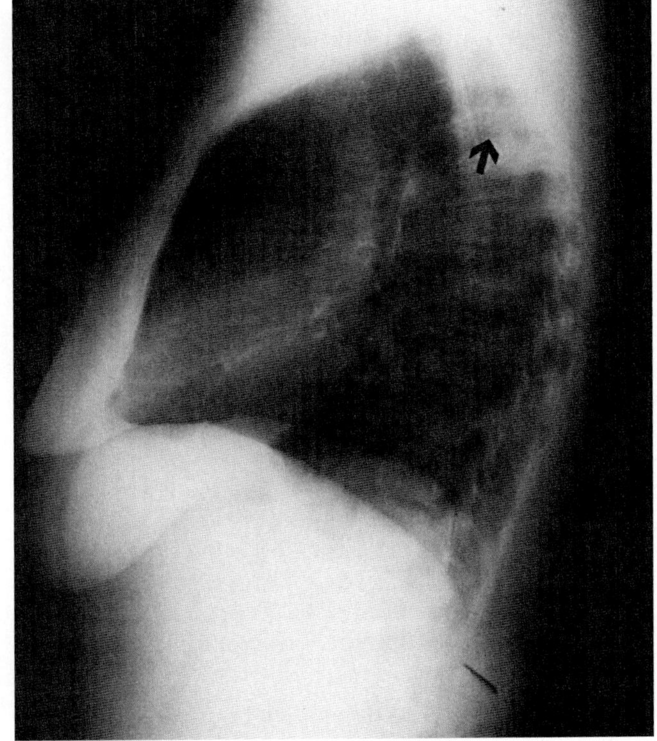

B

Figure 140–1. Chest x-ray with PA **(A)** and lateral **(B)** views showing a possible mass in the right upper lobe *(arrows)*.

Assessment

1. A 58 yo woman with new-onset hemoptysis is admitted for work-up of a possible lung mass.
2. She has anemia and a history of hyperlipidemia and hypertension.

▶ Clinical Course

The patient was further evaluated for lung cancer on an outpatient basis. A bronchoscopy (with biopsy) was performed that identified squamous cell carcinoma. The chest CT scan revealed a 2.5-cm × 2-cm right lung mass (see Figure 140–2). A mediastinoscopy was performed to determine the resectability of the tumor. The mediastinoscopy and biopsy revealed unresectable Stage IIIB NSCLC with metastasis to the contralateral mediastinal nodes. PFTs included FEV_1 1.49 L, FVC 1.9 L. An echocardiogram showed mild LVH with an LVEF of 55%.

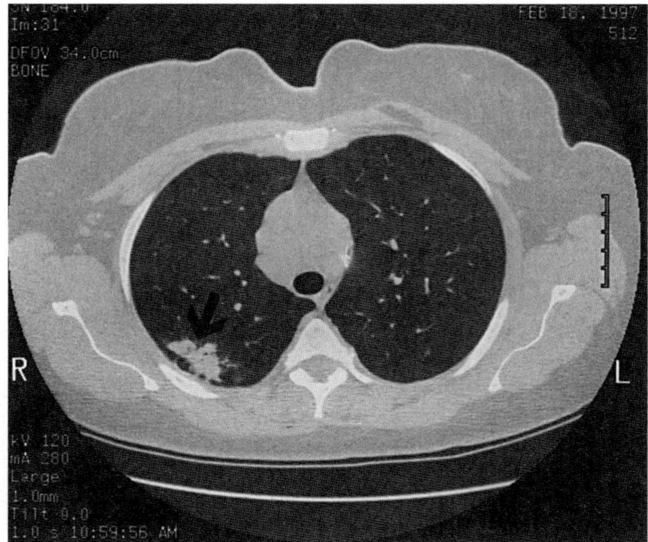

Figure 140–2. CT scan of the chest revealing a 2.5-cm × 2-cm right lung mass *(arrow)*.

▶ Questions

Problem Identification

1. a. Identify the patient's drug therapy problems.
b. What signs, symptoms, and other information indicate the presence of NSCLC in this patient?

Desired Outcome

2. What is the goal for treatment of NSCLC in this patient? What is the likelihood of achieving this goal?

Therapeutic Alternatives

3. a. What chemotherapeutic regimens may be considered for NSCLC?
b. What nondrug therapies may be used for NSCLC?

Optimal Plan

4. a. Design a specific chemotherapeutic regimen to treat this patient and explain why you chose this regimen.
b. What additional measures should be taken to ensure the tolerability of the regimen and to prevent adverse effects?
c. What additional laboratory and clinical information is needed prior to administration of the chemotherapy?
d. Calculate the patient's BSA, creatinine clearance, and the amount of each drug to be administered based on the regimen chosen.

Outcome Evaluation

5. What clinical and laboratory parameters are necessary to evaluate the therapy for achievement of the desired therapeutic outcome and the occurrence of adverse effects?

Patient Education

6. What information should be provided to the patient to optimize therapy and minimize adverse effects?

▶ Clinical Course

The patient's subsequent courses were further complicated by the occurrence of DVT, CVA, weight loss, neutropenic fever, anemia, nausea/vomiting, and infections. At one point, the patient presented with a serum calcium level of 11.5 mg/dL and an albumin of 2.0 g/dL with symptoms of weakness, confusion, nausea, and vomiting.

▶ Follow-Up Questions

1. Calculate the patient's corrected calcium level and provide an interpretation of that value.
2. What treatment modalities may be used to correct hypercalcemia?

▶ Clinical Course

A repeat chest CT prior to cycle 3 of carboplatin/paclitaxel shows an increase in the size of the initial mass and several new suspicious lesions.

▶ Follow-Up Questions

3. What treatment options are available for the patient at this time?
4. Design a specific chemotherapeutic regimen to treat this patient.

▶ Clinical Course

Six weeks after beginning the new chemotherapy regimen, the patient presents to the ED with complaints of headache and mental status changes as per the patient's husband and caregiver. An MRI of the head reveals multiple lesions, most likely brain metastases.

▶ Follow-Up Questions

5. *Briefly discuss options (drug and nondrug) to treat brain metastases.*
6. *What is the role of antiepileptic agents in the setting of brain metastases?*

▶ Self-Study Assignments

1. Review clinically important drug interactions for cancer patients started on phenytoin. Include appropriate monitoring parameters. Extend your review beyond the medications this patient is currently receiving.
2. The oncologist has decided to place this patient on gefitinib. Design a patient education session for this new drug therapy.

▶ Clinical Pearl

More than 90% of lung cancers are attributable to cigarette smoking. Smoking cessation is the only method proven to decrease the risk of lung cancer.

References

1. Clinical practice guidelines for the treatment of unresectable non-small cell lung cancer. Adopted on May 16, 1997 by the American Society of Clinical Oncology. J Clin Oncol 1997;15:2996–3018.
2. Sause W, Kolesar P, Taylor S, et al. Final results of phase III trial in regionally advanced unresectable non-small cell lung cancer: Radiation Therapy Oncology Group, Eastern Cooperative Oncology Group, and Southwest Oncology Group. Chest 2000;117:358–364.
3. Dillman RO. Concurrent chemoradiation in unresectable stage III non-small cell lung cancer: Too much pain for no gain. Cancer J Sci Am 1996;2:76.
4. Pritchard RS, Anthony SP. Chemotherapy plus radiotherapy compared with radiotherapy alone in the treatment of locally advanced, unresectable, non-small-cell lung cancer. A meta-analysis. Ann Intern Med 1996;125:723–729.
5. Smit EF, VanMeerbeeck JP, Lianes, P, et al. Three-arm randomized study of two cisplatin-based regimens and paclitaxel plus gemcitabine in advanced non-small-cell lung cancer: A phase III trial of the European Organization for Research and Treatment of Cancer Lung Cancer Group—EORTC 08975. J Clin Oncol 2003;21:3909–3917.
6. Solomon B, Ball DL, Richardson G, et al. Phase I/II study of concurrent twice-weekly paclitaxel and weekly cisplatin with radiation therapy for stage III non-small cell lung cancer. Lung Cancer 2003;41:353–361.
7. Furuse K, Fukuoka M, Kawahara M, et al. Phase III study of concurrent versus sequential thoracic radiotherapy in combination with mitomycin, vindesine, and cisplatin in unresectable stage III non-small-cell lung cancer. J Clin Oncol 1999;17:2692–2699.
8. Curran WJ, Scott C, Langer C, et al. Phase III comparison of sequential vs concurrent chemoradiation for patients with unresected stage III non-small cell lung cancer (NSCLC). Initial Report of Radiation Therapy Oncology Group (RTOG) 9410.Proc Am Soc Clin Oncol 2000;19:1891. Abstract.
9. Fukuoka M, Yano S, Giaccone G, et al. Multi-institutional randomized phase II trial of gefitinib for previously treated patients with advanced non-small-cell lung cancer. J Clin Oncol 2003;21:2237–2246.

141 COLON CANCER

▶ Improving the Odds for Cure (Level I)

Elizabeth Gray Paulson, PharmD, BCOP

▶ After completing this case study, students should be able to:

- Discuss the therapeutic alternatives for treating colon cancer.
- Describe the treatment for adverse effects associated with colon cancer therapy.
- Develop an optimal chemotherapy treatment and monitoring plan for patients with colorectal cancer.
- Discuss important issues about chemotherapy regimens for colorectal cancer with patients.

PATIENT PRESENTATION

Chief Complaint

"I'm here for chemotherapy."

HPI

Janice Halsey is a 50 yo woman diagnosed with colon cancer 2 months ago. She had been asymptomatic until the onset of RLQ discomfort. Two days after the initial symptom onset, she experienced extreme abdominal pain and presented to the ED. An abdominal CT scan showed a large tumor in the ascending colon. A 6-cm tumor was subsequently resected, and all gross disease was removed. A diverting colostomy was performed at that time. The liver was clear on CT scan and examination by surgeons. The pathology report on the colon tumor was consistent with adenocarcinoma. Final staging was Duke's stage C (T3, N2 M0) or Stage III using TNM.

PMH

None

FH

Father age 81 alive and well, mother age 76 has type 2 DM but is otherwise in good health. Patient has five siblings, two with HTN. No family history of cancer. She is married and has three children, all alive and well.

SH

Worked as a manager at the local grocery store for 25 years. She smoked 1 ppd for 30 years until she quit 10 years ago; drinks two glasses of wine/week.

All
NKDA

ROS
She recently lost weight. Is finally getting her strength back after surgery. No chest pain, palpitations, SOB, DOE, or wheezing. Complains of mild irritation around the colostomy site but states that the colostomy is working well, with no current malodorous problems. Has a few aches and pains, which are normal for her.

Meds
Temazepam 15 mg po at bedtime PRN sleep

PE

VS
P 120/70, P 75, RR 18, T 36.9°C; Ht 5′5″, Wt 52.2 kg; BSA 1.55m^2

HEENT
PERRLA, EOMI

Neck/LN
Neck supple; no thyromegaly or palpable lymph nodes

Thorax
No crackles or wheezing

CV
RRR; normal heart sounds; no murmurs or cardiomegaly

Abd
Diverting colostomy in RLQ. She is tender at both costal margins. No masses are palpable

Genit/Rect
Heme (–) stool

Ext
Pulses intact; no CCE

Neuro
A & O × 3; CNs intact; reflexes 2+ and symmetric. No focal neurologic deficits

Labs

Na 135 mEq/L	Hgb 13.3 g/dL	AST 15 IU/L
K 3.9 mEq/L	Hct 38.5%	ALT 30 IU/L
Cl 102 mEq/L	RBC 4.41 × 10^6/mm^3	LDH 543 IU/L
CO_2 25 mEq/L	Plt 213 × 10^3/mm^3	Alb 2.5 g/dL
BUN 20 mg/dL	WBC 6.87 × 10^3/mm^3	Ca 7.2 mg/dL
SCr 0.8 mg/dL	ANC 4.14 × 10^3/mm^3	Phos 2.1 mg/dL
Glu 95 mg/dL		Uric acid 2.2 mg/dL

Assessment
Patient with Dukes Stage C adenocarcinoma of the colon. Patient presented to the cancer center for chemotherapy. Because she is 50 years old and has had resection of all bulky disease, aggressive treatment is warranted for cure.

▶ Questions

Problem Identification

1. *Create a list of the patient's drug therapy problems.*

Desired Outcome

2. *What are the desired outcomes for chemotherapy in this patient?*

Therapeutic Alternatives

3. *What chemotherapeutic options are available for this patient?*

Optimal Plan

4. *Design a chemotherapy regimen for treating this patient's colon carcinoma.*

Outcome Evaluation

5. *What parameters should be monitored to evaluate the efficacy and adverse effects of the regimen you recommended?*

Patient Education

6. *What information should be provided to the patient to ensure the safety and efficacy of your regimen?*

▶ Self-Study Assignments

1. Develop standardized, written, patient counseling information on the treatment of chemotherapy-induced diarrhea for regimens containing 5-FU.

References

1. Cassidy J, Scheithauer W, McKendrick J, et al. Capecitabine (X) vs bolus 5-FU/leucovorin (LV) as adjuvant therapy for colon cancer (the X-ACT study): positive efficacy results of a phase III trial. Proceedings of the 40th annual meeting of the American Society of Clinical Oncology, New Orleans LA: 2004; Abstract #3509.
2. Andre T, Boni C, Mounedji-Boudiaf L, et al. Multicenter International Study of Oxaliplatin/5-Fluorouracil/Leucovorin in the Adjuvant Treatment of Colon Cancer (MOSAIC) Investigators. Oxaliplatin, fluorouracil, and leucovorin as adjuvant treatment for colon cancer. N Engl J Med 2004;350:2343–2351.

142 PROSTATE CANCER

▶ For Men Only (Level II)

Judith A. Smith, PharmD, BCOP

▶ After completing this case study, students should be able to:

- Describe the typical symptoms associated with prostate cancer at initial diagnosis and at disease progression.
- Compare and contrast the hormone therapy options for first-line treatment of metastatic prostate cancer.
- Recommend a pharmacotherapeutic plan for patients with hormone-refractory metastatic prostate cancer.
- Recommend an appropriate pain management plan for a patient with bony metastatic disease.
- Educate patients about the common toxicities associated with the hormonal and chemotherapeutic agents used in prostate cancer treatment.

PATIENT PRESENTATION

Chief Complaint

"I'm having difficulty with urination and have had pains in my back and thighs that is getting worse lately. I used to be able to run 10 miles easily now I cannot make it past 1 mile."

HPI

Harvey Jones is a 57 yo man who has been complaining over the past year of an increasing frequency and intensity of pain in his lower back and legs. He has attributed this pain to "getting older" and has only sought out prescriptions from his PCP. He takes Celebrex daily and Lortab 5 mg/500 mg as needed for significant pain. HJ reports that recently it seems he has needed to use the Lortab at least twice a day. During a routine annual physical, his PCP noted an abnormally large prostate; laboratory resulted showed a PSA level of 58 ng/mL. He was referred to a urologist and ultimately a medical oncologist for additional work-up.

PMH

HTN
GERD
Mild osteoarthritis involving the hands and knees

FH

Father died from MI at age 67; mother died of colon cancer at age 70.

SH

Active financial analyst from New York City area. He is married and has one son and two daughters, both in good health. He has four brothers; one has colon cancer, and the others are alive and well. He denies any history of tobacco or alcohol use.

ROS

Patient reports that he has problems when he goes to the bathroom. He says it takes him a long time to start to urinate and then dribbles come out. He does not ever feel like he has completely emptied his bladder so it seems like he is making frequent trips to the bathroom. He states that this seems to have gotten worse over the past year and is now interrupting his work. The patient noted significant more pain in his back and legs that has interfered with his jogging routine. The stiffness and pain in his back is so bad that he now requires Lortab frequently to make it through the day.

Meds

Lortab 5 mg/500 mg 1 tablet po Q 4 to 6 H PRN pain
Celebrex 200 mg po once daily
Zestril 20 mg po once daily
Aspirin (enteric coated) 325 mg daily

All

Penicillin → hives

PE

Gen

The patient is a middle aged, physically fit white man in considerable pain and discomfort

VS

BP 140/80, P 70, RR 18, T 36.9°C; Ht 6′1″, Wt 79.5 kg, BSA 2.02 m^2

Skin

Non-abraded, normal

HEENT

PEERLA, EOMI, disks flat, TMs intact, no hemorrhages or exudates

Neck/LN

Supple, no nodes palpated

Chest

Clear, good breath sounds

CV

Normal rate and rhythm; no m/r/g

Abd

Soft, non-tender, bowel sounds present in all quadrants; no hepatosplenomegaly

Genit/Rect

Normal male genitalia; enlarged boggy prostate on rectal exam with multiple firm nodules in the anterior lobe

MS/Ext

Extreme pain noted when lower back examined and mild pain in both lower extremities. Limited ROM in bilateral knee joints. Pulses 2+

Neuro

A & O × 3, CN II–XII intact, sensory and motor levels intact, Babinski (−), DTRs 2+

Labs

Na 137 mEq/L	Hgb 12.5 g/dL	AST 25 IU/L
K 4.6 mEq/L	Hct 38%	ALT 12 IU/L
Cl 104 mEq/L	Plt 200 × 10^3/mm^3	Alk Phos 1875 IU/L
CO_2 22 mEq/L	WBC 5.4 × 10^3/mm^3	T. bili 0.2 mg/dL
BUN 10 mg/dL		PSA 58 ng/mL
SCr 0.9 mg/dL		Testosterone 10 ng/dL
Glu 97 mg/dL		

Bone Scan

Increased uptake in the lower spine, pelvis, and the left & right femurs.

Ultrasound-Guided Transrectal Prostate Biopsy

Positive for adenocarcinoma, Gleason score 4 + 3 = 7

Assessment

57 yo man with newly-diagnosed metastatic prostate cancer here for consideration of initial treatment options. Suspected metastatic sites include lower spine, pelvis and bilateral femurs.

Questions

Problem Identification

1. *What signs, symptoms, and other information are consistent with metastatic prostate cancer in this case?*

Desired Outcome

2. *Considering this patient's disease stage and treatment history, what are reasonable therapeutic goals?*

Therapeutic Alternatives

3. *Create a list of the feasible treatment options for this man's initial therapy, including the advantages, potential adverse effects, and complications associated with each option.*

Optimal Plan

4. *Design an optimal pharmacotherapeutic plan for the treatment of this patient's metastatic prostate cancer.*

Outcome Evaluation

5. *How should the therapy you recommended be monitored for efficacy and adverse effects?*

Patient Education

6. *What information should be provided to the patient about his new therapy?*

Clinical Course

Mr. Jones responded well to the initial therapy you recommended. On routine follow up 18 months later, he presents with new symptoms. The pain in his back has worsened, and he also developed significant shoulder, hip, and rib pain. His PSA is 253 ng/mL. His pain medications were adjusted, but he is still experiencing considerable pain whenever he tries to get up out of a chair. His oncologist suspects that the patient has new metastatic disease. The patient states that he does not want to "give up" and would like to seek out more treatment options.

Follow-Up Questions

1. *Given the patient's motivation to seek further treatment and his reasonable physical condition, what therapeutic options are available for him at this time?*
2. *What therapeutic options are available for appropriate pain management for this patient?*

Self-Study Assignments

1. Outline the effective treatment options for localized prostate cancer.
2. Provide the rationale for and identify patients who are appropriate candidates for neoadjuvant androgen ablative therapy prior to surgery or radiation for locally advanced prostate cancer.
3. Locate information resources that are available to prostate cancer patients and their families.
4. Identify information sources you can use to find clinical studies that are available for patients with prostate cancer.

Clinical Pearl

Because prostate cancer often metastases to bone, an important supportive care intervention is to adequately assess, monitor, and modify pain management regimens to help improve the patient's quality of life.

References

1. Kuyu H, Lee WR, Bare R, et al. Recent advances in the treatment of prostate cancer. Ann Oncol 1999;10:891–898.
2. Koch M, Steidle C, Brosman S, et al. An open-label study of abarelix in men with symptomatic prostate cancer at risk of treatment with LHRH agonists. Urology 2003;62:877–882.
3. Culine S, Droz JP. Chemotherapy in advanced androgen-independent prostate cancer 1990–1999: A decade of progress? Ann Oncol 2000;11:1523–1530.
4. Hudes G. Estramustine-based chemotherapy. Semin Urol Oncol 1997;15:13–19.
5. Tannock IF, Osoba D, Stockler MR, et al. Chemotherapy with mitoxantrone plus prednisone or prednisone alone for symptomatic hormone-resistant prostate cancer: A Canadian randomized trial with palliative end points. J Clin Oncol 1996;14:1756–1764.
6. Heidenreich A, Hofmann R, Engelmann UH. The use of bisphosphonate for the palliative treatment of painful bone metastasis due to hormone refractory prostate cancer. J Urol 2001;165: 136–140.

143 NON-HODGKIN'S LYMPHOMA

▶ When the Deck is Stacked Against You (Level II)

Keith A. Hecht, PharmD

▶ After completing this case study, students should be able to:

- Identify and describe the components of the staging work-up and the corresponding staging and classification systems for non-Hodgkin's lymphoma (NHL).
- Describe the pharmacotherapeutic treatment of choice and the alternatives available for the treatment of NHL.
- Identify acute and chronic toxicities associated with the drugs used to treat NHL and the measures used to prevent or treat these toxicities.
- Identify monitoring parameters for response and toxicity in patients with NHL.
- Provide detailed patient education for the chemotherapeutic regimen.

PATIENT PRESENTATION

Chief Complaint

"What's the next step for my lymphoma?"

HPI

Brian Jacobson is a 62 year-old man who presents to the oncologist's office for recommendations about treatment of a newly diagnosed diffuse, large B-cell lymphoma. He had been in relatively good health since his heart attack five years ago. Two weeks ago he began experiencing night sweats and fevers up to 100.6°F. His wife states that the night sweats are so severe that he drenches the sheets at night. He thought he was developing pneumonia and called his physician. His PCP issued a prescription for an antibiotic. His symptoms persisted despite completion of a 10 day course of levofloxacin. The patient then saw his PCP for evaluation. On physical exam, he had an enlarged, painless, golf-ball sized inguinal lymph node on the left side. Splenomegaly was also noted. Complete work-up ruled out non-malignant etiologies. The patient was referred for excisional biopsy of the inguinal lymph node, and pathologic evaluation revealed large B-cell lymphoma. He has now been referred to the oncologist for further evaluation and treatment recommendations.

PMH

HTN ×15 years
Type 2 DM × 7 years
CAD s/p MI 5 years ago
Occasional GERD for "many years"

FH

The patient is the oldest of 7 children (4 sisters and 2 brothers), all are alive and well. He has 3 children, all are in good health. No family history of malignancies.

SH

The patient is a Blackjack dealer in a local casino. He does not smoke but complains about all the tourists who smoke while they play at his table. He claims no illicit drug use. He drinks 1 to 2 glasses of red wine nightly. Diet is mostly buffet food. He states that he does not eat much vegetables, as he must save room for "the good stuff" on the buffet. He has been married for 34 years. His wife is with him today in the clinic.

ROS

The patient reports continuing night sweats and fever. Additionally, he describes an unexplained weight loss of approximately 25 pounds over the last 3 months. He denies headaches, changes in vision, or fainting episodes. He reports no lesions in his mouth, difficulty swallowing, or nosebleeds. He denies chest pain, tachycardia, or swelling in the extremities. The patient denies wheezing, shortness of breath, or cough. He also denies burning on urination, frequency, dribbling, or blood in the urine. He has not noticed any bleeding or bruising. He has not received any prior transfusions.

Meds

Lisinopril 10 mg po once daily
Metoprolol XL 50 mg po once daily
Aspirin 81 mg po once daily
Metformin 500 mg po twice daily
Famotidine 20 mg po PRN heartburn
Hydrocodone/Acetaminophen 5/500 1 to 2 tablets Q 4–6 H PRN pain

Allergies

Penicillin: Rash

PE

Gen
The patient is an elderly white man in no apparent distress.

VS
BP 140/95, P 95, RR 14, T 98.9°F; Ht 6′0″, Wt 80 kg

Skin
No rashes or moles noted

HEENT
PERRLA. TMs clear. No masses in the tonsils, palate, or floor of the mouth; no stomatitis. Several missing teeth, but no gingival inflammation is noted.

Neck
Supple, no masses

Chest
Lungs are CTA & P

CV
RRR, no m/r/g

Abd
Soft and non-tender, non-distended. The spleen is palpable just below the costal margin. No hepatomegaly. Bowel sounds are normoactive.

Genit/Rect
Normal male genitalia

Ext
Without edema, warm to the touch, pulses palpable bilaterally

Neuro
Symmetric cranial nerve function. Symmetric facial muscle movement, and the tongue is midline. The palate is symmetric. Balance and coordi-

nation of the upper extremities are intact with no evidence of tremor. There is symmetric coordination of rapidly alternating movements. Motor strength in the upper and lower extremities is normal and symmetric.

LN Survey

The lymph node survey is negative for any palpable peripheral nodes in the preauricular, postauricular, cervical, supraclavicular, infraclavicular, or axillary areas. No palpable inguinal nodes present. Small scar noted from excisional biopsy of left inguinal node.

Labs

Na 140 mEq/L	Hgb 14.2 g/dL	AST 29 IU/L	Phos 4.0 mg/dL
K 4.5 mEq/L	Hct 41.5%	ALT 27 IU/L	Uric acid 7.6 mg/dL
Cl 102 mEq/L	Plt 254 × 10^3/mm^3	Alk phos 75 IU/L	PT 12.2 sec
CO_2 30 mEq/L	WBC 9.2 × 10^3/mm^3	LDH 1242 IU/L	aPTT 21.7 sec
BUN 20 mg/dL	70% Neutros	T. bili 0.6 mg/dL	B_2-microglobulin 4.8 mg/dL
SCr 1.0 mg/dL	2% Bands	T. prot 6.3 g/dL	
Glu 156 mg/dL	18% Lymphs	Alb 3.7 g/dL	
	9% Monos		
	1% Eos		

CT Abdomen/Pelvis

Spleen is enlarged. Liver appears normal.

Chest X-Ray

No adenopathy in the hilum or mediastinum.

Tumor Pathology

Diffuse large cell lymphoma, B-cell type.
CD20+, CD45+, CD3

Initial Assessment

Large cell lymphoma. Further staging will include bilateral BM biopsies, gallium scan or PET scan, HIV test, CT of the chest, and a baseline cardiac assessment in light of the patient's history of HTN and CAD.

▶ Clinical Course

- Bone marrow biopsies are negative for lymphoma.
- PET scanning revealed multiple foci of increased FDG (fluorodeoxyglucose) uptake; increased uptake noted in the spleen and left side inguinal lymph nodes; increased uptake also seen in 3 mesenteric lymph nodes
- HIV test is negative.
- CT of the chest shows slightly enlarged lymph nodes in the left axilla representing hyperplastic changes. Mediastinal adenopathy is not noted.
- MUGA scan reveals a LVEF of 48% with moderate septal left ventricular hypokinesis.

Assessment

Large B-cell lymphoma, stage IISB.

▶ Questions

Problem Identification

1. a. *Identify all of the drug therapy problems of this patient.*
   b. *What clinical and other information is consistent with the diagnosis of non-Hodgkin's lymphoma?*
   c. *Explain what system of staging was used and how his stage of disease was determined.*
   d. *What laboratory and clinical features does this patient have that may affect his prognosis?*

Desired Outcome

2. *What are the goals of therapy in this case?*

Therapeutic Alternatives

3. *What alternative drug therapies are available for the treatment of this non-Hodgkin's lymphoma?*

Optimal Plan

4. a. *What drug, dosage form, schedule, and duration of therapy are best for treating this patient's non-Hodgkin's lymphoma?*
   b. *What other interventions should be made to maintain control of the patient's other concurrent diseases?*
   c. *What nondrug therapies might be useful for this patient?*

Outcome Evaluation

5. a. *How is the response to the treatment regimen for the non-Hodgkin's lymphoma assessed?*
   b. *What acute adverse effects are associated with the chemotherapy regimen, and what parameters should be monitored?*
   c. *What pharmacologic measures should be instituted to treat or prevent the acute toxicities associated with the chemotherapy regimen?*
   d. *What are potential late complications of the chemotherapy regimen, and how can they be detected and prevented?*

Patient Education

6. *What information would you provide to the patient about the agents used to treat the non-Hodgkin's lymphoma?*

▶ Clinical Course

The patient tolerated therapy very well without nausea or vomiting. He experienced some chills and fever with the treatment. His antihypertensive medication was modified, increasing his lisinopril to 20 mg daily and his metoprolol XL to 100 mg daily, achieving average systolic BPs in the 120s and average diastolic BPs in the 70s. He was also started on simvastatin 20 mg daily. Renal function remained stable and tumor lysis syndrome was not observed. Elevated blood glucose levels were problematic, and the patient was covered with sliding-scale insulin. The patient achieved a complete response to his therapy. Six months after completing therapy, follow-up PET scans showed recurrent disease in the mesenteric and inguinal lymph nodes, and he was found to have relapsed disease.

▶ Follow-Up Question

1. *What therapeutic options are available for patients with relapsed diffuse large B-cell lymphoma?*

▶ Clinical Course

The patient was presented with various treatment options. He and his wife decided they did not want to undergo aggressive, high-dose chemotherapy and decided to attempt treatment with radioimmunotherapy.

▶ Self-Study Assignments

1. What is the role of bone marrow or stem cell transplantation for aggressive non-Hodgkin's lymphoma?
2. What is the role of dexrazoxane, an anthracycline cardioprotector, in the treatment of malignancy?
3. If the patient experienced tumor lysis syndrome, what options are there for treating the hyperuricemia?

▶ Clinical Pearl

The diagnosis of non-Hodgkin's lymphoma must be established by an appropriate biopsy (an excisional biopsy, not an aspiration biopsy) to provide tissue for pathologic review. The prognosis and treatment of non-Hodgkin's lymphoma is dependent on the histologic type and the presence of certain adverse clinical features.

References

1. The International Non-Hodgkin's Lymphoma Prognostic Factors Project. A predictive model for aggressive non-Hodgkin's lymphoma. N Engl J Med 1993;329: 987–994.
2. Rodriguez J, Cabanillas F, McLaughlin P, et al. A proposal for a simple staging system for intermediate grade lymphoma and immunoblastic lymphoma based on the "tumor score." Ann Oncol 1992;3:711–717.
3. Fisher RI, Gaynor ER, Dahlberg S, et al. Comparison of a standard regimen (CHOP) with three intensive chemotherapy regimens for advanced non-Hodgkin's lymphoma. N Engl J Med 1993;328:1002–1006.
4. Vose JM, Link BK, Grossbard ML, et al. Phase II study of rituximab in combination with CHOP chemotherapy in patients with previously untreated, aggressive non-Hodgkin's lymphoma. J Clin Oncol 2001;19:389–397.
5. Coiffier B, Lepage E, Briere J, et al. CHOP chemotherapy plus rituximab compared with CHOP alone in elderly patients with diffuse large-B-cell lymphoma. N Engl J Med 2002;346:235–242.
6. Basser RL, Green MD. Strategies for prevention of anthracycline cardiotoxicity. Cancer Treat Rev 1993;19:57–77.
7. Ganz WI, Sridhar KS, Ganz SS, et al. Review of tests for monitoring doxorubicin-induced cardiomyopathy. Oncology 1996;53:461–470.

Acknowledgment: This case was modified and updated based on the case written for the fifth edition by Krista M. King, PharmD, BCOP.

144 HODGKIN'S DISEASE

▶ The Young G.I. (Level I)

Cindy L. O'Bryant, PharmD, BCOP

▶ After completing this case study, students should be able to:

- Identify and describe the tests performed as part of the staging work-up and the corresponding staging and classification systems for Hodgkin's Disease (HD).
- Describe the pharmacotherapeutic treatment of choice and the alternatives available for the treatment of HD.
- Identify acute and chronic toxicities associated with the medications used to treat HD and the measures used to prevent or treat these toxicities.
- Identify monitoring parameters for response and toxicity in patients with HD.
- Provide detailed patient education corresponding to the chemotherapeutic regimen.

PATIENT PRESENTATION

Chief Complaint

"I'm here for a second opinion about the treatment of my Hodgkin's disease."

HPI

Jack Riley is a 24 yo man who presents for recommendations about treatment of newly diagnosed Hodgkin's Disease. Two months ago he started having drenching night sweats, fevers, and a 9.1-kg weight loss. He also complained of difficulty swallowing and shortness of breath with wheezing on exertion. He was seen by the physician on his military base, who performed a chest x-ray that showed a large left pleural effusion and a mediastinal mass that was 48% of the thoracic diameter. He had an excisional biopsy of mediastinal nodes that demonstrated nodular sclerosing Hodgkin's disease.

PMH

None

FH

The patient has two brothers, both in good health. None of his relatives have any history of malignancy.

SH

The patient was born in Texas. He has been serving in the military for the past 6 years. He drinks about two glasses of alcoholic beverages/day. He does not use street drugs. He smokes one pack of cigarettes a day. He started smoking at the age of 18. The patient is recently married and wishes to have a family.

ROS

He describes fevers, drenching night sweats, and weight loss of about 9.1 kg over the past 2 months. He denies any vision changes or headaches. The patient reports shortness of breath with wheezing on exertion and a cough. He denies any chest pain. He notes recent dysphagia but denies diarrhea, constipation, or urinary symptoms. His performance status is 1 on the Zubrod scale.

Meds

Ibuprofen 400 mg po Q 4–6 H PRN for fevers

All

NKDA

PE

Gen

The patient is a young-appearing, thin male in no apparent distress

VS

BP 120/68, P 114, RR 18, T 37.2°C; Ht 6′, Wt 72.6 kg

Skin

No rashes or moles

LN

Not palpable in the preauricular, postauricular, submandibular, submental, cervical, infraclavicular, axillary, epitrochlear or inguinal areas bilaterally. Supraclavicular nodes are palpable bilaterally.

HEENT

No scleral icterus, thrush, mucositis, or tonsillar enlargement

Chest

Decreased breath sounds on the left, half the way up; faint wheezing

CV

RRR; no JVD, murmurs, or gallops

Abd

The abdomen is soft and non-tender. The spleen is enlarged, extending 4 cm below the left costal margin. Bowel sounds are normoactive.

Genit/Rect

Normal male genitalia; stool is guaiac (–)

Ext

Without edema

Neuro

Patient is A & O × 3. CN II–XI intact; remainder of exam is non-focal

Labs

Na 142 mEq/L	Hgb 12.1 g/dL	ALT 27 IU/L	PT 13.1 sec
K 4.2 mEq/L	Hct 37.1%	ALT 32 IU/L	aPTT 28.4 sec
Cl 101 mEq/L	Plt 355 × 10^3/mm^3	Alk phos 224 IU/L	Phos 3.7 mg/dL
CO_2 27 mEq/L	WBC 6.4 × 10^3/mm^3	LDH 571 IU/L	Uric acid 5.0 mg/dL
BUN 13 mg/dL	81% Neutros	T. bili 0.7 mg/dL	
SCr 0.9 mg/dL	5% Lymphs	T. prot 8.1 g/dL	
Glu 101 mg/dL	11% Monos	Alb 3.6 g/dL	
	3% Eos		

Chest X-Ray

Marked anterior mediastinal adenopathy is seen. This extends into the left hilar region with suggestion of narrowing in the left mainstem bronchus (see Figure 144–1). A left pleural effusion is noted that fills 50% of the volume of the left hemithorax. Possible nodular intraparenchymal lung nodule left base. The right lung is clear.

CT Chest

There is adenopathy in the lower neck and mediastinum. The mediastinal disease extends into the prevascular space, right paratracheal and subcarinal space. There is involvement of the hila bilaterally. There is mass effect on the tracheobronchial tree. Narrowing of the lingular bronchus is seen. Maximal transverse diameter of the mediastinal mass is 12 cm. There is a large left pleural effusion. The left lung is compressed in its entirety with the exception of a tiny amount of aerated lung seen in the upper lobe. The effusion is the predominant cause of the atelectasis, but in the lingula, an obstructive component may be present. The mediastinum is shifted toward the right side by the effusion. The right lung is aerated with no evidence of parenchymal involvement.

Tumor Pathology

Identification of lacunar cells (a variant of Reed-Sternberg cells) classifying this as Hodgkin's disease, nodular sclerosis (NS)

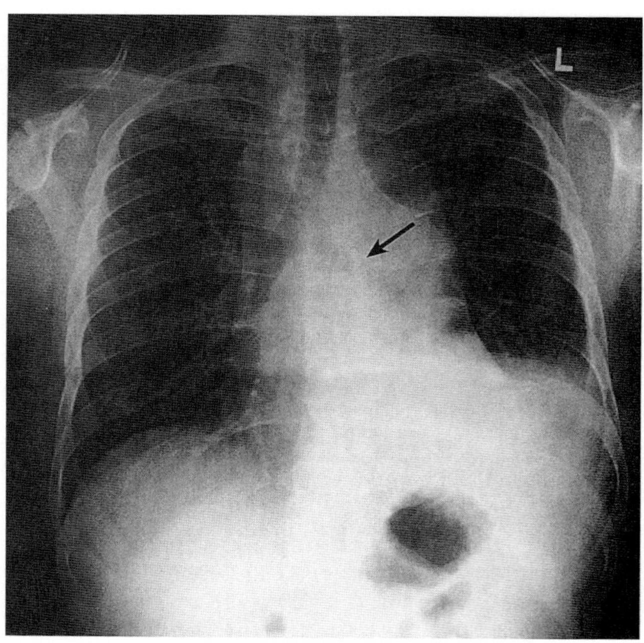

Figure 144–1. Chest x-ray showing anterior mediastinal adenopathy. This extends into the left hilar region with suggestion of narrowing in the left mainstem bronchus *(arrow)*. A left pleural effusion is noted that fills 50% of the volume of the left hemithorax. Possible nodular intraparenchymal lung nodule at left base. The right lung is clear.

Initial Assessment

Nodular sclerosis Hodgkin's disease with bulky mediastinal mass. Further staging will include bilateral BM biopsies, gallium scan or PET scan, and CT scans of the neck, abdomen, and pelvis.

▶ Clinical Course

- Bone marrow biopsies are negative for Hodgkin's disease.
- PET scan reveals bilateral supraclavicular adenopathy and extensive mediastinal adenopathy. There appears to be discrete foci of uptake in the region of the upper-mid-abdomen consistent with possible celiac nodes in the abdomen. There is diffuse enlargement of the spleen. The rest of the tracer distribution appears to be within normal limits.
- CT of the neck reveals large right paratracheal adenopathy/superior mediastinal adenopathy, including prevascular adenopathy. The mediastinal adenopathy is quite large. There is also necrotic adenopathy seen within the left lower neck lateral to the internal jugular vein measuring 2 cm × 1 cm. The right paratracheal lymphadenopathy measures 3 cm × 1.5 cm. There is also a left-sided pleural effusion.
- CT of the abdomen and pelvis reveals splenomegaly. There is no evidence of adenopathy in the mesentery, retroperitoneum, or pelvis. The liver is normal. The pancreas, adrenals, and kidneys are normal.

Assessment

Nodular sclerosis Hodgkin's disease, stage IIIB

▶ Questions

Problem Identification

1. a. *What clinical and other information is consistent with the diagnosis of Hodgkin's disease?*
   b. *Explain what system of staging was used and how his stage of disease was determined.*

Desired Outcome

2. *What are the goals of therapy in this case?*

Therapeutic Alternatives

3. *What therapeutic treatment options are available for managing this patient's Hodgkin's disease?*

Optimal Plan

4. *What drug, dosage form, schedule, and duration of chemotherapy are best for treating this patient's Hodgkin's disease?*

Outcome Evaluation

5. a. *How is the response to the treatment regimen for Hodgkin's disease assessed?*
   b. *What acute adverse effects are associated with the chemotherapy regimen, and what parameters should be monitored?*
   c. *What pharmacologic measures should be instituted to treat or prevent the acute toxicities associated with the chemotherapy regimen?*
   d. *What acute adverse effects are associated with radiotherapy, and how should they be monitored and treated?*
   e. *What are potential late complications of the chemotherapy/radiotherapy regimen, and how can they be detected and prevented?*

Patient Education

6. *What information would you provide to the patient about the chemotherapy agents?*

▶ Clinical Course

The patient was admitted to the hospital for treatment. He was also having trouble eating because of the mediastinal mass pressing on his esophagus. Because of the large left pleural effusion, thoracic surgery was consulted and a left chest tube was inserted to drain the pleural effusion. The effusion was consistent with chylothorax and was found to be negative for Hodgkin's disease. The patient received his first cycle of chemotherapy and experienced acute nausea and vomiting. He experienced severe pain from the chest tube and was placed on morphine PCA. His chest tube output was monitored closely by thoracic surgery, and the tube was removed after the output was < 250 mL/24h. His pain was much improved with the chest tube removed, and he was discharged on oral morphine. His oral intake gradually improved with the assistance of a dietitian. He returned to the clinic for his next cycle of chemotherapy, which was administered in an outpatient setting.

▶ Self-Study Assignments

1. What is the antiemetic regimen of choice to prevent acute nausea and vomiting for highly emetogenic chemotherapy?
2. What is the role of bone marrow or stem cell transplantation for Hodgkin's disease?
3. What are the salvage therapy options for patients with relapsing Hodgkin's disease?

▶ Clinical Pearl

Hodgkin's disease can be cured with chemotherapy, even if it is in advanced stages.

References

1. Tesch H, Sieber M, Diehl V. Treatment of advanced stage Hodgkin's disease. Oncology 2001;60:101–109.
2. Duggan DB, Petroni GR, Johnson JL, et al. Randomized comparison of ABVD and MOPP/ABV hybrid for the treatment of advanced Hodgkin's disease: Report of an Intergroup trial. J Clin Oncol 2003;21:607–614.

3. Chronowski GM, Wilder RB, Levy LB, et al. Second malignancies after chemotherapy and radiotherapy for Hodgkin disease. Am J Clin Oncol 2004;27:73–80.
4. Reece DE. Hematopoietic stem cell transplantation in Hodgkin disease. Curr Opin Oncol 2002;14:165–170.

Acknowledgement: This chapter is based on the case written for the Fifth Edition by Krista M. King, PharmD, BCOP.

145 OVARIAN CANCER

▶ Perspectives and Future Developments in Ovarian Cancer (Level II)

William C. Zamboni, PharmD
Laura L. Jung, PharmD
Margaret E. Tonda, PharmD

▶ After completing this case study, students should be able to:

- Recognize the signs and symptoms of ovarian cancer.
- Describe the genetic factors associated with ovarian cancer.
- Recommend a pharmacotherapeutic plan for the chemotherapeutic treatment of newly diagnosed and relapsed ovarian cancer.
- Recognize the dose-limiting and most commonly occurring toxicities associated with the chemotherapeutic agents used in the treatment of ovarian cancer.

PATIENT PRESENTATION

Chief Complaint

"This is my first cycle of chemotherapy and I am worried about getting sick."

HPI

Julia Erving is a 53 yo woman who presented to the ED 9 weeks ago with a 3-day history of acute abdominal pain. She also reported a weight gain of about 9 kg over the previous 3 months. CT scans of the abdomen and pelvis showed a large, soft-tissue pelvic mass. Exploratory laparotomy revealed a 20 × 10 cm mass near the left ovary, positive microscopic disease in the omentum, and positive bilateral external iliac nodes. A 3-cm mass in the liver was also found. A TAH and left oophorectomy were performed at that time. The CA-125 was 380 IU/mL. Tumor biopsies from the ovary and liver were positive for epithelial ovarian cancer with serous histology. Bulky residual disease persists in the mesenteric lymph nodes, presacral spine (1.5 cm), and para-aortic region (2.2 cm). She is now admitted to undergo her first cycle of consolidative chemotherapy.

PMH

Right-sided oophorectomy for ruptured ectopic pregnancy 12 years ago
S/P conjugated estrogens and progesterone × 5 years for HRT
Type 2 DM ×10 years
HTN × 5 years
Bilateral numbness in feet

FH

Divorced with no children; mother, maternal aunt, and cousin all have ovarian cancer; father is alive and well.

SH

Denies smoking; social alcohol use.

Meds

Nifedipine XL 60 mg po daily
Glipizide 10 mg po daily

All

Penicillin → seizures
Aspirin → stomach cramps

ROS

Stomach area feels heavy and painful; she sometimes feels nauseated.

PE

Gen
The patient is an African-American woman appearing to be her stated age.

VS
BP 130/80, P 110, RR 22, T 37.6°C; Wt 60 kg, Ht 5′4″

Skin
No erythema, rash, ecchymosis, petechiae, or breakdown

LN
No cervical or axillary lymphadenopathy

HEENT
PERRLA, EOMI; TMs intact; fundus benign; OP with dry mucus membranes

Breasts
Without masses, discharge, or adenopathy. No nipple or skin changes

Cor
RRR; no murmurs, rubs, or gallops

Pulm
Lungs are clear to auscultation with a slight decrease at the left base; mainly resonant throughout all lung fields

Abd
Soft and non-tender without hepatosplenomegaly

Genit/Rect
Normal female genitalia; heme (–) dark brown stool; no rectal wall tenderness or masses

Ext

No C/C/E

Neuro

Speech: no dysarthria, rate normal. CN II–XII intact. Motor: normal strength throughout; tone normal. Sensation decreased to light touch and pinprick below the knees bilaterally. Vibration sense diminished at the great toes bilaterally. Reflexes 2+ and symmetric throughout. Babinski negative bilaterally. Cerebellar: finger-to-nose and heel-to-shin are without dysmetria. Rapid alternate movements are normal as are gross and fine motor coordination. Good sitting and standing balance without an assistive device. Gait: able to toe and tandem walk without difficulty. Gait normal in speed and step length. Cognition: alert and oriented × 3. Able to do serial 7s. Able to abstract. Short- and long-term memories are intact

Labs

Na 137 mEq/L	Hgb 13.6 g/dL	AST 21 IU/L
K 3.1 mEq/L	Hct 38%	ALT 24 IU/L
Cl 99 mEq/L	Plt 150 × 10^3/mm^3	T. bili 0.8 mg/dL
CO_2 22 mEq/L	WBC 5.2 × 10^3/mm^3	Amylase 129 IU/L
BUN 20 mg/dL	60% Neutros	Lipase 62 IU/L
SCr 1.5 mg/dL	3% Bands	CA-125 140 IU/mL
Glu 180 mg/dL	30% Lymphs	
	5% Monos	
	1% Eos	
	1% Basos	

UA

WBC 5–10/hpf, RBC 1/hpf, 1+ ketones, 1+ protein, pH 5.0

Genetic Results (from DNA analysis of a blood sample)

BRCA1 positive

▶ Questions

Problem Identification

1. a. *What are the patient's drug therapy problems?*
   b. *What information (signs, symptoms, laboratory values) indicates the presence and severity of ovarian cancer?*
   c. *What stage of ovarian cancer does this patient have, and how does the stage of disease affect the choice of therapy?*
   d. *What is the significance of the size of residual tumor after primary cytoreductive surgery?*

Desired Outcome

2. *What are the goals of therapy for this patient?*

Therapeutic Alternatives

3. a. *How do her genetic results influence the choice of therapy and prognosis?*
   b. *What are the consolidative chemotherapy options for this patient?*

Optimal Plan

4. a. *Which consolidative chemotherapy regimen and ancillary treatment measures would you recommend for this patient?*
   b. *Use the Calvert equation[7] to calculate the carboplatin dose required to achieve a target AUC of 5 mg/mL min.*

Outcome Evaluation

5. *How would you monitor the therapy for efficacy and adverse effects?*

Patient Education

6. *What information would you provide to the patient about this therapy?*

▶ Clinical Course

Ms. Erving completed 6 cycles of docetaxel and carboplatin. Her serum CA-125 level slowly declined over the treatment course (110 IU/mL, 95 IU/mL, 85 IU/mL, 60 IU/mL, and 45 IU/mL after the first, second, third, fourth, and fifth cycles, respectively) and was 30 IU/mL 2 weeks after her sixth cycle. Because of the slow reduction in CA-125, the decision was made to continue docetaxel and carboplatin for 4 more cycles. However, after her third additional cycle (ninth overall cycle), she began to complain of increased numbness in her toes. Therapy was continued for one more cycle, and her CA-125 levels continued to decrease to 12 IU/mL 4 weeks after the fourth additional cycle (tenth overall cycle). Based upon her CA-125 levels and negative CT scans, Ms. Erving was defined as a clinical complete response. Treatment was discontinued and CA-125 levels were followed monthly.

Over the next 4 months the CA-125 levels were as follows: 20 IU/mL, 30 IU/mL, 43 IU/mL, and 88 IU/mL. Five months after completing the last cycle of chemotherapy, a CT scan of the abdomen and pelvis revealed a mass (5 × 6 × 6 cm) arising from the retroperitoneum and a 2-cm mass in the head of the pancreas. Biopsies of the pancreas and abdominal/pelvic mass were positive for recurrent epithelial ovarian cancer. Laboratory data were normal except for a CA-125 level of 150 IU/mL. Ms. Erving is now admitted for her first cycle of chemotherapy for her relapsed ovarian cancer.

▶ Follow-Up Questions

1. *What chemotherapeutic options are available for this patient's relapsed ovarian cancer?*
2. *Which of the chemotherapeutic regimens would you suggest for the patient's locally relapsed ovarian cancer? Why?*
3. *What are the potential toxicities of pegylated liposomal doxorubicin? How can they be prevented and treated?*

▶ Clinical Course

After four cycles of salvage chemotherapy with pegylated liposomal doxorubicin 40 mg/m^2 every 28 days, CA-125 levels were decreasing and radiographic findings showed no progression of disease. However, the patient complained of having trouble putting on her shoes and her feet hurt when she walked. On physical exam, the patient's feet were red, swollen, and cracked. The fifth cycle of pegylated liposomal doxorubicin therapy was delayed for 2 weeks and the redness on her feet resolved. The pegylated liposomal doxorubicin was restarted at 30 mg/m^2 every 28 days.

After 3 additional cycles of pegylated liposomal doxorubicin, the pain, redness, and swelling in Ms. Erving's feet returned. In addition, her CA-125 levels over this 3 month period where 92 IU/mL, 150 IU/mL, and 182 IU/mL.

Considering the poor prognosis and aggressive nature of her disease, she was enrolled on a Phase I trial of gemcitabine and topotecan. Even though gemcitabine and topotecan are approved for clinical use, the combination has not been evaluated in patients. Thus, a Phase I trial of the combination was developed to determine the maximum tolerated dose of gemcitabine in combination with a fixed dose of topotecan. She was treated with topotecan 0.75 mg/m^2/day IV over 30 minutes on days 1 to 4, gemcitabine 1,000 mg/m^2/day IV over 1 hour on day 1, repeated every 21 days. Filgrastim 5 mcg/kg/day was started 24 hours after the last dose of chemotherapy and continued until the ANC was $> 1.0 \times 10^3$/mm^3 for two consecutive days. Her treatment is ongoing.

▶ Self-Study Assignments

1. How is carboplatin dosing calculated?
2. What is the probable cause of the paclitaxel and docetaxel hypersensitivity?
3. What are the issues related to maintenance therapy in patients with advanced ovarian cancer after complete response to consolidative chemotherapy?
4. How does the polymorphism in cytochrome P450 3A4 potentially affect docetaxel therapy in the treatment of ovarian cancer?

▶ Clinical Pearl

The objective of Phase I clinical trials is to determine the maximum tolerated dose and dose-limiting toxicities. In Phase I trials, the dose of a chemotherapeutic agent is increased in cohorts of patients until dose-limiting toxicity is achieved.

References

1. Boyd J, Sonoda Y, Federici MG, et al. Clinicopathologic features of BRCA-linked and sporadic ovarian cancer. JAMA 2000;283:2260–2265.
2. McGuire WP, Hoskins WJ, Brady MF, et al. Cyclophosphamide and cisplatin compared with paclitaxel and cisplatin in patients with stage III and stage IV ovarian cancer. N Engl J Med 1996;334:1–6.
3. Ozols RF, Bundy BN, Greer BE, et al. Phase III trial of carboplatin and paclitaxel compared with cisplatin and paclitaxel in patients with optimally resected stage III ovarian cancer: A Gynecological Oncology Group study. J Clin Oncol 2003;21:3194–3200.
4. du Bois A, Luck HJ, Meier W, et al. A randomized clinical trial of cisplatin/paclitaxel versus carboplatin/paclitaxel as first-line treatment of ovarian cancer. J Natl Cancer Inst 2003;95;1320–1329.
5. Morgan RJ, Copeland L, Gershenson D, et al. NCCN ovarian cancer practice guidelines. The National Comprehensive Cancer Network. Oncology (Huntingt) 1996;10(11 Suppl):293–310.
6. Vasey P. Role of docetaxel in the treatment of newly diagnosed advanced ovarian cancer. J Clin Oncol 2003;21(10 Suppl):136–144.
7. Calvert AH, Newell DR, Gumbrell LA, et al. Carboplatin dosage: Prospective evaluation of a simple formula based on renal function. J Clin Oncol 1989;7:1748–1756.
8. Parmar MK, Ledermann J, Colombo N, et al. ICON and AGO Collaborators. Paclitaxel plus platinum-based chemotherapy versus conventional platinum-based chemotherapy in women with relapsed ovarian cancer: The ICON4/AGO-OVAR-2.2 trial. Lancet 2003;361:2099–2106.
9. Alberts DS, Liu PY, Hannigan EV, et al. Intraperitoneal cisplatin plus intravenous cyclophosphamide versus intravenous cisplatin plus intravenous cyclophosphamide for stage III ovarian cancer. N Engl J Med 1996;335:1950–1955.
10. Safra T, Muggia F, Jeffers S, et al. Pegylated liposomal doxorubicin (Doxil): Reduced clinical cardiotoxicity in patients reaching or exceeding cumulative doses of 500 mg/m^2. Ann Oncol 2000;11:1029–1033.

146 ACUTE LYMPHOCYTIC LEUKEMIA

▶ Jenny's Long Battle (Level II)

Mark T. Holdsworth, PharmD, BCOP

▶ After completing this case study, students should be able to:

- Identify common drug-induced diseases in children with acute lymphocytic leukemia (ALL).
- Design effective prophylactic and treatment strategies for drug-induced diseases in children with ALL.
- Describe a contemporary management strategy for tumor lysis syndrome.
- Interpret the laboratory values that signify the response of ALL to chemotherapy.
- Discuss key information that should be presented to a child's family when educating them about the chemotherapy agents used for ALL.
- Describe the ancillary medications and supportive care measures that are necessary when administering intermediate-dose methotrexate.
- Discuss current controversies regarding use of intermediate-dose methotrexate in children with ALL.
- Discuss the influence of pharmacogenetics on the dynamics of pharmacotherapy during treatment of ALL.

PATIENT PRESENTATION

Chief Complaint

Fatigue and low-grade temperature.

HPI

Jenny Martinez is a 3 yo girl brought to the pediatric clinic by her parents, who report that for the past week she has been quite fatigued and has had fevers, easy bruising, and puffiness of the extremities.

PMH

Up-to-date on immunizations; no prior surgeries or serious medical problems.

FH

No family history of cancer. Resides near a site with a history of radioactive contamination.

SH

Not applicable

ROS

Noncontributory

Meds

None

All

NKDA

PE

Gen

Alert, interactive, well-developed but ill-appearing child

VS

BP 130/83, P 95, RR 34, T 36.8°C; Ht 38″, Wt 17.3 kg, BSA 0.6 m^2

Skin

Diffuse pallor; random tan macular bruises just inferior to the hairline, face, and over the proximal upper extremity, with a petechial-appearing rash over the buttocks and lower left flank.

HEENT

Head is NC/AT; PERRLA; EOMI; nares are clear bilaterally; throat shows no erythema. Question of petechial hemorrhage of mucous membranes.

Neck/LN

Neck is supple and non-tender with shotty cervical and submandibular lymphadenopathy

Lungs/Thorax

CTA bilaterally without wheezes or crackles, and there is good air movement throughout

Breasts

Undeveloped

CV

Heart has RRR without murmur

Abd

Soft and non-tender, without distention. There are good bowel sounds and no masses present. Hepatosplenomegaly is noted.

Genit/Rect

No tenderness, bruising, or blood observed.

MS/Ext

Shotty lymphadenopathy in the inguinal area; femoral pulses are 2+ bilaterally. Extremities display no CCE, and there is no bone pain elicited with palpation.

Neuro

Without dysmorphic features or deformities. Frequent rapid eye blinking (R > L); eyes seemed briefly dysconjugate when asked to focus. Fixes and follows well with conjugate eye movements. Hearing appears intact. Motor exam shows normal muscle tone and bulk. Gait is normal. DTRs are normal. General muscle strength is symmetric and normal. Facial strength appears symmetric and normal.

Labs

Hgb 5.7 g/dL	AST 93 IU/L	SCr 1.0 mg/dL
Hct 17.2%	ALT 60 IU/L	PT 12 sec
WBC 37.5 × $10^3/mm^3$	LDH 1875 IU/L	aPTT 24 sec
2% Segs	T. bili 0.7 mg/dL	Varicella titer (+)
0% Bands	T. prot 6.9 g/dL	Anti-HAV (–)
85% Lymphs	Alb 3.5 g/dL	HBsAg (–)
4% Monos	Ca 8.3 mg/dL	Anti-HBs (–)
1% Myelos	Phos 5.1 mg/dL	Anti-HCV (–)
8% Blasts	Uric acid 12.1 mg/dL	

BM Aspirate

90% blasts, 3% erythroid precursors, 2% lymphocytes, 2% metamyelocytes, 1% promyelocytes, 2% myelocytes. DNA index 1.0. Early pre-B cell ALL with L1 morphology. RT-PCR positive for TEL-AML 1 fusion transcript and negative for E2A-PBX1.

Chest X-Ray

Normal with no mediastinal mass noted.

LP

Glucose 55 mg/dL, T. protein 15 mg/dL, no blasts present.

Assessment

Acute lymphocytic leukemia with pancytopenia and replacement of normal bone marrow elements.

► Clinical Course

The patient was admitted to the pediatric subacute care unit. Medications and treatments upon admission included the following:

Day 1 (day of admission):

- 1 unit of irradiated/filtered platelets
- 1 unit PRBCs

- D_5 0.9% NS IV at 2,000 mL/m²/day
- Rasburicase 3.5 mg IV x 1 dose

On day 1 of admission, the patient developed a fever of 38.5°C.

Day 2 induction chemotherapy orders:

- Vincristine 1 mg IV Q week × 4 (on days 1, 8, 15, and 22)
- Prednisone 10 mg po TID × 28 days
- Asparaginase 3,600 units IM on chemotherapy days 2, 5, 8, 12, 15, and 19
- Intrathecal therapy (IT) with methotrexate 12 mg on chemotherapy days 1 and 15

Four hours after the first chemotherapy, she developed moderate nausea and vomiting with 4 vomiting episodes.

Week 1 of induction therapy:

The patient remained in the hospital for the first 8 days. On day 2, serum uric acid was 0.2 mg/dL, and remained below the normal range during the first week of therapy. She became afebrile after day 3. Hematology tests obtained during the following 2 weeks of induction therapy were as follows:

Parameter (units)	Week 2 (Day 7)	Week 3 (Day 15)
Hgb (g/dL)	8.7	11.7
Hct (%)	25.1	35.3
Plt (× 10³/mm³)	22.0	70.0
WBC (× 10³/mm³)	0.670	2.35
Segs (%)	5	18
Bands (%)	0	0
Lymphs (%)	92	68
Monos (%)	1	12
Myelos (%)	0	2
Blasts (%)	2	0
Uric Acid (mg/dL)	2.1	2.5

On day 15 of chemotherapy, a second BM aspirate revealed 1% blasts; 4% promyelocytes; 2% myelocytes; 4% metamyelocytes; 63% erythroblasts and other erythroid precursors; 9% lymphocytes; 4% plasma cells; 10% bands; 1% neutrophils; 0% eosinophils; 0% basophils; 1% reticulum cells; and 1% monocytes. Day 15 LP showed CSF glucose 47 mg/dL, T. prot 14 mg/dL, no blasts present.

Questions

Problem Identification

1. a. *Identify the patient's drug therapy problems during the first week of induction therapy.*
   b. *Since vincristine and the IT methotrexate are to be administered on the same day, what precautions must be observed to avoid severe drug toxicity?*

Desired Outcome

2. a. *What are the initial goals of pharmacotherapy in this patient, and were they achieved?*
   b. *What are the long-term treatment goals in this patient?*

Therapeutic Alternatives

3. *List the therapeutic alternatives for the drug therapy problems that developed during induction therapy and discuss the risks and benefits of each.*

Optimal Plan

4. *Outline the optimal treatment schedule and duration for the drug therapy problems described in the previous answer. What therapeutic alternatives should be considered if initial therapy fails?*

Outcome Evaluation

5. *What key laboratory parameters are indicative of an adequate response to induction therapy?*

Patient Education

6. a. *What information should be provided to the patient's parents about the potential beneficial and adverse effects from the chemotherapy agents used during induction therapy?*
   b. *Jenny's parents are concerned that their residence near a radioactive site may have resulted in their child's illness. Discuss any evidence to support an environmental link with this malignancy.*

Clinical Course–Induction Week 3

During week 3, Jenny develops abdominal pain and constipation. Despite the use of laxatives, after 2 days Jenny's abdominal pain worsens and she develops severe malaise and vomiting. Her parents bring her into the clinic, and the PE reveals an ill-appearing child with altered consciousness and severe abdominal pain. Vital signs are BP 70/30, P 140, RR 45, and T 37°C. The remainder of her PE is WNL. The following laboratory values are reported:

Hgb 11.7 g/dL
Hct 35.3%
Plt 70 × 10³/mm³
WBC 2.35 × 10³/mm³
Segs 18%
Bands 0%
Lymphs 68%
Monos 12%
Myelos 2%
Blasts 0%

Glu 785 mg/dL
Lactate 440 mg/dL
AST 53 IU/L
ALT 35 IU/L
LDH 170 IU/L
T. bili 2.5 mg/dL
T. prot 7.3 g/dL
Alb 4.1 g/dL

Ca 9.7 mg/dL
Phos 5.2 mg/dL
Uric acid 2.3 mg/dL
PT 14 sec
aPTT 27 sec
D. Bili 2.1 mg/dL

She is hospitalized, blood cultures are drawn, and broad-spectrum antibiotics are initiated. She is scheduled to receive day 19 of chemotherapy on the following day, and orders are written to continue chemotherapy on the current schedule.

▶ Follow-Up Questions–Induction Week 3

1. *Is this current hospitalization likely the result of a drug- or disease-related problem? What additional laboratory tests should be obtained at this time?*
2. *What modifications in the therapeutic plan should be made?*

▶ Clinical Course–Induction Week 4

On day 28 of chemotherapy (end of induction), her laboratory values are:

Hgb 12.8 g/dL	WBC $11.0 \times 10^3/mm^3$
Hct 38.2%	86% Segs
Plt $326 \times 10^3/mm^3$	0% Bands
	10% Lymphs
	4% Monos
	0% Myelos
	0% Blasts

The results of the day 28 BM aspirate showed 2% blasts; 3% promyelocytes; 5% myelocytes; 7% metamyelocytes; 8% bands; 8% neutrophils; 56% erythroblasts and other erythroid precursors; 5% lymphocytes; 1% monocytes; and 5% eosinophils and precursors.

▶ Clinical Course–Consolidation Phase

After completion of induction therapy and resolution of her acute illness, she entered a consolidation phase (weeks 5 through 24), which consisted of the following:

- Mercaptopurine 50 mg/m^2 po daily
- Methotrexate 1 g/m^2 IV $\times$ 1 dose on weeks 7, 10, 13, 16, 19, and 22
- Vincristine 2 mg/m^2 IV $\times$ 1 dose on weeks 8, 9, 17, and 18
- Prednisone 10 mg po TID $\times$ 7 days on weeks 8 and 17
- IT with methotrexate 12 mg $\times$ 1 dose on weeks 5, 6, 9, 12, 15, and 18

During week 6 of consolidation, Jenny develops severe pancytopenia as illustrated by the following CBC:

Hgb 7.5 g/dL	WBC $0.3 \times 10^3/mm^3$
Hct 22.2%	46% Segs
Plt $25 \times 10^3/mm^3$	0% Bands
	50% Lymphs
	2% Monos
	1% Eos
	1% Basos

The oncologists are concerned that Jenny may be experiencing a relapse and have ordered a bone marrow biopsy.

▶ Follow-Up Questions–Consolidation (Week 6)

3. *What other possible explanations are there for the pancytopenia?*
4. *After a several week delay in chemotherapy, week 7 of consolidation is initiated. Jenny is scheduled to receive her first course of intermediate-dose methotrexate (1 g/m^2). Which additional medications and supportive measures will be necessary for administration of this dose of methotrexate?*
5. *What laboratory tests and examinations must be performed prior to the methotrexate administration?*
6. *After the methotrexate administration, the 24-hour peak concentration is 8.7 μmol. The 48-hour concentration is 0.3 μmol. What is the significance of these findings, and what additional changes in therapy should be made based on these concentrations?*

▶ Clinical Course–Week 62

After completing the consolidation phase on week 62, the plan is for her to receive maintenance therapy for 2.5 years. The resident in charge of her case prepares the following schedule of orders:

- Mercaptopurine 10 mg/m^2 po three times a week
- Methotrexate 20 mg/m^2 po $\times$ 1 dose weekly
- Vincristine 2 mg/m^2 IV daily $\times$ 7 days, every 15 weeks
- Prednisone 50 mg/m^2 po $\times$ 7 days, every 15 weeks
- IT with methotrexate $\times$ 1 dose every 8 weeks

▶ Follow-Up Questions

7. *Identify any problems with the preceding medication schedule of maintenance therapy. Are there any explanations for the altered dosing for one of these medications?*
8. *During the maintenance phase of her chemotherapy protocol, which laboratory test is closely monitored to gauge the adequacy of her chemotherapy doses?*
9. *What is the target value for this laboratory measurement, and how will the chemotherapy doses be changed if the laboratory test is above the target range?*

▶ Clinical Course

Jenny experiences two grand mal seizures during week 97 of chemotherapy. A CT scan of her brain reveals areas of white matter hypodensity and cerebral calcification.

▶ Follow-Up Questions–Week 97

10. *Explain whether these CNS findings are likely the result of chemotherapy and what is known about this problem and the risks associated with it.*
11. *What modifications in chemotherapy should be made as a consequence of these CNS findings?*
12. *Based upon these recent CNS findings, explain what is known regarding Jenny's long-term outlook.*

▶ Self-Study Assignments

1. Discuss the current controversies regarding the use of intermediate-dose methotrexate as standard therapy in female children with ALL.
2. Provide evidence to support the value of maintaining adequate dose intensity in the maintenance phase of ALL therapy (focus on trials that report the actual received-dose intensity).
3. Discuss the value of colony-stimulating factors in the prophylaxis or treatment of therapy-related complications in children with ALL.

▶ Clinical Pearl

Although a DNA index = 1.0 generally is a high-risk feature for childhood ALL, the TEL-AML 1 fusion transcript [associated with t(12;21)] in this patient indicates a good prognosis case of B-ALL. However, relapses can still occur and tend to occur late in children with this translocation. For this reason, it is still not recommended to reduce the intensity of chemotherapy for children with this translocation.

References

1. Holdsworth MT, Raisch DW, Winter SS, et al. Assessment of the emetogenic potential of intrathecal chemotherapy and response to prophylactic treatment with ondansetron. Support Care Cancer 1998;6:132–138.
2. Holdsworth MT, Nguyen P. Role of i.v. allopurinol and rasburicase in tumor lysis syndrome. Am J Health-Syst Pharm 2003;60:2213–2224.
3. Holdsworth MT, Mathew P. Efficacy of colony-stimulating factors in acute leukemia. Ann Pharmacother 2001;35:92–108.
4. ASHP Commission on Therapeutics. ASHP therapeutic guidelines on the pharmacologic management of nausea and vomiting in adult and pediatric patients receiving chemotherapy or radiation therapy or undergoing surgery. Am J Health-Syst Pharm 1999;56:729–764.
5. Evans WE, Hon YY, Bomgaars L, et al. Preponderance of thiopurine S-methyltransferase deficiency and heterozygosity among patients intolerant to mercaptopurine or azathioprine. J Clin Oncol 2001;19:2293–2301.
6. Mahoney DH, Shuster JJ, Nitschke R, et al. Acute neurotoxicity in children with B-precursor acute lymphoid leukemia: An association with intermediate-dose intravenous methotrexate and intrathecal triple therapy—A Pediatric Oncology Group study. J Clin Oncol 1998;16:1712–1722.

147 CHRONIC MYELOGENOUS LEUKEMIA

▶ Philadelphia Freedom? (Level II)

R. Donald Harvey III, PharmD, BCPS, BCOP
Christine Walko, PharmD

▶ After completing this case study, students should be able to:

- Identify the presenting signs and symptoms of chronic myelogenous leukemia (CML).
- Identify important prognostic indicators for CML.
- Construct treatment options for CML.
- List appropriate parameters to monitor efficacy and potential adverse effects of treatment for CML.
- Educate patients on treatment complications and the most common side effects of current therapy for CML.

PATIENT PRESENTATION

Chief Complaint

"I've been really tired lately."

HPI

John Pella is a 46 yo man who complains of shortness of breath on exertion, an unintentional weight loss of 6.4 kg, and fatigue beginning 4 months ago. He also notes fullness in his left upper quadrant and early satiety.

PMH

Appendectomy (1974) complicated with infection
Tonsillectomy (1965)
Hernia repair (1997)

FH

Father died of pulmonary embolism at age 54. Mother is 73 yo with type 2 diabetes. His 47 yo sister and 23 yo old son are in good health. Grandparents may have had CAD. No history of cancer.

SH

Married and lives with his wife of 25 years. He works full-time in the maintenance department of a local packaging company. Smoked ½ to ¾ pack of cigarettes/day for more than 20 years until he quit 4 years ago. Denies alcohol consumption.

ROS

Increased weakness and tiredness. Occasional fever, chills, and night sweats; shortness of breath on exertion. Denies bleeding, headaches, nausea, vomiting, chest pain, or urinary symptoms.

Meds

None

All

Penicillin (skin rash—31 years ago)

PE

Gen

WDWN white man in NAD who appears his stated age

VS

BP 120/88, P 84, RR 18, T 37°C, actual weight 90.9 kg, Ht 6′1″

Skin

Warm, dry, with good turgor. No evidence of rash, ecchymoses, petechiae, or cyanosis

HEENT

PERRLA, EOMI, sclerae anicteric, TMs clear. No sinus discharge or tenderness. Oral mucosa moist and intact

Neck

Supple without masses. No carotid bruits auscultated. No thyromegaly appreciated.

LN

Approximately 1-cm, non-tender palpable node in right inguinal area. No other lymphadenopathy noted.

Chest

CTA; no rales or rhonchi

CV

NSR; normal S_1 and S_2 without murmur

Abd

Soft, symmetric, and non-tender. Spleen palpable 8 cm below costal margin. Normoactive bowel sounds. No hepatomegaly noted. Well-approximated abdominal surgical scar noted.

Rect

Deferred

MS/Ext

No joint deformities or peripheral edema. ROM and muscle strength symmetrical throughout

Neuro

CN II-XII intact. DTRs 1+ throughout. Gait steady. A & O × 3

Labs

Na 143 mEq/L	Hgb 12.1 g/dL	AST 30 IU/L	Ca 8.9 mg/dL
K 4.4 mEq/L	Hct 32%	ALT 86 IU/L	Mg 3.0 mEq/L
Cl 109 mEq/L	Plt 456 × 10^3/mm^3	Alk phos 29 IU/L	Phos 4.8 mg/dL
CO_2 24 mEq/L	WBC 97.0 × 10^3/mm^3	LDH 325 IU/L	Uric acid 0.9 mg/dL
BUN 50 mg/dL	24% Segs	T. bili 4.9 mg/dL	LAP absent
SCr 0.7 mg/dL	8% Bands	T. prot 2.9 g/dL	
Glu 148 mg/dL	64% Lymphs	Alb 1.6 g/dL	
Retic 2.3%	3% Myelos		
	1% Monos		

Bone Marrow Biopsy

Cytogenetic studies revealed a translocation involving the long arms of chromosomes 9 and 22 [t(9q;22q)] (Philadelphia chromosome), with 95% of malignant cells analyzed found to be Ph-positive. The marrow was hypercellular and consisted of 2% to 3% myeloblasts, but showed no other blastic abnormalities. This information is consistent with the characteristics of CML in chronic phase (CML-CP).

▶ Questions

Problem Identification

1. a. *What information in the patient's history is consistent with a diagnosis of CML-CP (see Figure 147–1)?*
   b. *Describe the natural progression of CML.*
   c. *List factors that signal a poor prognosis for CML patients in chronic phase.*

Desired Outcome

2. *What are long-term therapy goals for this patient?*

Therapeutic Alternatives

3. *What nonpharmacologic and pharmacologic alternatives should be considered for this patient?*

Optimal Plan

4. *Considering all patient factors, describe the optimal initial treatment plan for this patient.*

Outcome Evaluation

5. *Describe parameters for monitoring disease response and toxicity for the treatment option you recommended.*

Patient Education

6. *What information should be given to the patient prior to treatment?*

▶ Clinical Course

The regimen you recommended was initiated. At the 2-week follow-up visit, the patient's WBC count was 28 × 10^3/mm^3. At the 4-week follow-up visit,

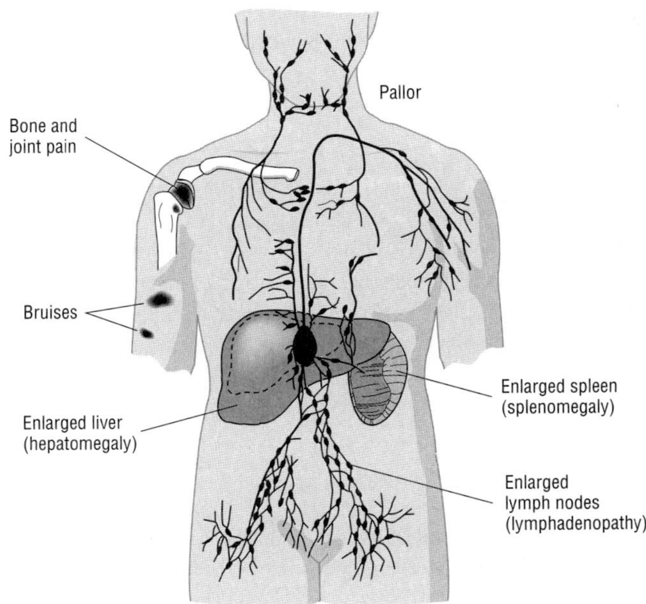

Figure 147–1. Common signs and symptoms of chronic myelogenous leukemia.

his WBC count had decreased to 8.0 × 10^3/mm^3. After 6 months of treatment, his WBC count remained stable at 7.6 × 10^3/mm^3, and a bone marrow biopsy revealed no positive metaphases for the Philadelphia chromosome. The patient discussed further treatment options with his physician. An allogeneic BMT from a matched-related sibling was chosen, using busulfan (4 mg/kg/day) for 4 days followed by cyclophosphamide (50 mg/kg/day) for 2 days as the BMT preparative regimen.

▶ Follow-Up Questions

1. *What is the goal of therapy for allogeneic BMT in the management of CML-CP?*
2. *Is this CML patient an optimal candidate for a BMT? Why or why not?*
3. *List common complications of allogeneic BMT and this preparative regimen.*
4. *Identify important laboratory and clinical values to monitor during the BMT course.*
5. *When the patient is discharged after BMT, what important information should be relayed to him?*
6. *If relapse occurs after allogeneic BMT, what treatment alternatives remain for this patient?*
7. *If the patient progresses to CML-blast crisis despite BMT, what is the best treatment option for him?*

▶ Self-Study Assignments

1. Describe the hematologic and cytogenetic response criteria (complete, partial, minor, and no response) for therapy in patients with CML, including WBC count, splenomegaly, and percent of Ph+ marrow cells.
2. How does the treatment of a Ph– CML patient differ from Ph+ disease?
3. Discuss the role of hydroxyurea, homoharringtonine, decitabine, tipifarnib, and antisense oligonucleotides in the treatment of CML-CP.

▶ Clinical Pearl

Fluorescence *in situ* hybridization (FISH) and quantitative polymerase chain reaction (PCR) enable the use of peripheral blood samples to monitor molecular remission and minimal residual disease in patients receiving imatinib.

References

1. Savage DG, Antman KH. Imatinib – a new oral targeted therapy. N Engl J Med 2002;346:683–693.
2. O'Brien SG, Guilhot F, Larson RA, et al. IRIS Investigators. Imatinib compared with interferon and low-dose cytarabine for newly diagnosed chronic-phase chronic myeloid leukemia. N Engl J Med 2003;348:994–1004.
3. Devergie A, Apperley JF, Labopin M, et al. European results of matched unrelated donor bone marrow transplantation for chronic myeloid leukemia. Impact of HLA class II matching. Bone Marrow Transplant 1997;20:11–19.
4. Deininger MW, O'Brien SG, Ford JM, et al. Practical management of patients with chronic myeloid leukemia receiving imatinib. J Clin Oncol 2003;21:1637–1647.

148 MELANOMA

▶ Remember Your ABCDE's (Level I)

J. Michael Vozniak, PharmD
Rowena N. Schwartz, PharmD, BCOP

▶ After completion of this case study, one should be able to:

- Identify risk factors for developing melanoma.
- Outline appropriate pharmacotherapeutic management for metastatic melanoma.
- Educate patients with the diagnosis of melanoma on the adverse effects of aldesleukin.

PATIENT PRESENTATION

Chief Complaint

"I'm here for my first IL-2 treatment."

HPI

Allen Nelson is a 43 year old white man who had been referred to the dermatology clinic by his PCP after discovering a recent change in a mole on his left scapula (see Figure 148–1). The mole was removed by excisional biopsy and was found to be a superficial spreading melanoma. The patient underwent a surgical excision of the primary tumor and a sentinel lymphadenectomy. The tumor was found to be 2.4-mm thick without ulceration and involving 2 lymph nodes without satellitosis. Laboratory studies revealed an elevated LDH of 754 IU/L. Work-up for metastatic disease included a CT scan of the chest, abdomen and pelvis. A solitary lung lesion was found and was consistent with metastatic disease. Based on the presence of metastasis, the patient has Stage IV (T3aN2M1c) melanoma. He presents to the hospital today for his first cycle of high-dose aldesleukin therapy.

PMH

Diabetes mellitus (type 2)
Hypertension

FH

Mother, 69, alive with DM; father, 73, alive with HTN and gout. One brother, 39, and one sister, 37, alive and healthy. No known family history of cancer, familial atypical multiple mole syndrome, or hereditary dysplastic nevus syndrome.

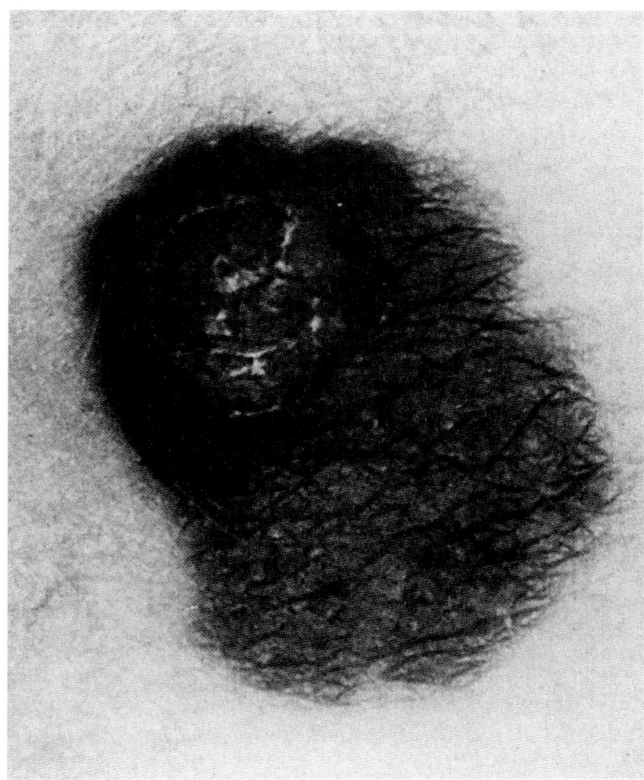

Figure 148–1. Superficial spreading melanoma developing in contiguity with a dysplastic nevus. *(Reprinted with permission from Lejeune FJ, Chaudhuri PK, Das Gupta TK, eds. Malignant Melanoma: Medical and Surgical Management. New York, McGraw-Hill, 1994: Plate 5b)*

SH

Currently employed as a sheet metal worker and previously worked as a roofer for 20 years. Lives with his wife, who is a hair stylist, and one son, age 15 years old. History of numerous severe blistering sunburns during summers as a child. No history of smoking. Drinks socially.

ROS

No changes in vision or hearing; no headaches, cough, fevers, chills, night sweats, nausea, or vomiting; no changes in bowel or bladder habits.

All

Erythromycin caused GI upset.

Meds

Enalapril 10 mg po every day
Glipizide 10 mg po every day

PE

Gen

WDWN white man, appearing anxious

VS

BP 124/78, P 76, RR 16, T 37.1°C; Ht 6′1″, Wt 126kg

Skin

Slightly diaphoretic, fair in complexion, left scapula wound apparent, scattered multiple nevi

HEENT

PERRLA, EOMI; sclera non icteric; throat without lesions or erythema

Neck/LN

Supple, no lymphadenopathy, thyroid without masses

Lungs

CTA bilaterally without wheezes, rales, or rhonchi

CV

RRR; S_1, S_2 normal; no m/r/g; no JVD

Abd

Soft, non-tender; (+) BS; no rebound, guarding, or distention; no HSM

Rect

Normal sphincter tone, heme (–), prostate normal size without nodules

Ext

No CCE, distal pulses 2+ bilaterally

Neuro

A & O × 3; CN II–XII intact; DTRs 2+ and symmetric throughout; cerebellar function intact; sensory levels grossly intact; 5/5 motor strength throughout; Babinski downgoing bilaterally

Labs

Na 140 mEq/L	Hgb 15.1 g/dL	AST 27 IU/L
K 4.4 mEq/L	Hct 44%	ALT 31 IU/L
Cl 99 mEq/L	Plt 325 × 10^3/mm^3	Alk phos 113 IU/L
CO_2 25 mEq/L	WBC 7.4 × 10^3/mm^3	LDH 754 IU/L
BUN 11 mg/dL	PMNs 68%	T. bili 0.8 mg/dL
SCr 0.9 mg/dL	Bands 2%	T. prot 6.5 g/dL
Glu 134 mg/dL	Eos 3%	Alb 4.1 g/dL
	Basos 1%	Ca 8.2 mg/dL
	Lymphs 22%	Mg 1.9 mg/dL
	Monos 4%	PO_4 3.9 mg/dL

Assessment

43 yo man with newly-diagnosed metastatic melanoma s/p excision of a cutaneous lesion presenting to the hospital to initiate his first cycle of high-dose aldesleukin therapy.

Questions

Problem Identification

1. a. *Create a list of the patient's drug therapy problems.*
   b. *What risk factor(s) does this patient have for developing melanoma?*
   c. *What are the characteristics of Stage IV melanoma, in terms of tumor size/thickness, nodal involvement, and metastases?*

Desired Outcome

2. *What are the goals of using high-dose aldesleukin in this patient?*

Therapeutic Alternatives

3. *If high-dose aldesleukin therapy was not chosen for this patient, what are other feasible pharmacotherapeutic options available?*

Optimal Plan

4. *As the first step in developing a treatment plan for this patient, determine the dose of aldesleukin.*

Outcome Evaluation

5. a. *Outline a plan to assess the efficacy and adverse effects of aldesleukin therapy.*
   b. *What supportive measures may be used to minimize adverse effects of aldesleukin therapy?*
   c. *For which parameters or conditions would you consider withholding a dose of aldesleukin?*
   d. *If a dose was withheld, how would you determine if the patient should receive subsequent doses?*
   e. *When should a course of aldesleukin therapy be prematurely discontinued?*

Patient Education

6. a. *Describe in non-technical terms the drug information the patient should receive prior to initiating aldesleukin therapy.*
   b. *What information would you give to the patient regarding sun exposure?*

Clinical Course

Prior to receiving his fifth dose of aldesleukin, his vital signs are noted to be:

BP 92/54, P 120, RR 18, Temp 38.0°C, Wt 140kg (13-kg increase from baseline)

On physical exam, he is diaphoretic, edematous (2+ pitting edema), and crackles are heard in his lungs bilaterally.

Follow-Up Questions

1. *What other information would you like to know prior to determining if the patient should receive further doses of aldesleukin?*
2. *What is the mechanism of the aldesleukin-related toxicities seen in this patient? Describe these adverse effects.*

Self-Study Assignments

1. Outline the chemotherapy and other options available to patients for the treatment of non-metastatic melanoma.
2. List expected or possible adverse effects associated with the chemotherapy used to treat melanoma.
3. Perform a literature search using MedLine and the Internet. Outline other treatment approaches that are currently being investigated for the treatment of melanoma.

Clinical Pearl

Clinical features of pigmented lesions that suggest melanoma include *A*symmetry of lesion, *B*order irregularity, *C*olor variation, *D*iameter > 6 mm, and *E*volution or enlargement of the mole (the ABCDEs of melanoma).

References

1. Greene FL, Page DL, Fleming ID, et al (eds). AJCC Cancer Staging Manual, 6th ed. Springer-Verlag, New York: 2002.
2. Atkins MB, Kunkel L, Sznol M, et al. High-dose recombinant interleukin-2 therapy in patients with metastatic melanoma: Long-term survival update. Cancer J Sci Am 2000;6(Suppl 1):S11–S14.
3. Middleton MR, Grob JJ, Aaronson N, et al. Randomized phase III study of temozolomide versus dacarbazine in the treatment of patients with advanced metastatic malignant melanoma. J Clin Oncol 2000;18:158–166.
4. Rosenberg SA, Yang JC, Topalian SL, et al. Treatment of 283 consecutive patients with metastatic melanoma or renal cell cancer using high-dose bolus interleukin-2. JAMA 1994;271:907–913.
5. Schwartz RN, Stover L, Dutcher J. Managing toxicities of high-dose interleukin-2. Oncology (Huntingt) 2002;16(11 Suppl 13);11–20.

149 HEMATOPOIETIC STEM CELL TRANSPLANTATION

A Dilemma in Antibiotic Therapy (Level III)

Simon Cronin, PharmD, MS

After completing this case study, students should be able to:

- Understand the difference between autologous and allogeneic bone marrow transplantation (BMT).
- Differentiate peripheral stem cell transplantation (PSCT) from BMT.
- Discuss the therapy of vancomycin-resistant enterococcal (VRE) infection with special emphasis on the BMT arena.
- Provide drug information to patients being treated for VRE.

PATIENT PRESENTATION

Chief Complaint

Unobtainable, as the patient was intubated and sedated when examined.

HPI

Keith Jameson is a 23 yo man who was admitted 18 days ago for an autologous PSCT for NHL Stage IIB. He is now +10 days post-PSCT. A triple lumen central catheter had been placed prior to this admission. His transplant preparative regimen consisted of high-dose cyclophosphamide (1800 mg/m^2/day) and etoposide (200 mg/m^2 Q 12 H) administered together each day × 4 days. The fifth day of chemotherapy consisted of a single dose of carmustine (450 mg/m^2).

The patient was having night sweats on admission and had experienced a 10-kg weight loss over the previous 6 months. He had also completed a course of ganciclovir therapy for CMV viremia. The medical team discontinued the ganciclovir prior to the transplant admission. A baseline chest x-ray on admission was suspicious for bilateral LL pneumonia. The admission ANC was 5.7 × 10^3/mm^3. Cefepime 2 g IV Q 8 H was initiated. On the following day the patient complained of pain at the central venous catheter site. Vancomycin 1 g IV Q 12 H was added, and antifungal prophylaxis with fluconazole 100 mg po once daily was begun.

The patient received his PSCT without any sequelae (cell dose 3.7 × 10^6/kg CD 34+ cells) despite persistent fevers. On day +4 post-transplant the patient began to complain of severe esophagitis/mucositis necessitating continuous narcotic analgesia. The WBC at this time was 0.2 × 10^3/mm^3.

On day +7 the patient developed laryngeal stridor and required intubation for 3 days to protect the airway. A repeat CXR showed a bilateral "white-out" process indicative of a worsening pneumonic process. Antibiotic therapy was broadened empirically by discontinuing cefepime and adding meropenem 500 mg IV Q 6 H plus levofloxacin 500 mg IV Q 24 H. Vancomycin and fluconazole were continued, but the fluconazole dose was increased to a treatment level of 400 mg/day.

On day +9 he developed watery diarrhea. Stool cultures were sent for *Clostridium difficile* toxin. The culture was negative for *C. difficile* but positive for vancomycin-resistant *Enterococcus faecium*. The patient was placed on reverse barrier nursing.

On day +10 (today), the patient's temperature is 38.3°C and *Enterococcus faecium* has been identified from the blood drawn through one lumen of the CVC. The latest chest x-ray is significantly worse, suggestive of a viral process. Antibiotic therapy has been modified today.

PMH

- Diagnosed with NHL 18 months ago and was treated with five courses of CHOP. He achieved a CR, but a follow up CT scan 3 months later showed disease progression with mediastinal involvement (Stage IIB). He then received two courses of ESHAP, and after each course he was hospitalized for IV antibiotics because of prolonged neutropenia and fever. After placement of a triple lumen catheter, he received high-dose cyclophosphamide followed by G-CSF for peripheral stem cell mobilization. The stem cells were then harvested by apheresis and stored in liquid nitrogen containing dimethylsulfoxide in readiness for the transplant.
- S/P DVT 6 months PTA.
- S/P 4-week course of ganciclovir prior to admission
- Hx severe back pain related to NHL
- Hx Herpes simplex infections on the mouth corners during winter months

FH

Married with one child. Both parents are alive; his father has prostate cancer that is currently in remission.

Meds

Fluconazole 400 mg IV daily
Famotidine 20 mg IV Q 12 H
Fentanyl patch 50 mcg Q 3 days
Meropenem 500mg IV Q 6 H
Levofloxacin 500 mg IV daily
Vancomycin 1 g IV Q 12 H

All

Morphine → intense pruritus
IV contrast dye → body rash

ROS

Unobtainable; patient is intubated

PE

Gen

Patient is a WDWN African-American man

VS

BP 115/68, P 86, T 38.3°C, currently intubated with FiO2 of 50% and saturating at 93%. Wt 97 kg (admission wt 95.6 kg), Ht 5′8″

HEENT

Face edematous; the oral-pharynx is red with some sloughing of the mucus membrane (grade II–III oral/esophageal mucositis)

Skin

Warm, dry; no rash

Neck/LN

Supple; no thyromegaly; a left cervical LN was palpable but was smaller than before the high-dose cyclophosphamide

Lungs

Bilateral decreased breath sounds

Heart

RRR; no murmurs, rubs, or gallops; normal heart sounds

Abd

Slight distention, RUQ tenderness, mild hepatomegaly

Ext

Bilateral edema grade I–II in both LE

Neuro

Sedated on respirator

Labs

Na 136 mEq/L	Hgb 8.6 g/dL	AST 22 IU/L
K 4.2 mEq/L	Hct 25%	ALT 29 IU/L
BUN 4.0 mg/dL	Plt 9.0 × 10^3/mm^3	Alk Phos 141 IU/L
SCr 0.5 mg/dL	WBC 0.200 × 10^3/mm^3	LDH 138 IU/L
Glu 98 mg/dL		T. bili 2.1 mg/dL

Plasma CMV DNA 1020 copies/mL by PCR

Blood Cultures

E. faecium (2/2 containers)
E. faecium (2/2 containers)

MICs

Ampicillin > 64 mcg/mL
Ciprofloxacin > 4 mcg/mL
Gentamicin > 500 mcg/mL
Doxycycline > 4 mcg/mL
Imipenem > 16 mcg/mL
Vancomycin > 16 mcg/mL
Erythromycin > 8 mcg/mL
Quinupristin/dalfopristin > 1.0 mcg/mL
Levofloxacin > 8 mcg/mL
Linezolid < 0.5 mcg/mL

Other Cultures

All other culture sites (urine, sputum, central venous catheter) are negative.

Assessment

New bacteremia with VRE, CMV viremia, and probable pneumonia in a neutropenic host who is day +10 post-autologous PSCT for NHL.
Patient is hemodynamically stable.

Questions

Problem Identification

1. a. *What risk factors did this patient have for developing VRE sepsis?*
   b. *What risk factors are there for developing CMV pneumonia?*
   c. *What other potential drug therapy problems does this patient have?*

Desired Outcome

2. *What are the therapeutic goals in this patient?*

Therapeutic Alternatives

3. *What alternative antibiotic(s) would effectively treat the VRE infection in this patient?*

Optimal Plan

4. a. *Outline an appropriate antibiotic regimen for treating this patient's VRE infection.*
   b. *What other pharmacotherapeutic measures should be implemented?*
   c. *What antibiotics are currently under investigation that hold promise for treatment of VRE?*

Outcome Evaluation

5. *What parameters should you monitor to assess the response to therapy and to detect adverse effects?*

Patient Education

6. *How will you explain to the patient's family that he has an antibiotic-resistant infection?*

Clinical Course

One of the antibiotic regimens you suggested was initiated intravenously. The patient continued to have low-grade fevers without chills but was hemodynamically stable. On day +12 post-transplant facial swelling was still evident, and there were new findings of LUQ abdominal tenderness and a 2-kg weight gain. At this time, the patient did not show signs of engraftment (WBC $0.2 \times 10^3/mm^3$), and other labs included Hgb 8.8 g/dL; BUN 5 mg/dL; SCr 0.5 mg/dL; T. bili 3.9 mg/dL; AST 32 IU/L; ALT 16 IU/L; LDH 138 IU/L; and alk phos 144 IU/L.

By day +14, the facial swelling and oral mucositis had dramatically improved and the WBC was $1.6 \times 10^3/mm^3$. On day +15, the bilirubin was 2.0 mg/dL and the alk phos was 130 IU/L. He continued to remain febrile with positive cultures for the same organism. Meropenem, levofloxacin, and fluconazole were discontinued. The first antibiotic you suggested for this bacteremia was discontinued and your second choice was initiated intravenously. After 5 days, blood cultures became negative. A repeat plasma PCR for CMV was <600 copies (negative). The patient was afebrile at this time, and all lab values were within normal limits. He was successfully extubated.

Follow-Up Questions

1. *Review the clinical and laboratory data on day +12 and suggest a possible reason for the change in liver function tests.*
2. *Assume that the LFT changes are not related to infection. Outline a therapeutic plan aimed at treating this new problem, should it progress.*

Self-Study Assignments

1. What is the difference between autologous bone marrow and peripheral stem cell (PSC) transplantation and what is the significance of the cell count in the transplanted PSCs?
2. Aside from the complications reviewed in this case, derive a list of potential problems that could occur after an allogeneic marrow transplant.

Clinical Pearl

Decreasing the duration of neutropenia reduces the risk of post-transplant fever and infection and therefore reduces the duration of antibiotic therapy.

References

1. Murray BE. Vancomycin-resistant enterococci. Am J Med 1997;102:284–293.
2. Allington DR, Rivey MP. Quinupristin/dalfopristin: A therapeutic review. Clin Ther 2001;23:24–44.
3. Batts DH. Linezolid—A new option for treating gram-positive infections. Oncology (Huntingt) 2000;14(8 Suppl 6):23–29.
4. Jorgensen JH, Crawford SA, Kelly CC, et al. In vitro activity of daptomycin against vancomycin-resistant enterococci of various Van types and comparison of susceptibility testing methods. Antimicrob Agents Chemother 2003;47: 3760–3763.
5. McNeil SA, Clark NM, Chandrasekar PH, et al. Successful treatment of vancomycin-resistant *Enterococcus faecium* bacteremia with linezolid after failure of treatment with Synercid (quinupristin/dalfopristin). Clin Infect Dis 2000; 30:403–404.
6. Terra S, Spitzer TR, Tsunoda SM. A review of tissue plasminogen activator in the treatment of veno-occlusive disease after bone marrow transplantation. Pharmacotherapy 1997;17:929–937.
7. Bianco JA, Applebaum FR, Nemunaitis J, et al. Phase I-II trial of pentoxifylline for the prevention of transplantation related toxicities following bone marrow transplantation. Blood 1991;78:1205–1211.
8. Richardson PG, Murakami C, Jin Z, et al. Multi-institutional use of defibrotide in 88 patients after stem cell transplantation with severe veno-occlusive disease and multisystem organ failure: Response without significant toxicity in a high-risk population and factors predictive of outcome. Blood 2002;100:4337–4343.

SECTION 18

Nutrition and Nutritional Disorders

150 PARENTERAL NUTRITION

▶ More Is Not Better (Level III)

Michael D. Kraft, PharmD

▶ After completing this case study, students should be able to:

- Describe how Crohn's disease and its attendant complications can cause malnutrition.
- Characterize the specific type and severity of malnutrition based on subjective and objective data.
- Identify potential complications related to TPN in patients with malnutrition (e.g., Refeeding Syndrome) and steps to avoid or manage such complications.
- Design a patient-specific total parenteral nutrition (TPN) prescription based on the nutritional diagnosis.
- Construct and evaluate appropriate monitoring parameters for a hospitalized patient receiving TPN.

PATIENT PRESENTATION

Chief Complaint

"The vomiting is getting worse along with the pain in my belly."

HPI

Diana Cummings is a 45 yo woman with a 30-year h/o Crohn's disease who returned to the GI Clinic and is being admitted to the hospital because of persistent disease symptoms, dehydration, decreased oral intake, unintentional weight loss, and malnutrition. The GI clinic staff has cared for her for 2 months (see Chapter 32, *Crohn's Disease*, in this casebook). When last seen as an outpatient in the GI Clinic 4 weeks ago, her major complaints were anorexia, postprandial abdominal pain, and distension for which an outpatient small-bowel follow-through (SBFT) study was recommended. Since that visit, the patient states that she was unable to pursue the test because of her worsening symptoms. She continued to have intermittent diarrhea, decreased food intake due to pain, weight loss and recently had to quit her job because of her illness.

Currently, her abdominal pain is constant, worse with eating, and localized to the periumbilical region. In addition, she vomits yellowish-green contents three to four times daily. Because of the abdominal pain, she has minimal oral intake and is having difficulty keeping a clear liquid diet down. Oral supplements such as Boost or Ensure were suggested at the last clinic visit, but she states that she could not afford to purchase them and has relied on a modified diet as tolerated. She relates a 7.3-kg weight loss in the last 4 weeks. Diarrheal stools occur every 3 to 4 days, but she denies any blood per rectum, fever, or chills. Upon admission, an abdominal x-ray and an SBFT study will be ordered.

PMH

Crohn's disease diagnosed in 1970 (weight loss, diarrhea, vomiting, abdominal pain) with episodes of disease exacerbation
Steroid dependency based on Cortrosyn stimulation test results
Osteopenia based on DEXA scan results
Hypertension
Depression with associated insomnia
Psychosis

PSH

Portion of jejunum resected 20 years ago (Crohn's scarring/stricture leading to obstruction)

Portion of small bowel resected 11 years ago (stricture/acute inflammation)

Portion of small bowel resected 7 years ago (Crohn's stricture leading to obstruction) leaving 180 cm of small intestine beyond the Ligament of Treitz with an intact ileocecal valve and colon

FH

Remarkable for DM, HTN, and CAD in her mother. No Family history of IBD.

SH

Formerly worked as an assistant in a home for the mentally handicapped; lives alone. Drinks alcohol socially; has a 23 pack-year history of smoking.

ROS

Constant abdominal pain, vomiting three to four times daily, moderately distended abdomen with one or two diarrheal stools every 3 or 4 days. She reports a 16 lb. weight loss over 4 weeks. Increased thirst sensation, fatigued, and is lightheaded upon rising. Decreased visual acuity attributed to old corrective lenses. Denies headache, vertigo, tinnitus, CP, SOB, cough, joint pain, aphthous ulcers, and skin rashes.

Meds

Prednisone 5 mg po once daily
Mesalamine 1,000 mg po TID
Trazodone 100 mg po at bedtime for sleep
Triavil 4–50 mg po BID
Vitamin B_{12} 1,000 mcg IM every month
Hydrochlorothiazide/triamterene 1 po daily (patient recently ran out)
Tramadol 50 mg po Q 6 H PRN

All

NKDA

PE

Gen

African-American woman, anxious and uncomfortable because of abdominal pain, Cushingoid appearing

VS

BP lying down 136/72, P 72, RR 15, T 37.9°C; Ht 5′2″, Wt 63 kg
BP standing 120/60, P 86

Skin

Dry skin with flakiness

HEENT

PERRLA, EOMI, anicteric sclerae, normal conjunctivae, mouth is dry, pharynx is clear

Lungs/Thorax

CTA and percussion bilaterally

CV

RRR, with no murmurs

Abd

Distended; high-pitched bowel sounds; diffuse tenderness throughout all quadrants with greater intensity in periumbilical region; well-healed surgical scar

Genit/Rect

An external skin tag is present, but no other perianal lesions are noted. No internal masses. Stool is guaiac negative

MS/Ext

(–) Cyanosis, (–) edema, 2+ dorsalis pedis and posterior tibial pulses bilaterally

Neuro

A & O × 3; CN II–XII intact; Motor 5/5 upper and lower extremity bilaterally; sensation intact and reflexes symmetric with downgoing toes

Labs

Na 129 mEq/L	Hgb 9.1 g/dL	AST 18 IU/L	Ca 7.1 mg/dL
K 2.8 mEq/L	Hct 38.2%	ALT 19 IU/L	Mg 0.8 mEq/dL
Cl 92 mEq/L	Plt 197 × 10^3/mm^3	Alk phos 140 IU/L	Phos 2.1 mg/dL
CO_2 36 mEq/L	WBC 11.6 × 10^3/mm^3	GGTP 98 IU/L	PT 14.2 sec
BUN 5 mg/dL		T. bili 0.3 mg/dL	INR 1.2
SCr 1.1 mg/dL		T. prot 5.8 g/dL	
Glu 76 mg/dL		Alb 2.1 g/dL	

Radiology

Abdominal x-ray shows dilated loops of proximal small intestine; SBFT with Gastrografin contrast shows filling of the jejunum, dilated up to 7–8 cm, followed by irregular narrowing, mucosal ulcerations and variably thickened folds within the proximal ileum; abnormal delay of contrast to reach the colon.

Assessment/Plan

1. Acute flare of Crohn's disease within the proximal ileum causing a partial SBO.
2. An NGT will be inserted and placed to low intermittent suction to aid in decompressing or removing the contents of the proximal GI tract.
3. A percutaneous triple lumen central venous catheter will be placed and ordered to receive an IVF of 5% dextrose and 0.9% NaCl with KCl 40 mEq/L at 100 mL/h.
4. Initiate hydrocortisone 100 mg IV Q 8 H and Pentasa 500 mg via NGT QID (clamp NGT for 60 minutes after each dose).
5. A surgical consult is requested in the event that the patient fails to respond to conservative medical management and develops an acute abdomen requiring surgical intervention.

Questions

Problem Identification

1. a. *Based on the data presented, classify the severity of this patient's Crohn's disease. Explain the rationale for this decision and how it guides the approach to treatment of this patient.*
   b. *What are the mechanisms whereby active Crohn's disease results in malnutrition?*
   c. *What clinical and laboratory data indicate the presence of malnutrition in this patient? Characterize the type and severity of malnutrition in this patient and describe why she is at nutritional risk.*
   d. *Create a list of this patient's problems related to nutrition, fluid, and electrolytes.*
   e. *What additional nutritional assessment data should you request and why?*

Desired Outcome

2. *What are the goals of specialized nutrition support in this patient?*

Therapeutic Alternatives

3. *What are the therapeutic options for specialized nutrition intervention in this patient?*

Optimal Plan

4. a. *What are the ranges of estimated daily goals for calories (kcal/kg/day), protein (g/kg/day), and hydration (mL/kg/day) for this patient?*
   b. *Design a TPN formulation for the first day of treatment that includes the volume and rate (mL/h), final amino acids (g/L), dextrose (g/L), lipid emulsion (g/L), electrolytes (mEq/day or μmol/day), vitamins, trace elements, and other additives. How quickly would you advance to goal infusion rate in this patient? Why?*
   c. *What other order(s) would you suggest at the initiation of the TPN?*

Outcome Evaluation

5. *What monitoring parameters and frequency are required for monitoring the TPN regimen?*

Patient Education

6. *What information should be provided to the patient and family during her hospitalization regarding the parenteral nutrition?*

Clinical Course

Ms. Cummings' signs and symptoms of intestinal obstruction resolve over the next week. On hospital day 9 the NGT is removed. The patient is initiated and slowly advanced to an oral diet over the next 3 to 4 days as tolerated.

Follow-Up Question

1. *How should the parenteral nutrition be weaned from the patient's care plan?*

Self-Study Assignments

1. This patient is at moderate to high risk for a condition called Refeeding Syndrome in the setting of initiating specialized nutrition support. What is the Refeeding Syndrome? What are its potential complications? How can it be prevented?
2. Explain how hypochloremic metabolic alkalosis can develop if a patient has long-standing chronic vomiting. How does hypokalemia develop during the same condition?
3. Calculate how many mL/day of a 20% lipid emulsion are needed to compound the daily TPN prescription you determined for this patient.
4. Calculate how many mL/day of dextrose 70% and amino acids 10% stock solutions are needed to compound the daily TPN prescription you determined for this patient.

Clinical Pearls

1. The Refeeding Syndrome can lead to serious complications, including death. It is one of the few true nutritional emergencies. A good rule of thumb is to "start low and go slow" with nutrition support (TPN or enteral nutrition) to avoid complications.
2. Glycemic control in the range of 70–150 mg/dL is acceptable during TPN infusion. Achieving tight glycemic control and avoiding hyperglycemia may reduce complications, including mortality.

References

1. Brooks MJ, Melnik G. The refeeding syndrome: An approach to understanding its complications and preventing its occurrence. Pharmacotherapy 1995;15:713–726.
2. ASPEN Board of Directors and the Clinical Guidelines Task Force. Guidelines for the use of parenteral and enteral nutrition in adult and pediatric patients. J Parenter Enteral Nutr 2002;26:73SA–74SA.
3. American Gastroenterological Association. AGA technical review on parenteral nutrition. Gastroenterology 2001;121:970–1001.
4. National Institutes of Health. Clinical guidelines on the identification, evaluation, and treatment of overweight and obesity in adults—The evidence report. Obes Res 1998(6 Suppl 2):51S–209S.
5. National Advisory Group on Standards and Practice Guidelines for Parenteral Nutrition. Safe practices for parenteral nutrition formulations. J Parenter Enteral Nutr 1998;22:49–66.
6. Clark CL, Sacks GS, Dickerson RN, et al. Treatment of hypophosphatemia in patients receiving specialized nutrition support using a graduated dosing scheme: Results from a prospective clinical trial. Crit Care Med 1995;23:1504–1511.

Acknowledgment: This chapter is based on the case written for the Fifth Edition by Douglas D. Janson, PharmD, BCNSP, and Kerry A. Cholka, PharmD.

151 ADULT ENTERAL NUTRITION

▶ Down the Tube (Level III)

Carol J. Rollins, MS, RD, PharmD, BCNSP
Elizabeth J. Ewing, PharmD

▶ After completing this case study, students should be able to:

- Calculate the protein, calorie, and fluid requirements for a patient who is to receive enteral nutrition therapy.
- Recommend an appropriate enteral formula and feeding route.
- Implement an appropriate monitoring plan to achieve the desired nutritional endpoints and avoid complications.
- Design an appropriate regimen for administering medications via a feeding tube, including recommending alternate dosage forms for medications that cannot be crushed.

PATIENT PRESENTATION

Carlos Ruiz is a 72 yo Hispanic man referred to your home health care company for initiation of tube feedings. During your conversation with him, he states to you, "I've lost a lot of weight since I started chemo. Food tastes bad." The physician's orders read: "Fiber-containing 1 kcal/cc formula, 2,300–2,400 kcal/day via enteral pump. Receiving cycle 2 of etoposide plus 5-FU today for gastric/esophageal cancer. The doses were decreased 25% today because of grade III mucositis/stomatitis with the first cycle." The patient's insurance coverage is Medicare, Parts A and B.

▶ Questions

Problem Identification

1. a. *What other information is necessary or would be helpful to evaluate the orders and provide recommendations for a feeding plan?*
   b. *How can you obtain this information for your home health care company, which is located across town from the clinic and hospital?*
   c. *Is insurance coverage an issue in this situation?*

▶ Clinical Course

After following appropriate procedures, you obtain the following additional information about the patient.

HPI

Mr. Ruiz saw his PCP 6 months ago with a chief complaint of persistent LUQ pain for 3 months. Weight at that time was 79 kg and height was 72 inches. He was slightly anemic (Hgb 11.6 g/dL). Pantoprazole was initiated for PUD. Four weeks later, Mr. Ruiz was seen for c/o worsening LUQ pain, early satiety, and "feeling full" all the time. Hgb was 10.1 g/dL at that time. An upper GI endoscopy revealed a tumor in the cardia of the stomach. CT scans of the chest, abdomen, and pelvis confirmed a gastric mass and gastrohepatic adenopathy.

Three weeks later, Mr. Ruiz underwent a near-total gastrectomy with distal pancreatectomy, splenectomy, and partial esophagectomy with a gastroesophageal anastomosis in the right chest. A feeding jejunostomy was also placed during surgery. Tissue pathology subsequently revealed a poorly differentiated gastric adenocarcinoma with transmural invasion and tumor present on the serosal margin. There was involvement of the esophageal wall and continuous spread to the peripancreatic soft tissue including neural invasion. Ten of 16 lymph nodes were positive for metastasis.

Three cycles of FCE (5-FU, cisplatin, etoposide) were given, with the third cycle reduced by 25% because of stomatitis, vomiting, dehydration, and renal dysfunction associated with previous courses. Therapy was also complicated by anorexia and severe hypomagnesemia, requiring IV replacement and continued oral magnesium supplementation. Dietary education for anorexia was provided. Cisplatin was to be dropped from the remaining three cycles of chemotherapy, and radiotherapy was to follow completion of the chemotherapy.

PMH

Superior vena cava syndrome
DVT
PUD
Hypothyroidism

FH

No family history available, patient was raised by family friends after his parents were killed in a car accident when he was an infant. No contact with relatives still in Central America.

SH

Married, 4 grown children; office worker; 35 pack-year tobacco use, quit 4 years ago; occasional alcohol use, average of two beers/week.

ROS

From clinic visit today:

Constitutional: Moderate fatigue, weakness, poor appetite, dysphagia

ENT: No vision changes or eye pain. No tinnitus or ear pain. No throat pain, but increasing difficulty swallowing over the last two weeks with poor tolerance to solid foods and inability to take large tablets

CV: No SOB, DOE, chest pain

Resp: No cough or sputum production

GI: Continued persistent abdominal and back pain; slightly improved with increased morphine dose and more frequent breakthrough coverage plus cyclobenzaprine use. No emesis or diarrhea; complains of intermittent nausea and mild/moderate constipation

GU: Increased urinary frequency and (+) dysuria for 3 days. No nocturia or hematuria.

MS: (+) Abdominal and back pain; no other muscle aches or bone pain
Skin: No rashes, nodules, or itching
Neuro: No headaches, dizziness, unsteady gait, or seizures
Endo: No symptoms of hypothyroidism
Heme/LN: No recent blood transfusions or swollen glands

Meds

Morphine sulfate sustained-release tablet, 90 mg po BID
Morphine sulfate solution (20 mg/5 mL), 20 mg po Q 2–3 H PRN pain
Protonix 40 mg po every morning
Megestrol acetate 40 mg, 5 tablets po QID
Magnesium oxide 400 mg po TID
Coumadin 7.5 mg po once daily
Docusate sodium 100 mg po at bedtime
Synthroid 0.125 mg po every morning
Cyclobenzaprine 10 mg po TID PRN back spasms
Cephalexin 500 mg po QID × 10 days (completed today)
Ciprofloxacin 500 mg po BID × 7 days (to start today)

All

NKDA; food allergy to Chinese food and tofu (hives, wheezing)

PE

Gen

Thin, pale-appearing Hispanic man; alert and conversant

VS

BP 122/71, P 88, RR 16; W 52.5 kg

Skin

No nodules, masses, or rash; no ecchymoses or petechiae; stage I pressure ulcer, 2 cm, right buttocks. Redness at edges of implantable venous access device that is very prominent on upper left chest wall

HEENT

PERRLA; EOMs intact. Eyes anicteric. Distinct temporal wasting. No mouth lesions; tongue normal size

Neck

Neck supple but thin; no thyromegaly or masses

LN

No cervical, supraclavicular, axillary, or inguinal adenopathy

Heart

RRR with no gallop, rubs, or murmur

Lungs

Basilar crackling rales, which clear with cough. A poorly-healed surgical incision is visible on the left posterior chest wall

Abd

Abdomen flat. Jejunostomy tube with slight erythema around the exit site, no drainage. Midline, LUQ, and RUQ incisions erythematous and incompletely healed with mild tenderness to palpation in the RUQ and epigastric area. No masses palpable.

Genit/Rect

Normal male genitalia; non-distended bladder; hard stool in rectal vault

MS/Ext

No clubbing or cyanosis; 2+ bilateral ankle to mid-calf edema; no spine or CVA tenderness

Neuro

Cranial nerves intact; DTRs active and equal

Endoscopy Report

From 2 days ago. Endoscope inserted to distal esophagus; stopped at the anastomosis by stricture. Biopsies from site of stricture were negative for adenocarcinoma. Tissue friable; stricture dilation not attempted due to risk of perforation. Possible stricture dilation will be reconsidered in 6 to 9 months if tissue friability is improved at that time.

Labs

Na 138 mEq/L	Hgb 9.6 g/dL	WBC 10.5 × 10^3/mm^3	AST 19 IU/L	T. chol 173 mg/dL
K 3.7 mEq/L	Hct 28.4%	66% Segs	ALT 24 IU/L	Trig 365 mg/dL
Cl 102 mEq/L	RBC 2.85 × 10^6/mm^3	9% Bands	Alk phos 55 IU/L	Ca 7.7 mg/dL
CO_2 26 mEq/L	Plt 100 × 10^3/mm^3	18% Lymphs	LDH 100 IU/L	Mg 2.8 mg/dL
BUN 21 mg/dL	MCV 105 μm^3	7% Monos	T. bili 0.9 mg/dL	Phos 3.8 mg/dL
SCr 1.0 mg/dL			D. bili 0.3 mg/dL	TSH 2.3 mIU/L
Glu 110 mg/dL			T. prot 4.2 g/dL	Thyroxine (free) 1.1 ng/dL
			Alb 2.1 g/dL	

Other

Peripheral blood smear: anisocytosis 2+, poikilocytosis 2+, macrocytosis 2+

Assessment

Continued weight loss related to esophageal stricture and chemotherapy with no evidence of cancer recurrence at the stricture.

Assessment

d. Create a drug therapy problem list for this patient.

e. What information indicates the presence or severity of malnutrition?

f. What type and degree of malnutrition does this patient exhibit? What evidence supports your assessment?

Desired Outcome

2. a. *What are the goals of nutrition support in this patient?*
   b. *What outcomes should be considered for the patient's other medical problems?*

Therapeutic Alternatives

3. a. *What are the potential alternatives for improving nutritional status in this patient other than initiating specialized nutrition support?*
   b. *What are the potential routes for specialized nutrition support and the reason(s) why each is or is not appropriate for this patient?*
   c. *A major economic issue is Medicare coverage for home enteral therapy. Based on the information now available to you, does this patient meet the necessary criteria?*

Optimal Plan

4. a. *Estimate the protein, calorie, and fluid requirements for this patient.*
   b. *What type of formula (e.g., polymeric, monomeric) is most appropriate for this patient?*
   c. *What administration regimen should be used for tube feedings?*
   d. *Assuming that the patient is to continue his current medications during tube feedings, how should each of these be administered?*

Outcome Evaluation

5. a. *What clinical and laboratory parameters are necessary to evaluate the therapy for detection and/or prevention of adverse effects and to evaluate achievement of the desired response?*
   b. *Should a food-grade dye be added to the enteral formula to monitor for aspiration? Explain the potential benefits and risks.*

Patient Education

6. *What information should be provided to the patient or his caregiver to enhance compliance, ensure successful therapy, and minimize adverse effects of enteral nutrition therapy?*

▶ Clinical Course

Feeding was initiated about 24 hours after the initial orders were sent to your home infusion company. A 1.06 calorie/mL, 0.044 g protein/mL, 310 mOsm/kg polymeric fiber containing formula was started using an enteral infusion pump via jejunostomy tube at 40 mL/h for 18 hours/day with plans for laboratory evaluation on day 3. Feedings would be advanced to 65 mL/h on day 4 if electrolytes and fluid status were acceptable. Basic metabolic panel results on day 3 revealed K 3.1 mEq/L and other electrolyte values WNL. Other laboratory results included Phos 2.0 mg/dL and Mg 1.9 mg/dL. The WBC count was $1.5 \times 10^3/\text{mm}^3$ with 30% neutrophils. The physician was notified of the laboratory results. Because the patient had a temperature of 39.1°C during the night, the physician decided to admit him to the hospital with neutropenic fever as the admitting diagnosis. Electrolytes were monitored daily during the 5 days of hospitalization and replaced intravenously as needed. Tube feedings were advanced to 65 mL/h after 12 hours of hospitalization, then to the goal of 95 mL/h by continuous infusion in another 12 hours. No further electrolyte replacement was needed after day 4 of hospitalization. The patient was changed to an 18-hour infusion of tube feeding at 130 mL/h on hospital day 4, and then discharged home on day 5. He has shown improvement in nutritional status at home, gaining 10 kg over the past 3 months. There have been no further electrolyte abnormalities despite chemotherapy and radiotherapy.

▶ Self-Study Assignments

1. Select a current patient you are following and design an appropriate regimen for administering medications via a feeding tube, including alternate dosage forms for medications that cannot be crushed and proper dosage adjustments for different forms where necessary.
2. Educate an actual patient or do a mock education with a classmate about medication administration through a feeding tube.
3. Determine the potential for various enteral formulas to interfere with anticoagulation using warfarin sodium.
4. Identify the metabolic changes associated with Refeeding Syndrome and the characteristics that increase the risk of this complication.

▶ Clinical Pearl

Medications administered through a feeding tube frequently clog the tube; evaluate the medication regimen for alternate dosage forms that do not require crushing or administration through the tube. When a tube clogs, a buffered pancreatic enzyme preparation may be used for declogging the tube.

References

1. Rollins CJ. Home care issues in nutrition support. In: Pharmacotherapy Self-Assessment Program, Module 8: Gastroenterology, Nutrition. Kansas City, MO; American College of Clinical Pharmacy, 2000.
2. ASPEN Board of Directors and the Clinical Guidelines Task Force. Guidelines for the use of parenteral and enteral nutrition in adult and pediatric patients. JPEN 2002;26(1 Suppl):1SA–138SA.
3. McClave SA, DeMeo MT, DeLegge MH, et al. North American Summit on Aspiration in the Critically Ill Patient: Consensus statement. JPEN 2002;26(6 Suppl): S80–S85.
4. Rollins CJ. Basics of enteral and parenteral nutrition. In: Wolinsky I, Williams L, (eds). Nutrition in Pharmacy Practice. Washington, DC: American Pharmaceutical Association, 2002:213–306.
5. Brooks MJ, Melnick G. The Refeeding Syndrome: An approach to understanding its complications and preventing its occurrence. Pharmacotherapy 1995; 15(6): 713–726.
6. Maloney JP, Halbower AC, Fouty BF, et al. Systemic absorption of food dye in patients with sepsis. N Engl J Med 2000;343:1047–1048. Letter.
7. Marcuard SP, Stegall KL, Trogdon S. Clearing obstructed feeding tubes. JPEN 1989;13(1):81–83.

152 OBESITY

▶ Girth Control (Level II)

Dannielle C. O'Donnell, PharmD, BCPS

▶ After completing this case study, students should be able to:

- Identify common obesity-related comorbidities.
- Calculate body mass index (BMI) and use waist circumference to determine a patient's risk of obesity-related morbidity.
- Develop a pharmacotherapeutic plan and treatment strategy for obese patients.
- Provide patient education on the expected benefits, possible adverse effects, and drug interactions with prescription weight loss medications.

PATIENT PRESENTATION

Chief Complaint

"I'm starving myself but I just can't seem to lose any weight. I want stomach staples and a tummy tuck!"

HPI

Madeline Bonsera is a 46 yo woman who states that she had maintained her ideal weight, which she feels is 58 kg, until her total hysterectomy at the age of 32. She says that the "hormones" she took for the first year after her hysterectomy caused her to gain weight, although the weight gain continued after stopping the hormones. She has previously tried OTC diet pills, prescription "water pills" and thyroid hormones, and most recently "one in a series of those low carb–high protein" diets. She relates that with most of these approaches she has initial modest success followed by weight regain. She is tearful as she talks about her weight struggles, attributing physical and marital problems to her weight. She states that her goal is to get back to what she weighed and the clothes she wore at age 25 before having children.

PMH

Hypercholesterolemia for approximately 6 years
Gallstones 4 years ago treated with lithotripsy and 2 years of ursodeoxycholic acid
Bilateral osteoarthritis of the knees
Asthma
Depression

PSH

TAH 14 years ago
Trigger-finger release bilaterally last year

FH

Mother had an MI at the age of 64 years; father died in an MVA at the age of 67. Maternal grandmother died at age 62 with diabetes. She states that her mother and grandmother were "a little heavy, but not obese." No other family members have a significant medical history, although she states that her sons are "big boys" and do "need to watch their weight."

SH

She is a married housewife who cares for her mother-in-law and has two sons who lives out of state. She has never smoked and denies IVDA. She previously enjoyed walking for exercise, but this is now limited by her knee pain and need to supervise her mother-in-law. She states, "I'm no couch potato. I'm busy all the time caring for my house and mother-in-law, and that's good exercise."

Diet

She had instruction on a low-fat, low-cholesterol diet several years ago, to which she initially says she is adhering, although with further prompting, she states that she is somewhat "bored" with her current food plan and is frustrated because she feels she must cook two different meals, one for her and one for her husband and mother-in-law since "they won't eat that boring stuff." Consequently, she has cut down on the number of meals she eats to one daily each evening that includes larger portion sizes and a dessert she generally bakes. She does admit to some snacking throughout the evening and often tasting or "finishing off" what she prepares for her mother-in-law's breakfast and lunch.

Meds

Antacid PRN indigestion
Simvastatin 10 mg po at bedtime
Acetaminophen 500 mg po PRN knee pain
Intra-articular cortisone injection, left knee 4 months ago
Albuterol inhaler PRN (uses about 2 canisters a year)

All

Adhesive tape produces rash.

ROS

She complains of general fatigue, "feeling blue," chronic bilateral knee pain, and a constant gnawing in her stomach and preoccupation with food and her weight. She denies symptoms of cold or heat intolerance; changes in skin, hair, or nails; nervousness; irritability; lethargy; muscle pain or weakness; palpitations; diarrhea or constipation; polyuria; polydipsia; chest pain; shortness of breath; recent head trauma; or thoughts of harming herself or others.

PE

Gen

The patient is a pleasant, but tearful, obese white woman in NAD. She is dressed neatly and appropriately for the weather.

VS

BP 138/88, P 80, RR 16, T 36.4°C Ht 5′4″, Wt 80 kg, waist 102 cm, hip 129 cm

Skin

Warm, with normal distribution of body hair. No significant lesions or discolorations

HEENT
NC/AT; PERRLA; EOMI; TMs intact

CV
RRR, S_1 and S_2 normal; no murmurs, rubs, or gallops

Pulm
CTA & P bilaterally

Abd
Obese with multiple striae; NT; ND; (+) BS; no palpable masses; hysterectomy scar present and well healed

Genit/Rect
Pelvic and rectal exams deferred

Ext
LE varicosities present. Palpation of knees reveals bony hypertrophy, and limited ROM elicits bony crepitus and patient discomfort bilaterally. Pedal pulses 2+ bilaterally

Neuro
A & O × 3; CN II–XII intact; Romberg test (–); sensory and motor levels intact; 2+ triceps tendons and DTR; Babinski (–)

Labs (Fasting)

Na 138 mEq/L	AST 24 IU/L
K 3.9 mEq/L	T. chol 241 mg/dL
Cl 96 mEq/L	LDL-C 141 mg/dL
CO_2 26 mEq/L	HDL-C 39 mg/dL
BUN 13 mg/dL	Trig 305 mg/dL
SCr 1.0 mg/dL	TSH 0.9 mIU/L
Glu 108 mg/dL	

▶ Questions

Problem Identification

1. a. *Create a drug therapy problem list for this patient.*
   b. *Calculate the patient's BMI. By using the BMI and any other markers of adiposity, categorize her obesity and stratify her risk.*
   c. *What information (signs, symptoms, laboratory values) indicates the presence or severity of obesity?*
   d. *Could any of the patient's problems have been caused by her drug therapy?*
   e. *What other medical conditions should be considered to exclude primary causes of her obesity?*

Desired Outcome

2. *What are the goals of therapy for the patient's obesity?*

Therapeutic Alternatives

3. a. *What nondrug therapies should be recommended for this patient?*
   b. *What prescription pharmacotherapeutic alternatives are available for this patient's obesity? Describe their pharmacology, indications, and potential for tolerance development.*

Optimal Plan

4. a. *What drug(s), dosage form(s), dose(s), schedule(s), and duration is/are appropriate to treat this patient's obesity and why?*
   b. *What alternatives would be appropriate if initial therapy fails?*

Outcome Evaluation

5. *What clinical and laboratory parameters are necessary to evaluate the therapy for achievement of the desired therapeutic outcome and to detect or prevent adverse effects?*

Patient Education

6. *What general and medication-specific information should be provided to the patient to enhance adherence, ensure successful therapy, and minimize adverse effects?*

▶ Clinical Course

Ms. Bonsera has joined Weight Watchers and the YWCA and shows progress at each of her 2-week weigh-ins, averaging a 1- to 2-kg weight loss at each visit through the end of week 8. Her blood pressure is stable, and she denies any adverse effects of her medication. However, at her 10-week visit she had lost only an additional 0.5 kg. Today at her 12-week visit, she has not lost any additional weight. She weighs 72.5 kg and her waist circumference is 98 cm. Her FBG is now 102 mg/dL and her lipid profile includes total cholesterol 212 mg/dL, LDL-C 120 mg/dL, HDL-C 45 mg/dL, and triglycerides 235 mg/dL. Her blood pressure has improved to 134/82.

She states that she is as compliant with her lifestyle modifications as in previous weeks and overall is in much better spirits. She has noticed an improvement in her clothing fit, but she is starting to become frustrated again. She wants to know if she should add on one of her previous OTC or herbal weight loss aids to "get things going again." Although she is pleased with the improvement in her blood pressure, glucose, and lipids, she continues to complain of knee pain while taking her acetaminophen on a PRN basis and wonders if she should have something stronger.

▶ Follow-Up Questions

1. *What changes, if any, should be made in her weight loss regimen?*
2. *How would you educate her regarding her question about restarting an over-the-counter or herbal product?*
3. *What, if anything, would you suggest to improve her knee symptoms?*
4. *What, if any, pharmacotherapeutic changes should be made for her lipids, glucose and/or blood pressure at this time?*

► Self-Study Assignments

1. List the limitations of height-weight charts or BMI determinations. What are the most accurate methods for quantifying body fat, and why are they not routinely employed?
2. Assume that you are a member of a pharmacy and therapeutics committee for a managed care corporation. Justify whether anti-obesity drugs should be a covered benefit, and if so, which specific agent(s) should be added to the formulary.
3. Identify the weight loss medications (Rx and OTC) withdrawn from the US market in the last decade and the reasons for withdrawal.
4. Compile a compendium of common herbal and dietary supplements that claim weight loss benefits, and make a list of the evidence for their safety and efficacy.
5. Identify the control schedule for the various prescription weight loss medications. What are the legal requirements for dispensing the various scheduled weight loss agents in your state?

► Clinical Pearl

Intermittent use of anorectic agents (i.e., for 4 weeks every few months, over the holidays, during vacations, or during periods of stress) may be effective in preventing weight regain in the later maintenance phase.

References

1. Campbell ML, Mathys ML. Pharmacologic options for the treatment of obesity Am J Health Syst Pharm 2001;58:1301–1308.
2. Halpern A, Mancini MC. Treatment of obesity: An update on anti-obesity medications. Obes Rev 2003;4:25–42.
3. American Gastroenterological Association. American Gastroenterological Association medical position statement on Obesity. Gastroenterology 2002;123:879–881.
4. Tuomilehto J, Lindstrom J, Eriksson JG, et al. Prevention of type 2 diabetes mellitus by changes in lifestyle among subjects with impaired glucose tolerance. N Engl J Med 2001;344:1343–1350.
5. Haller CA, Benowitz NL. Adverse cardiovascular and central nervous system events associated with dietary supplements containing ephedra alkaloids. N Engl J Med 2000;343:1833–1838.
6. American Diabetes Association and National Institute of Diabetes, Digestive and Kidney Diseases. The prevention or delay of type 2 diabetes. Diabetes Care 2002;25:742–749.

SECTION 19

Emergency Preparedness and Response

153 CHEMICAL EXPOSURE

▶ Terrorism or Freak Accident?

Colleen Terriff, PharmD

▶ After completing this case study, students should be able to:

- Identify potential toxins or chemical agents that could be used in a terrorist attack.
- Determine the proper antidote or treatments and the dosing regimens for a potential chemical weapon, based on patient signs and symptoms.
- Manage seizures that may occur during severe exposure to certain chemical agents.
- Learn how to access pharmaceutical supplies for one victim as well as many victims in their health-system and communities.

PATIENT PRESENTATION

Patient Scenario

Many patients present to your hospital's Emergency Department visibly teary, coughing, and having trouble breathing.

HPI

Patients arrive at the ED via car, taxi and ambulance. They were attending an all-day seminar at the downtown convention center when, after a loud explosion down the hall, they were exposed to smoke and "fumes." Paramedics also reported that patients complained of difficulty breathing and blurred vision. Patients were covering their eyes, coughing, crying, and even drooling.

Dozens of patients outside the ED are awaiting decontamination, and patients appear to be anxious and extremely concerned. Medical Alert has been activated for city and county, and the Regional Disaster Hospital has been notified of Alert. All local EDs are securing their perimeters and setting up decontamination units. Scene decontamination of patients is occurring before some are arriving via ambulance. Patients arriving by car or cab or by foot have not been decontaminated.

PMH, PSH, FH and SH

Not obtained.

ROS

Most patients can only nod to some questions, making individual interviews difficult. The ED lead physician instructs nurses to get patient vital signs and approximate age and weight. Medical residents are told to do brief triage physical exams on an estimated 25 patients each.

Summary of PE Findings

Gen

Patients appear anxious, breathing quickly. Some have required intubation.

VS

BP: A few patients have mildly elevated BP; P: Most have tachycardia, but a few have bradycardia; RR: Most patients are tachypneic; T: most are normal; Pain: Most patients indicate that they do not have significant pain

Skin

Some patients are profusely sweaty; no cyanosis, clubbing or edema present

HEENT

Bilateral pinpoint pupils, non-reactive to light, profuse rhinorrhea, and hypersalivation

Neck/lymph nodes:
Exam not performed

Lungs/thorax:
Rapid respiratory rate, rhonchi present throughout; a few patients exhibit bronchoconstriction and excessive respiratory secretions

CV
Tachycardia for most patients; too noisy to listen for heart sounds for most patients

Abd
Some patients complain of nausea, a few experience emesis

Genital/Rect
DRE and stool guaiac not performed

MS/Ext
Facial muscle twitching noticed in a few patients who also had substantial rhinorrhea and complaints of severe vision changes

Neuro
Initially, 5 have flaccid paralysis and respiratory arrest requiring intubation; 3 of these 5 patients are seizing

Labs
Complete metabolic panel, CBC, toxicology screen: Pending
Serum cholinesterase, blood cyanide levels: Pending

Other
O2 sat ordered for patients in more severe respiratory distress. Blood gases ordered on intubated patients. Multiple chest x–rays: pending.

Lead Physician's Assessment
Based on feedback from the scene and the Regional Disaster Hospital, 1,000 people may have been affected by this chemical release, going to 4 area hospitals. The ED staff is also alerted to get information from victims and save patient belongings as evidence for FBI. Scene fire chief acting as Incident Commander asks for assistance (request relayed from combined communications center to hospitals) from healthcare providers triaging victims at area hospitals to attempt to identify chemical agent based on symptomatology. An ED medical resident contacts the Regional Poison Control Center for guidance identifying the possible agent. The pharmacy department is also contacted for their assistance with antidote recommendations, including dosing and side effect monitoring.

▶ Questions

Problem Identification

1. a. *Create a list of potential chemical agents that the patients may have been exposed to based on presenting signs and symptoms.*
   b. *How serious is this exposure, and what could be some potential sequelae?*

Desired Outcome

2. a. *What are the goals of pharmacotherapy in this case?*
   b. *How do your goals change if there were 15 patients presenting with these symptoms and differing degrees of severity and exposure?*

Therapeutic Alternatives

3. a. *What nonpharmacologic measures are available to treat these patients?*
   b. *What feasible pharmacotherapeutic alternatives are available for treating these patients?*
   c. *Suppose there are 100 patients in your hospital's Emergency Department needing an antidote and you only have enough antidote to treat 25 patients. How do you decide who gets life-saving treatment?*

Optimal Plan

4. a. *What antidotes are required for this chemical exposure? Provide the adult doses, routes, and repeat dosing information for each antidote.*
   b. *There are special dosing kits and administration devices available for these antidotes (see Figures 153–1 and 153–2). Describe how these kits should be administered.*
   c. *If a patient's condition worsens and seizure activity occurs, what class of medications should be used for this chemical-induced seizure?*

Outcome Evaluation

5. *Outline a monitoring plan to assess if the pharmacotherapy treatment for these patients is successful.*

Patient Education

6. a. *What information would you share with the patients about immediate side effects of each of the antidotes?*
   b. *How long might it take for patients to recover from the ocular effects of the chemical exposure? Incorporate this information into your educational efforts.*

▶ Clinical Course

(Students: Your instructor can provide you with the outcome of this incident).

▶ Follow-Up Questions

1. *If your pharmacy department runs out of antidotes and more are needed emergently, where can you obtain additional antidote supplies: locally, regionally, nationally?*

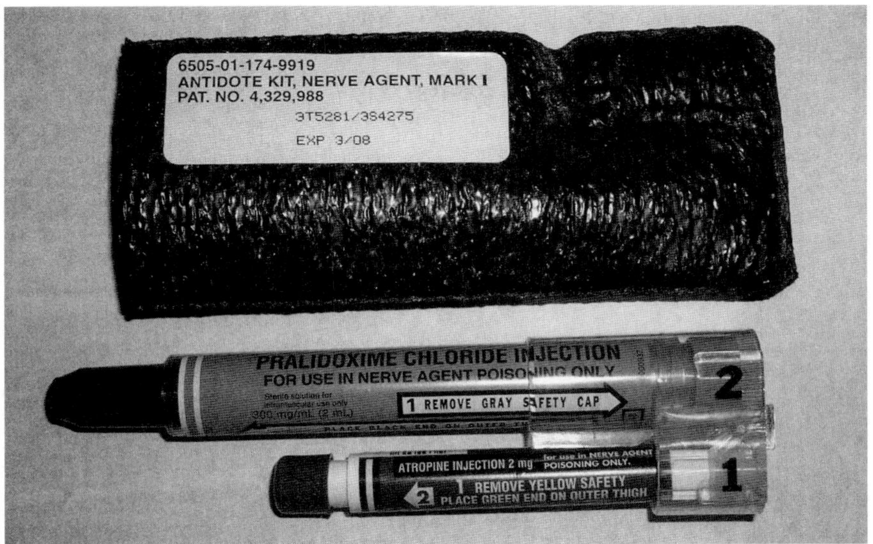

Figure 153–1. The Mark-I autoinjector, consisting of two antidotes to be used after exposures to a nerve or organophosphate agent in a disaster situation. The kit contains an atropine autoinjector (2 mg/0.7 mL) and a pralidoxime chloride (2-PAM) autoinjector (600 mg/2 mL).

▶ Clinical Pearl

Most chemical agents that could be used for a terrorist attack would likely be exploded or released as a gas in order to increase respiratory exposure and allow for rapid systemic entry into victims. Therefore, clinicians need to quickly triage patients, classify symptoms for identification, and administer appropriate treatment if available.

▶ Self Study Assignments

1. Research information on the Strategic National Stockpile Program and the CHEMPACK program. Look into issues such as response time, types of antidotes, and treatment available with each program.
2. Review and describe the limitations of a Mark-I auto-injector for administration of nerve agent antidotes to children, especially infants.

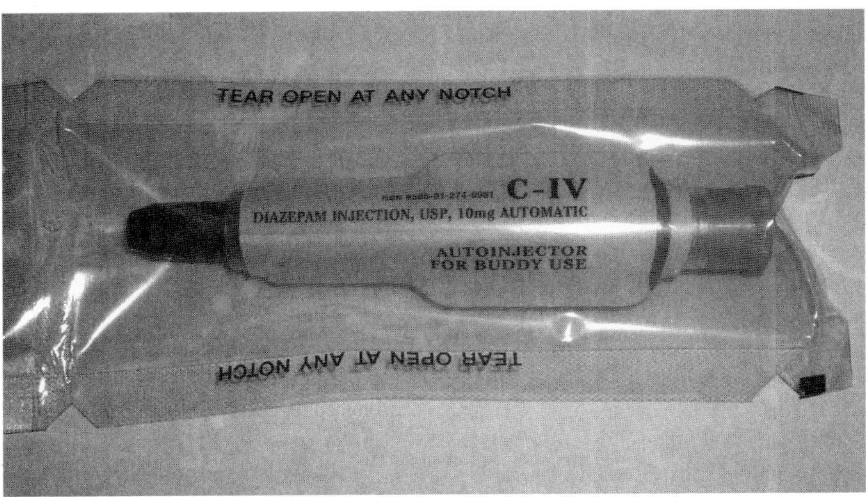

Figure 153–2. Diazepam provided as a 10-mg dose in a military-designed autoinjector.

References

1. North Carolina Statewide Program for Infection Control and Epidemiology (SPICE). Chemical terrorism agents and syndromes. Available on the Internet at: www.unc.edu/depts/spice/chemical-generic.pdf. Accessed August 8, 2004.
2. Field Management of Chemical Casualties Handbook, 2nd ed. US Army Medical Research Institute of Chemical Defense (USAMRICD). July 2000. Available on the Internet at: www.vnh.org/FieldManChemCasu/. Accessed August 8, 2004.
3. Centers for Disease Control and Prevention. Emergency preparedness and response: Chemical Agents. Available on the Internet at: www.bt.cdc.gov/agent/agentlistchem.asp. Accessed August 8, 2004.
4. Bozeman WP, Dilbero D, Schauben JL. Biologic and chemical weapons of mass destruction. Emerg Med Clin N Amer. 2002;20:975–993.
5. Arnold JL. CBRNE—Chemical warfare agents. Available on the Internet at: www.emedicine.com/emerg/topic852.htm. Accessed August 8, 2004.
6. Bartlett JG, Sifton DW, Gwynned LK. PDR Guide to Biological and Chemical Warfare Response, 1st ed. Montvale, NJ: Thomson Healthcare; 2002:79–86;94;101–102;126–127.
7. Pediatric Preparedness for Disasters and Terrorism: A National Consensus Conference. National Center for Disaster Preparedness, Columbia University Mailman School of Public Health; 2003. Available on the Internet at www.childrenshealthfund.org/CHF2286VFinal_adj.2.pdf. Accessed August 28, 2004.
8. Meridian Medical Technologies. Overview of homeland security auto-injectors. Available on the Internet at: www.domesticpreparedness.com/onlineexhibits/meridian/autoinjectors.html. Accessed August 31, 2004.

SECTION 20

Complementary and Alternative Therapies (Level III)

Charles W. Fetrow, PharmD
Maria B. Yaramus, PharmD

To the Reader:

With the recent surge in the promotion and use of complementary and alternative medicine (CAM), patients have increased their desire for knowledge on the potential benefits of these therapies. The purpose of this section is to provide additional questions related to currently used dietary supplements. Nine case examples are included in this section.

Each of the nine fictitious patient vignettes below is directly related to a patient case that was presented earlier in this book. Each scenario involves one or more questions asked by a patient about a specific remedy. Additional follow-up questions are then asked to help students provide a scientifically-based answer to the patient's question(s). Students will need to refer to additional references other than the *Pharmacotherapy* textbook in order to answer these questions satisfactorily. Be sure that they rely on reputable sources to support their answers. You may wish to have them cite the literature references that they used to answer the questions. Medical literature references are provided at the end of each of these vignettes.

Here is the first general question to get you started:

1. *What general questions might be asked of patients before you provide a recommendation for or against the use of any herbal or dietary supplement?*

CASE 21

▶HYPERLIPIDEMIA: SECONDARY PREVENTION—GARLIC AND OMEGA-3 FATTY ACIDS

▶ Clinical Course

While attending a wellness fair, Mr. Harper engages in a discussion with a pharmacist about the safety and efficacy of natural products. The pharmacist comments that natural products are often tried for hyperlipidemia, but few possess reproducible efficacy data.

Mr. Harper states that he is interested in making significant lifestyle changes after reading several nutrition guides. He is concerned about getting control of his health and preventing complications related to high cholesterol. He doesn't know where to start and how to put all of the information together. His daughter-in-law, a registered dietician, notes that his lipid panel is not within NCEP guidelines and suggests "natural approaches" to aggressively lower his lipids. She recommends a regimen consisting of garlic, gugulipid, and omega-3 fatty acids along with exercise.

▶ Follow-Up Questions

Garlic

1. *Based on available data, what are the postulated antihyperlipidemic mechanisms of garlic?*
2. *Briefly review and critique one major clinical trial that compared the efficacy of garlic on human serum lipoprotein profiles.*
3. *Given this patient's medical and personal situation, would you recommend self treatment with garlic? Why or why not?*
4. *What education should be provided to patients who choose to use this alternative therapy?*

Omega-3 Fatty Acids

5. *Based on available data, what are the postulated antihyperlipidemic mechanisms of omega-3 fatty acids?*
6. *Briefly review and critique one major clinical trial that compared the efficacy of omega-3 fatty acids on human serum lipoprotein profiles.*

7. *Given this patient's medical and personal situation, would you recommend self-treatment with fish oil? Why or why not?*

8. *What education should be provided to patients who choose to use this alternative therapy?*

9. *Are there any other dietary supplements that are claimed to be useful for hyperlipidemia?*

CASE 68

▶ ALZHEIMER'S DISEASE AND GINKGO BILOBA EXTRACT

▶ Clinical Course

One month later, Mrs. Dale's daughter phones the clinic with a question about her mother's therapy. After attending an Alzheimer's support group, the daughter reveals that she was given literature on the medicinal use of Ginkgo biloba extract (GbE) for improving memory and mental function. Now convinced that botanical medicine offers distinct advantages over conventional therapies for dementia, the daughter asks if her mother could be titrated off the current medication and started on Ginkgo biloba with the same expected therapeutic effect. She also asks whether combination therapy with her current medication and ginkgo would be better than a single product for improving cognition, mood, memory, and behavior.

▶ Follow-Up Questions

1. *Based on available data, what is the postulated mechanism of action for GbE?*

2. *Briefly review and critique one major clinical trial that compared the efficacy of GbE with conventional therapies for memory loss and impaired cognition associated with Alzheimer's disease.*

3. *Given this patient's medical and personal situation, would you recommend self treatment with GbE? Why or why not?*

4. *What education should be provided to patients who choose to use this alternative therapy?*

5. *Are there any other dietary supplements that are claimed to be useful for improving memory and cognition?*

CASE 72

▶ MAJOR DEPRESSION AND ST. JOHN'S WORT

▶ Clinical Course

Approximately 2 months after starting treatment, the patient returns to your pharmacy for a refill of her antidepressant medication. She questions you about taking St. John's Wort because she feels the antidepressant isn't working well enough. Furthermore, she believes that she had felt a little better on St. John's Wort when she tried it before. She adds that all her "previously troubled friends" have tried it and professed its value. She believes that it is truly safer than her current medication because it's "natural."

▶ Follow-Up Questions

1. *Based on the available data, what is the postulated mechanism of action for St. John's wort (SJW)?*

2. *Briefly review and critique one major clinical trial that compared efficacy of SJW with conventional therapies for depression.*

3. *Given this patient's medical and personal situation, would you recommend self-treatment with SJW? Why or why not?*

4. *What education should be provided to patients who choose to use this alternative therapy?*

5. *Are there any other dietary supplements that are claimed to be useful for depression?*

CASE 74

▶ GENERALIZED ANXIETY DISORDER AND KAVA KAVA

▶ Clinical Course

Ms. Long begins the prescribed course of therapy for anxiety. After 2 weeks, she calls her family practitioner and reveals that her restlessness is somewhat greater and she is not sleeping. Subsequently, her physician increases the dose and prescribes alprazolam 0.25 mg po at bedtime. One week later, she discontinues the initial anti-anxiety agent due to continued nausea and worsening of her insomnia but continues the alprazolam. A friend recommends that she try an herbal tea whose main ingredient is kava as a natural remedy to calm her nerves and allow her to sleep. Feeling that the tea made her less jittery, Ms. Long calls her local pharmacy to explore the possibility of taking kava on a regular basis in an attempt to ease her restlessness and help her sleep, thereby allowing her to be more productive during the day and attentive in class. She would like to continue the alprazolam at night and try kava for daytime anxiety. She is also concerned about the addictive and daytime sedation potential of Kava. If effective, she would like to discontinue the evening alprazolam.

▶ Follow-Up Questions

1. *Based on available data, what is the postulated mechanism of action for kava?*

2. *Briefly review and critique one major clinical trial that compared the efficacy of kava with conventional therapies for anxiety symptoms.*

3. *Given this patient's medical and personal situation, would you recommend self-treatment with kava? Why or why not?*

4. *What education should be provided to patients who choose to use this alternative therapy?*

5. *Are there any other dietary supplements that are claimed to be beneficial in patients with generalized anxiety of nonpsychotic origin?*

CASE 76

▶ INSOMNIA AND VALERIAN (*VALERIANA OFFICINALIS*)

▶ Clinical Course

Ms. Parker's daughter, a nurse, associates with a local herbalist and has accumulated literature on natural products as a psychotherapeutic alternative for her mother. She requests that the clinician consider valerian to help her mother sleep. Having investigated the natural products section of her pharmacy, she came across a combination of herbals touted as nature's sleep aid (Kava/Valerian combination). The daughter requests information about the safety of this combination product and its addiction potential.

▶ Follow-Up Questions

1. *Based on available data, what is the postulated mechanism of action for Valerian root?*

2. *Briefly review and critique one major clinical trial that compared the efficacy of valerian root with conventional therapies on sleep structure in patients with psychophysiological insomnia.*

3. *Given this patient's medical and personal situation, would you recommend self-treatment with valerian root? Why or why not?*

4. *What education should be provided to patients who choose to use this alternative therapy?*

5. *Are there any other dietary supplements that are claimed to have positive effects on sleep structure and that can be recommended for mild psychophysiological insomnia?*

CASE 87

▶ MANAGING MENOPAUSAL SYMPTOMS AND BLACK COHOSH

▶ Clinical Course

Having heard some "bad press" on hormone replacement therapy on her local television news station, the patient asks about the use of dietary supplements "that might not be as harmful for me." Specifically, she is interested in "something called black cohosh."

▶ Follow-Up Questions

1. *Based on the available data, what is the postulated mechanism of action for black cohosh?*

2. *Briefly review and critique one pivotal trial that evaluated efficacy of black cohosh for post-menopausal vasomotor complaints.*

3. *Given this patient's medical and personal situation, would you recommend self-treatment with black cohosh? Why or why not?*

4. *What education should be provided to patients who choose to use this alternative therapy?*

5. *Are there any other dietary supplements that are claimed to be useful for postmenopausal vasomotor symptoms?*

CASE 89

▶ BENIGN PROSTATIC HYPERPLASIA AND SAW PALMETTO

▶ Clinical Course

After several months on the recommended treatment with good but not total symptom relief, the patient read an article in a magazine about the potential benefits of saw palmetto for relief of BPH symptoms. He comes to you now to ask your professional opinion about this supplement.

▶ Follow-Up Questions

1. *Based on available data, what is the postulated mechanism of action for saw palmetto (SP)?*

2. *Briefly review and critique one major clinical trial that compared efficacy of SP with conventional therapies for benign prostatic hyperplasia (BPH).*

3. *Given this patient's medical and personal situation, would you recommend self-treatment with SP? Why or why not?*

4. *What education should be provided to patients who choose to use this alternative therapy?*

5. *Are there any other dietary supplements that are claimed to be useful for BPH?*

CASE 95

▶ OSTEOARTHRITIS AND GLUCOSAMINE

▶ Clinical Course

After 2 weeks on a scheduled dose of her new medication, Ms. Webster decides that she has waited long enough for resolution of her symptoms. Inadequate pain relief has driven her to call the doctor's office and request something else. The physician assistant who answers the phone recommends that she go to her local pharmacy and "pick up a bottle of glucosamine."

▶ Follow-Up Questions

1. *Based on the available data, what is the postulated mechanism of action for glucosamine?*

2. *Briefly review and critique one major clinical trial that compared the efficacy of glucosamine with conventional therapies for osteoarthritis (OA).*

3. *Given this patient's medical and personal situation, would you recommend self-treatment with glucosamine? Why or why not?*

4. *What education should be provided to patients who choose to use this alternative therapy?*

5. *Are there any other dietary supplements that are claimed to be useful for OA?*

CASE 114

▶ RHINOSINUSITIS AND ECHINACEA

▶ Clinical Course

After experiencing bothersome diarrhea and abdominal cramps from the treatment regimen, Ms. Schuele questions you about the use of echinacea. She states that "it has to be safer than the antibiotics" she had used previously, and that she is "sick of taking antibiotics anyway because they obviously won't work for me in this case."

▶ Follow-Up Questions

1. *Based on the available data, what is the postulated mechanism of action for echinacea?*

2. *Briefly review and critique one major clinical trial that compared efficacy of echinacea with conventional therapies for upper respiratory tract infections.*

3. *Given this patient's medical and personal situation, would you recommend self-treatment with echinacea? Why or why not?*

4. *What education should be provided to patients who choose to use this alternative therapy?*

5. *Are there any other dietary supplements that are claimed to be useful for upper respiratory tract infections?*

APPENDIX A
CONVERSION FACTORS AND ANTHROPOMETRICS[1]

CONVERSION FACTORS

SI Units

SI units *(le Systéme International d'Unités)* are used in many countries to express clinical laboratory and serum drug concentration data. Instead of employing units of mass (such as micrograms), the SI system uses moles (mol) to represent the amount of a substance. A molar solution contains 1 mole (the molecular weight of the substance in grams) of the solute in 1 liter of solution. The following formula is used to convert units of mass to moles (μg/mL to μmol/L or, by substitution of terms, mg/mL to mmol/L or ng/mL to nmol/L).

Micromoles per Liter (μmol/L)

$$\mu\text{mol/L} = \frac{\text{Drug concentration } (\mu\text{g/mL}) \times 1000}{\text{Molecular weight of drug (g/mol)}}$$

Milliequivalents

An equivalent weight of a substance is that weight which will combine with or replace 1 g of hydrogen; a milliequivalent is 1/1000 of an equivalent weight.

Milliequivalents per Liter (mEq/L)

$$\text{MEq/L} = \frac{\text{Weight of salt (g)} \times \text{Valence of ion} \times 1000}{\text{Molecular weight of salt}}$$

$$\text{Weight of salt (g)} = \frac{\text{mEq/L} \times \text{Molecular weight of salt}}{\text{Valence of ion} \times 1000}$$

Approximate Milliequivalents—Weights of Selected Ions

SALT	mEq/g SALT	mg SALT/mEq
Calcium Carbonate ($CaCO_3$)	20.0	50.0
Calcium Chloride ($CaCl_2 \cdot 2H_2O$)	13.6	73.5
Calcium Gluceptate ($Ca[C_7H_{13}O_8]_2$)	4.1	245.2
Calcium Gluconate ($Ca[C_6H_{11}O_7]_2 \cdot H_2O$)	4.5	224.1
Calcium Lactate ($Ca[C_3H_5O_3]_2 \cdot 5H_2O$)	6.5	154.1
Magnesium Gluconate ($Mg[C_6H_{11}O_7]_2 \cdot H_2O$)	4.6	216.3
Magnesium Oxide (MgO)	49.6	20.2
Magnesium Sulfate ($MgSO_4$)	16.6	60.2
Magnesium Sulfate ($MgSO_4 \cdot 7H_2O$)	8.1	123.2
Potassium Acetate ($K[C_2H_3O_2]$)	10.2	98.1
Potassium Chloride (KCl)	13.4	74.6
Potassium Citrate ($K_3[C_6H_5O_7] \cdot H_2O$)	9.2	108.1
Potassium Iodide (KI)	6.0	166.0
Sodium Acetate ($Na[C_2H_3O_2]$)	12.2	82.0

[1] This appendix contains information from Appendices 1 and 2 from Anderson PO, Knoben JE, Troutman WG, et al. (eds. Handbook of clinical drug data, 10th ed. New York. McGraw-Hill, 2002:1053–1058, with permission.

Approximate Milliequivalents—Weights of Selected Ions (continued)

SALT	mEq/g SALT	mg SALT/mEq
Sodium Acetate ($Na[C_2H_3O_2] \cdot 3H_2O$)	7.3	136.1
Sodium Bicarbonate ($NaHCO_3$)	11.9	84.0
Sodium Chloride (NaCl)	17.1	58.4
Sodium Citrate ($Na_3[C_6H_5O_7] \cdot 2H_2O$)	10.2	98.0
Sodium Iodide (NaI)	6.7	149.9
Sodium Lactate ($Na[C_3H_5O_3]$)	8.9	112.1
Zinc Sulfate ($ZnSO_4 \cdot 7H_2O$)	7.0	143.8

Valences and Atomic Weights of Selected Ions

SUBSTANCE	ELECTROLYTE	VALENCE	MOLECULAR WEIGHT
Calcium	Ca^{++}	2	40.1
Chloride	Cl^-	1	35.5
Magnesium	Mg^{++}	2	24.3
Phosphate	$HPO^=_4$ (80%)	1.8	96.0*
(pH = 7.4)	$H_2PO^-_4$ (20%)		
Potassium	K^+	1	39.1
Sodium	Na^+	1	23.0
Sulfate	$SO^=_4$	2	96.0*

*The molecular weight of phosphorus only is 31; that of sulfur only is 32.1.

Anion Gap

The anion gap is the concentration of plasma anions not routinely measured by laboratory screening. It is useful in the evaluation of acid-base disorders. The anion gap is greater with increased plasma concentrations of endogenous (eg. phosphate, sulfate, lactate, ketoacids) or exogenous (eg. salicylate, penicillin, ethylene glycol, ethanol, methanol) species. The formulas for calculating the anion gap follow:

$$\text{(A) Anion Gap} = (Na^+ + K^+) - (Cl^- + HCO^-_3)$$

or

$$\text{(B) Anion Gap} = Na^+ - (Cl^- + HCO^-_3)$$

where

the expected normal value for A is 11–20 mmol/L;
the expected normal value for B is 7–16 mmol/L.*

*Note that there is a variation at the upper and lower limits of the normal range.

Temperature

Fahrenheit to Centigrade: (°F – 32) × 5/9 = °C
Centigrade to Fahrenheit: (°C × 9/5) + 32 = °F
Centigrade to Kelvin: °C + 273 = °K

Weights and Measures

Metric Weight Equivalents

1 kilogram (kg) = 1000 grams
1 gram (g) = 1000 milligrams
1 milligram (mg) = 0.001 gram
1 microgram (mcg, μg) = 0.001 milligram
1 nanogram (ng) = 0.001 microgram

1 picogram (pg) = 0.001 nanogram
1 femtogram (fg) = 0.001 picogram

Metric Volume Equivalents

1 liter (L) = 1000 milliliters
1 deciliter (dL) = 100 milliliters
1 milliliter (mL) = 0.001 liter
1 microliter (μL) = 0.001 milliliter
1 nanoliter (nL) = 0.001 microliter
1 picoliter (pL) = 0.001 nanoliter
1 femtoliter (fL) = 0.001 picoliter

Apothecary Weight Equivalents

1 scruple (℈) = 20 grains (gr)
60 grains (gr) = 1 dram (ʒ)
8 drams (ʒ) = 1 ounce (℥)
1 ounce (℥) = 480 grains
12 ounces (℥) = 1 pound (lb)

Apothecary Volume Equivalents

60 minims (♏) = 1 fluidram (fl ʒ)
8 fluidrams (fl ʒ) = 1 fluid ounce (fl ℥)
1 fluid ounce (fl ℥) = 480 minims
16 fluid ounces (fl ℥) = 1 pint (pt)

Avoirdupois Equivalents

1 ounce (oz) = 437.5 grains
16 ounces (oz) = 1 pound (lb)

Weight/Volume Equivalents

1 mg/dL = 10 μg/mL
1 mg/dL = 1 mg%
1 ppm = 1 mg/L

Conversion Equivalents

1 gram (g) = 15.43 grains
1 grain (gr) = 64.8 milligrams
1 ounce (℥) = 31.1 grams
1 ounce (oz) = 28.35 grams
1 pound (lb) = 453.6 grams
1 kilogram (kg) = 2.2 pounds
1 milliliter (mL) = 16.23 minims
1 minim (♏) = 0.06 milliliter
1 fluid ounce (fl oz) = 29.57 mL
1 pint (pt) = 473.2 mL
0.1 mg = 1/600 gr
0.12 mg = 1/500 gr
0.15 mg = 1/400 gr
0.2 mg = 1/300 gr
0.3 mg = 1/200 gr
0.4 mg = 1/150 gr
0.5 mg = 1/120 gr
0.6 mg = 1/100 gr
0.8 mg = 1/80 gr
1 mg = 1/65 gr

ANTHROPOMETRICS

Creatinine Clearance Formulas

FORMULAS FOR ESTIMATING CREATININE CLEARANCE IN PATIENTS WITH STABLE RENAL FUNCTION

Adults [Age 18 Years and Older][1]

$$CI_{cr}\ (\text{Males}) = \frac{(140 - \text{Age}) \times (\text{Weight})}{Cr_s \times 72}$$

$$Cl_{cr}\ (\text{Females}) = 0.85 \times \text{Above value*}$$

where

Cl_{cr} = creatinine clearance in mL/min
Cr_s = serum creatinine in mg/dL
Age is in years
Weight is in kg.

*Some studies suggest that the predictive accuracy of this formula for women is better *without* the correction factor of 0.85.

Children [Age 1–18 Years][2]

$$Cl_{cr} = \frac{0.48 \times (\text{Height}) \times (\text{BSA})}{Cr_s \times 1.73}$$

where

BSA = body surface area in m^2
Cl_{cr} = creatinine clearance in mL/min
Cr_s = serum creatinine in mg/dL
Height is in cm.

FORMULA FOR ESTIMATING CREATININE CLEARANCE FROM A MEASURED URINE COLLECTION

$$Cl_{cr}\ (\text{mL/min}) = \frac{U \times V^*}{P \times 1}$$

where

U = concentration of creatinine in a urine specimen (in same units as P)
V = volume of urine in mL
P = concentration of creatinine in serum at the midpoint of the urine collection period (in same units as U)
T = time of the urine collection period in minutes (eg, 6 hr = 360 min; 24 hr = 1440 min).

*The product of U × V equals the production of creatinine during the collection period and, at steady state, should equal 20–25 mg/kg/day ideal body weight (IBW) in males and 15–20 mg/kg/day IBW in females. If it is less than this, inadequate urine collection may have occurred and Cl_{cr} will be underestimated.

Ideal Body Weight

IBW is the weight expected for a nonobese person of a given height. The IBW formulas below and various life insurance tables can be used to estimate IBW. Dosing methods described in the literature may use IBW as a method in dosing obese patients.

Adults [Age 18 Years and Older][3]

IBW (Males = 50 + (2.3 × Height in inches over 5 feet)
IBW (Females = 45.5 + (2.3 × Height in inches over 5 feet)

where IBW is in kg.

Children [Age 1–18 Years][2]

Under 5 Feet Tall:

$$IBW = \frac{(Height^2 \times 1.65)}{1000}$$

where

IBW is in kg;
Height is in cm.

5 Feet or Taller:

$$IBW\ (Males) = 39 + (2.27 \times \text{Height in inches over 5 feet})$$
$$IBW\ (Females) = 42.2 + (2.27 \times \text{Height in inches over 5 feet})$$

where IBW is in kg

References

1. Cockcroft DW, Gault MH. Prediction of creatinine clearance from serum creatinine. *Nephron* 1976;16:31–41.
2. Traub SL, Johnson CE. Comparison of methods of estimating creatinine clearance in children. *Am J Hosp Pharm* 1980;37:195–201.
3. Devine BJ. Gentamicin therapy. *Drug Intell Clin Pharm* 1974;8:650–5.

APPENDIX B
COMMON LABORATORY TESTS

The following table is an alphabetical listing of common laboratory tests and their reference ranges for adults as measured in plasma or serum (unless otherwise indicated). Reference values differ among laboratories, so readers should refer to the published reference ranges used in each institution. Values are reported in traditional units only.

Laboratory Test	Reference Range for Adults
Acid phosphatase	0 to 0.8 IU/L
Activated partial thromboplastin time (aPTT)	25 to 40 sec
Adrenocorticotropic hormone (ACTH)	15 to 80 pg/mL
Alanine aminotransferase (ALT)	5 to 35 IU/L
Albumin	3.5 to 5.0 g/dL
Albumin:creatinine ratio (urine)	Normal: < 30 mg/g; Microalbuminuria 30–300 mg/g; Proteinuria: > 300 mg/g
Alkaline phosphatase	30 to 120 IU/L
Alpha-fetoprotein (AFP)	0 to 20 ng/mL
Amikacin, therapeutic	15 to 30 mg/L peak; ≤ 8 mg/L trough
Ammonia	15 to 45 mcg/dL
Amylase	0 to 130 IU/L
Anion gap	8 to 16 mEq/L
Antidouble-stranded DNA (anti-ds DNA)	Negative
Anti-HAV	Negative
Anti-HBc	Negative
Anti-HBs	Negative
Anti-HCV	Negative
Anti-Sm antibody	Negative
Antinuclear antibody (ANA)	Negative at 1:20 dilution
Aspartate aminotransferase (AST)	5 to 40 IU/L
β_2-microglobulin	0.6 to 2.0 mg/dL
Bilirubin, direct	0.1 to 0.3 mg/dL
Bilirubin, indirect	0.1 to 1.0 mg/dL
Bilirubin, total	0.1 to 1.2 mg/dL
Bleeding time	3 to 7 min
Blood gases, arterial (ABG)	
pH	7.35 to 7.45
pco_2	35 to 45 mm Hg
po_2	80 to 100 mm Hg
HCO_3	22 to 26 mEq/L
O_2 saturation (Sao_2)	≥ 95%
Blood urea nitrogen (BUN)	5 to 25 mg/dL
Brain Natriuretic Peptice (BNP)	< 100 pg/mL
BUN-to-creatinine ratio	10:1 to 20:1
CA-125	< 35 IU/mL
CA 15–3	< 22 U/mL
CA 27.29	< 38 U/mL
Calcium, ionized	4.4 to 5.9 mg/dL; 2.2 to 2.5 mEq/L

Laboratory Test	Reference Range for Adults
Calcium, total	9 to 11 mg/dL; 4.5 to 5.5 mEq/L
Carbamazepine, therapeutic	4 to 12 mg/L
Carboxyhemoglobin	< 3%
Carcinoembryonic antigen (CEA)	< 3 ng/mL non-smokers; 0 to 6 ng/mL smokers
Cardiac Troponin I	0.00 to 0.50 ng/mL
CD4 lymphocyte count	31 to 61% of total lymphocytes
CD8 lymphocyte count	18 to 39% of total lymphocytes
Cerebrospinal fluid (CSF)	
Pressure	75 to 175 mm H_2O
Glucose	30 to 80 mg/dL
Protein	15 to 45 mg/dL
WBC	< 10/mm^3
Chloride	95 to 105 mEq/L
Cholesterol, HDL	< 40 mg/dL low, ≥ 60 mg/dL high
Cholesterol, LDL	< 100 mg/dL desirable
	100 to 129 mg/dL near or above optimal
	130 to 159 mg/dL borderline high
	160 to 189 mg/dL high
	≥ 190 mg/dL very high
Cholesterol, total	< 200 mg/dL desirable
	200 to 239 mg/dL borderline high
	≥ 240 mg/dL high
CO_2 content	22 to 30 mEq/L
Complement component 3 (C3)	70 to 160 mg/dL
Complement component 4 (C4)	20 to 40 mg/dL
Copper	70 to 150 mcg/dL
Cortisol (serum)	
8:00 AM to 10:00 AM	5 to 23 mcg/dL
4:00 PM to 6:00 PM	3 to 13 mcg/dL
Cortisol, free (urine)	10 to 110 mcg/24 h
C-reactive protein (CRP)	< 0.8 mg/dL or < 8 mg/L
Creatine (phospho)kinase (CPK, CK)	30 to 180 IU/L
CK-MB	> 5% in myocardial infarction
Creatinine clearance (CLcr, urine)	85 to 135 mL/min
Creatinine, serum	0.5 to 1.5 mg/dL
Cryptococcal antigen	< 1:8
D-dimers	< 200 ng/mL
Dexamethasone suppression test	8:00 AM cortisol < 10 mcg/dL
DHEAS	1 to 12 μmol/L
Digoxin, therapeutic	> 0.8 ng/mL
Erythrocyte sedimentation rate (ESR)	
Westergren	0 to 20 mm/h men; 0 to 30 mm/h women
Wintrobe	0 to 9 mm/h men; 0 to 15 mm/h women
Erythropoietin	2 to 25 IU/L; 2 to 25 mIU/mL
Estradiol, serum (women)	5 to 25 pg/mL
Ethanol, legal intoxication	≥ 50 to 100 mg/dL; ≥ 0.05 to 0.1%
Ethosuccimide, therapeutic	40 to 100 mg/L
Ferritin	2 to 20 mcg/dL; 20 to 200 ng/mL
Fibrin degradation products (FDP)	2 to 10 mg/L
Fibrinogen	200 to 400 mg/dL

Laboratory Test	Reference Range for Adults
Folic acid	0.2 to 1.0 mcg/dL; 2 to 10 ng/mL
Folic acid (RBC)	165 to 760 ng/mL
Follicle-stimulating hormone (FSH)	30 to 100 mIU/mL (postmenopausal women)
	5 to 22 mIU/mL (women, midcycle)
Free thyroxine index (FT_4I)	6.5 to 12.5
Gamma glutamyl transferase (GGT)	0 to 30 IU/L
Gentamicin, therapeutic	4 to 10 mg/L peak; ≤ 2 mg/L trough
Globulin	2.3 to 3.5 g/dL
Glucose, fasting (FBG)	70 to 110 mg/dL
Glucose, two-hour postprandial blood (PPBG)	< 140 mg/dL
Haptoglobin	60 to 270 mg/dL
HBeAg	Negative
HBsAg	Negative
HBV DNA	Negative
Hematocrit	40 to 54% men
	36 to 46% women
Hemoglobin	13.5 to 17.5 g/dL men
	12 to 16 g/dL women
Hemoglobin A_{1c} (HbA_{1c})	3.8 to 6.4%
Homocysteine	5 to 14 μmol/L
Imipramine, therapeutic	100 to 300 ng/mL
International normalized ratio (INR), therapeutic	2.0 to 3.0 (2.5 to 3.5 for some indications)
Iron, serum	50 to 160 mcg/dL men
	40 to 150 mcg/dL women
Lactate	0.5 to 1.5 mEq/L
Lactate dehydrogenase (LDH)	100 to 190 IU/L
Lidocaine, therapeutic	1.5 to 6.0 mg/L
Lipase	20 to 180 IU/L
Lithium, therapeutic	0.5 to 1.25 mEq/L
Luteinizing hormone (LH)	24 to 105 mIU/mL (midcycle peak)
Magnesium	1.8 to 3.0 mg/dL; 1.5 to 2.5 mEq/L
Mean corpuscular hemoglobin (MCH)	26 to 34 pg
Mean corpuscular hemoglobin concentration (MCHC)	31 to 37 g/dL
Mean corpuscular volume (MCV)	80 to 100 μm^3
Nortriptyline, therapeutic	50 to 140 ng/mL
Osmolality (serum)	280 to 300 mOsm/kg
Osmolality (urine)	200 to 800 mOsm/kg
Parathyroid hormone (PTH), intact	10 to 65 pg/mL
Parathyroid hormone (PTH), N-terminal	8 to 24 pg/mL
Parathyroid hormone (PTH), C-terminal	50 to 330 pg/mL
Phenobarbital, therapeutic	15 to 40 mg/L
Phenytoin, therapeutic	10 to 20 mg/L
Phosphorus	2.5 to 4.5 mg/dL; 1.7 to 2.6 mEq/L
Platelet count	150 to 400 × $10^3/mm^3$
Potassium	3.5 to 5.0 mEq/L
Prealbumin (transthyretin)	10 to 40 mg/dL
Primidone	5 to 20 mg/L
Procainamide, therapeutic	3 to 14 mg/L
Procainamide, therapeutic	3 to 14 mg/L
Prolactin	< 20 ng/mL or mcg/L

Laboratory Test	Reference Range for Adults
Prostate-specific antigen (PSA)	0 to 4 ng/mL
Protein, total	6.0 to 8.0 g/dL
Prothrombin time (PT)	10 to 12 sec
Quinidine, therapeutic	2 to 6 mg/L
Radioactive iodine uptake (RAIU)	< 6% in 2 hours
Red blood cell (RBC) count, total	4.6 to 6.0 × 10^6/mm^3 men 4.0 to 5.0 × 10^6/mm^3 women
Red blood cell (RBC) folic acid	165 to 760 ng/mL
Red cell distribution width (RDW)	11.5 to 14.5%
Reticulocyte count	0.5 to 1.5% of total RBC count
Retinol-binding protein (RBP)	2.7 to 7.6 mg/dL
Rheumatoid factor (RF) titer	< 1:20
Salicylate, therapeutic	150 to 300 mg/L
Sodium	135 to 145 mEq/L
Testosterone, total	3 to 10 ng/mL men 0.3 to 1.0 ng/mL women
Testosterone, free	> 40 pmol/L men 2.4 to 12.5 pmol/L women
Theophylline, therapeutic	5 to 20 mg/L
Thrombin time	20 to 24 sec
Thyroid-stimulating hormone (TSH)	0.3 to 5.0 mIU/L
Thyroid-binding globulin (TBG)	10 to 26 mcg/dL
Thyroxine (T_4), free	0.8 to 2.8 ng/dL
Thyroxine (T_4), total	4.5 to 11.5 mcg/dL
Thyroxine-binding prealbumin (transthyretin)	10 to 40 mg/dL
Thyroxine index, free (FT_4I)	6.5 to 12.5
Tobramycin, therapeutic	4 to 10 mg/L peak; ≤ 2 mg/L trough
Total iron-binding capacity (TIBC)	250 to 450 mcg/dL
Transferrin	200 to 430 mg/dL
Transferrin saturation	30 to 50%
Transthyretin (thyroxine-binding prealbumin)	10 to 40 mg/dL
Triglycerides	< 150 mg/dL normal 150 to 199 mg/dL borderline high 200 to 499 mg/dL high ≥ 500 mg/dL very high
Triiodothyronine (T_3)	75 to 200 ng/dL
Triiodothyronine (T_3) resin uptake	25 to 35%
Troponin-I (cardiac)	0.00 to 0.50 ng/mL
TSH receptor antibodies (TSH Rab)	0 to 1 U/mL
Uric acid	3.5 to 8.0 mg/dL
Urinalysis (urine)	
pH	4.5 to 8.0
Specific gravity	1.005 to 1.030
Protein	Negative
Glucose	Negative
Ketones	Negative
RBC	1 to 2 per low-power field (lpf)
WBC	3 to 4 per low-power field (lpf)
Casts	Occasional hyaline
Urobilinogen (urine)	0.5 to 4.0 Ehrlich Units/24 h

Laboratory Test	Reference Range for Adults
Valproic acid, therapeutic	50 to 150 mg/L
Vancomycin, therapeutic	15 to 30 mg/L peak
Vitamin A (retinol)	30 to 95 mcg/dL
Vitamin B_{12}	200 to 900 pg/mL
Vitamin D_3, 1,25-dihydroxy	20 to 76 pg/mL
Vitamin D_3, 25-hydroxy	10 to 50 ng/mL
Vitamin E (alpha tocopherol)	5 to 20 mg/L
White blood cell (WBC) count, total	4.5 to 10.0 $\times 10^3/mm^3$
WBC differential (peripheral blood)	
Polymorphonuclear neutrophils (PMNs)	50 to 65%
Bands	0 to 5%
Eosinophils	0 to 3%
Basophils	1 to 3%
Lymphocytes	25 to 35%
Monocytes	2 to 6%
WBC differential (bone marrow)	
Polymorphonuclear neutrophils (PMNs)	3 to 11%
Bands	9 to 15%
Metamyelocytes	9 to 25%
Myelocytes	8 to 16%
Promyelocytes	1 to 8%
Myeloblasts	0 to 5%
Eosinophils	1 to 5%
Basophils	0 to 1%
Lymphocytes	11 to 23%
Monocytes	0 to 1%
Zinc	60 to 150 mcg/dL

APPENDIX C
PART I: COMMON MEDICAL ABBREVIATIONS

Note: Many of the medical abbreviations contained in Part I of this appendix are used in the casebook. A more extensive list of abbreviations is available on the Internet at www.pharma-lexicon.com.

A & O	Alert and oriented
A & P	Auscultation and percussion, anterior and posterior, assessment and plan
A & W	Alive and well
aa	Of each (ana)
AA	Aplastic anemia, Alcoholics Anonymous
AAA	Abdominal aortic aneurysm
AAL	Anterior axillary line
AAO	Awake, alert, and oriented
Abd	Abdomen
ABG	Arterial blood gases
ABP	Arterial blood pressure
ABW	Actual body weight
AC	Before meals (*ante cibos*)
ACEI	Angiotensin-converting enzyme inhibitor
ACLS	Advanced cardiac life support
ACT	Activated clotting time
ACTH	Adrenocorticotropic hormone
AD	Alzheimer's disease, right ear (*auris dextra*)
ADA	American Diabetes Association, adenosine deaminase
ADE	Adverse drug effect (or event)
ADH	Antidiuretic hormone
ADHD	Attention-deficit hyperactivity disorder
ADL	Activities of daily living
ADR	Adverse drug reaction
AED	Antiepileptic drug(s)
AF	Atrial fibrillation
AFB	Acid-fast bacillus
AFP	α-Fetoprotein
A/G	Albumin-globulin ratio
AI	Aortic insufficiency
AIDS	Acquired immunodeficiency syndrome
AKA	Above-knee amputation
ALD	Alcoholic liver disease
ALL	Acute lymphocytic leukemia
ALP	Alkaline phosphatase
ALS	Amyotrophic lateral sclerosis
ALT	Alanine aminotransferase
AMA	Against medical advice; American Medical Association
AMI	Acute myocardial infarction
AML	Acute myelogenous leukemia
Amp	Ampule
ANA	Antinuclear antibody
ANC	Absolute neutrophil count
ANLL	Acute non-lymphocytic leukemia
AODM	Adult onset diabetes mellitus
AOM	Acute otitis media
AP	Anterior-posterior
APACHE	Acute Physiology and Chronic Health Evaluation
APAP	Acetaminophen (acetyl-*p*-aminophenol)
aPTT	Activated partial thromboplastin time
ARC	AIDS-related complex
ARDS	Adult respiratory distress syndrome
ARF	Acute renal failure
AROM	Active range of motion
AS	Left ear (*auris sinistra*)
ASA	Aspirin (acetylsalicylic acid)
ASCVD	Arteriosclerotic cardiovascular disease
ASD	Atrial septal defect
ASH	Asymmetric septal hypertrophy
ASHD	Arteriosclerotic heart disease
AST	Aspartate aminotransferase
ATG	Antithymocyte globulin
ATN	Acute tubular necrosis
AU	Each ear (*auris uterque*)
AV	Arteriovenous, atrioventricular
AVM	Arteriovenous malformation
AVR	Aortic valve replacement
AWMI	Anterior wall myocardial infarction
BAL	Bronchioalveolar lavage
BBB	Bundle branch block, blood-brain barrier
BC	Blood culture
BCG	Bacillus Calmette Guerin
BCNP	Board Certified Nuclear Pharmacist
BCNSP	Board Certified Nutrition Support Pharmacist
BCNU	Carmustine

BCP	Birth control pill
BCPS	Board Certified Pharmacotherapy Specialist
BE	Barium enema
BID	Twice daily *(bis in die)*
BKA	Below-knee amputation
BM	Bone marrow, bowel movement
BMD	Bone mineral density
BMR	Basal metabolic rate
BMT	Bone marrow transplantation
BNP	Brain natriuretic peptide
BP	Blood pressure
BPD	Bronchopulmonary dysplasia
BPH	Benign prostatic hyperplasia
BPRS	Brief Psychiatric Rating Scale
bpm	Beats per minute
BR	Bedrest
BRBPR	Bright red blood per rectum
BRM	Biological response modifier
BRP	Bathroom privileges
BS	Bowel sounds, breath sounds, blood sugar
BSA	Body surface area
BSO	Bilateral salpingo-oophorectomy
BTFS	Breast tumor frozen section
BUN	Blood urea nitrogen
Bx	Biopsy
C & S	Culture and sensitivity
CA	Cancer, calcium
CABG	Coronary artery bypass graft
CAD	Coronary artery disease
CAH	Chronic active hepatitis
CAM	Complementary and alternative medicine
CAPD	Continuous ambulatory peritoneal dialysis
CBC	Complete blood count
CBD	Common bile duct
CBG	Capillary blood gas, corticosteroid binding globulin
CBT	Cognitive-behavioral therapy
CC	Chief complaint
CCA	Calcium channel antagonist
CCB	Calcium channel blocker
CCE	Clubbing, cyanosis, edema
CCK	Cholecystokinin
CCMS	Clean catch midstream
CCN	Lomustine
CCPD	Continuous cycling peritoneal dialysis
CCU	Coronary care unit
CDAD	*Clostridium difficile*-associated diarrhea
CEA	Carcinoembryonic antigen
CF	Cystic fibrosis
CFS	Chronic fatigue syndrome
CFU	Colony-forming unit
CHD	Coronary heart disease
CHF	Congestive heart failure
CHO	Carbohydrate
CHOP	Cyclophosphamide, hydroxydaunorubicin (doxorubicin), Oncovin (vincristine), prednisone
CI	Cardiac index
CK	Creatine kinase
CKD	Chronic kidney disease
CLL	Chronic lymphocytic leukemia
CM	Costal margin
CMG	Cystometrogram
CML	Chronic myelogenous leukemia
CMV	Cytomegalovirus
CN	Cranial nerve
CNS	Central nervous system
C/O	Complains of
CO	Cardiac output, carbon monoxide
COLD	Chronic obstructive lung disease
COPD	Chronic obstructive pulmonary disease
CP	Chest pain, cerebral palsy
CPA	Costophrenic angle
CPAP	Continuous positive airway pressure
CPK	Creatine phosphokinase
CPP	Cerebral perfusion pressure
CPR	Cardiopulmonary resuscitation
CR	Complete remission
CRF	Chronic renal failure, corticotropin-releasing factor
CRH	Corticotropin-releasing hormone
CRI	Chronic renal insufficiency, catheter-related infection
CRNA	Certified Registered Nurse Anesthetist
CRNP	Certified Registered Nurse Practitioner
CRP	C-reactive protein
CRTT	Certified Respiratory Therapy Technician
CS	Central Supply
CSA	Cyclosporine
CSF	Cerebrospinal fluid, colony-stimulating factor
CT	Computed tomography, chest tube
CTB	Cease to breathe
cTnI	Cardiac troponin I
CTZ	Chemoreceptor trigger zone
CV	Cardiovascular
CVA	Cerebrovascular accident
CVAT	Costovertebral angle tenderness
CVC	Central venous catheter
CVP	Central venous pressure
Cx	Culture
CXR	Chest x-ray
D & C	Dilatation and curettage
d4T	Stavudine
D_5W	5% Dextrose in water
DBP	Diastolic blood pressure
D/C	Discontinue, discharge
DCC	Direct current cardioversion

ddC Zalcitabine
ddI Didanosine
DES Diethylstilbestrol
DI Diabetes insipidus
DIC Disseminated intravascular coagulation
Diff Differential
DIP Distal interphalangeal
DJD Degenerative joint disease
DKA Diabetic ketoacidosis
dL Deciliter
DM Diabetes mellitus
DMARD Disease-modifying antirheumatic drug
DNA Deoxyribonucleic acid
DNR Do not resuscitate
DO Doctor of Osteopathy
DOA Dead on arrival
DOB Date of birth
DOE Dyspnea on exertion
DOT Directly observed therapy
DPGN Diffuse proliferative glomerulonephritis
DRE Digital rectal examination
DRG Diagnosis-related group
DS Double strength
DSHEA Dietary Supplement Health and Education Act (1994)
DST Dexamethasone suppression test
DTIC Dacarbazine
DTP Diphtheria-tetanus-pertussis
DTR Deep-tendon reflex
DVT Deep-vein thrombosis
Dx Diagnosis
EBV Epstein-Barr virus
EC Enteric-coated
ECF Extended care facility
ECG Electrocardiogram
ECMO Extracorporeal membrane oxygenator
ECOG Eastern Cooperative Oncology Group
ECT Electroconvulsive therapy
ED Emergency Department
EEG Electroencephalogram
EENT Eyes, ears, nose, throat
EF Ejection fraction
EGD Esophagogastroduodenoscopy
EIA Enzyme immunoassay
EKG Electrocardiogram
EMG Electromyogram
EMT Emergency Medical Technician
Endo Endotracheal, endoscopy
EOMI Extraocular movements (or muscles) intact
EPO Erythropoietin
EPS Extrapyramidal symptoms
ER Estrogen receptor
ERCP Endoscopic retrograde cholangiopancreatography
ERT Estrogen replacement therapy
ESLD End-stage liver disease
ESR Erythrocyte sedimentation rate
ESRD End-stage renal disease
ESWL Extracorporeal shockwave lithotripsy
ET Endotracheal
EtOH Ethanol
FB Finger-breadth, foreign body
FBS Fasting blood sugar
FDA Food and Drug Administration
FDP Fibrin degradation products
FEM-POP Femoral-popliteal
FEV_1 Forced expiratory volume in one second
FFP Fresh frozen plasma
FH Family history
Fio_2 Fraction of inspired oxygen
fl Femtoliter
FM Face mask
FOBT Fecal occult blood test
FOC Fronto-occipital circumference
FPG Fasting plasma glucose
FPIA Fluorescence polarization immunoassay
FSH Follicle-stimulating hormone
FTA Fluorescent treponemal antibody
F/U Follow-up
FUDR Floxuridine
FUO Fever of unknown origin
Fx Fracture
G-CSF Granulocyte colony-stimulating factor
G6PD Glucose-6-phosphate dehydrogenase
GAD Generalized anxiety disorder
GB Gall bladder
GBS Group B *Streptococcus,* Guillain-Barre syndrome
GC Gonococcus
GDM Gestational diabetes mellitus
GE Gastroesophageal, gastroenterology
GERD Gastroesophageal reflux disease
GFR Glomerular filtration rate
GGT Gamma-Glutamyl transferase
GGTP Gamma-Glutamyl transpeptidase
GI Gastrointestinal
GM-CSF Granulocyte-macrophage colony-stimulating factor
GN Glomerulonephritis, graduate nurse
gr Grain
GT Gastrostomy tube
gtt Drops (guttae)
GTT Glucose tolerance test
GU Genitourinary
GVHD Graft-versus-host disease
GVL Graft-versus-leukemia

Gyn	Gynecology
H & H	Hemoglobin and hematocrit
H & P	History and physical examination
H/A	Headache
HAART	Highly-active antiretroviral therapy
HAV	Hepatitis A virus
Hb, hgb	Hemoglobin
HbA_{1c}	Glycosylated hemoglobin (hemoglobin A1c)
HBIG	Hepatitis B immune globulin
HBP	High blood pressure
HBsAg	Hepatitis B surface antigen
HBV	Hepatitis B virus
HC	Hydrocortisone, home care
HCG	Human chorionic gonadotropin
HCO_3	Bicarbonate
Hct	Hematocrit
HCTZ	Hydrochlorothiazide
HCV	Hepatitis C virus
Hcy	Homocysteine
HD	Hodgkin's disease, hemodialysis
HDL	High-density lipoprotein
HEENT	Head, eyes, ears, nose, and throat
HEPA	High-efficiency particulate air
HGH	Human growth hormone
HH	Hiatal hernia
Hib	*Haemophilus influenzae* type b
HIV	Human immunodeficiency virus
HJR	Hepatojugular reflux
HLA	Human leukocyte antigen
HMG-CoA	Hydroxy-methylglutaryl coenzyme A
H/O	History of
HOB	Head of bed
HPA	Hypothalamic-pituitary axis
hpf	High-power field
HPI	History of present illness
HR	Heart rate
HRT	Hormone replacement therapy
HS	At bedtime *(hora somni)*
HSM	Hepatosplenomegaly
HSV	Herpes simplex virus
HTN	Hypertension
Hx	History
I & D	Incision and drainage
I & O	Intake and output
IABP	Intra-arterial balloon pump
IBD	Inflammatory bowel disease
IBW	Ideal body weight
ICP	Intracranial pressure
ICS	Intercostal space
ICU	Intensive care unit
ID	Identification, infectious disease
IDDM	Insulin-dependent diabetes mellitus
IFN	Interferon
IHD	Ischemic heart disease
IJ	Internal jugular
IM	Intramuscular, infectious mononucleosis
IMV	Intermittent mandatory ventilation
INH	Isoniazid
INR	International normalized ratio
IOP	Intraocular pressure
IP	Intraperitoneal
IPG	Impedance plethysmography
IPN	Interstitial pneumonia
IPPB	Intermittent positive pressure breathing
IRB	Institutional Review Board
ISA	Intrinsic sympathomimetic activity
ISDN	Isosorbide dinitrate
ISH	Isolated systolic hypertension
ISMN	Isosorbide mononitrate
IT	Intrathecal
ITP	Idiopathic thrombocytopenic purpura
IU	International unit
IUD	Intrauterine device
IV	Intravenous
IVC	Inferior vena cava, intravenous cholangiogram
IVDA	Intravenous drug abuse
IVF	Intravenous fluids
IVIG	Intravenous immunoglobulin
IVP	Intravenous pyelogram, intravenous push
IVSS	Intravenous Soluset
IWMI	Inferior wall myocardial infarction
JODM	Juvenile-onset diabetes mellitus
JRA	Juvenile rheumatoid arthritis
JVD	Jugular venous distention
JVP	Jugular venous pressure
kcal	Kilocalorie
KCL	Potassium chloride
KOH	Potassium hydroxide
KUB	Kidney, ureters, bladder
KVO	Keep vein open
L	Liter
LAD	Left anterior descending, left axis deviation
LAO	Left anterior oblique
LAP	Leukocyte alkaline phosphatase
LBBB	Left bundle branch block
LBP	Low back pain
LCM	Left costal margin
LDH	Lactate dehydrogenase
LDL	Low-density lipoprotein
LE	Lower extremity
LES	Lower esophageal sphincter
LFT	Liver function test
LHRH	Luteinizing hormone-releasing hormone
LIMA	Left internal mammary artery

LLE	Left lower extremity
LLL	Left lower lobe
LLQ	Left lower quadrant
LLSB	Left lower sternal border
LMD	Local medical doctor
LMP	Last menstrual period
LOC	Loss of consciousness, laxative of choice
LOS	Length of stay
LP	Lumbar puncture
LPN	Licensed Practical Nurse
LPO	Left posterior oblique
LPT	Licensed Physical Therapist
LR	Lactated Ringer's
LS	Lumbosacral
LTCF	Long-term care facility
LUE	Left upper extremity
LUL	Left upper lobe
LUQ	Left upper quadrant
LVH	Left ventricular hypertrophy
MAP	Mean arterial pressure
MAR	Medication administration record
mcg	Microgram
MCH	Mean corpuscular hemoglobin
MCHC	Mean corpuscular hemoglobin concentration
MCL	Midclavicular line
MCP	Metacarpophalangeal
MCV	Mean corpuscular volume
MD	Medical Doctor
MDI	Metered-dose inhaler
MEFR	Maximum expiratory flow rate
mEq	Milliequivalent
mg	Milligram
MHC	Major histocompatibility complex
MI	Myocardial infarction, mitral insufficiency
MIC	Minimum inhibitory concentration
MICU	Medical intensive care unit
mL	Milliliter
MM	Multiple myeloma
MMA	Methylmalonic acid
MMEFR	Maximal midexpiratory flow rate
MMR	Measles-mumps-rubella
MMSE	Mini mental status exam
MOM	Milk of magnesia
MPV	Mean platelet volume
m/r/g	Murmur/rub/gallop
MRI	Magnetic resonance imaging
MRSA	Methicillin-resistant *Staphylococcus aureus*
MS	Mental status, mitral stenosis, musculoskeletal, multiple sclerosis, morphine sulfate
MSE	Mental status exam
MSW	Master of Social Work
MTD	Maximum tolerated dose
MTP	Metatarsophalangeal
MTX	Methotrexate
MUD	Matched unrelated donor
MUGA	Multiple gated acquisition
MVA	Motor vehicle accident
MVI	Multivitamin
MVR	Mitral valve replacement
N & V	Nausea and vomiting
NAD	No acute (or apparent) distress
N/C	Non-contributory, nasal cannula
NC/AT	Normocephalic, atraumatic
NG	Nasogastric
NGT	Nasogastric tube
NHL	Non-Hodgkin's lymphoma
NIDDM	Non–insulin-dependent diabetes mellitus
NKA	No known allergies
NKDA	No known drug allergies
NL	Normal
NNRTI	Non-nucleoside reverse transcriptase inhibitor
NOS	Not otherwise specified
NPH	Neutral protamine Hagedorn, normal pressure hydrocephalus
NPN	Non-protein nitrogen
NPO	Nothing by mouth (*nil per os*)
NRTI	Nucleoside reverse transcriptase inhibitor
NS	Neurosurgery, normal saline
NSAID	Nonsteroidal anti-inflammatory drug
NSCLC	Non-small cell lung cancer
NSR	Normal sinus rhythm
NSS	Normal saline solution
NTG	Nitroglycerin
NT/ND	Non-tender, non-distended
NVD	Nausea/vomiting/diarrhea, neck vein distention
NYHA	New York Heart Association
O & P	Ova and parasites
OA	Osteoarthritis
OB	Obstetrics
OBS	Organic brain syndrome
OCD	Obsessive-compulsive disorder
OCG	Oral cholecystogram
OD	Right eye (*oculus dexter*), overdose, Doctor of Optometry
OGT	Oral glucose tolerance test
OHTx	Orthotopic heart transplantation
OLTx	Orthotopic liver transplantation
OOB	Out of bed
OPD	Outpatient department
OPG	Ocular plethysmography
OPV	Oral poliovirus vaccine
OR	Operating room
OS	Left eye (*oculus sinister*)
OSA	Obstructive sleep apnea

OT	Occupational therapy
OTC	Over-the-counter
OU	Each eye (*oculus uterque*)
P	Pulse, plan, percussion, pressure
P & A	Percussion and auscultation
P & T	Peak and trough
PA	Physician Assistant, posterior-anterior, pulmonary artery
PAC	Premature atrial contraction
$Paco_2$	Arterial carbon dioxide tension
Pao_2	Arterial oxygen tension
PAT	Paroxysmal atrial tachycardia
PBI	Protein-bound iodine
PBSCT	Peripheral blood stem cell transplantation
PC	After meals (*post cibum*)
PCA	Patient-controlled analgesia
PCI	Percutaneous coronary intervention
PCKD	Polycystic kidney disease
PCN	Penicillin
PCOS	Polycystic ovarian syndrome
PCP	*Pneumocystis carinii* pneumonia, phencyclidine
PCWP	Pulmonary capillary wedge pressure
PDA	Patent ductus arteriosus
PE	Physical examination, pulmonary embolism
PEEP	Positive end-expiratory pressure
PEFR	Peak expiratory flow rate
PEG	Percutaneous endoscopic gastrostomy, polyethylene glycol
PERLA	Pupils equal, react to light and accommodation
PERRLA	Pupils equal, round, and reactive to light and accommodation
PET	Positron emission tomography
PFT	Pulmonary function test
pH	Hydrogen ion concentration
PharmD	Doctor of Pharmacy
PI	Principal investigator, protease inhibitor
PID	Pelvic inflammatory disease
PIP	Proximal interphalangeal
PKU	Phenylketonuria
PMD	Private medical doctor
PMH	Past medical history
PMI	Point of maximal impulse
PMN	Polymorphonuclear leukocyte
PMS	Premenstrual syndrome
PNC-E	Postnecrotic cirrhosis-ethanol
PND	Paroxysmal nocturnal dyspnea
PNH	Paroxysmal nocturnal hemoglobinuria
po	By mouth *(per os)*
POAG	Primary open-angle glaucoma
POD	Postoperative day
POS	Polycystic ovarian syndrome
PP	Patient profile
PPBG	Postprandial blood glucose
ppd	packs per day
PPD	Purified protein derivative
PPH	Past Psychiatric History
PPI	Proton pump inhibitor
PPN	Peripheral parenteral nutrition
pr	Per rectum
PR	Progesterone receptor, partial remission
PRA	Panel-reactive antibody, plasma renin activity
PRBC	Packed red blood cells
PRN	When necessary, as needed *(pro re nata)*
PSA	Prostate-specific antigen
PSCT	Peripheral stem cell transplant
PSE	Portal systemic encephalopathy
PSH	Past surgical history
PT	Prothrombin time, physical therapy, patient
PTA	Prior to admission
PTCA	Percutaneous transluminal coronary angioplasty
PTH	Parathyroid hormone
PTT	Partial thromboplastin time
PTU	Propylthiouracil
PUD	Peptic ulcer disease
PVC	Premature ventricular contraction
PVD	Peripheral vascular disease
Q	Every *(quaque)*
QA	Quality assurance
QD	Every day *(quaque die)*
QI	Quality improvement
QID	Four times daily *(quater in die)*
QNS	Quantity not sufficient
QOD	Every other day
QOL	Quality of life
QS	Quantity sufficient
R & M	Routine and microscopic
RA	Rheumatoid arthritis, right atrium
RAIU	Radioactive iodine uptake
RAO	Right anterior oblique
RBBB	Right bundle branch block
RBC	Red blood cell
RCA	Right coronary artery
RCM	Right costal margin
RDA	Recommended daily allowance
RDP	Random donor platelets
RDW	Red cell distribution width
REM	Rapid eye movement
RES	Reticuloendothelial system
RF	Rheumatoid factor, renal failure, rheumatic fever
RHD	Rheumatic heart disease
RLE	Right lower extremity
RLL	Right lower lobe
RLQ	Right lower quadrant
RML	Right middle lobe

RN	Registered nurse
RNA	Ribonucleic acid
R/O	Rule out
ROM	Range of motion
ROS	Review of systems
RPGN	Rapidly progressive glomerulonephritis
RPh	Registered Pharmacist
RPR	Rapid plasma reagin
RR	Respiratory rate, recovery room
RRR	Regular rate and rhythm
RRT	Registered Respiratory Therapist
RSV	Respiratory syncytial virus
RT	Radiation therapy
RT-PCR	Reverse transcriptase-polymerase chain reaction
RTA	Renal tubular acidosis
RTC	Return to clinic
RUE	Right upper extremity
RUL	Right upper lobe
RUQ	Right upper quadrant
SA	Sinoatrial
SAH	Subarachnoid hemorrhage
Sao_2	Arterial oxygen percent saturation
SBE	Subacute bacterial endocarditis
SBFT	Small bowel follow-through
SBO	Small bowel obstruction
SBP	Systolic blood pressure
SC	Subcutaneous, subclavian
SCID	Severe combined immunodeficiency
SCLC	Small cell lung cancer
SCr	Serum creatinine
SDP	Single donor platelets
SEM	Systolic ejection murmur
SG	Specific gravity
SGOT	Serum glutamic oxaloacetic transaminase
SGPT	Serum glutamic pyruvic transaminase
SH	Social history
SIADH	Syndrome of inappropriate antidiuretic hormone secretion
SIDS	Sudden infant death syndrome
SIMV	Synchronized intermittent mandatory ventilation
SJS	Stevens-Johnson syndrome
SL	Sublingual
SLE	Systemic lupus erythematosus
SMBG	Self-monitoring of blood glucose
SNRI	Serotonin-norepinephrine reuptake inhibitor
SOB	Shortness of breath
S/P	Status post
SPEP	Serum protein electrophoresis
SPF	Sun protection factor
SQ	Subcutaneous
SRI	Serotonin reuptake inhibitor
SSKI	Saturated solution of potassium iodide
SSRI	Selective serotonin reuptake inhibitor
STAT	Immediately, at once
STD	Sexually transmitted disease
SVC	Superior vena cava
SVRI	Systemic vascular resistance index
SVT	Supraventricular tachycardia
SW	Social worker
SWI	Surgical wound infection
Sx	Symptoms
T	Temperature
T & A	Tonsillectomy and adenoidectomy
T & C	Type and crossmatch
TAH	Total abdominal hysterectomy
TB	Tuberculosis
TBG	Thyroid-binding globulin
TBI	Total body irradiation, traumatic brain injury
T/C	To consider
TCA	Tricyclic antidepressant
TCN	Tetracycline
TED	Thromboembolic disease
TEN	Toxic epidermal necrolysis
TENS	Transcutaneous electrical nerve stimulation
TFT	Thyroid function test
TG	Triglyceride
THA	Total hip arthroplasty
THC	Tetrahydrocannabinol
TIA	Transient ischemic attack
TIBC	Total iron-binding capacity
TID	Three times daily (*ter in die*)
TIH	Tumor-induced hypercalcemia
TIPS	Transjugular intrahepatic portosystemic shunt
TLC	Therapeutic lifestyle changes
TLI	Total lymphoid irradiation
TLS	Tumor lysis syndrome
TM	Tympanic membrane
TMJ	Temporomandibular joint
TMP-SMX	Trimethoprim-sulfamethoxazole
TnI	Troponin I (cardiac)
TnT	Troponin T
TNTC	Too numerous to count
TOD	Target organ damage
TPN	Total parenteral nutrition
TPR	Temperature, pulse, respiration
TSH	Thyroid-stimulating hormone
TSS	Toxic shock syndrome
TTP	Thrombotic thrombocytopenic purpura
TUIP	Transurethral incision of the prostate
TURP	Transurethral resection of the prostate
Tx	Treat, treatment
UA	Urinalysis, uric acid
UC	Ulcerative colitis

UCD	Usual childhood diseases
UE	Upper extremity
UFC	Urinary free cortisol
UGI	Upper gastrointestinal
UOQ	Upper outer quadrant
UPT	Urine Pregnancy Test
URI	Upper respiratory infection
USP	United States Pharmacopeia
UTI	Urinary tract infection
UV	Ultraviolet
VA	Veterans' Affairs
VAMC	Veterans' Affairs Medical Center
VDRL	Venereal Disease Research Laboratory
VF	Ventricular fibrillation
VLDL	Very low-density lipoprotein
VNA	Visiting Nurses' Association
VO	Verbal order
VOD	Veno-occlusive disease
VP-16	Etoposide
V/Q	Ventilation/perfusion
VRE	Vancomycin-resistant *Enterococcus*
VS	Vital signs
VSS	Vital signs stable
VT	Ventricular tachycardia
VTE	Venous thromboembolism
WA	While awake
WBC	White blood cell
W/C	Wheelchair
WDWN	Well-developed, well-nourished
WHO	World Health Organization
WNL	Within normal limits
W/U	Work-up
Y-BOCS	Yale-Brown Obsessive-Compulsive Scale
yo	Year-old
ZDV	Zidovudine

PART II: Prevent Medication Errors by Avoiding These Dangerous Abbreviations or Dose Designations

Abbreviation or Dose Expression	Intended Meaning	Misinterpretation	Correction
Apothecary symbols	dram, minim	Misunderstood or misread (symbol for dram misread for "3" and minim misread "mL").	Use the metric system.
AU	aurio uterque (each ear)	Mistaken for OU (oculo uterque—each eye).	Don't use this abbreviation.
D/C	discharge, discontinue	Premature discontinuation of medications when D/C (intended to mean "discharge") has been misinterpreted as "discontinued" when followed by a list of drugs.	Use "discharge" and "discontinue."
Drug names			
ARA-A	vidarabine	cytarabine (ARA-C)	Use the complete spelling
AZT	zidovudine (RETROVIR)	azathioprine	for drug names.
CPZ	COMPAZINE (prochlorperazine)	chlorpromazine	
DPT	DEMEROL-PHENERGAN-THORAZINE	diphtheria-pertussis-tetanus (vaccine)	
HCl	hydrochloric acid	potassium chloride (The "H" is misinterpreted as "K.")	
HCT	hydrocortisone	hydrochlorothiazide	
HCTZ	hydrochlorothiazide	hydrocortisone (seen as HCT250 mg)	
$MgSO_4$	magnesium sulfate	morphine sulfate	
MSO_4	morphine sulfate	magnesium sulfate	
MTX	methotrexate	mitoxantrone	
TAC	triamcinolone	tetracaine, ADRENALIN, cocaine	
$ZnSO_4$	zinc sulfate	morphine sulfate	
Stemmed names			
"Nitro" drip	nitroglycerin infusion	sodium nitroprusside infusion	
"Norflox"	norfloxacin	NORFLEX (orphenadrine)	

Abbreviation or Dose Expression	Intended Meaning	Misinterpretation	Correction
μg	microgram	Mistaken for "mg" when *handwritten.*	Use mcg
o.d. or OD	once daily	Misinterpreted as "right eye" (OD—oculus dexter) and administration of oral medications in the eye.	Use "daily."
TIW or tiw	three times a week	Mistaken as "three times a day."	Don't use this abbreviation.
per os	orally	The "os" can be mistaken for "left eye."	Use "PO," "by mouth," or "orally."
q.d. or QD	every day	Mistaken as q.i.d., especially if the period after the "q" or the tail of the "q" is misunderstood as an "i."	Use "daily" or "every day."
qn	nighty or at bedtime	Misinterpreted as "qh" (every hour).	Use "nightly."
qhs	nightly at bedtime	Misread as every hour.	Use "nightly."
q6PM, etc.	every evening at 6 PM	Misread as every six hours.	Use 6 PM "nightly."
q.o.d. or QOD	every other day	Misinterpreted as "q.d." (daily) or "q.i.d. (four times daily) if the "o" is poorly written.	Use "every other day."
sub q	subcutaneous	The "q" has been mistaken for "every" (e.g., one heparin dose ordered "sub q 2 hours before surgery" misunderstood as every 2 hours before surgery).	Use "subcut." or write "subcutaneous."
SC	subcutaneous	Mistaken for SL (sublingual).	Use "subcut." or write "subcutaneous."
U or u	unit	Read as a zero (0) or a four (4), causing a 10-fold overdose or greater (4U seen as "40" or 4u seen as 44").	"Unit" has no acceptable abbreviation. Use "unit."
IU	international unit	Misread as IV (intravenous)	Use "units."
cc	cubic centimeters	Misread as "U" (units).	Use "mL."
x3d	for three days	Mistaken for "three doses."	Use "for three days."
BT	bedtime	Mistaken as "BID" (twice daily).	Use "hs."
ss	sliding scale (insulin) or 1/2 (apothecary)	Mistaken for "55."	
> and <	greater than and less than	Mistakenly used opposite of intended.	Use "greater than" or "less than."
/ (slash mark)	separates two doses or indicates "per"	Misunderstood as the number 1 ("25 unit/10 units" read as "110" units.	Do not use a slash mark to separate doses. Use "per."
Name letters and dose numbers run together (e.g., Inderal40 mg)	Inderal 40 mg	Misread as Inderal 140 mg.	Always use space between drug name, dose, and unit of measure.
Zero after decimal point (1.0)	1 mg	Misread as 10 mg if the decimal point is not seen.	Do not use terminal zeros for doses expressed in whole numbers.
No zero before decimal dose (.5 mg)	0.5 mg	Misread as 5 mg.	Always use zero before a decimal when the dose is less than a whole unit.

Reprinted with permission from the Institute of Safe Medication Practices *(www.ismp.org).* Originally printed in: Cohen MR. Medication Errors. Washington, DC, The American Pharmaceutical Association, 1999. To report real or potential medication errors, contact the ISMP by telephone (215-947-7797), fax (215-914-1492), or e-mail (ismpinfo@ismp.org).

APPENDIX D
SAMPLE RESPONSES TO CASE QUESTIONS

37 PEDIATRIC GASTROENTERITIS

▶ Dihydrogen Monoxide and Other Critical Elements (Level II)

William McGhee, PharmD
Basil J. Zitelli, MD, FAAP

A 5-day history of vomiting, diarrhea, and other symptoms causes a young mother to seek medical attention at the Emergency Department for her 5-month-old son. The patient has signs of moderate dehydration on physical and laboratory examination. The presumed diagnosis is viral gastroenteritis probably caused by rotavirus. Students should understand that replacement of fluid and electrolyte losses is critical to the effective treatment of acute diarrhea. Oral rehydration therapy with carbohydrate-based solutions is the primary treatment of diarrhea in children with mild to moderate dehydration. When caregivers are properly instructed, therapy can begin at home. Intravenous fluids may be needed for cases of severe dehydration. Early feeding of patients with an age-appropriate diet helps to reduce stool volume after completion of rehydration therapy. Although antidiarrheal and antiemetic products are available, they have limited effectiveness, can cause adverse effects, and may divert attention from appropriate fluid and electrolyte replacement. Families should have a commercially available oral rehydration solution at home to start treatment as soon as diarrhea begins.

▶ Questions

Problem Identification

1. a. Create a list of the patient's drug therapy problems.

This patient has typical viral gastroenteritis and diarrhea, a common pediatric problem in the United States, where it is estimated that 16.5 million children younger than 5 years of age experience 21 to 37 million episodes of diarrhea annually.[1] Peak incidence is in the 6 to 24 month age group. Viral gastroenteritis is usually caused by rotavirus infection, which is characterized by the acute onset of emesis, progressing to watery diarrhea with diminishing emesis. Rotavirus is the most common cause of pediatric gastroenteritis in the United States, accounting for 25% of cases, with the majority of cases occurring in otherwise healthy children. Other common viruses include Norwalk-like viruses and adenovirus.[2] Rotavirus is transmitted by the fecal–oral route, and spread of the virus is common in hospitals and similar settings such as day care. Infection occurs when ingested virus infects enterocytes in the small intestine, leading to cell death and loss of brush border digestive enzymes. Approximately 48 hours after exposure, infected children develop fever, vomiting, and watery diarrhea. Fever and vomiting usually subside in 1 to 2 days, but diarrhea can continue for several days leading to significant dehydration. Dehydration and corresponding electrolyte losses are the primary causes of morbidity in gastroenteritis. Approximately 65% of hospitalizations and 85% of diarrhea-related deaths occur in the first year of life.

The patient has moderate dehydration (acute weight loss of 8%, from 7.1 kg [15.65 lb] to 6.5 kg [14.33 lb]) as well as clinical and laboratory evidence of dehydration with metabolic acidosis.

b. What information (signs, symptoms, laboratory values) indicates the presence or severity of gastroenteritis?

The most accurate indicator of the degree of dehydration is actual weight loss. Fortunately for the patient, he had a physician's office visit 7 days earlier where he was weighed. An actual weight loss of 0.6 kg (1.32 lb or 8%) was documented.

By history, the patient had a 5-day history of fever, vomiting, and diarrhea of acute onset; he had a reported decrease in the number of wet diapers; and his lips appeared to be dry.

He has a social history of day care attendance, where several of his day care mates had similar illnesses recently, as well as a 2-year-old sibling with a recent history of diarrhea for 3 days. This is a typical history in pediatric gastroenteritis.

On physical exam, his skin turgor was decreased and the capillary refill was increased at 2 to 3 seconds. His tongue was dry with cracked and dry lips. His anterior fontanelle was sunken and he had sunken eyes, and he was tachycardic and tachypneic.

His labs indicated metabolic acidosis (total CO_2 13 mEq/L and Cl 110 mEq/L) and his urinalysis showed a specific gravity of 1.028 (indicating moderate dehydration). Ketones in the urine indicate fat breakdown in a hypocaloric diet. His dehydration was isotonic (defined as serum sodium between 130 and 150 mEq/L).

See Table 37–1 for clinical assessment guidelines for dehydration.

Desired Outcome

2. What are the goals of pharmacotherapy in this case?

Reversing dehydration, restoring normal urine output, and maintenance of adequate nutrition are the goals of appropriate pharmacotherapy of dehydration. Replacement of fluid and electrolyte losses is the critical element of effective treatment. This is necessary to prevent excessive water,

TABLE 37–1. Clinical Assessment Guidelines for Dehydration in Children of All Ages[3,4]

Parameter	Mild	Moderate	Severe
Weight loss	3% to 5%	6% to 9%	≥10%
Body fluid loss	30–50 mL/kg	50–100 mL/kg	>100 mL/kg
Stage of shock	Impending	Compensated	Uncompensated
Heart rate	Normal	Increased	Increased
Blood pressure	Normal	Normal	Normal to reduced
Respiratory rate	Normal	Normal	Increased
Skin turgor	Normal	Decreased	"Tenting"
Anterior fontanelle	Normal	Sunken	Sunken
Capillary refill	<2 seconds	2–3 seconds	>3 seconds
Mucous membranes	Slightly dry	Dry	Dry
Tearing	Normal/absent	Absent	Absent
Eye appearance	Normal	Sunken orbits	Deeply sunken orbits
Mental status	Normal	Normal to listless	Normal to lethargic to comatose
Urine volume	Slightly decreased	<1 mL/kg/h	<1 mL/kg/h
Urine specific gravity	1.020	1.025	>1.035
BUN	Upper normal	Elevated	High
Blood pH	7.40–7.22	7.30–6.92	7.106.8
Thirst	Slightly increased	Moderately increased	Very thirsty or too lethargic to indicate

electrolyte, and acid–base disturbances. Reinstitution of an age-appropriate diet is essential to assure adequate nutrition and to reduce stool volume. Further morbidity and unnecessary hospitalization may be prevented.

Other secondary goals may include providing symptomatic relief and treating any curable causes of diarrhea.

Therapeutic Alternatives

3. a. What nondrug therapies might be useful for this patient?

Oral rehydration therapy (ORT) with carbohydrate-based solutions is the mainstay of treatment of fluid and electrolyte losses caused by diarrhea in children with mild to moderate dehydration. ORT can be used regardless of the patient's age, causative pathogen, or initial serum sodium concentration. The basis for the effectiveness of ORT is the phenomenon of glucose–sodium cotransport, where sodium ions given orally are absorbed along with glucose (and other organic molecules) from the lumen of the intestine into the bloodstream.[2] Once these molecules are absorbed, free water will naturally follow. Any of the commercially available oral rehydration solutions (ORS) can successfully be used to rehydrate otherwise healthy children with mild to moderate dehydration (refer to textbook Chapter 36 for more detailed product information). These products are formulated on physiologic principles and should be close to isotonic to avoid unnecessary shifts in fluid. They are to be distinguished from other nonphysiologic clear liquids that are commonly but inappropriately used to treat dehydration. Clear liquids to be avoided include colas, ginger ale, apple juice, chicken broth, and sports beverages.[4] This patient was inappropriately treated because in addition to an ORS (Pedialyte), the pediatrician recommended a variety of clear liquids including water, Jell-O water, and cola. These liquids have unacceptably low electrolyte concentrations, and cola beverages are hypertonic because of the high glucose concentrations, with osmolalities greater than 700 mOsm.[4]

Early feeding of age-appropriate foods. Although carbohydrate-based ORT is highly effective in replacing fluid and electrolyte losses, it has no effect on stool volume or duration of diarrhea, which can be discouraging to parents. To overcome this limitation, cereal-based ORT (e.g., rice flour-based ORT) has been used investigationally and can reduce stool volume by 20% to 30%. However, there are no commercial products available in the United States. Another ORT product based on rice-syrup solids (Infalyte) was equivalent to carbohydrate-based ORT. Nonetheless, early feeding of patients as soon as oral rehydration is completed may provide similar reductions in stool volume.[5] Therefore, children with diarrhea requiring rehydration should be fed with age-appropriate diets immediately after completing ORT. Optimal ORT incorporates early feeding of age-appropriate foods. Unrestricted diets generally do not worsen the symptoms of mild or moderate diarrhea and decrease the stool output compared with ORT alone.

ORT is well established as the appropriate therapy for prevention and treatment of diarrhea with mild to moderate dehydration associated with pediatric gastroenteritis. The principles of ORT include early rehydration with an appropriate ORS, replacement of ongoing fluid losses from diarrhea and vomiting with an ORS, and reintroduction of age-appropriate diets as soon as rehydration is complete. As simple as this sounds, the majority of health care providers, contrary to the guidelines of the American Academy of Pediatrics (AAP) and the recommendations of the CDC, overuse IV hydration, prolong rehydration, delay reintroduction of age-appropriate diets, and withhold ORT inappropriately, especially in children who are vomiting.[5] Continuing education of health care workers and reemphasizing the value of oral rehydration versus IV rehydration is essential for the future success of ORT.

b. What feasible pharmacotherapeutic alternatives are available for treatment of this patient's diarrhea?

Antidiarrheal compounds have been used to treat pediatric gastroenteritis. Their use is intended to shorten the course of diarrhea and to relieve discomfort by reducing stool output and electrolyte losses. However, their usefulness remains to be proven, and antidiarrheal compounds generally should not be used to treat pediatric gastroenteritis. These agents have a variety of proposed mechanisms; their possible benefits and limitations are outlined below.

Antimotility agents (opioids and opioid/anticholinergic combination products) delay GI transit and increase gut capacity and fluid retention. *Loperamide* with ORT significantly reduces the volume of stool losses, but this reduction is not clinically significant. Loperamide also may have an unacceptable rate of side effects (lethargy, respiratory depression, altered mental status, ileus, abdominal distention). Anticholinergic agents (e.g., *atropine* or *mepenzolate bromide*) may cause dry mouth that can alter the clinical evaluation of dehydration. Infants and children are especially susceptible to toxic effects of anticholinergics. Antimotility agents can worsen the course of diarrhea in shigellosis, antibiotic-associated pseudomembranous colitis, and *E. coli* 0157:H7-induced diarrhea. *Importantly, reliance on antidiarrheal compounds may shift the focus of treatment away from appropriate ORT and the early feeding of the child.* They are not recommended by the AAP to treat acute diarrhea in children because of the modest clinical benefit, limited scientific evidence of efficacy, and concern for toxic effects.

Antisecretory agents (bismuth subsalicylate) may have an adjunctive role for acute diarrhea. Bismuth subsalicylate decreases intestinal secretions secondary to cholera and *E. coli* toxins, decreases frequency of unformed stools, decreases total stool output, and reduces the need for ORT. However, the benefit is modest, and it requires dosing every 4 hours. Also, pediatric patients may absorb salicylate (but the effect on Reye's syndrome is unknown). This treatment is also not recommended by the AAP because of modest benefit and concern for toxicity.

Adsorbent drugs (kaolin and pectin; polycarbophil) may bind bacterial toxins and water, but their effectiveness remains unproven. There is no conclusive evidence of decreased duration of diarrhea, number of stools, or total stool output. Major toxicity is not a concern with these products, but they may adsorb nutrients, enzymes, and drugs. The FDA recognizes only polycarbophil as an effective adsorbent. These products are not recommended by the AAP because of lack of efficacy.

Colonic microflora replacement products (Lactobacillus acidophilus, L. bulgaricus) supposedly replace microflora loss secondary to previous antibiotic therapy. These probiotics purportedly suppress growth of pathogenic microorganisms, restoring normal intestinal function. However, there is no consistent evidence that microflora replacement improves diarrhea. *Lactobacillus GG* (or LGG) is a bacterial strain that was isolated from humans by Drs. Gorbach and Goldin (hence the name LGG) in the 1980s. Recently, when LGG was given in combination with ORT, there were no significant reductions in diarrhea duration or stool output.[6] Any beneficial effects of probiotics may be limited to prophylactic usage in high-risk populations or in the presence of bacterial colonization. Lactobacillus-containing compounds are not recommended by the AAP because of limited evidence of efficacy.

Antiemetic drugs have been used in dehydrated patients who are vomiting. However, the benefit of these agents is questionable and they are unnecessary. *Promethazine* and *trimethobenzamide* are the most commonly prescribed agents. Side effects of these medications include sedation that can interfere in the evaluation of patients with worsening dehydration and drowsiness. Their use is not recommended.

Optimal Plan

4. What drug(s), dosage forms, schedule, and duration of therapy are best for this patient?

Treatment of a child with dehydration is directed primarily by the degree of dehydration present.[2] This patient had diarrhea with moderate dehydration (6% to 9% loss of body weight). There are four treatment situations:[4]

Diarrhea without dehydration. ORT may be given in doses of 10 mL/kg to replace ongoing stool losses. Some children may not take the ORT because of its salty taste. For these few patients, freezer pops are available in a variety of flavors. ORT may not be necessary if fluid consumption and age-appropriate feeding continues. Infants should continue to breast-feed or take regular-strength formula. Older children can usually drink full-strength milk.

Diarrhea with mild dehydration (3% to 5% weight loss). Correct dehydration with ORT 50 mL/kg over a 4-hour period. Reassess the status of dehydration and volume of ORT at 2-hour intervals. Concomitantly replace continuing losses from stool or emesis at 10 mL/kg for each stool; estimate emesis loss and replace with fluid. Children with emesis can usually tolerate ORT, but it is necessary to administer ORT in small 5- to 10-mL aliquots (1 to 2 teaspoonfuls) every 1 to 2 minutes. Feeding should start immediately after rehydration is complete, using the feeding guidelines described above.

Diarrhea with moderate dehydration (6% to 9% weight loss). Because the patient presented to the ED this treatment was performed there, but it can usually be accomplished at home. Correct the dehydration with ORT 100 mL/kg plus replacement of ongoing losses (10 mL/kg for each stool, plus estimated losses from emesis as above) during the first 4 hours. Assess rehydration status hourly and adjust the amount of ORT accordingly. Close supervision is required, but this can be continued at home. Rapid restoration of blood volume helps to correct acidosis and to increase tissue perfusion. Resume feeding of age-appropriate diet as soon as rehydration is completed.

Diarrhea with severe dehydration (≥10% weight loss). Severe dehydration and uncompensated shock should be treated aggressively with IV isotonic fluids to restore intravascular volume. Poorly treated pediatric gastroenteritis, especially in infants, can cause life-threatening severe dehydration and should be considered a medical emergency. The patient may be in shock and should be referred to an ED. Administer 20 mL/kg aliquots of normal saline or Ringer's lactate solution over 15 to 30 minutes (even faster in uncompensated shock). Reassess the patient's status after each completed fluid bolus. Repeat boluses of up to 80 mL/kg total fluid may be used. Isotonic fluid replacement may be discontinued when blood pressure is restored, heart rate is normalized, peripheral pulses are strong, and skin perfusion is restored. Urine output is the best indicator of restored intravascular volume and should be at least 1 mL/kg/hr. If the patient does not respond to rapid IV volume replacement, other underlying disorders should be considered, including septic shock, toxic shock syndrome, myocarditis, cardiomyopathy, pericarditis, and other underlying diseases. ORT may be instituted to complete rehydration when the patient's status is satisfactory. Estimate the degree of remaining dehydration and treat according to the above guidelines. The IV line should be kept in place until it is certain that IV therapy will not be reinstituted. After ORT is complete, resume age-appropriate feeding following the guidelines outlined previously.

Outcome Evaluation

5. What clinical and laboratory parameters should be monitored to evaluate therapy for achievement of the desired therapeutic outcome?

Vital signs should normalize with appropriate therapy, but they may be unreliable in patients with fever, agitation, pain, or respiratory illnesses. Tachycardia is usually the first sign of mild dehydration (see Table 37–1 of this *Instructor's Guide*). With increasing acidosis and fluid loss, the respiratory rate increases and breathing becomes deeper (hyperpnea). Hypotension is usually a sign of severe dehydration.

Any existing CNS alterations should be reversed. No CNS changes occur in mild dehydration; some patients may appear listless with moderate dehydration, and severely dehydrated patients appear quite ill with lethargy or irritability.

Skin changes should be normalized. Mucous membranes should appear moist (previously dry in all degrees of dehydration). Capillary refill is normally <2 seconds and usually is not altered in mild dehydration. Capillary refill in moderately dehydrated patients is 2 to 3 seconds and >3 seconds in severe dehydration. Skin turgor (elasticity) should be normal. There is no change in mild dehydration; but it decreases in moderate dehydration, with "tenting" occurring in patients with severe dehydration. The anterior fontanelle should no longer be sunken, which is seen in moderate to severe dehydration.

The eyes should appear normal. No change occurs in mild dehydration, but in moderate to severe dehydration, tearing will be absent and the eyes will appear sunken.

Laboratory tests should be assessed appropriately. Most dehydration occurring with pediatric gastroenteritis is isotonic, and serum electrolyte determinations are unnecessary. However, some patients with moderate dehydration (those whose histories and physical examinations are inconsistent with routine gastroenteritis), those with prolonged inappropriate intake of hypotonic or hypertonic solutions, and all severely dehydrated patients should have serum electrolytes determined and corrected.

Urine volume and specific gravity should be normalized. Progressive decreases in urine volume and increases in specific gravity are expected with increasing severity of dehydration. Urine output will be decreased to <1 mL/kg/h in moderate dehydration and <1 mL/kg/h in severe dehydration (see Table 37–1 of this *Instructor's Guide*). Specific gravity will be 1.020 in mild dehydration, 1.025 in moderate dehydration, and maximal in patients with severe dehydration. Adequate rehydration should normalize both urine output and specific gravity.

Patient Education

6. What information should be provided to the child's parents to enhance compliance, to ensure successful therapy, and to minimize adverse effects?

Treatment of diarrhea due to gastroenteritis in your child should begin at home.[2] It is a good idea for you to keep ORT at home at all times (especially in rural areas and poor urban neighborhoods where access to health care may be delayed), and to use it as instructed by your doctor. Sometimes doctors instruct new parents about this treatment at the first newborn visit. Be careful of information obtained from sources on the Internet. Much of the information available does not concur with the American Academy of Pediatrics guidelines for the use of ORT in pediatric gastroenteritis.[7]

However, infants with diarrhea should receive a medical evaluation for diarrhea. Additionally, any child with diarrhea and fever should be evaluated to rule out serious illness.[8]

Early home management will result in fewer complications such as severe dehydration and poor nutrition, as well as fewer office or emergency room visits.

Any of the commercial oral rehydration products can be used to effectively rehydrate your child. However, rehydration alone does not reduce the duration of diarrhea or the volume of stool output. Early feeding after rehydration is necessary and can reduce the duration of diarrhea by as much as one-half day.

Effective oral rehydration always combines early feeding with an age-appropriate diet after rehydration. This will correct dehydration, improve nutritional status, and reduce the volume of stool output.

Vomiting usually does not preclude the use of oral rehydration. Consistent administration of small amounts (1 to 2 teaspoonfuls) of an oral rehydration solution every 1 to 2 minutes can provide as much as 10 ounces per hour of rehydration fluid. Parents must resist the child's desires for larger amounts of liquid. Otherwise, further vomiting may occur.

If the child does not stop vomiting after the appropriate administration of oral rehydration (as above) and appears to be severely dehydrated, contact your doctor, who may refer you to the emergency room for intravenous rehydration therapy.

Oral rehydration is insufficient therapy for bloody diarrhea (dysentery). Contact your doctor if this occurs.

Additional treatments, including antidiarrheal compounds and antimicrobial therapy, are almost never necessary in the treatment of pediatric gastroenteritis. Most children can be successfully rehydrated with ORS without the use of antiemetic medication.

Proper handwashing technique, diaper-changing practices, and personal hygiene can help to prevent spread of the disease to other family members. The child should be kept out of day care until the diarrhea stops.

References

1. Glass RI, Lew JF, Gangarosa RE, et al: Estimates of morbidity and mortality rates for diarrheal diseases in American children. *J Pediatr* 1991;118(4, [Pt 2]): S27–S33.
2. Duggan C, Santosham M, Glass RI. The management of acute diarrhea in children: Oral rehydration, maintenance, and nutritional therapy. *MMWR Morb Mortal Wkly Rep* 1992;41(RR-16):1–20.
3. Provisional Committee on Quality Improvement, Subcommittee on Acute Gastroenteritis. Practice parameter: The management of acute gastroenteritis in young children. *Pediatrics* 1996;97:424–435.
4. Snyder J. The continuing evolution of oral therapy for diarrhea. *Semin Pediatr Infect Dis* 1994;5:231–235.
5. Santosham M. Oral rehydration therapy: Reverse transfer of technology. *Arch Pediatric Adolesc Med* 2002;156:1177–1179. Editorial.
6. Costa-Ribeiro H, Ribeiro TC, Mattos AP, et al: Limitations of probiotic therapy in

acute, severe dehydrating diarrhea. *J Pediatr Gastroenterol Nutr* 2003;36:112–115

7. McClung HJ, Murray RD, Heitlinger LA. The Internet as a source for current patient information. *Pediatrics* 1998;101:1065. Abstract.
8. Centers for Disease Control and Prevention. Managing acute gastroenteritis among children: Oral rehydration, maintenance, and nutritional therapy. *MMWR Morb Mortal Wkly Rep* 2003;52, (RR-16):1–16.

51 CHRONIC GLOMERULONEPHRITIS

▶ An Ongoing Battle With Lupus (Level III)

Melanie S. Joy, PharmD

A 23-year-old woman with a history of diffuse proliferative glomerulonephritis (DPGN) secondary to systemic lupus erythematosus (SLE) presents with hematuria and renal biopsy features characteristic of advanced DPGN. In addition to requiring immunosuppressive therapy for DPGN, the patient also needs evaluation for possible treatment of hypertension, dyslipidemia, edema, anemia, and corticosteroid-induced osteoporosis. Cyclophosphamide and azathioprine are potent immunosuppressive agents that may be useful either as single agents or combined with prednisone for DPGN. Cyclophosphamide should probably be avoided at this time because the patient received it on two previous occasions and relapsed after treatment and because of the risk of toxicity. Other potential alternatives include cyclosporine, mycophenolate mofetil, fludarabine, methotrexate, immune globulins, plasma exchange, total lymphoid irradiation, and investigational agents. This is a complex case because it requires students to develop pharmacotherapeutic plans for all of the patient's medical problems.

▶ Questions

Problem Identification

1. a. *Create a list of this patient's drug therapy problems.*

DPGN requiring immunosuppressive drug therapy

HTN inadequately treated with present doses of atenolol and clonidine

Hypercholesterolemia that is currently untreated

Edema that is currently untreated

Osteoporosis/osteopenia in need of treatment to prevent fractures (*Note:* T score is the SD below or above the expected mean peak BMD obtained)

Anemia that is currently untreated

b. *What information obtained from the medical history, physical examination, and laboratory analysis indicates the presence of glomerulonephritis?*

Elevated serum creatinine to 2.2 mg/dL

Renal biopsy results

Urinalysis (hematuria, casts, nephrotic range proteinuria)

Arthralgias, fatigue, and anemia are symptoms of SLE

Gross proteinuria, edema, elevated cholesterol, and decreased serum albumin are evidence of the nephrotic syndrome

c. *What information indicates complications from the disease itself or long-term treatment?*

Osteoporosis/osteopenia caused by long-term corticosteroid treatment

Oligomenorrhea secondary to treatment with cyclophosphamide and corticosteroids

HTN, which may be a consequence of either loss of renal function or by corticosteroid therapy

Dyslipidemia, which may be secondary to corticosteroid therapy and the nephrotic syndrome

Edema, which is secondary to the nephrotic syndrome and subsequent hypoalbuminemia

Anemia, which may be a result of renal insufficiency, iron deficiency, chronic disease (SLE), and/or bleeding

d. *Calculate the patient's measured creatinine clearance (CLcr)/glomerular filtration rate (GFR) from the present 24-hour urine collection and the MDRD equation and compare these to the measured CLcr 6 months ago to assess the rate of progression of chronic kidney disease.*

Measured CLcr at Present Time ($CLcr_{present}$)

$$CLcr_{present} = \frac{Ucr \times U\ vol}{SCr \times Time} \quad \frac{54.5\ mg/dL \times 2151\ mL}{2.2\ mg/dL \times 1440\ min}$$

$$CLcr_{present} = 37\ mL/min$$

Estimated GFR at Present Time ($GFR_{present}$) Using the MDRD Equation

$$GFR_{present} = 170 \times [SCr]^{-0.999} \times [Age]^{-0.176} \times [0.762\text{ if female}] \times [1.180\text{ if black}] \times [BUN]^{-0.170} \times [Alb]^{+0.318}$$

$$GFR_{present} = 28\ mL/min/1.73m2$$

Measured CLcr 6 Months Ago ($CLcr_{past}$)

$$CLcr_{past} = \frac{81\ mg/dL \times 1200\ mL}{1.2\ mg/dL \times 1440\ min}$$

$$CLcr_{past} = 56.3\ mL/min$$

With a decline in renal function of at least 20 mL/min over 6 months, this patient needs aggressive therapy to slow her development to end-stage kidney disease (ESKD), given findings on renal biopsy demonstrating active proliferative glomerulonephritis. Regarding the staging of CKD, this patient remains unchanged in Stage 3 (GFR 30 to 59 mL/min) if using the 24-hour CLcr collection estimate of GFR. However, the patient moved from Stage 3 to Stage 4 if using the MDRD calculation. These conflicting results demonstrate the variability in measurements between the two calculated methods. The MDRD equation has not been adequately validated in patients without kidney diseases, and patients with type 1 diabetes mellitus, older than 70 years, pregnant women, serious comorbid conditions, transplant recipients, and patients with extreme values of serum albumin. Also, the MDRD has not been validated in patients with rapidly changing serum creatinine or urea nitrogen concentrations.[1]

e. *What other risk factors for renal disease progression does this patient have?*

Uncontrolled hypertension. HTN has been associated with vascular and glomerular damage to the kidneys. The presence of elevated pressure transferred to both renal arterioles and glomeruli leads to sclerosis of the intrarenal arterioles and glomeruli. The ischemia that results from the vascular lesions in the afferent arterioles leads to elevated pressures within the glomerulus and glomerulosclerosis. This results in further basement membrane injury and worsening proteinuria. The MDRD study demonstrated that strict BP control (MAP of 92 mmHg) in patients with baseline proteinuria >1 g/day and GFR of 25 to 55 mL/min had a protective effect against progressive renal disease.[1]

Hypercholesterolemia. Some data suggest that elevated lipid levels may lead to LDL cholesterol binding to mesangial cells in the glomerulus. Oxidation of these bound cells by macrophages results in foam cell formation. This oxidized LDL acts as a cytotoxic agent to the glomerulus, causing cell damage.

f. *Describe the possible glomerular lesions attributable to SLE in this patient.*

Renal disease develops in up to 75% of patients with SLE. Renal biopsy changes may be present in 95% of all lupus patients. On the contrary, only 10% to 15% of patients progress to end-stage renal disease. Although tubulointerstitial disease may be the only manifestation of renal disease, glomerular disease is more commonly the case. It has been suggested that the glomerular manifestations of the disease occur because of the deposition of IgG antidouble-stranded DNA antibodies in the glomerulus, bound to the antigen. The subsequent glomerular damage occurs as a result of the activation of complement and damage to tissues. Although the initial damage occurs in the mesangium, increased antigen/antibody complexes lead to enhanced damage to other areas of the glomerulus as well.

Mesangial disease is the mildest and earliest form of lupus nephritis. It is manifest as increased mesangial proliferation and matrix expansion. Patients present with mild proteinuria, microscopic hematuria, and red cell casts.

Focal proliferative disease involves mesangial and endothelial proliferation in a focal, segmental pattern involving <50% of the glomeruli. Thickening of the basement membrane may occur in the affected areas. Patients present with mild proteinuria, microscopic hematuria, and red cell casts. In addition, nephrotic syndrome, hypertension, or mild renal insufficiency may be present.

Diffuse proliferative disease is more severe than the focal proliferative form. Crescent formation may be present. Immunoglobulins (IgG, IgM, IgA) and complement (C3 and C4) are found in the glomeruli. The mesangial and endothelial deposits are more prominent than in the focal proliferative form. Patients may present similarly to the focal proliferative form. However, patients may also present with acute renal failure, nephritic sediment, nephrotic range proteinuria, edema, and HTN.

Membranous disease is associated with diffuse basement membrane thickening without prominent hypercellularity. Patients usually present with the nephrotic syndrome.[2–4]

g. *What is the typical clinical presentation of SLE, and which attributes are present in this patient?*

Female-to-male disposition 9:1; this patient is female.

Black-to-white race incidence of 3:1; this patient is black.

High probability for therapy resistance and relapse in black versus white patients; this patient is black.

Peak onset of disease between ages 15 and 40 years; this patient was diagnosed at age 15.

Signs and symptoms of SLE: Arthralgias, arthritis, malaise, malar rash, fatigue, Raynaud's, pleuritis, pericarditis, anemia, renal involvement. This patient currently has arthralgias, fatigue, anemia, and renal involvement.

Laboratory abnormalities in SLE: Elevated ANA titer, circulating antibodies to double-stranded DNA, hypocomplementemia. This patient has hypocomplementemia, positive anti-DS DNA, decreased hemoglobin, increased serum creatinine, active urinary sediment, proteinuria, and hypoalbuminemia.[5]

Desired Outcome

2. *What are the pharmacotherapy goals for this patient's lupus nephritis?*

Arrest and/or slow the rapid rate of renal function deterioration as demonstrated by improvement in proteinuria and urinary sediment.

Prevent renal and cardiovascular complications by achieving a goal MAP of 92 mm Hg in this patient with proteinuria of >3 g/day.

Treat concurrent hypercholesterolemia to prevent long-term renal and cardiovascular complications. The LDL should be reduced from 204 to <100 mg/dL in a patient with established chronic kidney disease, as these patients are considered to be in the highest risk group.

Treat the bone complications (osteoporosis of spine and osteopenia of hip) of long-term corticosteroid therapy in order to increase or stabilize bone mineral density.

Treat the mild anemia to achieve a hemoglobin of 11 to 12 g/dL and hematocrit of 33% to 36% in a premenopausal woman with moderate renal insufficiency according to the K/DOQI guidelines for the treatment of anemia.

Therapeutic Alternatives

3. *What treatment alternatives are available for achieving the goals related to lupus nephritis and its complications?*

Glomerulonephritis

High-dose oral prednisone (1 mg/kg/day) has been used as induction therapy with improvement in renal function in some patients. It is subsequently tapered to every-other-day low-dose therapy (0.25 mg/kg) for maintenance. Some clinicians also use this maintenance regimen after pulse IV methylprednisolone (usually a 3-day course of 1-gram doses)

Cyclophosphamide may be given orally as 2.5 mg/kg daily or IV as 0.5 to 1.0 g/m^2 BSA monthly for 6 consecutive months (and often every 3 months thereafter for another 3 to 6 months). The IV route may decrease the risk of hemorrhagic cystitis as a result of less cumulative exposure than with the oral route.

Azathioprine 2 mg/kg orally daily may be administered in place of cyclophosphamide if cytotoxic therapy is needed for longer than 3 to 6 months. Azathioprine is considered to be safer than cyclophosphamide for long-term therapy because of less gonadal and bladder toxicity. Azathioprine is associated with side effects (occurring infrequently) that include macrocytosis, leukopenia, pancreatitis, and hepatotoxicity.

The combination of one of the cytotoxic agents with prednisone is suggested for patients with a presumed poor prognosis (e.g., advanced renal disease on biopsy, African-American race). When prednisone is used in combination with cyclophosphamide, the oral prednisone dose is usually decreased to 0.5 mg/kg daily.

Methylprednisolone pulse therapy (250 to 1000 mg IV for 3 days) may be used in patients who present with acute renal failure, with subsequent conversion to standard doses of oral prednisone and cyclophosphamide. This high-dose aggressive therapy is usually limited to two courses because of an increased incidence of adverse effects.

Cyclosporine has been used as a single agent to avoid treatment with steroids during maintenance therapy. Dosages of 5 mg/kg/day have resulted in good responses in some patients. However, higher relapse rates have been reported in patients who are not also receiving combined therapy with corticosteroids. There is a risk of drug-induced nephrotoxicity with this agent.

Mycophenolate mofetil has been gaining acceptance for both the initial and maintenance treatment phases of lupus nephritis.[5–7] A recent randomized study showed equivalent effectiveness of a regimen of mycophenolate mofetil plus prednisolone given for 12 months as compared with a regimen of cyclophosphamide plus prednisolone given for 6 months followed by azathioprine plus prednisolone for 6 months. The lower long-term potential toxicity profile of mycophenolate over cyclophosphamide may also guide therapy selections.[6]

Other approved drugs undergoing evaluation as therapies for lupus nephritis include fludarabine, methotrexate, and immunoglobulins. Investigational agents currently being evaluated include anti-CD40 ligand antibody and CTLA4-Ig. These agents are designed to decrease B cell activation by blocking costimulatory signals from T-helper cells. Plasma exchange and total lymphoid irradiation are investigational nondrug therapies currently being evaluated for lupus-nephritis. For additional discussion of treatment options, refer to the textbook chapter on glomerulonephritis and references 2 and 3.

Hypertension

The dosage of atenolol and/or clonidine could be titrated to achieve blood pressure control. Maximum doses are atenolol 100 mg and clonidine 1 mg.

Alternatively, because this patient is exhibiting progressive renal insufficiency, the most reasonable alternative may be to change to an agent that has been demonstrated to slow progressive renal disease caused by HTN (e.g., primarily the *ACE inhibitors or the angiotensin receptor blockers (ARBs)* or secondarily the *nondihydropyridine calcium channel blockers diltiazem* or *verapamil*). The ACE inhibitors/ARBs selectively dilate the efferent arterioles, thus decreasing glomerular capillary pressure and shear forces on the glomerular basement membrane. They reduce urinary protein excretion and decrease the rate of progression of the renal failure, possibly by exerting an independent protective effect on the glomerulus. The ACE inhibitors have been used to prevent progressive renal disease that is a result of nondiabetic as well as diabetic causes. Although initial studies demonstrated renal protective effects of captopril, other ACE inhibitors have been reported to have benefits as well.[8] Initial daily dosages of selected agents include ramipril 2.5 to 5 mg; lisinopril 10 mg; enalapril 5 mg; benazepril 20 mg; fosinopril 10 mg; or quinapril 10 mg. Dosage titration for these agents is based on the blood pressure response, reduction in proteinuria, and elevation in serum creatinine.

Most of the current data using ARBs is from clinical trials in patients with diabetes. Initial daily dosages of selected agents include candesartan 8 mg, irbesartan 150 mg, losartan 25 mg, valsartan 80 mg. Similar to the ACE inhibitors, the dosage should be titrated based on blood pressure and proteinuria response.

The patient should be advised to limit usage of traditional NSAIDs and COX-2 selective inhibitors because of their antagonism of HTN control, as well as their negative kidney effects secondary to inhibition of renal prostaglandins.

Hyperlipidemia

There is an increase in early onset hyperlipidemia and coronary heart disease in patients with SLE. Also, as proteinuria progresses, the serum cholesterol often increases as the serum protein decreases. This patient may benefit from interventions to minimize additional damage to the glomerulus from oxidized LDL and to reduce the risk of premature cardiovascular death. Dietary instruction regarding avoidance of foods high in fat and cholesterol should be provided in addition to an exercise program.[9]

HMG-CoA reductase inhibitors (statins) are the agents of choice based on the percent reduction in LDL-C, their favorable side-effect profile, and the documented allergy to gemfibrozil in this patient. Because of the large reduction in LDL-C required (51%), a potent agent should be initiated (e.g., simvastatin, atorvastatin, rosuvastatin). The selection of rosuvastatin would require initiation and titration of therapy at a maximum dose of 5 mg and 40 mg daily, respectively, due to 10% of the parent drug being eliminated by the kidneys. Fluvastatin would provide inadequate therapy. Lovastatin and atorvastatin are metabolized by the cytochrome P450 3A4 isoenzyme, and simvastatin is an inducer of this enzyme system. Pravastatin and fluvastatin have not been documented to interact with cytochrome P450 isoenzymes. However, this patient is not taking any medications known to affect this enzyme system, so the potential for drug-drug interactions is limited in this case.

Ezetimibe selectively inhibits the intestinal absorption of cholesterol and related phytosterols. Although it is indicated for use as a single agent (in conjunction with dietary interventions), it was primarily designed to be added to statin therapy, which may result in an additional 17% reduction in total cholesterol and 25% reduction in LDL cholesterol.

Niacin is often not well tolerated, and this patient may be predisposed to GI problems because of long-term corticosteroid use.

Bile acid sequestrants (cholestyramine or *colestipol)* are also an option, because their efficacy is good and they may be preferred in younger patients. Refer to the textbook chapter on hyperlipidemia for a detailed discussion of the treatment of lipid disorders.

Edema

Treatment options to mobilize the edema of the lower extremities should be implemented. Although it is usually appropriate to wait until assessment of the results of dietary sodium restriction and treatment of the underlying condition prior to instituting pharmacotherapy, this patient has an ongoing glomerular disease process despite several courses of therapy. It is likely that dietary sodium restriction alone will not be effective given the severity of the nephrotic syndrome.

Diuretics are the main treatment options for this condition. Therapy with a *thiazide (hydrochlorothiazide, chlorothiazide)* diuretic is usually instituted first in patients with adequate renal function, whereas patients with reduced renal function are initiated on therapy with *loop diuretics (e.g., furosemide, torsemide)* with or without a thiazide (usually metolazone). Given the reduced CLcr and frequent resistance to diuretic therapy in nephrotic patients, loop diuretics are usually first-line therapy. Patients with allergies to sulfa drugs may require therapy with ethacrynic acid.

Assessments of therapy include evaluation of serum electrolytes, edema response, blood pressure, and symptoms of overdiuresis (postural hypotension, cramping).

Anemia

Diagnosis of the underlying cause of anemia in this patient is necessary to ensure appropriate treatment. Analysis of the CBC (and red blood cell indices), serum iron, total iron binding capacity, transferrin saturation, ferritin, folate, vitamin B12, and erythropoietin are needed.

Oral or parenteral iron therapy is necessary if iron stores are depleted. This is not applicable to this patient because the serum ferritin level is 200 ng/mL. If needed, oral therapy is usually initiated as an iron salt such as ferrous sulfate 325 mg once daily, which provides 65 mg of elemental iron. The dose should be slowly titrated according to GI tolerance to achieve a total daily intake of about 200 mg elemental iron per day (i.e., 1 tablet po TID) in patients with chronic kidney disease. The oral ferrous salts (e.g., sulfate, fumarate, gluconate, polysaccharide) contain different concentrations of elemental iron. Therefore, appropriate doses of elemental iron need to be considered when initiating a dosage regimen. Parenteral iron may be indicated if iron stores are found to be significantly depleted.

This patient exhibits an erythropoietin level of <2 mIU/mL in the presence of a hemoglobin and hematocrit of 10.4 g/dL and 31.7%, respectively. This erythropoietin level is severalfold lower than would be expected in the presence of anemia, suggesting a deficit at the level of the kidney in this patients with a reduced GFR. Decreased concentrations of erythropoietin may require once-weekly or every-other-week SQ *recombinant epoetin alfa* therapy or every 2- to 4-week therapy with *darbepoetin alfa*. These decreased concentrations, if present, are likely a result of underlying renal insufficiency.

Depressed serum concentrations of *folate* and *vitamin* B_{12} would require replacement therapy. These levels were not obtained in this patient, and RBC indices are also not available. Please refer to the textbook chapter on anemias for further details.

Osteoporosis

Although the patient exhibited osteoporosis of the lumbar spine and osteopenia of the hip, the need for continued long-term corticosteroid administration predisposes her to continued worsening of bone density, especially with aging. She should be instructed about the need to have an intake of 1500 mg of elemental calcium daily while on chronic corticosteroid therapy.[10]

If adequate intake is not possible, *calcium supplements* such as Os-Cal (500 mg elemental calcium) or TUMS (200 mg elemental calcium) should be prescribed.

To enhance calcium absorption in patients with chronic kidney disease, a *vitamin D* supplement should also be administered. The choice of vitamin D product may be dictated by the need for activated 1,25-dihydroxyvitamin D_3 *(calcitriol)* as indicated by reduced levels. Initiation of therapy with a nonactivated compound (ergocalciferol) may be sufficient if levels of 25-hydroxyvitamin D are adequate, with a change to 1,25 dihydroxyvitamin D_3 (calcitriol) when renal function declines further or when patients are resistant to therapy with 25-hydroxylated compounds. The newest published K/DOQI guidelines address the selection of therapies and monitoring for patients with abnormalities of calcium, phosphorus, and/or parathyroid hormone.[11]

Because the patient has osteoporosis of the spine and osteopenia of the hip, a trial of *nasal calcitonin* or *oral alendronate* or *risedronate* may help to prevent further bone resorption and gain additional bone mass. Alendronate and risedronate are FDA approved for treatment of glucocorticoid-induced osteoporosis in men and women receiving a daily dosage equivalent to ≥7.5 mg of prednisone and who have low bone mineral density.

Because the patient is premenopausal, conjugated estrogens or selective estrogen receptor modulators (SERMs) such as raloxifene would not be indicated. *Estrogen-containing oral contraceptives* would be a reasonable consideration. It is necessary to advise that estrogen-containing hormones may place patients with SLE at a higher risk of thrombosis than their healthy counterparts because of the presence of anticardiolipin antibodies in some of these patients. Also, some data have suggested that estrogens can cause an increase in SLE activity in some female patients.

Optimal Plan

4. Based on the available therapeutic options, design a pharmacotherapeutic plan for the management of lupus nephritis and its complications.

Glomerulonephritis

Because this patient has had two courses of cyclophosphamide in the past, she should not receive additional courses because of potential for long-term toxicity, unless other options are unavailable. These side-effect risks include sterility, osteoporosis, and secondary cancers. In addition, because she has had progressive kidney disease while on maintenance prednisone and exhibits long-term adverse effects (osteoporosis), her exposure to this agent should be decreased, if possible.

Both azathioprine and mycophenolate mofetil would spare her from further deterioration in bone mineral density. Azathioprine doses up to 4 mg/kg/day orally have been used. Given the past history of nonresponse to azathioprine, this is probably not the best option in this patient. A recent randomized study, published clinical observations, and case series have supported the role of mycophenolate mofetil as a treatment alternative for lupus nephritis. Mycophenolate mofetil dosing can begin at 250 mg twice daily and be increased at 2-week intervals to a maximum of 1500 mg twice daily. The slow titration upward helps to establish GI tolerance to therapy. Its short duration of action is an advantage; if toxicity occurs, it can be quickly reversed by prompt discontinuation of mycophenolate mofetil.

A lower dose of prednisone (5 to 10 mg daily) may be possible with combination therapy, thereby limiting further reduction in bone mass.

Cyclosporine therapy would be considered later in the treatment options because of its nephrotoxicity and lack of adequate data demonstrating sustained outcomes.

Other available and investigational drugs and therapies would be considered after the preferred options described above have failed.

Hypertension

An ACE inhibitor or ARB should be used because of the additional renal protective benefits of these drugs in glomerular diseases. The choice may depend on the need for enhanced compliance (i.e., a once-daily product). Ramipril 2.5 to 5 mg or lisinopril 10 mg po daily could be initiated. Because of data indicating the protective effects of ramipril in nondiabetic renal disease, it may be the preferred agent in this patient.[8] The ARBs losartan, irbesartan, and valsartan can all be administered as once-daily products. Initial dosages are 25 mg, 150 mg, 80 mg. The need to titrate the dose upward would depend on the BP reduction demonstrated and the response to proteinuria. It is standard clinical practice to attempt to titrate to the maximum approved doses for the maximal proteinuria reduction. The serum creatinine should be monitored weekly after therapy initiation and dosage changes to detect increases in serum creatinine. If this patient is unable to tolerate ACE inhibitors because of cough or allergy, an ARB may be substituted with caution.

If an acute reduction is desired because of the high current BP (160/115 mm Hg), a 0.1-mg dose of clonidine is the recommended oral therapy until the ACE inhibitor begins to reduce the pressure. Clonidine is probably not indicated in this patient, because there is no indication of symptoms, end-organ damage, or other urgency to necessitate rapid lowering of blood pressure.

Atenolol may be able to be discontinued after the efficacy of the ACE inhibitor therapy is determined. Because the data regarding calcium channel blockers and renal disease progression are not as well established as ACE inhibitor therapy, these agents are not considered first-line therapy.

Concomitant therapy with a diuretic for the management of edema may cause additional reductions in blood pressure. Aggressive diuresis should not be undertaken in this patient because of the possibility of further worsening of renal function.

Hyperlipidemia

Any of the reductase inhibitors (except fluvastatin) are capable of producing an acceptable reduction in LDL-C. Low initial and titration doses of rosuvastatin are necessary in patients with reduced GFR. The most cost-effective therapy should be instituted. Although pravastatin may be a preferred agent because of its lack of activity on the cytochrome P450 3A4 enzymes, this patient is not currently on medications that may interact. Atorvastatin 10 mg at bedtime could be initiated, with the possibility of increasing the dose to 80 mg for increased efficacy, if tolerated.

Because this patient needs a 51% LDL-C reduction to attain a goal of 100 mg/dL, the bile acid sequestrants or ezetimibe are not reasonable choices as single agents. However, either of these agents could be used as additive treatment if single-agent therapy with a statin provides inadequate control of dyslipidemia. The lack of significant drug interactions with ezetimibe may make this agent preferable to the bile acid sequestrants.

Edema

This patient requires therapy with a loop diuretic (e.g., furosemide 40 mg po daily in the morning). The response to therapy (reduction in lower extremity edema) and adverse events (cramping, dizziness, postural hypotension, low blood pressure) should be evaluated in a week. Follow-up blood work (electrolytes, BUN, and creatinine) should also be obtained to determine the need for potassium replacement therapy and dosage increases if indicated by assessment of edema. If a dose increase is warranted, furosemide 40 mg BID or 60 to 80 mg daily is reasonable. Metolazone can be added to therapy when the dosage of oral furosemide reaches approximately 600 mg daily or when there is no further increase in efficacy at the maximum attained dosage.

Anemia

The laboratory results suggest that reduced erythropoietin concentrations (< 2 mIU/mL) may be the cause of the anemia. Reduced renal function often leads to reduced erythropoietin secretion from the kidneys. This results in less stimulation for the differentiation of erythrocyte precursors into mature red blood cells. Therapy with subcutaneous epoetin alfa 100 units/kg weekly or darbepoetin alfa 60 mcg every two weeks may be initiated. Follow-up monitoring includes obtaining hemoglobin and hematocrit every two to four weeks. Changes (increases or decreases) in dosage of 20% to 25% are recommended based on the absolute hemoglobin/hematocrit and rate of rise. An alternative strategy to dosage reductions with darbepoetin alfa therapy is to extend the dosing interval beyond the starting interval of every two weeks. Based on the shorter half-life of epoetin alfa and the lack of adequate evidence to suggest the efficacy of extended intervals beyond once weekly, extended dosing of epoetin alfa cannot currently be recommended.

Oral iron is often initiated during erythropoietin therapy because accelerated red blood cell formation causes a depletion of iron stores as a consequence of its incorporation into red cells. Oral ferrous sulfate 325 mg (65 mg elemental iron) once daily is suggested as initial therapy. The dose should be titrated to 325 mg TID (about 200 mg elemental iron per day) over several weeks based on GI tolerance.

Oral iron therapy commonly causes GI side effects ranging from constipation to diarrhea. The patient should be educated about possible constipation, with stool softeners prescribed as indicated.

Osteoporosis

The patient should begin therapy with a calcium and vitamin D supplement. Os-Cal 250 mg with D is a reasonable combination product option. When administered as 2 tablets BID, the patient will receive 1000 mg elemental calcium and 500 IU vitamin D daily. Alternatively one could recommend one Os-Cal 500 mg with D twice daily. The advantage of the former formulation is the intake of more vitamin D. With the intake of an additional 500 mg of calcium in the diet, the patient will receive the recommended 1500 mg for patients receiving chronic glucocorticoid therapy.

The bisphosphonates such as alendronate are not good options because this patient has progressive renal insufficiency with an estimated CLcr of 37 mL/min. Bisphosphonates are eliminated primarily by the kidneys and are not recommended for patients with CLcr <30 mL/min.

Although intranasal calcitonin has demonstrated only a 1-year gain in BMD versus the 3-year gain with alendronate in glucocorticoid-treated patients, it is a reasonable option in this patient with osteoporosis of the spine and a contraindication to bisphosphonates. Calcitonin is administered once daily in the nostril with 1 spray delivering 200 IU calcitonin.

The patient should receive dietary instruction about the amount of calcium present in various foods, as well as some physical activity assessment and education to enhance weight bearing exercises to prevent worsening osteoporosis.

Outcome Evaluation

5. Outline a clinical and laboratory monitoring plan for each of the patient's drug therapy problems.

The patient should return to nephrology clinic in 2 weeks for assessment of progressive renal insufficiency and safety and efficacy of mycophenolate mofetil and ACE inhibitor therapy.

Laboratory assessment should include a CBC, liver enzymes, CPK, electrolytes, urea nitrogen and creatinine. Additional follow-up labs and visits should occur at 4- to 6-week intervals to closely follow this patient's rapidly progressive renal disease and ACE inhibitor and lipid-lowering therapy.

Urinalysis should be performed at each visit, as well as a spot urine protein-to-creatinine ratio.

Blood pressure measurements should be performed at each clinic visit. In addition, the patient should be taught to monitor her blood pressure at home.

Adverse effect questioning at each subsequent clinic visit and appropriate modification in therapy will enhance patient compliance and disease treatment.

A repeat DEXA scan should be performed 1 year after implementation of osteoporosis therapy to assess efficacy. A 24-hour urine collection to determine the amount of calcium eliminated may be performed to identify whether a thiazide diuretic is indicated to minimize urinary losses.

Patient Education

6. What should the patient be told regarding the drug therapy she is to receive to treat her condition and its complications?

Mycophenolate Mofetil (CellCept)

This drug acts to suppress your immune system in order to control your body's response to lupus. Take 1 tablet (250 mg) twice daily on an empty stomach for best absorption. The dose may be gradually increased every 2 weeks to minimize gastrointestinal side effects.

Use appropriate contraception and avoid becoming pregnant while taking this medication, because it may be harmful to a developing fetus.

You may experience some gastrointestinal side effects such as diarrhea and vomiting; notify your doctor if they become persistent or troublesome.

The number of white cells in your blood will be monitored monthly because low counts have been reported.

Prednisone

Prednisone is used to suppress your lupus disease activity. Take the prescribed dose with food to minimize stomach upset.

Prednisone can cause side effects including increased risk of infection, fluid gain or swelling, increased blood sugar, stomach ulcers, mood swings, and weight gain.

Ramipril (Altace)

This medication decreases blood pressure, and it may decrease the protein being spilled into your urine.

Dizziness or lightheadedness may occur if your blood pressure is lowered too much. This often decreases with chronic therapy. Contact your physician if this persists.

This drug may increase the concentration of potassium in your bloodstream or cause a nagging cough.

Contact your physician if you become pregnant because this medication (like mycophenolate mofetil) may harm your unborn child.

This medication should be taken on an empty stomach for best absorption.

Atorvastatin (Lipitor)

This drug is used to lower cholesterol levels. Take the prescribed 10-mg tablet once daily at bedtime. Bedtime is the preferred time to take the drug, because most cholesterol synthesis occurs while you are sleeping.

Contact your doctor if you experience muscle pain.

Furosemide

This drug is used to reduce the swelling in your legs. Because this drug will cause you to urinate more frequently, take the tablet in the morning instead of at bedtime.

Furosemide can cause a reduction in potassium concentrations in your body. Blood tests will be done periodically to monitor potassium concentrations.

Contact your doctor is you experience cramping or dizziness (especially when standing from a seated position).

Darbepoetin Alfa (Aranesp)

Darbepoetin alfa is prescribed to increase your red blood cell count.

It is given by subcutaneous injection and may cause stinging and burning when given.

It may also cause an elevation in your blood pressure.

Iron (e.g., Ferrous Sulfate)

Oral iron therapy is prescribed because you are receiving erythropoietin. Erythropoietin often causes iron deficiency. Iron will improve your response to erythropoietin therapy.

Iron is absorbed best if taken on an empty stomach.

Iron may cause a harmless darkening of the stools. Other common side effects are stomach upset, constipation, and/or diarrhea. Tell your doctor if these side effects become troublesome.

Calcium

Calcium is needed to make the bones strong and to prevent them from breaking.

You should ingest 1500 mg of elemental calcium daily because you are at high risk of worsening bone disease as a consequence of long-term prednisone therapy. This can be accomplished by taking 2 Os-Cal with D tablets twice daily. This will provide you with 1000 mg of your required calcium and 500 IU vitamin D.

You will need to supplement your diet with high calcium-containing foods such as milk, cheese, beans, yogurt, and ice cream to get the other 500 mg you need. This can be obtained from 2 glasses of milk, 3 to 5 ounces of cheese, 2 cups of yogurt, or 4 cups of ice cream.

Do not take the calcium with food, because the phosphorus in your diet may reduce its absorption.

Vitamin D

This vitamin will also prevent your bones from breaking. You need extra vitamin D because you have been taking prednisone for a long time.

You will receive close to the recommended daily requirement of 800 units by taking the Os-Cal with D.

Calcitonin (Miacalcin) Nasal Spray

This medication will prevent continuing bone loss. Administer 1 spray in 1 nostril daily. The spray should be alternated between nostrils on a daily basis to prevent irritation.

Prior to the first dose of medication, the pump should be primed by holding it upright and depressing the two white side arms of the pump until a full spray is produced.

The opened bottle may be stored at room temperature. Unopened bottles should be stored in the refrigerator.

References

1. Levey AS, Bosch JP, Lewis JB, et al: A more accurate method to estimate glomerular filtration rate from serum creatinine: A new prediction equation. Modification of Diet in Renal Disease Study Group. *Ann Intern Med* 1999;130: 461–470.
2. Austin HA, Balow JE. Treatment of lupus nephritis. *Semin Nephrol* 2000;20: 265–276.
3. Cameron JS. Lupus nephritis. *J Am Soc Nephrol* 1999;10:413–424.
4. Korbet SM, Lewis EJ, Schwartz MM, et al: Factors predictive of outcome in severe lupus nephritis. Lupus Nephritis Collaborative Study Group. *Am J Kidney Dis* 2000;35:904–914.
5. Mok CC, Lai KN. Mycophenolate mofetil in lupus glomerulonephritis. *Am J Kidney Dis* 2002;40:447–457.
6. Chan TM, Li FK, Tang CS, et al: Efficacy of mycophenolate mofetil in patients with diffuse proliferative lupus nephritis. Hong Kong-Guangzhou Nephrology Study Group. *N Engl J Med* 2000;343:1156–1162.
7. Kingdon EJ, McLean AG, Psimenou E, et al: The safety and efficacy of MMF in lupus nephritis: A pilot study. *Lupus* 2001;10:606–611.
8. Remuzzi G, Tognoni G, for the GI Group SEN. Randomised placebo-controlled trial of effect of ramipril on decline in glomerular filtration rate and risk of terminal renal failure in proteinuric, non-diabetic nephropathy. *Lancet* 1997;349: 1857–1863.
9. Wierzbicki AS. Lipids, cardiovascular disease and atherosclerosis in systemic lupus erythematosus. *Lupus* 2000;9:194–201.
10. Recommendations for the prevention and treatment of glucocorticoid-induced osteoporosis. American College of Rheumatology Task Force on Osteoporosis Guidelines. *Arthritis Rheum* 1996;39:1791–1801.
11. National Kidney Foundation. K/DOQI clinical practice guidelines for bone metabolism and disease in chronic kidney disease. *Am J Kidney Dis* 2003; 42(suppl 3):S1–S202.

116 DIABETIC FOOT INFECTION

► Watch Your Step (Level II)

Renee-Claude Mercier, PharmD
A. Christie Graham, PharmD

Accidentally stepping on a piece of metal results in erythema and swelling of the right foot in a 65-year-old Native-American woman with poorly controlled type 2 diabetes mellitus. Laboratory evaluation reveals leukocytosis with a left shift. The patient underwent incision and drainage of the lesion with removal of a 2-cm metallic foreign body from the foot. Empiric antimicrobial treatment must be initiated before results of wound culture and sensitivity testing are known. Because of this particular patient's condition, parenteral monotherapy with ampicillin/sulbactam, cefotetan, or cefoxitin would constitute appropriate therapy. Other alternatives include ticarcillin/clavulanate, piperacillin/ tazobactam, imipenem/cilastatin, ertapenem, or the combination of clindamycin plus either a third-generation cephalosporin or a fluoroquinolone. When tissue cultures are reported as positive for methicillin-resistant *Staphylococcus aureus* (MRSA), students are asked to change to more specific therapy, which include parenteral vancomycin (first-line) or the second-line agents linezolid, dalfopristin/quinupristin, or daptomycin. Although parenteral therapy may be completed as an outpatient, attention must be given to the patient's social and economic situation. Better glycemic control and education on techniques for proper foot care are important components of a comprehensive treatment plan for this patient.

▶ Questions

Problem Identification

1. a. Create a list of the patient's drug therapy problems.

Cellulitis and infection of the right foot in a patient with diabetes.

Poorly controlled type 2 diabetes mellitus, as evidenced by a HbA_{1c} of 11.8% (goal <7%) and recent episode of DKA.

Nonadherence with medication administration and home glucose monitoring.

Renal insufficiency secondary to diabetic nephropathy.

History of depression, which may be inadequately treated (the patient is described as having a "flat affect").

Fungal infection of toenails requiring treatment.

Language barrier requiring additional resources (i.e., translator) to optimize patient education.

b. What signs, symptoms, or laboratory values indicate the presence of an infection?

Swollen, sore, and red foot.

2+ edema of the foot increasing in amplitude.

WBC elevated ($16.4 \times 10^3/mm^3$) with increased PMNs and bands.

X-ray showing the presence of a foreign body in the right foot.

c. What risk factors for infection does the patient have?

Patient stepped on a foreign object

She is a poorly controlled diabetic patient.

Vascular calcifications in the foot per X-ray indicate a decreased blood supply.

Poor foot care (presence of fungus and overgrown toenails).

d. What organisms are most likely involved in this infection?

Aerobic isolates: *Staphylococcus aureus, Streptococcus spp., Enterococcus spp., Proteus mirabilis, Escherichia coli, Klebsiella spp., Pseudomonas aeruginosa.*

Anaerobic isolates: *Peptostreptococcus, Bacteroides fragilis.*[1,2]

Desired Outcome

2. What are the therapeutic goals for this patient?

Eradicate the bacteria.

Prevent the development of osteomyelitis and the need for amputation.

Preserve as much normal limb function as possible.

Improve control of diabetes mellitus.

Prevent further recurrence of foot infection.

Therapeutic Alternatives

3. a. What nondrug therapies might be useful for this patient?

Deep culture of the wound for both anaerobes and aerobes.

Appropriate wound care by experienced podiatrists (I & D, débridement of the wound, toenail clipping), nurses (wound care, dressing changes of wound, foot care teaching), and physical therapists (whirlpool treatments, wound débridement, teaching about minimal weight-bearing with a walker or crutches).

Bedrest, minimal weight-bearing, leg elevation, and control of edema.

Proper education about wound care and the importance of good diabetes control, glucometer use, and adherence with the medication regimens.[3]

b. What feasible pharmacotherapeutic alternatives are available for the empiric treatment of the foot infection?

Diabetic foot infections are classified into two categories:

Non–limb-threatening infections. Superficial, no systemic toxicity, minimal cellulitis extending less than 2 cm from portal of entry, ulceration not extending fully through skin, no significant ischemia.

Limb-threatening infections. More extensive cellulitis, lymphangitis, and ulcers penetrating through skin into subcutaneous tissues, prominent ischemia.

Oral antimicrobial therapy may be used in mild, uncomplicated diabetic foot infections *only*.[4] Suggested regimens include:

Amoxicillin/clavulanate monotherapy; or

Fluoroquinolone plus clindamycin combination.

Although these regimens cover the most likely causative organisms, it is important to note that *amoxicillin/clavulanate* does not cover *Pseudomonas aeruginosa*.

Treatment of limb-threatening infections must include IV antibiotic therapy. IV monotherapy may be used with:

Piperacillin/tazobactam;

Ticarcillin/clavulanate; or

Imipenem/cilastatin

These agents cover all of the most likely causative organisms, including anaerobes and *Pseudomonas aeruginosa*. However, imipenem/cilastatin is a potent β-lactamase inducer, so therapy with the other agents may be preferable.

The following agents could also be used as IV monotherapy, but they do not cover *Pseudomonas aeruginosa:*

Ampicillin/sulbactam;

Ertapenem;

Cefotetan;

Cefoxitin; or

Third generation cephalosporin (ceftriaxone/cefotaxime) plus IV clindamycin combination

Ertapenem has the additional benefit of once-daily dosing, but as a carbapenem it may lead to the induction of β-lactamase (this is yet to be established).

Clindamycin IV plus either *aztreonam* or an oral or IV *fluoroquinolone* could be used in patients with limb-threatening infections who are allergic to penicillin.

Vancomycin IV may be used in therapy if MRSA is a suspected causative organism. Persons who are at high risk for MRSA wound infection include those who: (a) have a previous history of MRSA infection/colonization, (b) have positive nasal cultures for MRSA, (c) have a recent history (within the last year) of prolonged hospitalization or ICU stay, or (d) receive frequent and/or prolonged courses of broad-spectrum antibiotics.[5–8] Should vancomycin be used empirically, gram-negative and anaerobic coverage will need to be added to provide adequate empiric coverage.

Aminoglycosides should be avoided in diabetic patients as they are at increased risk for the development of diabetic nephropathy and renal failure.

Becaplermin 0.01% Gel (Regranex) is FDA-approved for the treatment of diabetic ulcers on the lower limbs and feet. Becaplermin is a genetically engineered form of platelet-derived growth factor, a naturally occurring protein in the body that stimulates diabetic ulcer healing. It is to be used as adjunct therapy, *in addition to* infection control and wound care. In one clinical trial, becaplermin applied once daily in combination with good wound care significantly increased the incidence of complete healing when compared to placebo gel (50% vs. 35%, respectively). Becaplermin gel also significantly decreased the time to complete healing of diabetic ulcers by 32% (about 6 weeks faster). The incidence of adverse events including infection and cellulitis was similar in patients treated with becaplermin gel, placebo gel, or good diabetic wound care alone.[9] Further studies are needed to assess which patients might best benefit from becaplermin use.

c. *What economic and social considerations are applicable to this patient?*

A simplified drug regimen (monotherapy and less-frequent dosing, whenever possible) should be selected because of her history of poor medication adherence.

The patient receives her health care primarily at Shiprock Indian Health Services (IHS). This may become an important consideration in selecting her future therapeutic plan.

For this patient to receive appropriate wound care and home IV therapy if judged necessary, the healthcare team must establish that her daughter or a home health care nurse will be able to provide assistance.

Optimal Plan

4. *Outline a drug regimen that would provide optimal initial empiric therapy for the infection.*

This diabetic foot infection has significant involvement of the skin and skin structures with deep tissue involvement. Moreover, the area of cellulitis and induration exceeded 2 cm (4 × 5 cm). Even though this is her first foot infection and is more likely to be caused by a single organism, one cannot rule out the presence of a polymicrobial infection because of the extensive skin and skin structure involvement. Initial empiric IV therapy is appropriate in serious, limb-threatening diabetic foot infections such as this one.

As discussed, a number of treatment options are appropriate for empiric therapy of diabetic foot infections. The antimicrobial therapy selection may be based on institutional cost and drug availability through the formulary system. It should also be adjusted for the patient's renal function. This patient's calculated CLcr, based on adjusted body weight [IBW × 0.4(actual − ideal body weight)] is 39 mL/min. Any one of the following regimens is appropriate as monotherapy because each has good coverage of the most commonly involved organisms (including both aerobic and anaerobic bacteria) and a good safety profile.

Ampicillin/sulbactam 1.5 to 3 g IV Q 8 h; the higher dosage should be reserved for serious infections in patients with poor peripheral circulation:

Cefotetan 1 g IV Q 12 ;

Ertapenem 1 g Q 24 .

Other acceptable IV alternatives given as monotherapy, with dose adjustments appropriate for Ms. Littlehorse's renal function, include:

Ticarcillin/clavulanate 2.0 g IV Q 6 h;

Piperacillin/tazobactam 2.25 g IV Q 6 h; or

Imipenem/cilastatin 250 mg IV Q 6 h.

These agents should not be considered first-line therapy because they are often restricted for more severe/life-threatening nosocomial infections due to their broader spectrum of activity, to prevent the development of resistance, and to reduce treatment costs. Because the patient does not have a life-threatening infection, is not a nursing home resident, and has no previous history of pseudomonal infection or diabetic foot infection, she is at low risk for pseudomonal infection.

Clindamycin 900 mg IV Q 8 h in combination with levofloxacin 500 mg po/IV once daily (or another fluoroquinolone in equivalent dose) is also appropriate in this case. However, this two-drug regimen is less convenient than monotherapy and is more often associated with *Clostridium difficile* colitis because of clindamycin use.

The decision whether to use vancomycin empirically is a clinical judgment call in this case. Given the patient's single risk factor of previous hospitalization (the details of which are not available), it seems reasonable to hold off on recommending vancomycin at this time.

Outcome Evaluation

5. a. *What clinical and laboratory parameters are necessary to evaluate your therapy for achievement of the desired therapeutic outcomes and monitoring for adverse effects?*

Regardless of the drug chosen, improvement in the signs and symptoms of infection and healing of the wound with prevention of limb amputation are the primary end points.

Decreased swelling, induration, and erythema should be observed after 72 to 96 hours of appropriate antimicrobial therapy and surgical débridement. The response to therapy is often patient dependent, and in some cases, improvement may not be seen for as long as 7 to 10 days of treatment.

A decrease in cloudy drainage and formation of new scar tissue are signs of positive response to therapy that may take as long as 7 to 14 days to be seen.

A WBC count and differential should be performed every 48 to 72 hours for the first week or until normalization if less than 1 week, and weekly thereafter until the end of therapy. Monitoring should continue until therapy is completed because neutropenia is associated with many antibiotics (e.g., ampicillin/sulbactam, cefotetan, cefoxitin, vancomycin).

Vancomycin is not considered nephro- or hepatotoxic, in general. Routine weekly serum creatinine levels may be recommended to prevent vancomycin-associated ototoxicity that can develop with accumulation of the drug should Ms. Littlehorse's renal function worsen. It would be reasonable to order a weekly vancomycin trough level also to ensure that an adequate trough level (≥ 10 mg/L) is being achieved.

Question the patient to detect any unusual side effects related to the drug or infusion (e.g., rash, nausea, vomiting, diarrhea) daily for the first 3 to 5 days and then weekly thereafter.

b. What therapeutic alternatives are available for treating this patient once results of cultures are known to contain MRSA?

Once the culture results are available and the involved organism(s) is (are) considered pathogenic and responsible for the infectious process, therapy should be targeted at the specific organism(s).

Vancomycin given IV is the drug of choice for skin and soft tissue infections caused by MRSA, as it has established efficacy, is generally well-tolerated, and is inexpensive

Linezolid has the advantage of oral administration, but it is expensive and its use is typically restricted to prevent the development of resistance.

Dalfopristin/quinupristin is another alternative, but it has the drawback of being associated with significant side effects, including severe infusion site reactions and myalgias/arthralgias.

Daptomycin is a lipopeptide approved in late 2003 for use in skin and soft tissue infections due to susceptible organisms including MRSA. It may ultimately prove to be a useful therapeutic alternative in this setting.

c. Design an optimal drug treatment plan for treating the MRSA infection while she remains hospitalized.

The patient's therapy should be narrowed to vancomycin 1 g IV Q 24 h. After the third dose, a vancomycin trough level should be recommended and therapy adjusted to maintain a trough > 10 mg/L.

Because vancomycin only covers gram-positive bacterial infections, it is essential to monitor for efficacy since diabetic foot infections are frequently polymicrobial. As noted above, the patient's infection should be assessed daily for changes in swelling, induration, and erythema. Temperature should be assessed at least twice daily and a WBC obtained daily if it was initially increased. Improvements in these physical signs and laboratory parameters should be observed after 72 to 96 hours of appropriate antimicrobial therapy and surgical débridement. If the area of swelling and erythema increases, foul odor or drainage develops, or if response to therapy appears inadequate, it may be necessary to broaden therapy so that Gram-negative and anaerobic bacteria are covered as well. Response to therapy is often patient dependent, and in some cases improvement may not be seen until after 7 to 10 days of treatment.

The duration of therapy is controversial and based on the patient's personal situation. Therapy should be continued until all signs and symptoms disappear and for at least 2 to 4 weeks total. Some patients require longer therapy, and wound healing in diabetic patients is often very slow.

The patient should remain hospitalized until she is afebrile for 24 to 48 hours, has signs of improvement and positive response to therapy (decreased swelling, redness, purulent drainage; normalization of the WBC), and outpatient wound care has been established, either by proper teaching to the patient (and her daughter) or through home health care services.

d. Design an optimal pharmacotherapeutic plan for completion of her treatment after she is discharged from the hospital.

The decision about completion of therapy with IV versus oral therapy is often based on clinical experience, because few clinical trials have been performed on long-term treatment of diabetic foot infections.

In this patient, continued use of IV vancomycin would probably be the best choice. The drug could be either infused at home, most likely with the daughter's assistance and frequent nursing care visits, or the patient may be required to visit her local IHS clinic daily to receive therapy, depending on what is economically feasible. Discharge planning should be involved in this case to ensure a smooth transition to outpatient therapy.

The patient should be seen in clinic at least once weekly while on therapy to assess therapeutic efficacy and safety. At each visit, a CBC should be obtained to evaluate for vancomycin-associated neutropenia or thrombocytopenia. A SCr should be obtained as well, and, if any significant changes in renal function are observed, the vancomycin dose should be adjusted.

Treatment with oral antibiotics may be considered if the wound is healing well with disappearance of signs and symptoms of infection, if there is formation of new scar tissue, and if the infection is no longer limb-threatening. MRSA drug susceptibilities can guide oral therapy. MRSA is sometimes susceptible to clindamycin, sulfamethoxazole/trimethoprim, or minocycline. Linezolid is another option, but it is very expensive.

Patient Education

6. What information should be provided to the patient to enhance compliance, to ensure successful therapy, and to minimize adverse effects with IV vancomycin?

We will need to see you in the clinic each week to make sure the antibiotic is working. At these visits we will draw some blood so that we can check for side effects of the medication.

Vancomycin should be infused slowly, over 1 to 2 hours, to prevent flushing and blood pressure decreases that are associated with rapid infusion.

Contact your doctor or me if any unusual side effects such as rash, shortness of breath, diminished hearing or ringing in the ears, or decreased urine production occur while taking this medicine.

Contact your home health care provider if pain, redness, or swelling is observed at the IV site.

Note: The patient needs to be made aware that osteomyelitis and limb amputation are possible consequences of these infections in diabetic patients. She also needs to be provided with personnel resources (telephone numbers, addresses) to contact if unusual reactions occur while on therapy, if infection worsens, or if she has questions or concerns. Compliance with outpatient clinic follow-up visits is of prime importance for success in this case.

References

1. Lipsky BA, Pecoraro RE, Wheat LJ. The diabetic foot: Soft tissue and bone infection. *Infect Dis Clin North Am* 1990:4:409–432.
2. Gerding DN. Foot infections in diabetic patients: The role of anaerobes. *Clin Infect Dis* 1995;20(suppl 2):S283–S288.
3. Levin ME. Management of the diabetic foot: Preventing amputation. *South Med J* 2002;95(1):10–20.
4. Lipsky BA, Pecoraro RE, Larson SA, et al: Outpatient management of uncomplicated lower-extremity infections in diabetic patients. *Arch Intern Med* 1990;150: 790–797.
5. Boyce JM. Methicillin-resistant Staphylococcus aureus. Detection, epidemiology, and control measures. *Infect Dis Clin North Am* 1989;3:901–913.
6. Herwaldt LA. Control of methicillin-resistant *Staphylococcus aureus* in the hospital setting. *Am J Med* 1999;106:11S–18S; discussion 48S–52S
7. Asensio A, Guerrero A, Quereda C, et al: Colonization and infection with methicillin-resistant *Staphylococcus aureus:* Associated factors and eradication. *Infect Control Hosp Epidemiol* 1996;17:20–28.
8. Mulligan ME, Murray-Leisure KA, Ribner BS, et al: Methicillin-resistant *Staphylococcus aureus:* A consensus review of the microbiology, pathogenesis, and epidemiology with implications for prevention and management. *Am J Med* 1993; 94:313–328.
9. Wieman TJ, Smiell JM, Su Y. Efficacy and safety of a topical gel formulation of recombinant human platelet-derived growth factor-BB (becaplermin) in patients with chronic neuropathic diabetic ulcers. A phase III randomized placebo-controlled double-blind study. *Diabetes Care* 1998;21(5):822–827.